Chemistry and Biology
of β-Lactam Antibiotics

Volume 2

Chemistry and Biology of β-Lactam Antibiotics

Volume 2   Nontraditional β-Lactam Antibiotics

Edited by

ROBERT B. MORIN

Bristol Laboratories
Syracuse, New York

MARVIN GORMAN

Eli Lilly and Company
Indianapolis, Indiana

1982

ACADEMIC PRESS

A Subsidiary of Harcourt Brace Jovanovich, Publishers

New York   London

Paris   San Diego   San Francisco   São Paulo   Sydney   Tokyo   Toronto

ACADEMIC PRESS, INC.
111 Fifth Avenue, New York, New York 10003

United Kingdom Edition published by
ACADEMIC PRESS, INC. (LONDON) LTD.
24/28 Oval Road, London NW1 7DX

Library of Congress Cataloging in Publication Data

Main entry under title:

Chemistry and biology of B-lactam antibiotics.

Includes bibliographies and index.
1. Antibiotics--Synthesis. 2. Penicillin. 3. Cepha-
losporin. 4. Lactams. 5. Chemistry, Pharmaceutical.
I. Morin, Robert B. II. Gorman, Marvin.
QD375.C47   615'.329   82-6638
ISBN 0-12-506302-4 (v.2)

PRINTED IN THE UNITED STATES OF AMERICA

82 83 84 85   9 8 7 6 5 4 3 2 1

Contents

3. Nocardicins

Takashi Kamiya, Hatsuo Aoki, and Yasuhiro Mine

4. The Chemistry of Thienamycin and Other Carbapenem Antibiotics

Ronald W. Ratcliffe and Georg Albers-Schönberg

5. The Penems

Ivan Ernest

6. Clavulanic Acid

Peter C. Cherry and Christopher E. Newall

Contributors

Numbers in parentheses indicate the pages on which the author's contributions begin.

Georg Albers-Schönberg (227), Institute for Therapeutic Research, Rahway, New Jersey 07065

Hatsuo Aoki (165), Research Laboratories, Fujisawa Pharmaceutical Co., Ltd., Kashima, Yodogawa-ku, Osaka 532, Japan

Peter C. Cherry (361), Glaxo Research Ltd., Glaxo-Allenburys Research, Greenford, Middlesex, UB6 OHE, England

Ivan Ernest (315), Woodward Research Institute, Ciba-Geigy, Ltd., Basel, Switzerland

Kenneth G. Holden (99), Smith Kline and French Research Laboratories, Philadelphia, Pennsylvania 19101

Takashi Kamiya (165), Research Laboratories, Fujisawa Pharmaceutical Co., Ltd., Kashima, Yodogawa-ku, Osaka 532, Japan

Yasuhiro Mine (165), Research Laboratories, Fujisawa Pharmaceutical Co., Ltd., Kashima, Yodogawa-ku, Osaka 532, Japan

Wataru Nagata (1), Shionogi Research Laboratories, Shionogi and Co., Ltd., Fukushima-ku, Osaka, Japan

Masayuki Narisada (1), Shionogi Research Laboratories, Shionogi and Co., Ltd., Fukushima-ku, Osaka, Japan

Christopher E. Newall (361), Glaxo Research Ltd., Glaxo-Allenburys Research, Greenford, Middlesex, UB6 OHE, England

Ronald W. Ratcliffe (227), Merck Institute for Therapeutic Research, Rahway, New Jersey 07065

Tadashi Yoshida (1), Shionogi Research Laboratories, Shionogi and Co., Ltd., Fukushima-ku, Osaka, Japan

Preface

The increasing therapeutic role of β-lactam antibiotics and the discovery of significant new members of this series through synthetic chemical or fermentation screening programs has led to an exponential growth during the last decade in the literature describing the chemistry and biology of these substances. The present volume, the second of a three-part treatise, attempts to present recent scientific information concerning this broad class of antibiotics. Previous extended monographs on the subject have focused exclusively on penicillins or cephalosporins with relevant chemistry. The present volumes cover advances in these two members of the class and in addition, the chemistry and biology of a series of new synthetic or biosynthetic β-lactam antibiotics.

Volume 1 is devoted to reports of recent studies on the chemical, biological, physicochemical and computational aspects of the properties of penicillins and cephalosporins; including an extensive review of the cephamycins (7-methoxycephalosporins). Volume 3 concentrates on the general biological properties, including biosynthesis, fermentation, mode of inhibition and killing of bacteria, mechanisms of enzymatic degradation, and a clinical perspective of use. Also included in that volume is a description of recently described monobactam antibiotics and an appendix which provides data and experimental procedures relevant to all three volumes. This volume is concerned with the many β-lactam antibiotics, defined as β-lactams having antibacterial or β-lactamase-inhibitory properties, but differing from penicillins or cephalosporins in any of the following ways: (a) lacking a fused ring system; (b) having the penicillin or cephalosporin ring system modified in size or heteroatom substitution; or (c) lacking the amide side chain common to the established β-lactam antibiotics. Each chapter in this volume describes a recently reported class of β-lactam antibiotics and provides a comprehensive discussion of published biological and chemical characteristics of this class.

The rapid growth of interest in the nontraditional β-lactam antibiotics represents the convergence of three independent aspects of the research in the field: (a) development of sufficient knowledge of the necessary synthetic chemistry; (b) better understanding of the requirements for biological activity through biochemical and theoretical studies; and (c) the discovery through intensive fermentation screening of new members having unique structural and antibacterial properties. Chapter 1 details those analogs, particularly oxacephalosporins, obtained by partial synthesis from fermentation-derived starting materials. Chapter 2 describes nuclear analogs of penicillins and cephalosporins obtained by total synthesis. In some cases similar compounds have been obtained by both routes. The synthesis of acylamino penems directed by the late Professor Woodward was a further extension of the research described in these chapters. The synthesis of compounds having a penem ring system or the related carbapenems received impetus with the discovery of the antibiotic thienamycin and the lactamase inhibitor clavulanic acid which both lack the typical amide side chain. Progress in penems is described in Chapter 5, in carbapenems (thienamycin) in Chapter 4, and in oxapenems (clavulanic acid) in Chapter 6. The discovery of nocardicin (Chapter 3) and monobactams (Volume 3, Chapter 7) indicates that a fused bicyclic β-lactam ring structure is not necessary for antibacterial properties. In the former example a β-lactam structure may supplement the host defense systems. The topics discussed in this volume appear to be the areas of greatest potential for the development of new therapeutic agents in the field of β-lactam antibiotics. Some of the most active antibacterials presently known are described in the following pages. Attesting to this importance is the fact that, of the substances described in Volume 2, one is presently in clinical use and at least two others are being extensively evaluated as therapeutic agents in man.

R. B. Morin
M. Gorman

Contents of Other Volumes

Partial Synthesis of Nuclear Analogs of Cephalosporins

WATARU NAGATA, MASAYUKI NARISADA, AND TADASHI YOSHIDA

I. Introduction

Recent advances in the chemistry and biology of β-lactam antibiotics have created a better understanding of the mechanism of action and the

Chemistry and Biology of
β-Lactam Antibiotics, Vol. 2

structure–activity relationships of this important class of antibiotics and have led β-lactam chemists to undertake the challenge of modifying the nucleus of penicillins and cephalosporins. Research along these lines has been spurred by the recent isolation of new, naturally occurring β-lactam antibiotics with novel nuclei, such as nocardicins (this volume, Chapter 2), clavulanic acid (this volume, Chapter 6), and carbapenem derivatives such as thienamycins and olivanic acids (this volume, Chapter 3), since these newly isolated β-lactams have shown unique biological properties. Thus, a variety of nuclear analogs that can be classified as penam (1),

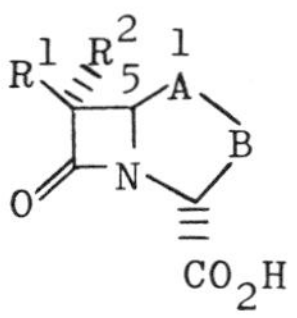

1a: A–B = OCH_2 or $OC(CH_3)_2$

1b: A–B = CH_2NAc

1c: A–B = CH_2CH_2

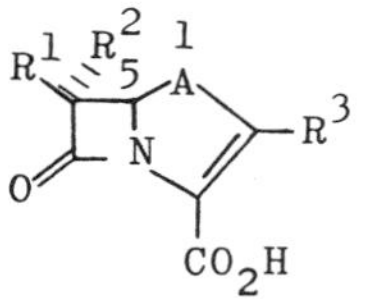

2a: A = S

2b: A = O

2c: A = CH_2

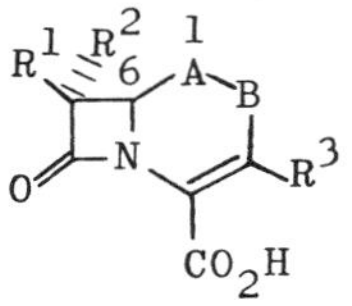

3a: A–B = S–S
      R^1 = $C_6H_5CH_2CONH$
      R^2 = R^3 = H

3b: A–B = OCH_2

3c: A–B =

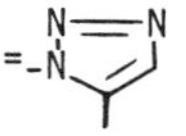

3d: A–B = CH_2CH_2

3e: A–B = CH_2O

3f: A–B = CH_2NCH_3 or $CH_2NCOOC_2H_5$

3g: A–B = CH_2S

penem (2), and cephem (3) analogs (A and B indicate S, O, NR, or CR^1R^2 in each formula) have been successfully prepared by both partial and total synthesis and tested for antibacterial activity. One of the first examples of this kind of cephalosporin analog was the 1,2-bisthiacephem derivative (3a) which showed increased biological activity and was discussed earlier (Heusler, 1972). Other synthetic nuclear analogs reported recently include 1-oxapenams (1a), 2-azaisopenams (1b), carbapenams (1c), 2-penems (2a), 1-oxa-2-penems (2b), 1-carba-2-penems (2c), 1-oxacephems (3b) (for nomenclature, see Narisada et al., 1979), 1-azacephems (3c), 1-carbacephems (3d), 2-oxaisocephems (3e), 2-azaisocephems (3f), and isocephems (3g).

Some of these compounds showed enhanced antibacterial activity, and some showed reduced activity as compared with that of their parent penicillin or cephalosporin. Because of the general difficulty in creating a C-5—A or C-6—A bond with the correct stereochemistry (β configuration) by partial synthesis starting from a penicillin or cephalosporin, most of these nuclear analogs were prepared by total synthesis as discussed in Chapter 2 of this volume. 2-Penems (**2a**), 1-oxa-2-penems (**2b**), 1-carba-2-penems (**2c**), 1-oxacephems (**3b**), and 1-azacephems (**3c**) were prepared by partial synthesis. Of these, compounds **2b** related to clavulanic acid, compounds **2c** related to thienamycins, and 2-penems (**2a**) are discussed separately in Chapters 6, 4, and 5, respectively of this volume.

This chapter treats nuclear analogs prepared by partial synthesis, excluding those treated in the other chapters, and thus focuses on partially synthetic 1-oxacephems (**3b**) with a brief mention of 1-azacephems (**3c**).

4a: A–B = S–S
4b: A–B = N–S

5a: A = CH₂
5b: A = O

6

Several cepham analogs (**4a**, **4b**, **5a**, and **5b**) have also been reported. However, since compounds **4a** and **4b** lack antibacterial activity and compounds **5a** and **5b** are prepared by total synthesis, they are not included in this chapter. Very recently partial synthesis of 3-azacephalosporin (**6**) from penicillin was announced (Aratani and Hashimoto, 1980).

Several excellent reviews on nuclear analogs of cephalosporins and penicillins have already appeared (Jaszberenyi and Gunda, 1975; Lowe, 1975; Mukerjee and Singh, 1975; Sammes, 1976; Webber and Ott, 1977; Gunda and Jaszberenyi, 1977; Cama and Christensen, 1978; Cooper, 1979; Jung *et al.*, 1980).

II. Synthesis of 1-Oxacephems and Other Nuclear Analogs

A. 1-Oxacephem Derivatives

1. *Introduction*

In 1974, Wolfe reported the synthesis of methyl 1-oxacephem-4-carboxylate (**7**) starting from penicillin. However, this ester (**7**) was not

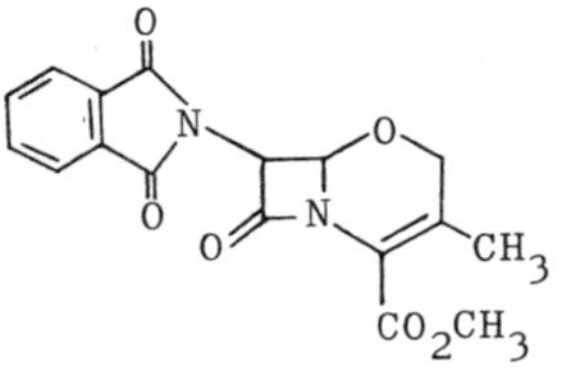

7

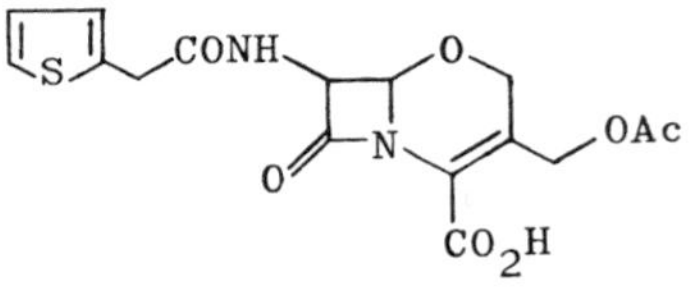

8

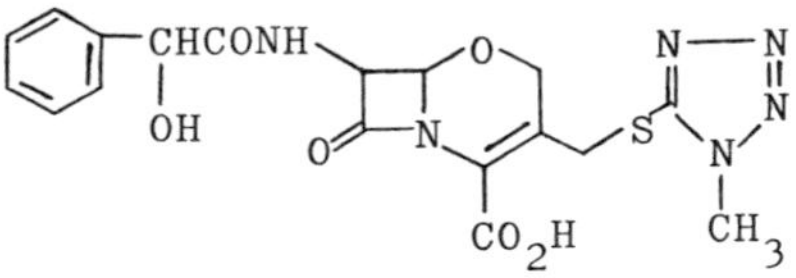

9

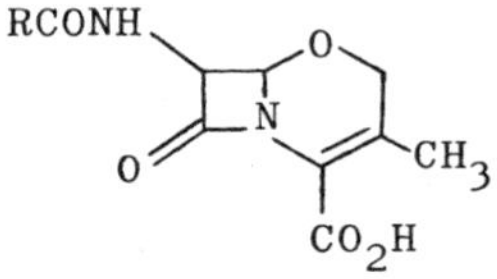

10a: R = $C_6H_5OCH_2-$

10b: R = $C_6H_5CH_2$ -

10c: R = C_6H_5CH-
                $|$
                CO_2H

converted into its free acid, thus it is not known whether such a nuclear analog exhibits antibacterial activity. In the same year Christensen and his associates at Merck & Company were successful in the synthesis of racemic 1-oxacephalothin (8). They demonstrated for the first time that this compound was biologically active and that its antibacterial spectrum and activity were parallel with those of cephalothin. This clearly demonstrated that the sulfur atom was not essential for the antibiotic activity of cephalosporins (Cama and Christensen, 1974). This finding was quite significant from the point of view of structure–activity relationships. It directed the interest of many β-lactam chemists toward the challenging synthesis of other nuclear analogs of cephalosporins. Later, the Merck group was also successful in synthesizing racemic 1-oxacefamandole (9) which was twice as active as cefamandole (Firestone *et al.*, 1977). In addition to clavulanic acid (Chapter 6, this volume), Beecham chemists were interested in structurally similar 1-oxacephems and reported synthesis of the 3-methyl-1-oxacephem derivative (10a) which was derived from penicillin and was therefore optically active (Brain *et al.*, 1977). Independent of the Beecham group, chemists of the Shionogi Research Laboratories were also successful in preparing optically active 10b starting from penicillin (Narisada *et al.*, 1977, 1979). They also found that, in contrast to the observations of the Merck group, the antibacterial activity of optically active 1-oxacephalothin (**8**) was 4 to 8 times higher than that of cephalothin. The Shionogi scientists found that the increase in activity was greatest with the 1-oxygen phenylmalonamido derivative (**10c**) which was 16 times as potent as the corresponding 1-thia congener. These findings gave an impetus to the Shionogi scientists to study

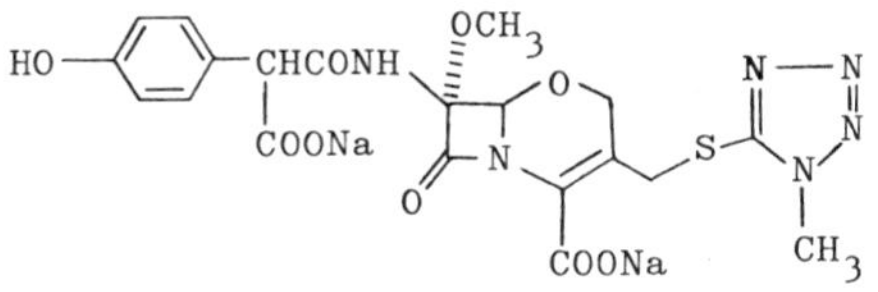

6059-S (LY 127935, moxalactam, latamoxef)

11

1-oxacephalosporins and led them to discover a new potent antibacterial agent, 6059-S (LY127935, moxalactam, latamoxef). The structure of 6059-S is shown by formula **11**. The antibacterial properties of this compound are described in Section V.

Extensive studies on structure–activity relationships in the 1-oxacephem series have indicated that the structural requirements necessary for exhibiting biological activity in 1-oxacephem derivatives are (1) R stereochemistry at C-6, (2) the Δ^3 double bond, and (3) the amido side

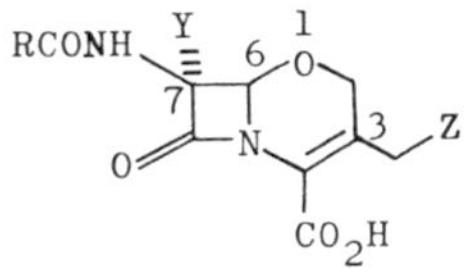

12

chain at C-7 with a β configuration. In order to meet these requirements, careful and well-considered plans are needed for the conversion of penicillins to 1-oxacephem derivatives (**12**). As is the case in other syntheses, chemoselective, regioselective, and stereoselective methods should be applied for efficient conversions. In performing the syntheses the following difficulties arise: (1) Applicable synthetic methods are limited, since azetidinone and bicyclic β-lactam intermediates are often unstable toward base and acid; (2) selection of a suitable protecting group is critical for obtaining a pure final product because of the increased instability of the 1-oxacephem nucleus; and (3) creation of the correct R stereochemistry at C-6 represents the most crucial step in the synthesis, since the 7β-acylamino side chain in azetidinone intermediates prevents the introduction of a C-6 β-oriented oxygen function at the same carbon.

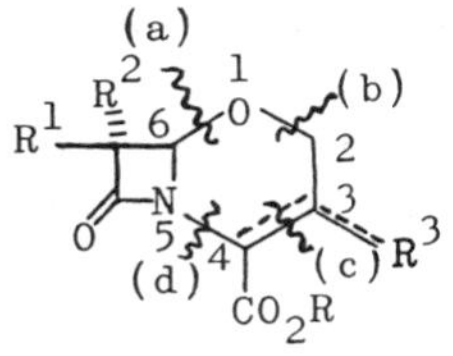

13

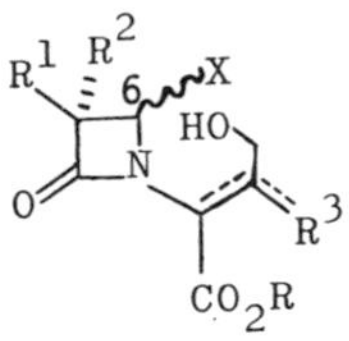

14a 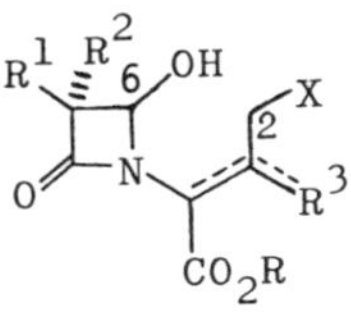   14b 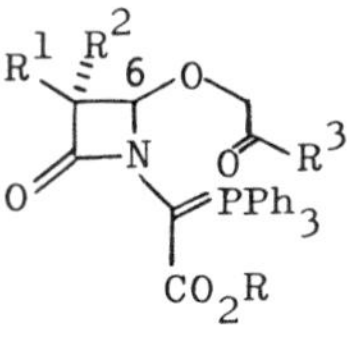   14c 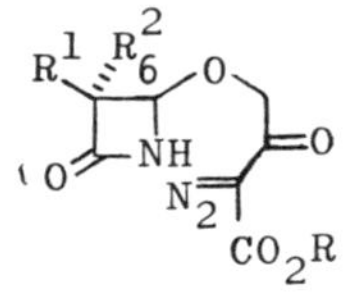   14d

A priori the following synthetic approaches via **14a–d** are feasible depending upon which bond must be formed for six-membered ring closure leading to the 1-oxacephem nucleus (**13**) (a = C-6—O, b = O—C-2, c = C-3—C-4, or d = C-4—N). Intermolecular acetalization (this reaction should be called an acetalization-type reaction, but for convenience we use the term "acetalization" in later discussions) at C-6 (C-4 in azetidinone numbering) is necessary before the cyclization in approaches via **14c** and **14d**, whereas the approach via **14a** involves direct, intramolecular acetalization. In these three cases stereocontrol during C-6—O bond formation provides a serious problem which was previously mentioned. In the approach via **14b** difficulties in the O—C-2 etherification bond formation may occur, and the intermediate **14b** may not be stable under these conditions. As indicated in the literature, the approach via **14c** was used often in both stereocontrolled and nonstereocontrolled syntheses. The approach via **14a** can provide a most efficient synthesis if the necessary functionalities in the hydroxymethyl butenoate side chain can be introduced and the C-6—O bond formation is stereospecific. The approach via **14b** is quite intriguing but so far has been unsuccessful, probably because of the reasons discussed above. No attempt at an approach via **14d** has been reported; however see Chapter 4, this volume. In the following sections the individual syntheses will be discussed in detail according to the type of approach used.

2.   *Synthesis via Wittig Cyclization: Nonstereocontrolled Syntheses*

   a.   General Remarks. In 1972, an interesting method for the conversion for penicillin-originated azetidinone (**15**) to cephems (**21**) was reported.

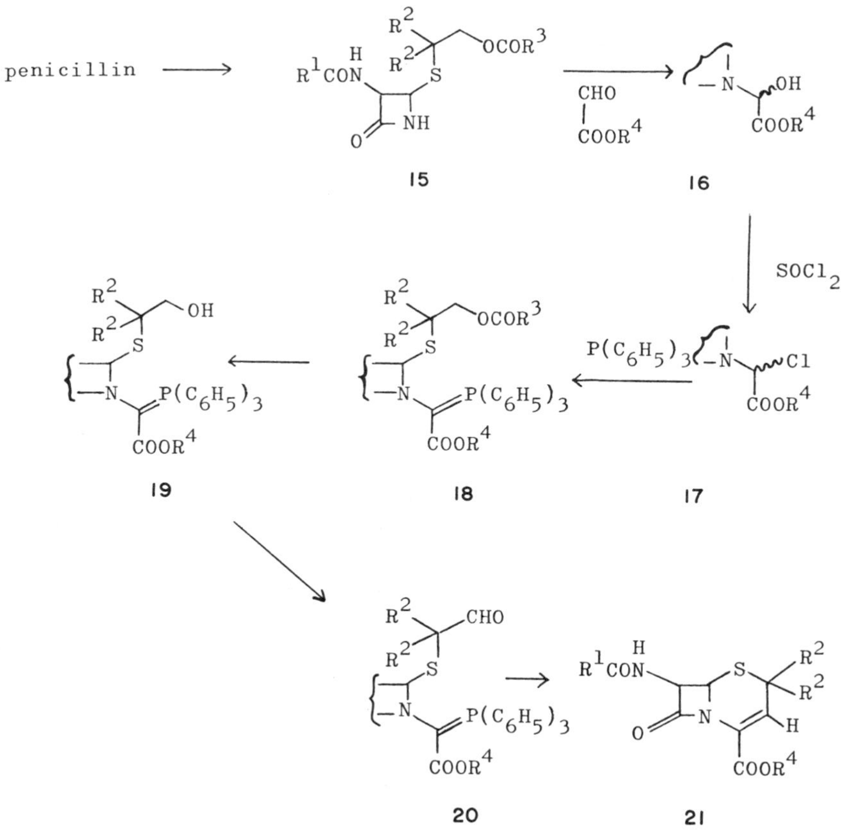

The method utilized the intramolecular Wittig reaction for construction of the cephem skeleton. The aldehyde group for this reaction was formed by oxidation of a primary alcohol, and the ylide moiety necessary for the Wittig reaction was introduced by a newly developed reaction sequence: condensation of 15 with glyoxalate which yields an epimeric mixture of glycolates (16), chlorination with thionyl chloride which produces an epimeric mixture of chlorides (17), and treatment with triphenylphosphine which gives the ylide (18) (Scartazzini *et al.*, 1972; Scartazzini and Bickel, 1972).

Soon thereafter, Beecham chemists also accomplished a synthesis of cephems (25) starting from penicillin (Nayler *et al.*, 1973a,b, 1976). In this case, an acetonyl group was derived through hydration of a propargyl group, whereas the N substituent on the β-lactam was introduced in a way similar to that discussed above.

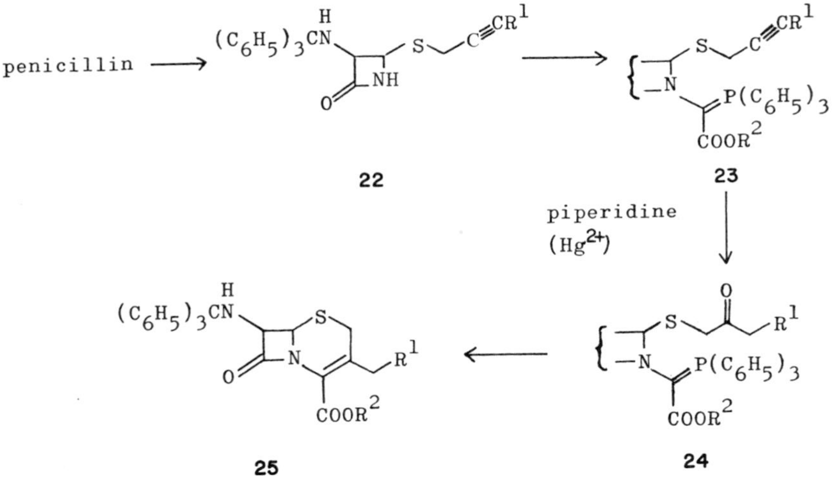

It was believed that these methods could be applied to the synthesis of 1-oxacephems if preparation of **14c** was accomplished. Thus, several syntheses of 1-oxacephems were initiated involving novel methods for the acetalization as well as for formation of the carbonyl group. Though all the syntheses treated in this section employ nonstereocontrolled inter-molecular acetalization and accordingly are not of industrial significance, they have been utilized effectively to prepare numerous derivatives for biological evaluation.

b. Synthesis by the Beecham Group. The first synthesis of optically active 7-acylamino-3-methyl 1-oxacephems (Branch and Pearson, 1979; Brain *et al.*, 1977) was accomplished by extending the synthetic method for (±)-1-oxacephem carboxylic acids. The latter compounds expected to exhibit β-lactamase inhibitory activity like clavulanic acid (Chapter 6, this volume). Later several C-3-modified 1-oxacephems were suc-cessfully prepared.

Replacement of an acetoxy group by a propargloxy group took place when an optically active azetidinone (**26**) prepared from penicillin was treated with propargyl alcohol in the presence of zinc acetate; a separable mixture of *cis*- and *trans*-acetals (**27**) was formed. After the N-substituent was introduced into the *cis*-acetal (**27**), the resulting **28** was hydrated using mercuric chloride in piperidine to produce **29**. An intramolecular Wittig reaction was effected smoothly in refluxing dioxane; compound **30** with the (6*S*,7*R*)-1-oxacephem skeleton was obtained in good yield. An attempt at *N*-bromosuccinimide-mediated bromination of **30** to obtain the bromomethyl compound (**31**), potentially useful for further modifi-cations at the C-3' position, failed.

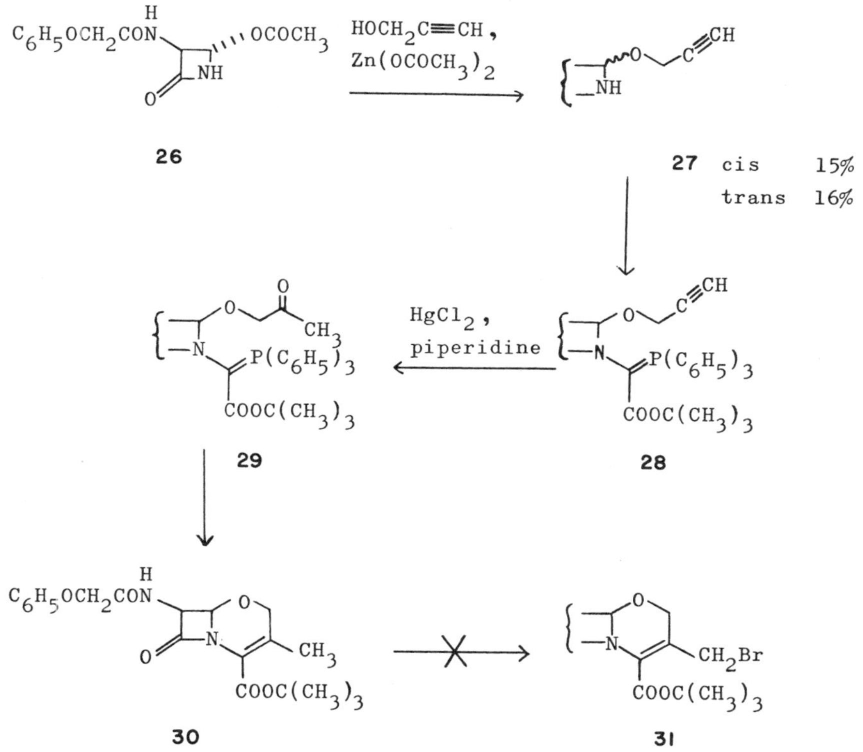

In a similar way, synthesis in the 7β-tritylamino series was also carried out. Optically active azetidinone **32** was acetalized with propargyl alcohol and zinc acetate to produce *cis*- and *trans*-acetals (**33**). Replacement of the methanesulfonyl group proceeded with an ease common to N-unsubstituted azetidinones. After introduction of the N-substituent into *cis*-acetal (**33**), a keto group was formed and then cyclized to **34** in a Wittig reaction. On treatment with *p*-toluenesulfonic acid monohydrate, **34** gave 7β-amino-1-oxacephem (**35**) suitable for further modifications of the amide side chain.

They also succeeded in obtaining new C-3 derivatives of 1-oxacephem. For the acetalization, various alcohols with different masked carbonyl groups were used. Reaction of sulfone **32** with 2-hydroxymethyl-1,3-dithiane and zinc acetate afforded *cis*-acetal **36** along with its trans epimer. Introduction of the N-substituent into **36** gave **37**. When the dithiane group was deprotected to form the aldehyde by heating with methyl iodide and barium carbonate, simultaneous cyclization occurred and 3'-demethyl-1-oxacephem (**38**) was obtained. The trityl group was then removed to form 7β-amino-1-oxacephem (**39**).

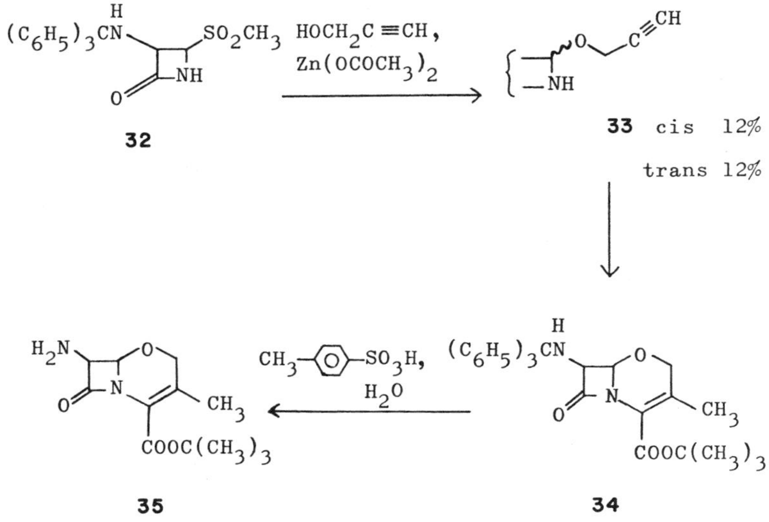
HOCH2C≡CH,
Zn(OCOCH3)2
32
33 cis 12%
trans 12%
CH3-⟨O⟩-SO3H,
H2O
35
34

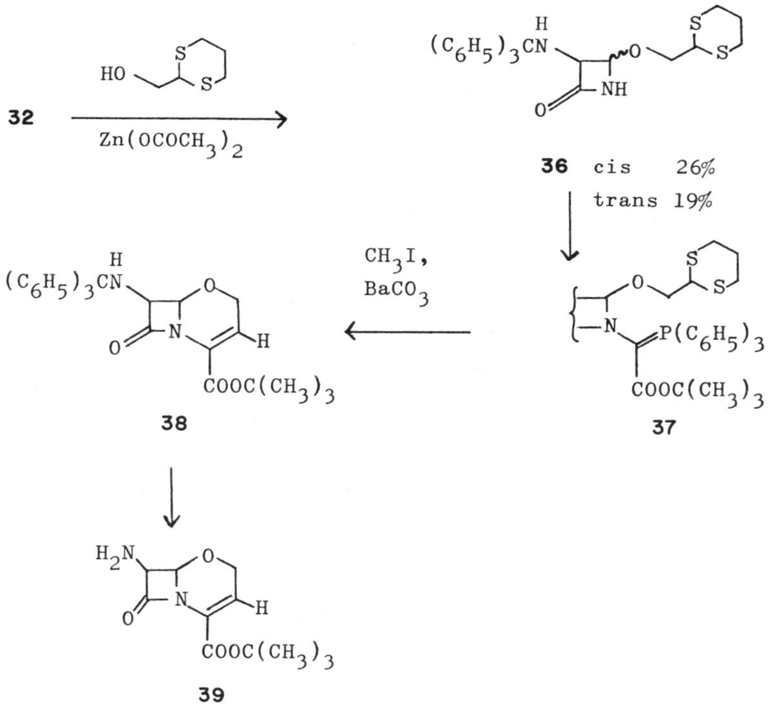
32
Zn(OCOCH3)2
36 cis 26%
trans 19%
CH3I,
BaCO3
38
37
39

Reaction of **32** with an allyl alcohol similarly afforded an epimeric mixture of acetals (**40**). The *cis*-acetal was converted to **41** by introduction of the N-substituent and further to **42** by ozonolysis of the olefinic group.

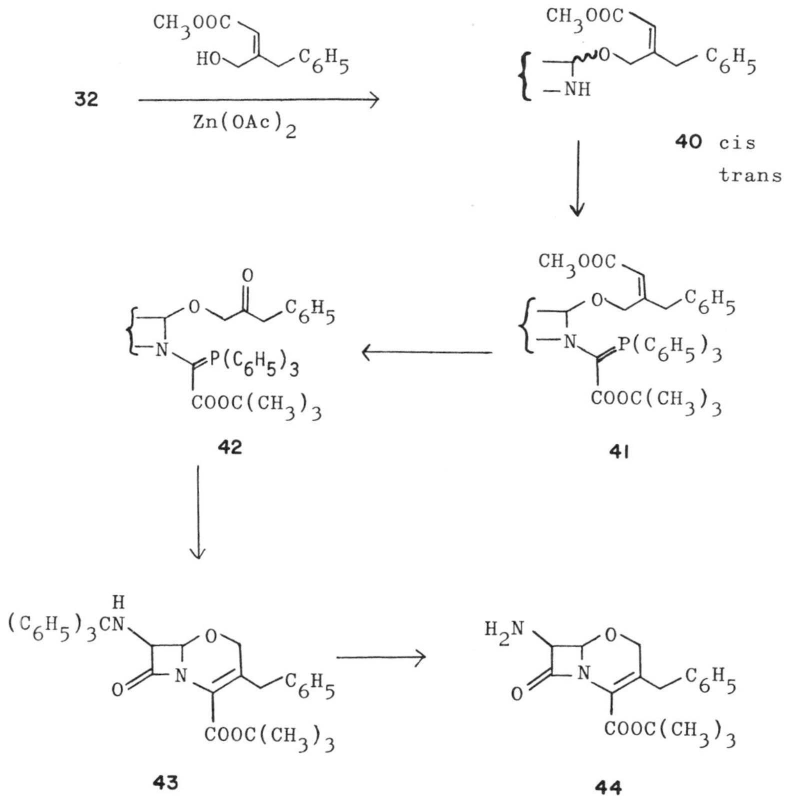

This was cyclized to 3-benzyl-1-oxacephem ester (**43**), from which the trityl group was removed to give the 7-amino compound (**44**).

Acylation of the amino derivatives **35**, **39**, and **44** and deprotection of the tertiary butyl group of the resulting acylamido derivatives including **30** proceeded smoothly as in conventional cephalosporin chemistry. Thus several C-3-modified 1-oxacephem carboxylic acids (**10a,d,e**; **45a,d**; **46a,d**) were obtained.

These 1-oxacephem carboxylates were reported to exhibit antibacterial activity that did not necessarily parallel that found in their 1-thia analogs. One of the most active 3-methylcephems is the phenylglycyl derivative, cephalexin; however, in the 1-oxa series, the corresponding compound

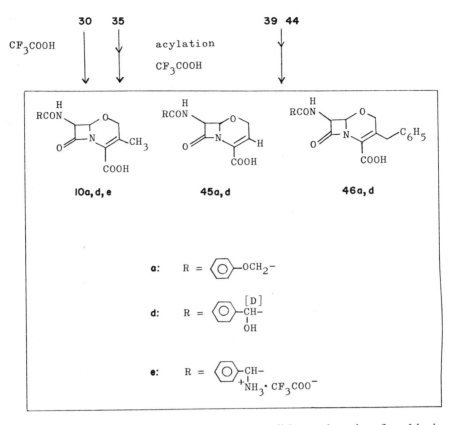

(10e) was the least active product. A possible explanation for this is discussed in Section II,A,2,c.

c. **Synthesis by the Shionogi Group (I).** Independent of the Beecham group, Shionogi chemists also synthesized optically active 3-methyl-1-oxacephems (Narisada *et al.*, 1977) according to the method mentioned in Section II,A,2,a. For formation of the N-substituent, they employed a modified method which had been developed at Shionogi for the synthesis of 3-trifluoromethyl cephems (Yamamoto *et al.*, 1977). In this procedure the glycolate group is formed by ozonolysis of the α-isopropylidene acetate moiety followed by reduction of the resulting oxalate group with zinc and acetic acid. The glycolate group is further transformed into the α-(triphenylphosphorylidene) acetate group by the procedures previously described for **18** (Section II,A,2,a).

Azetidinone **47**, a Beecham intermediate, was deprotected with *p*-toluenesulfonic acid monohydrate to give the salt (**48**), which was chlori-

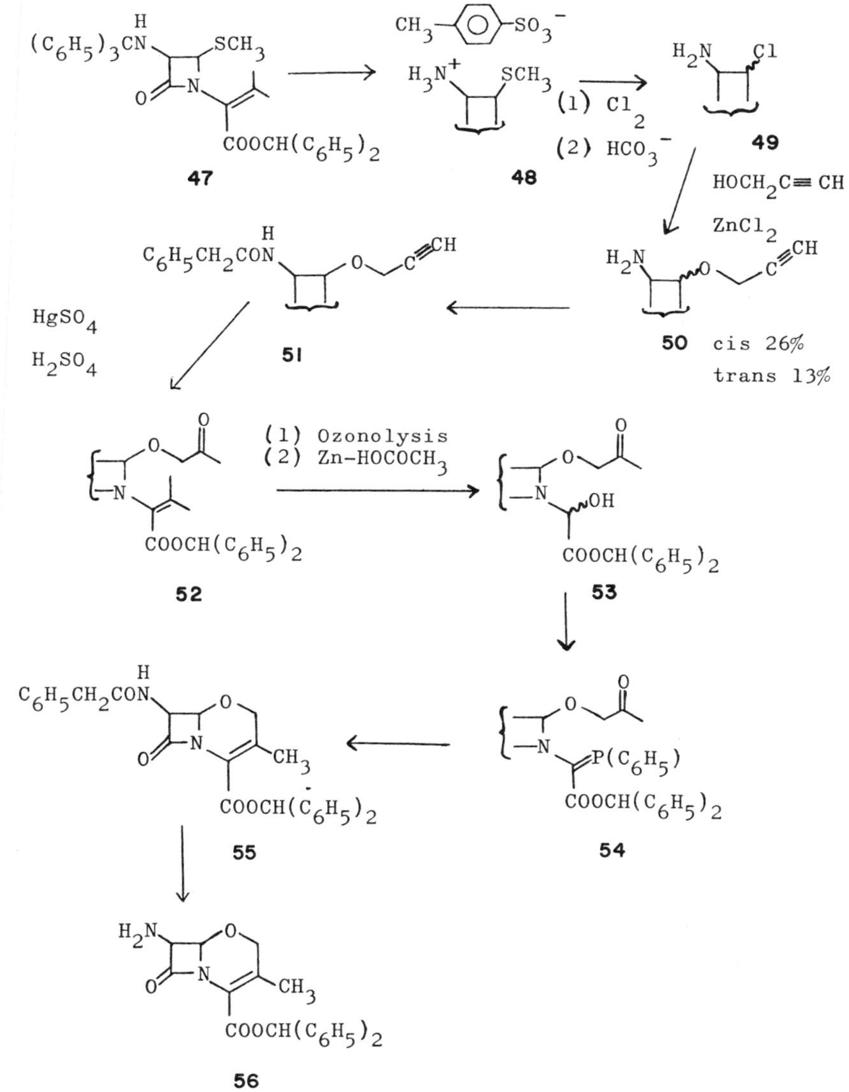

nated to yield a 4:1 mixture of *cis*- and *trans*-chlorides (**49**). The heavy-metal salt-mediated transformation of the chlorides into the desired *cis*-acetal with propargyl alcohol was extensively investigated. Zinc chloride, silver tetrafluoroborate, and stannous chloride were found to produce various mixtures of *cis*- and *trans*-acetals (**50**) with ratios of 2:1, 1:1, and 3:2 and in yields of 39, 38, and 14%, respectively. The mixture was separable by chromatography, however, the corresponding allyl ethers prepared similarly were separated with difficulty.

The propargyl group of phenylacetamide (51) was converted to the acetonyl moiety to give 52. Compound 52 was transformed into an epimeric mixture of 53 by ozonolysis of the isopropylidene group followed by reduction with zinc and acetic acid. Chlorination of 53 followed by reaction with triphenylphosphine gave ylide 54. Wittig reaction of 54 proceeded to afford 1-oxacephem ester 55. The amide side chain of 55 was cleaved easily by the conventional method of treatment with phosphorus pentachloride followed by methanol to yield 7β-amino derivative 56.

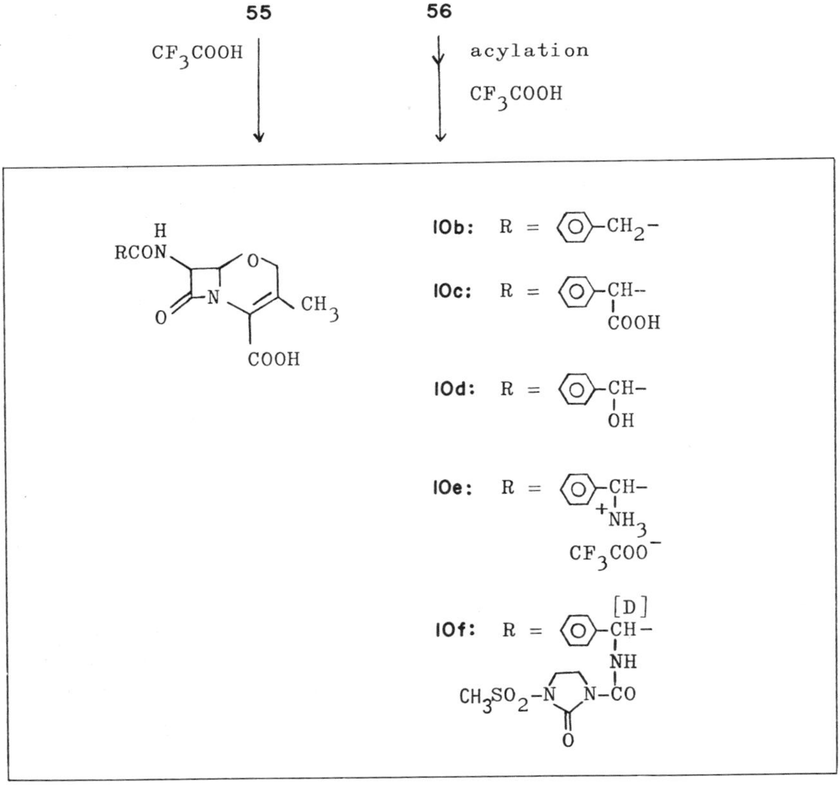

Introduction of various amide side chains and successive deprotection of the benzhydryl ester group with trifluoroacetic acid smoothly produced several (6S,7R)-3-methyl-1-oxacephem carboxylic acids (10b–f). Antibacterial activity of compounds 10b,c,d,f proved to be four to eight times higher than that of the 1-thia congeners; whereas **10e**, the cephalexin analog, was found to be almost devoid of *in vitro* antibacterial activity in accord with the observation of Beecham chemists. Although **10e** as its trifluoroacetate was stable, the free amine was unstable upon comparison of the hydrolysis rates of **10e** and cephalexin. It was suggested that **10e** might decompose during the assay by intramolecular aminolysis of the β-lactam ring activated by the O-1. Compounds (**10c,f**) with side chains useful on penicillins exhibited markedly enhanced antibacterial activity and a broad spectrum against gram-negative bacteria (Section IV,C,1).

   d.   Synthesis by Shionogi Group (II). The method used for 3-methyl derivatives could be improved to one more broadly applicable for the synthesis of C-3-substituted methyl 1-oxacephems (Narisada *et al.*, 1979; Japanese Kokai, 1977b, 1979a).

   Allyl acetal (**57**) obtained by partial hydrogenation of **51** was oxidized with peracid to an epimeric mixture of epoxides (**58**). Introduction of a functional group Z to be located at position C-3′ was performed in three ways. First, a regioselective cleavage reaction of the epoxide ring of **58** either with a mixture of HZ (**59a–f**) and its alkali metal salt or with HZ (HX) in the presence of an acid catalyst afforded **60a–f**, which were then oxidized to give **61a–f**. Compound **61g** was prepared from **58** in a slightly modified way. Second, **58** was cleaved with hydrogen chloride to give chlorohydrins **62**, which on oxidation to **63** and subsequent replacement with HZ (**59c**) in the presence of triethylamine furnished **61c** as well. Finally, conversion of the isopropylidene group into the ylide-one was carried out on **61a–g** by the previously described procedures to yield **64a–g**. In the third route, the conversion was performed in advance of cleavage of the epoxide ring. When the bromides (**65**) derived from **58** were treated with triphenylphosphine, the epoxide ring was simultaneously cleaved by the eliminated hydrogen bromide to yield bromohydrins **66**. These bromohydrins were then oxidized to give **67**. A replacement reaction involving **67** and the sodium salt of HZ (**59h**) afforded **64h**. The triazine derivative (**64h**) could best be synthesized by this route, as the sensitive hydroxy group of the triazine ring was affected by the treatment with thionyl halide. Wittig cyclization of **64a–h** was realized satisfactorily, 3-substituted methyl-1-oxacephems (**68a–h**) being obtained. The structure of a representative compound (**68d**) was confirmed rigorously by X-ray crystallographic analysis (Section III,B).

   Cleavage reaction of the phenylacetamide side chain of **68a–g** was carried out in the conventional way to give **69a–g**, whereas that of **68h** to give **69h** was accomplished after protection of the reactive hydroxyl

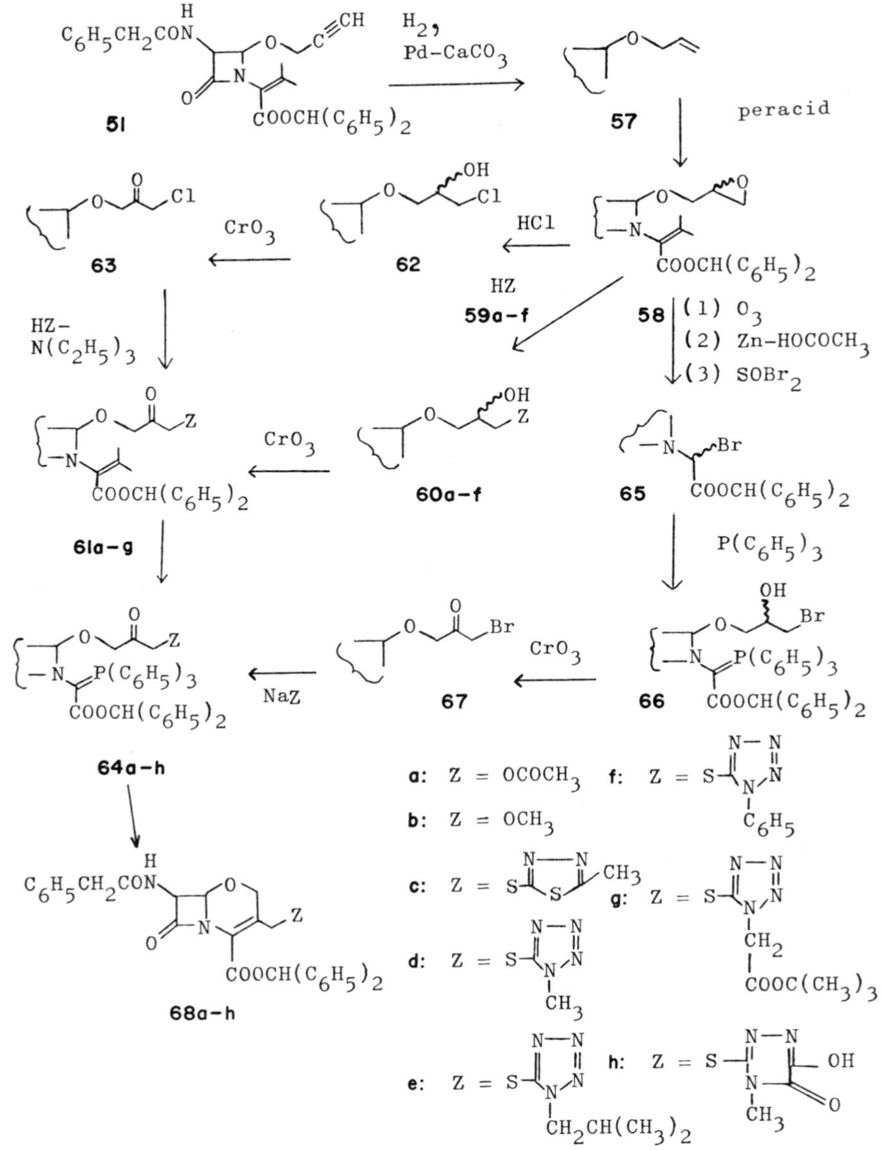

$C_6H_5CH_2CON$ ... $\equiv CH$　H_2, Pd-CaCO$_3$ →

51　COOCH(C_6H_5)$_2$　　**57**　peracid

CrO$_3$ ←　**62**　HCl ←

COOCH(C_6H_5)$_2$

63

HZ **59a–f**

58 (1) O$_3$ (2) Zn-HOCOCH$_3$ (3) SOBr$_2$

HZ–N(C_2H_5)$_3$

CrO$_3$ ←　**60a–f**

65　Br　COOCH(C_6H_5)$_2$

COOCH(C_6H_5)$_2$

61a–g

P(C_6H_5)$_3$

P(C_6H_5)$_3$　COOCH(C_6H_5)$_2$

NaZ ←　**67**　CrO$_3$ ←　**66**

COOCH(C_6H_5)$_2$

64a–h

$C_6H_5CH_2CON$

COOCH(C_6H_5)$_2$

68a–h

a: Z = OCOCH$_3$

b: Z = OCH$_3$

c: Z = S⎯(N—N / S)—CH$_3$

d: Z = S⎯(N—N / N,N) CH$_3$

e: Z = S⎯(N—N / N,N) CH$_2$CH(CH$_3$)$_2$

f: Z = S⎯(N—N / N,N) C$_6H_5$

g: Z = S⎯(N—N / N,N) CH$_2$ COOC(CH$_3$)$_3$

h: Z = S⎯(N—N / N) OH, CH$_3$, O

group as its silyl ether. Deprotection of the ester group of **68a–d** with trifluoroacetic acid afforded **70a–d**. Attempts to transform **70a** to **70d** under various conditions were unsuccessful. Decomposition preceded the conversion, and only an intractable mixture was formed.

(1) PCl$_5$-pyridine
(2) CH$_3$OH

68a–g $\longrightarrow$

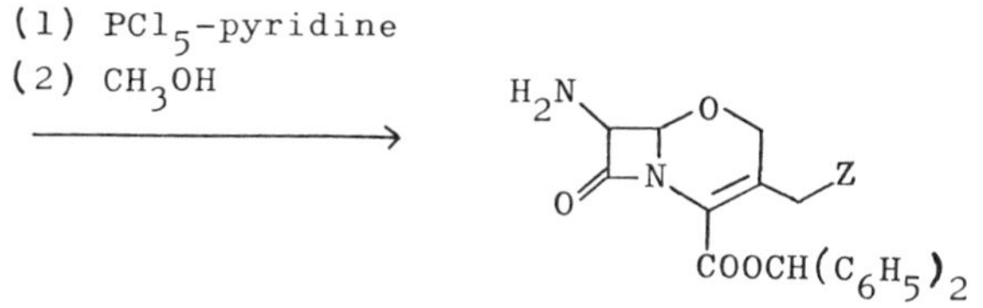

69a–g

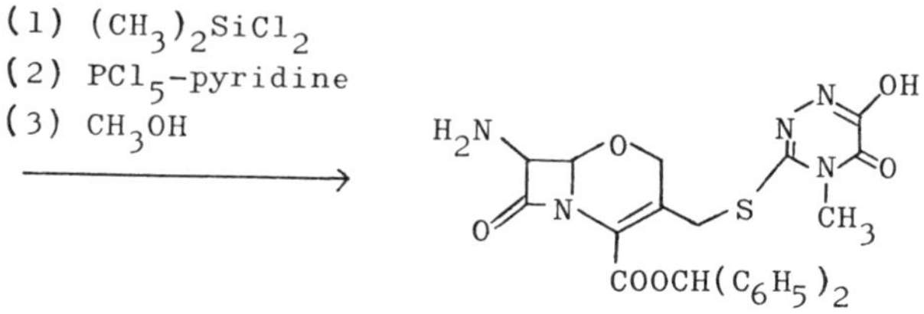

(1) (CH$_3$)$_2$SiCl$_2$
(2) PCl$_5$-pyridine
(3) CH$_3$OH

68h $\longrightarrow$

69h

CF$_3$COOH

68a–d $\longrightarrow$

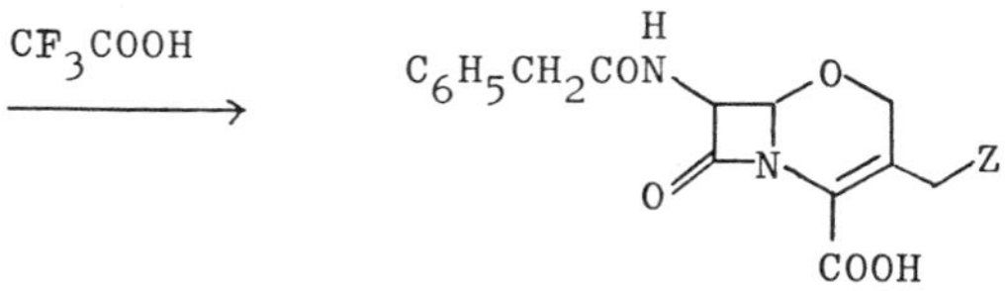

70a–d

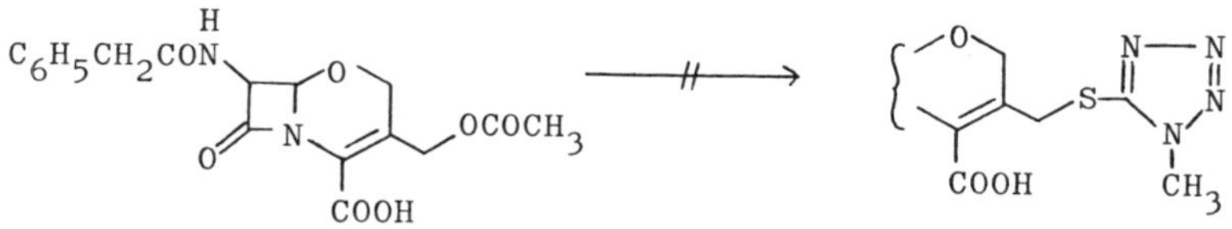

70a $\quad\quad$ // $\longrightarrow$ $\quad\quad$ **70d**

The 7α-methoxylation of **69d** was performed by a modification of the method developed for cephalosporins by Yanagisawa *et al.* (1976). It was condensed with 3,5-di-*tert*-butyl-4-hydroxybenzaldehyde to give **71d**, which was oxidized with nickel peroxide to a quinoid compound (**72d**). Addition of methanol followed by treatment with Girard T yielded 7α-methoxy-1-oxacephem (**74d**). The structure of the phenylacetyl derivative (**75d**) was confirmed by X-ray crystallographic analysis (Section III,B).

e. Synthesis by the Shionogi Group (III). The synthesis of 3-substituted 1-oxacephems was also performed at Shionogi (Hamashima *et al.*, 1979b). A urethane (**76**) prepared from the *cis*-acetal (**51**) was similarly converted to an epimeric mixture of epoxides (**77**). Acid-catalyzed hydration followed by acid hydrolysis of the partially formed acetonide yielded glycols (**78**). These were subjected to periodic acid oxidation to give aldehyde

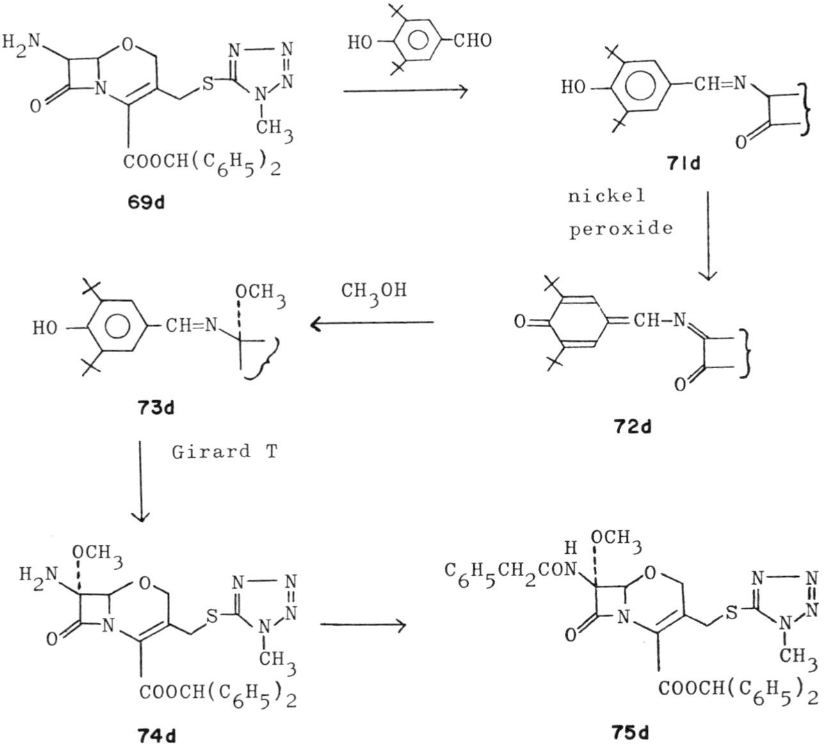

79, which was further converted to methyl ester **80** by chromic acid oxidation followed by treatment with diazomethane. After transformation of the isopropylidene group into the ylide-one, the methyl ester group was selectively hydrolyzed with sodium hydroxide to yield **82a**. A phenyl-acetamide derivative (**82b**) was similarly prepared. Attempts to cyclize the amide (**82b**) by a Wittig reaction in the presence of acetic anhydride (Woodward, 1977) gave an undesired tetrahydroxazine derivative (**83b**). On the other hand, the urethane (**82a**) was found to yield the desired **84** as well as a small amount of **83a** on heating in a mixture of acetic anhydride, toluene, and dimethylacetamide. Mild hydrolysis of **84** in aqueous pyridine afforded the 3-hydroxy-1-oxacephem (**85**) necessary for further modifications.

Methylation with diazomethane yielded **86a**, whereas treatment with a complex of chlorine and triphenylphosphine and mesylation afforded **86b** and **86c**, respectively. The latter two compounds were converted to either **86d** or **86e** by thiolation or chemical reduction, respectively. The resulting variously C-3-substituted 1-oxacephems (**86a–e**) were depro-

cis-5l ⟶

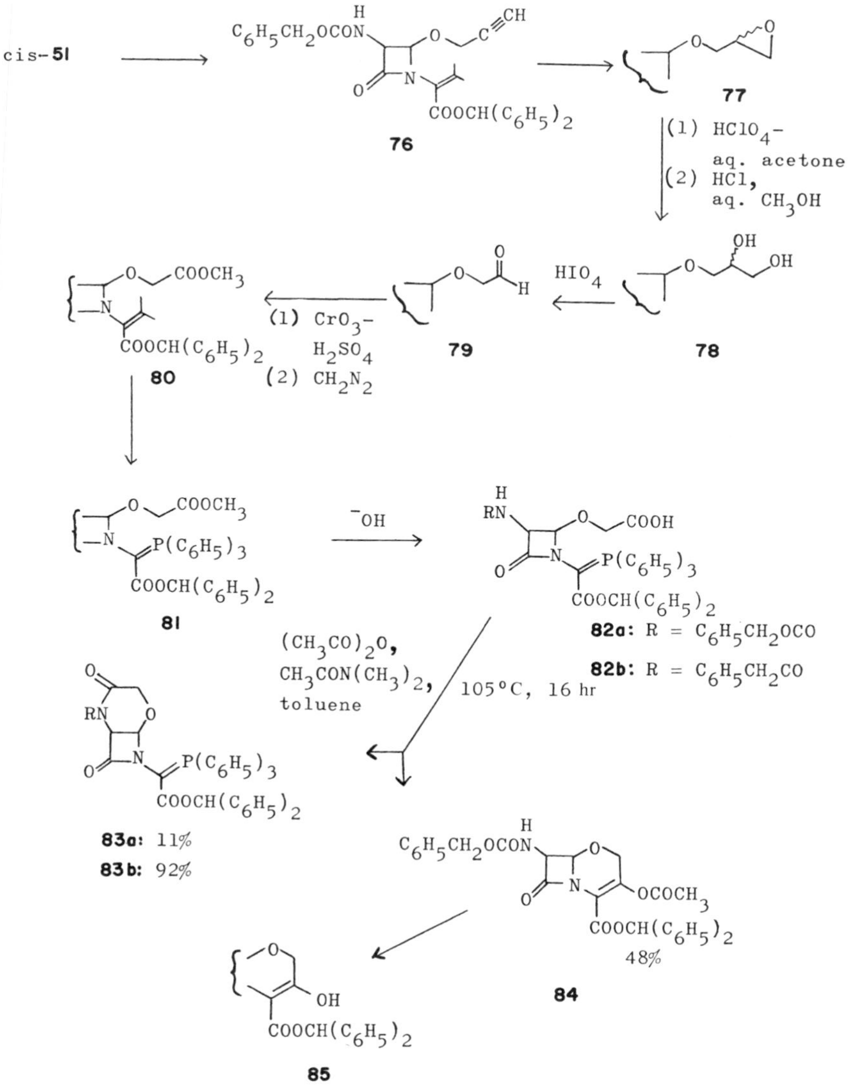

tected to yield amino acids **87a–e** by a method recently developed at Shionogi (Tsuji *et al.*, 1979) using aluminum trichloride and anisole. A 7α-methoxy derivative was also synthesized. Selective deprotection of the benzhydryl ester group of **86b** with trifluoroacetic acid and anisole and subsequent esterification with *p*-nitrobenzyl bromide afforded *p*-nitrobenzyl ester **88b**. The urethane group of **88b** was deprotected using aluminun trichloride and anisole to give **89b** which was methoxylated as described previously for **74d** to yield **90b**.

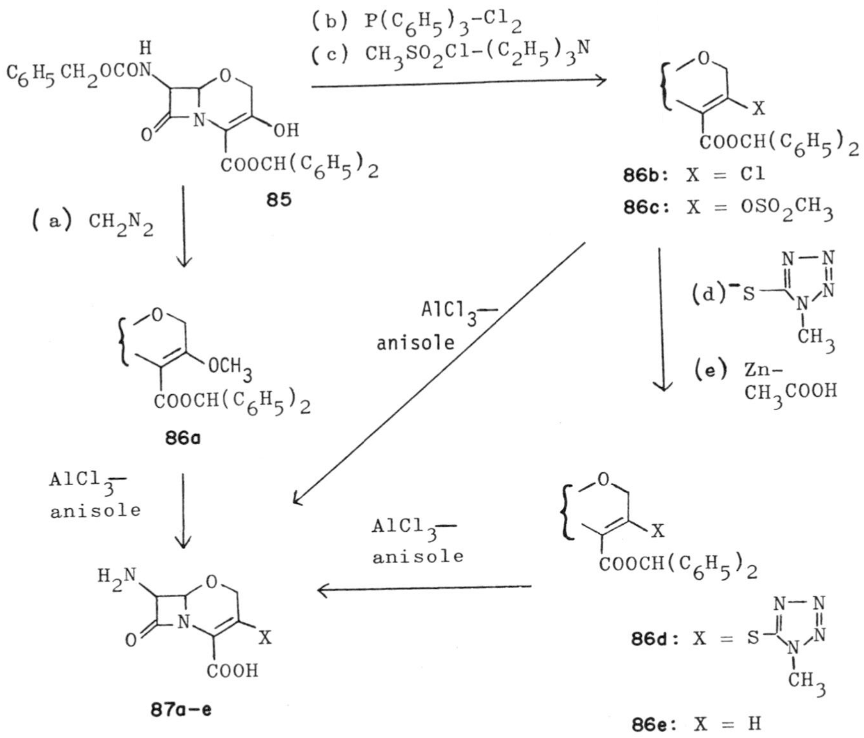

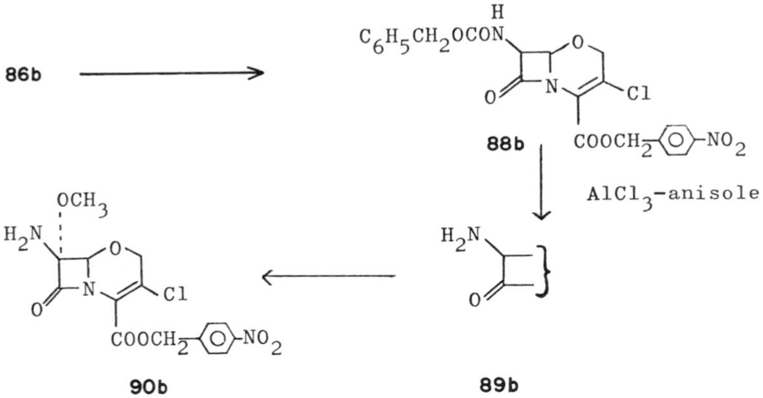

   f. Synthesis by the Shionogi Group (IV). Shionogi chemists synthesized several series of 7β-acylamino derivatives of 1-oxacephems **69** and

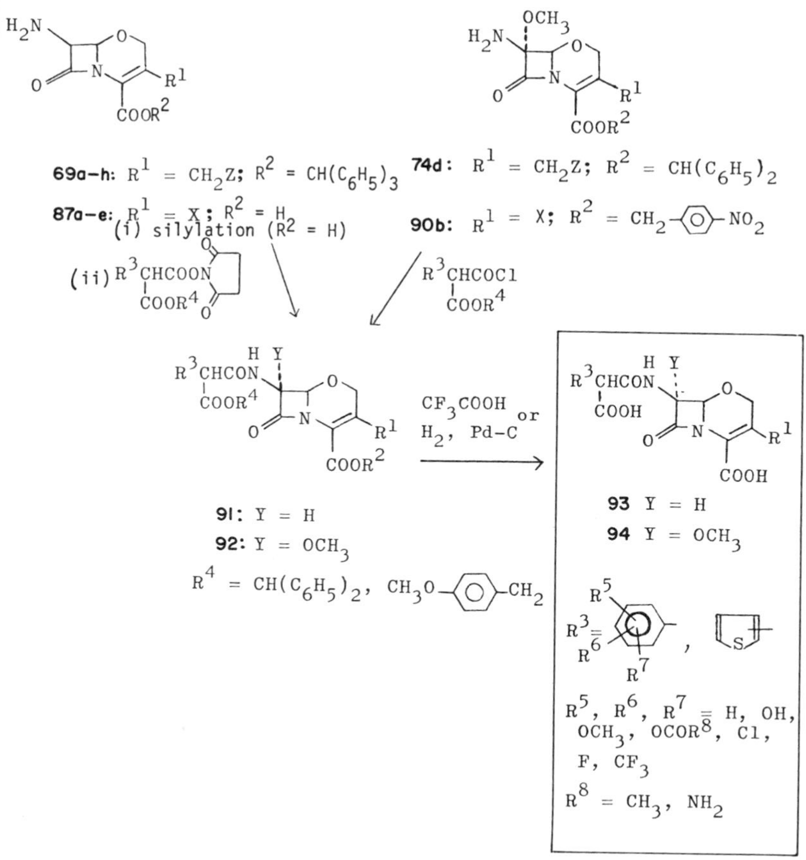

69a–h: $R^1 = CH_2Z$; $R^2 = CH(C_6H_5)_3$

87a–e: $R^1 = X$; $R^2 = H$
(i) silylation ($R^2 = H$)

(ii) $R^3CHCOON$ (with $COOR^4$ and succinimide)

74d: $R^1 = CH_2Z$; $R^2 = CH(C_6H_5)_2$

90b: $R^1 = X$; $R^2 = CH_2-\langle O \rangle-NO_2$

$R^3CHCOCl$
$COOR^4$

R^3CHCON / $COOR^4$

CF_3COOH or H_2, Pd–C $\longrightarrow$

R^3CHCON / $COOH$

91: Y = H
92: Y = OCH$_3$

$R^4 = CH(C_6H_5)_2$, $CH_3O-\langle O \rangle-CH_2$

93 Y = H
94 Y = OCH$_3$

R^5, R^6, $R^7 = $ H, OH, OCH$_3$, OCOR^8, Cl, F, CF$_3$

$R^8 = CH_3$, NH$_2$

87, as well as 7α-methoxy-1-oxacephems such as **74d** and **90b**. Syntheses of 7β-arylmalonamido and 7β-(2-acylamino-2-phenylacetamido) derivatives are discussed here, and their antibacterial activity is discussed in Section IV.

Acylation of 3-substituted methyl 1-oxacephems **69a–h** and trimethylsilyl derivatives of 3-substituted 1-oxacephems **87a–e** proceeded most smoothly with succinimino ester of arylmalonic monoester to give the desired **91**. Although the same reagents did not effect acylation satisfactorily on the 7α-methoxy-1-oxacephems **74d** and **90b**, acylation was carried out smoothly with the corresponding chlorides which were prepared *in situ* by reaction with oxalyl chloride and triethylamine. 1-Oxacephems with an arylmalonamido side chain (**92**) were produced in high yield. On deprotection of the ester groups by treatment with trifluoroacetic acid and anisole or by catalytic hydrogenation in the case of *p*-nitrobenzyl ester, **91** and **92** afforded numerous examples of aryl-malonamido-1-oxacephems (**93** and **94**) (Narisada *et al.*, 1979; Japanese Kokai, 1977c, 1978a,b,d, 1979a,b).

Introduction of a D-phenylglycine moiety into **69d** was most satisfac-

R^1—⟨O⟩—[D]CHCOON (with NH–CO–OC(CH$_3$)$_3$ and succinimide)

H$_2$N (β-lactam, O, N, Z) COOCH(C$_6$H$_5$)$_2$

69d

⟶

R^1—⟨O⟩—[D]CHCON—(β-lactam) NH–CO–OC(CH$_3$)$_3$

95d

CF$_3$COOH –anisole

ClOC(CH$_3$)$_3$, LiOCH$_3$, –65°C

R^1—⟨O⟩—[D]CHCON—(β-lactam, OCH$_3$) NH–CO–OC(CH$_3$)$_3$

97d

R^1—⟨O⟩—[D]CHCON—(oxacephem, Y, Z) $^+$NH$_3$ CF$_3$COO$^-$ O COOH

96d: Y = H
98d: Y = OCH$_3$

⟵ CF$_3$COOH –anisole

R^{2}COCl ↓

R^1—⟨O⟩—[D]CHCON—(oxacephem, Y, Z) NH–CO–R^2 COOH

99d: Y = H
100d: Y = OCH$_3$

R^1 = H, OH, NH$_2$COO–

R^2 = CH$_3$SO$_2$N⟩N–, C$_2$H$_5$N⟩N–, CH$_3$N(CH$_3$)N–,

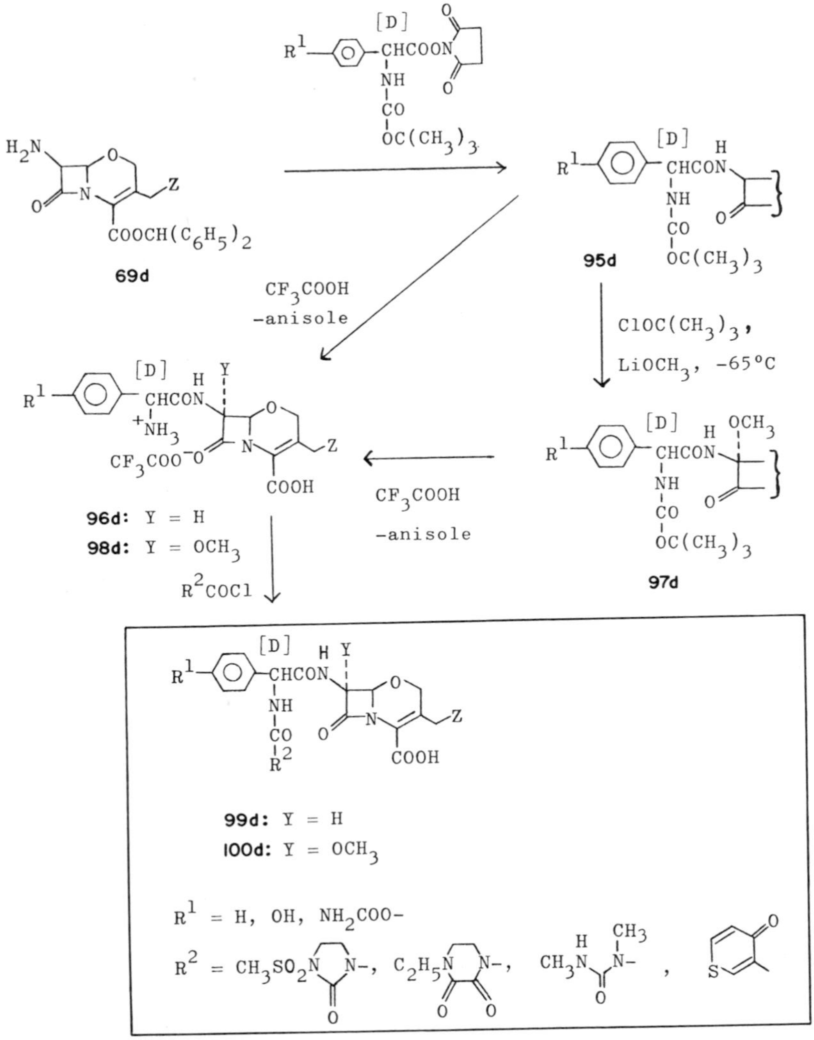

torily effected without racemization of the side chain by using succinimino D-phenylglycyl derivatives giving **95d**. As it was difficult to acylate 7α-methoxyamine (**74d**) without racemization of the side chain, methoxylation was first carried out on **95d** with *tert*-butyl hypochlorite and lithium methoxide (Koppel and Koehler, 1973), giving **97d**. Protecting groups of **95d** and **97d** were removed to produce the corresponding amino acid trifluoroacetates **96d** and **98d**, respectively. Treatment of **96d** and **98d** with various acylating agents used in penicillin and cephalosporin chemistry yielded the corresponding 7β-(2-ureido- or 2-acylamino-2-phenylacetamido)-1-oxacephems **99d** and **100d**, respectively (Japanese Kokai, 1978c, 1979a).

g. Synthesis by the Fujisawa Group (I). A synthesis of 3-unsubstituted 1-oxacephems was carried out at Fujisawa recently (Hemmi *et al.*, 1980;

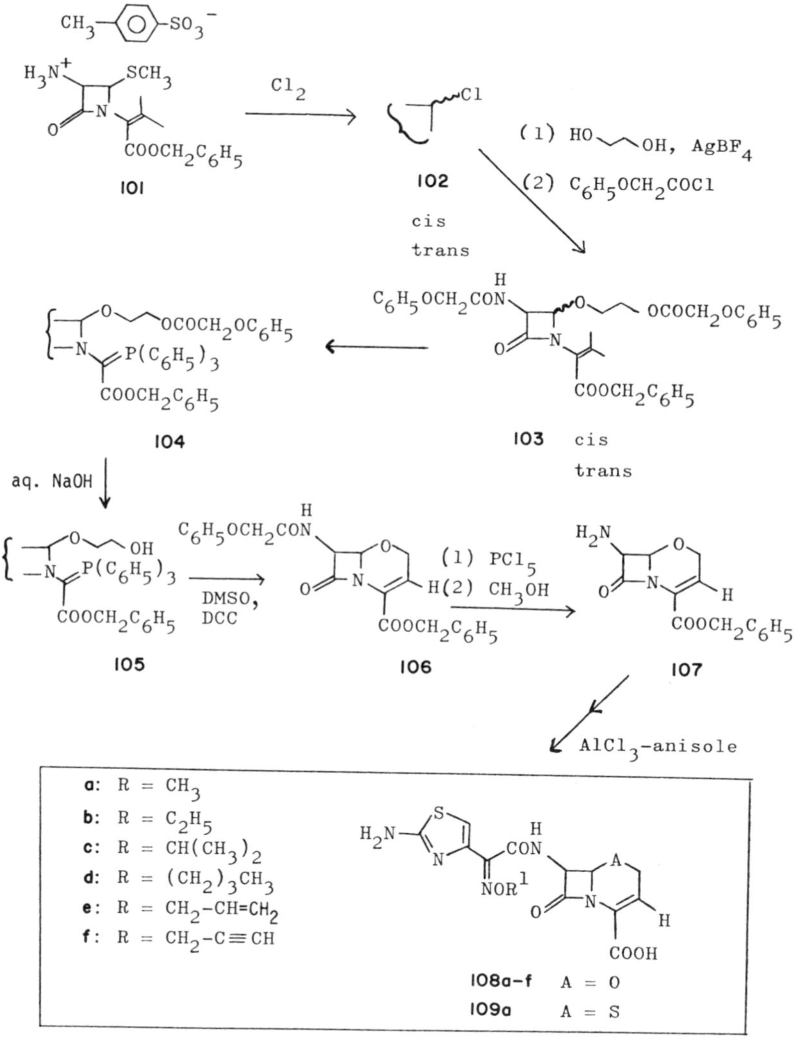

Japanese Kokai, 1979d). An epimeric mixture of cis- and trans-chlorides (102) was converted to a mixture of cis- and trans-acetals (103) by reaction with ethylene glycol in the presence of silver tetrafluoroborate and subsequent O,N-acylation. After formation of the N-substituent on the separated cis-acetal (103) in a way similar to that described previously (Section II,A,2,c), the hydroxy group was regenerated to give 105. Oxidation with dimethyl sulfoxide and dicyclohexyl carbodiimide afforded the desired aldehyde, which immediately cyclized to produce 3-unsubstituted 1-oxacephems (106). The amide group was cleaved in the usual way to afford amine 107. By acylation and subsequent deprotection with aluminum trichloride and anisole (Tsuji et al., 1979), several derivatives of 7β-[(2-aminothiazol-4-yl)-2-(Z)-alkoxyimino]acetamido-1-oxacephems (108a–f) were obtained. Antibacterial activity of the ethyl ether derivative (108b) was reported to be the highest and was almost equal to that of ceftizoxime (109a).

3. Syntheses via Wittig Cyclization: Stereocontrolled Syntheses

a. **General Remarks.** All the previously described synthetic methods clearly have a common drawback in that they involve a nonstereocontrolled acetalization step. Thus several alternatives were developed: One employed stereospecific acid-catalyzed acetalization of enantio-oxazolinoazetidinone, whereas the others solved the problem of cis-acetal formation by a cleavage reaction of oxazolidinoazetidinone without C—O bond rupture.

b. **Synthesis by the Shionogi Group (V).** Using a reductive cleavage, Shionogi chemists accomplished the conversion of oxazolinoazetidinone (110) obtained from methoxycarbonyl penicillin to the intermediate 52 common to the previous synthesis of 3-methyl-1-oxacephems (Section II,A,2,c) (Yoshioka et al., 1979). The transformation of 110 into intermediates for the synthesis of 3'-substituted methyl-1-oxacephems (Section II,A,2,d) was also accomplished.

Reduction of 110 with aluminum amalgam and subsequent phenylacetylation yielded oxazolidine ester (111), which was transformed into methyl ketone oxazolidine (112) by treatment with methylmagnesium bromide in the presence of an excess of triethylamine. Reductive cleavage of 112, possessing a 1,4-dicarbonyl system, was found to be effected best with zinc and hydrogen chloride. However, it was necessary to stop the reaction at an intermediate stage to avoid overreduction. A mixture of the desired 52 and 112 was obtained. A simple silica gel chromatography gave 52 in 50% yield with 42% recovery of 112.

Regioselective bromination of the separated methyl ketone (52) with cupric bromide under ketal formation conditions proceeded smoothly, giving **113** after deketalization. Direct substitution reactions of thiolate and acetate ions on **113** were carried out to produce **61d** and **61a**, respectively. The versatile intermediate **58** was derived by reduction with sodium borohydride followed by treatment with potassium tertiary butoxide. Compounds **52, 58, 61d**, and **61a** represent useful intermediates in the syntheses discussed previously (Section II,A,2,c and d).

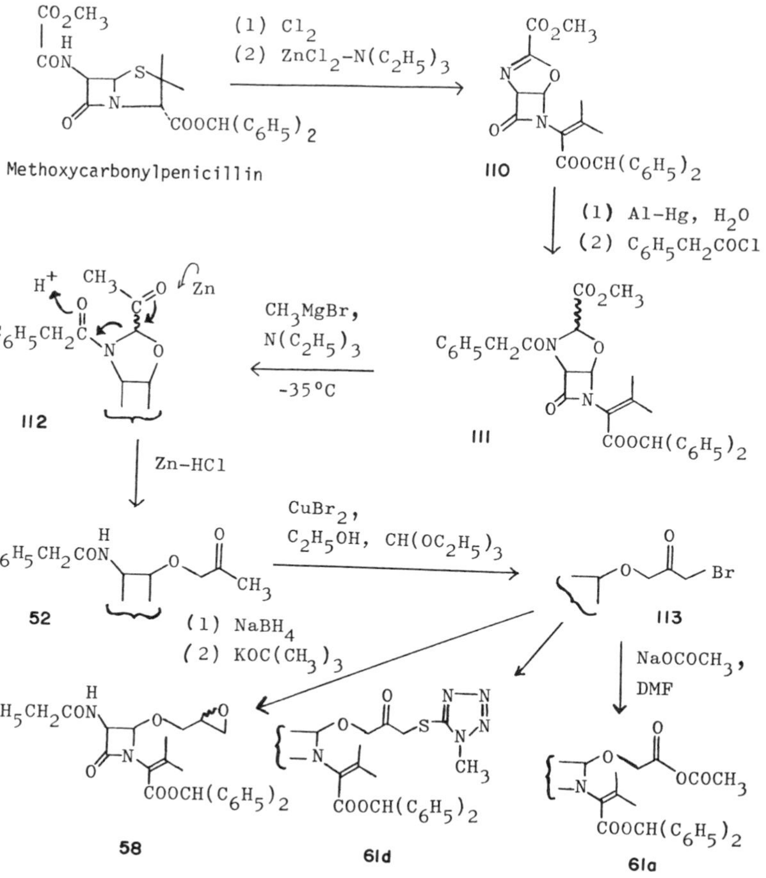

c. **Synthesis by the Shionogi Group (VI).** An interesting stereospecific cleavage reaction of an oxazolinoazetidinone with alcohols to give *trans*-acetal had been noted by Corbett and Stoodley (1974). By applying this method to *enantio*-oxazolinoazetidinone (**117**), Shionogi chemists were able to achieve stereocontrolled acetalization which leads to a very efficient method for the synthesis of 7α-methoxy-1-oxacephems (Uyeo *et al.*, 1979).

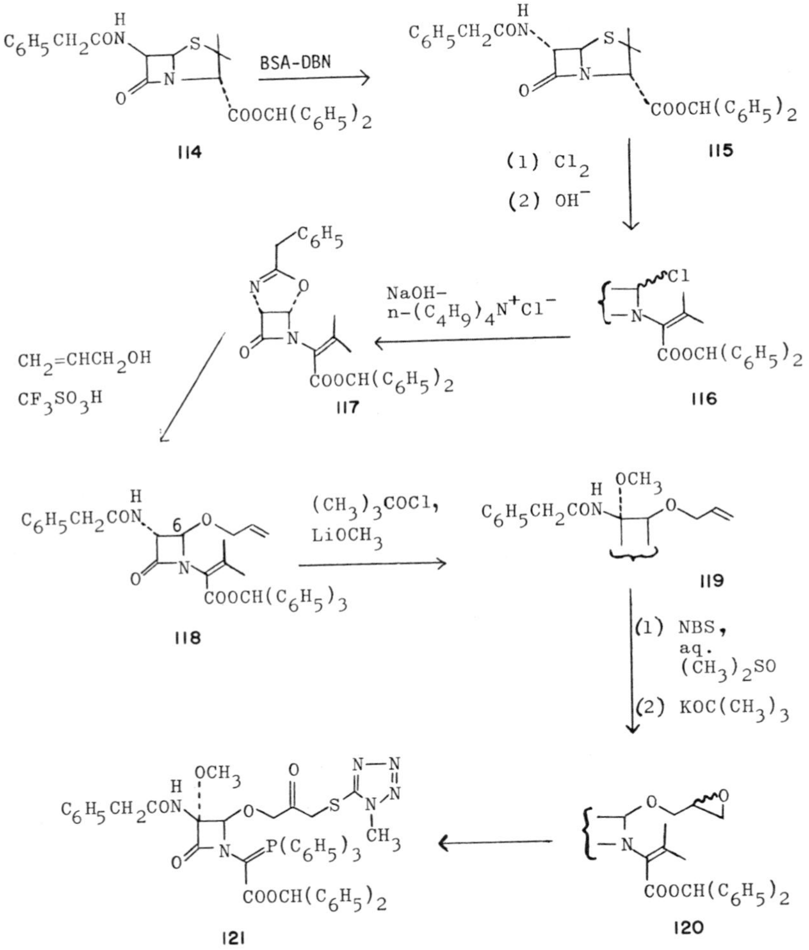

Epipenicillin (**115**) derived from **114** was converted to the *enantio-oxazolinoazetidinone* (**117**) by way of **116**. Stereospecific cleavage of **117** with allyl alcohol in the presence of a catalytic amount of trifluoro-methanesulfonic acid was effected as expected, producing *trans*-acetal **118** in high yield with the correct configuration at C-6 (cephem numbering). Although methoxylation with *tert*-butyl hypochlorite and lithium methoxide (Koppel and Koehler, 1973) could be carried out at any transformation step, methoxylation at the earliest step proved to be the most advantageous, **119** being prepared with high stereoselectivity. Epoxidation of **119** by successive treatments with *N*-bromosuccinimide in aqueous dimethyl sulfoxide and *tert*-butoxide yielded **120**. Further conversions to **121** were performed in a way similar to that described previously (Section II,A,2,d).

Alternatively, propargyl acetal (**122**) derived similarly from **117** was

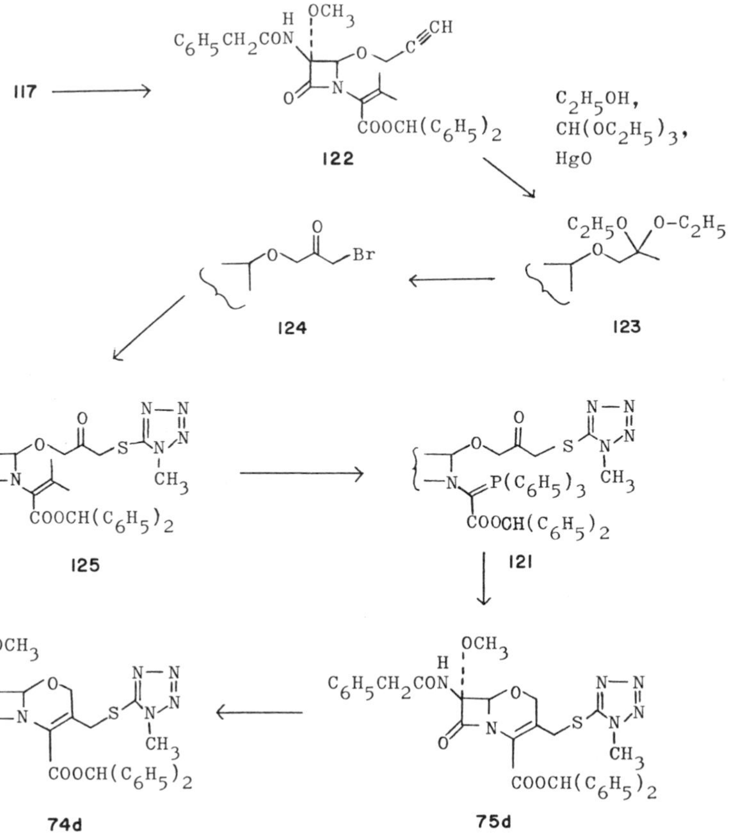

converted to ketal (**123**) by heating in a mixture of ethanol, *ortho*-ethylformate, and mercuric oxide. Bromination gave **124** which underwent the replacement reaction (Section II,A,3,b), yielding **125**. Conversion of the isopropylidene group to the ylide-one was carried out as previously described (Section II,A,2,d), the product (**121**) being obtained in comparable yield. It cyclized like the 7α-unsubstituted series and gave 7α-methoxy-1-oxacephem (**75d**). Lunn *et al.* (1974) reported that amide cleavage of 7α-methoxycephems was accompanied by C-7 epimerization. It was felt that this might be the case in the amide cleavage reaction of **75d**. However, it was found that, owing to stabilization by hydrogen bonding between the 7β-amino group and the oxygen atom at the 1-

position, no epimerization at C-7 was observed after successive treatments with phosphorous pentachloride, methanol, and diethylamine. Compound **74d** was formed as a single product, believed to be thermodynamically stable.

d. Synthesis by the Fujisawa Group (II). Recently, Fujisawa chemists were also successful in transformation of oxazolinoazetidinone (**128**) into 2-oxo-1-oxacephem compounds (Aratani *et al.*, 1980; Japanese Kokai,

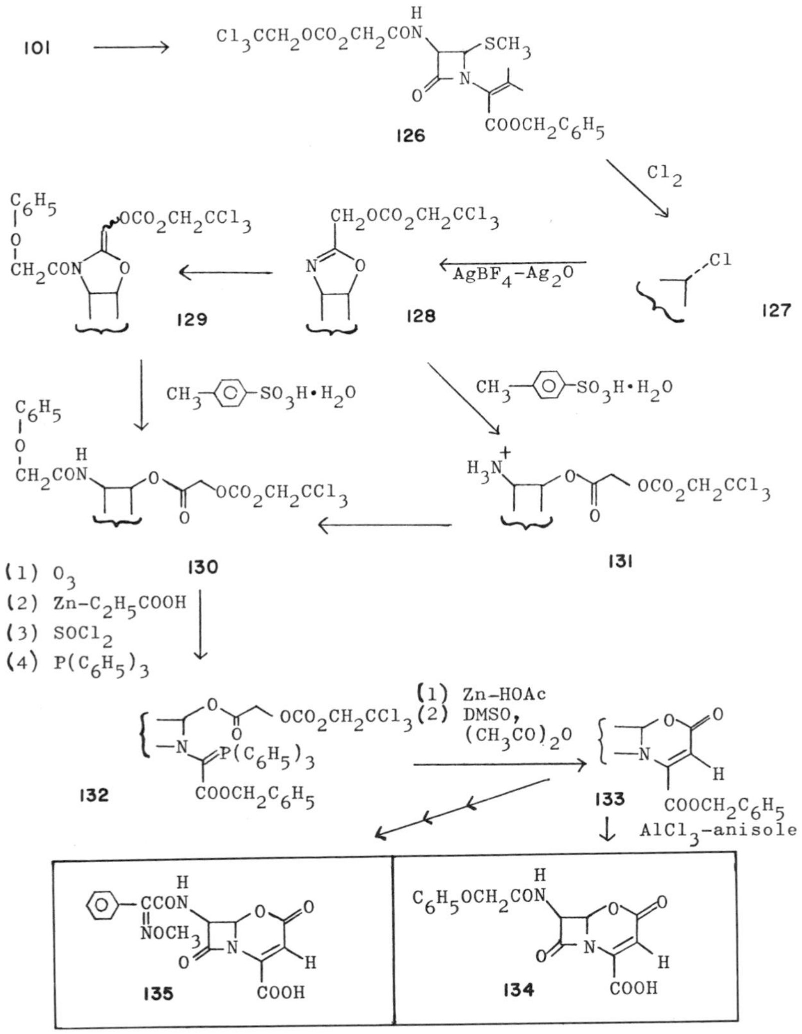

1980). They employed a method for hydrolytic cleavage of oxazolino-azetidinone developed by Wolfe *et al.* (1975).

trans-Chloride 127, derived fron penicillin by way of 126, was cyclized to 128. This compound was phenoxyactylated to yield 129, which was treated with *p*-toluenesulfonic acid monohydrate to give 130. Alternatively, 128 was cleaved to afford 131 and then converted further to 130 by acylation. A sequence of reactions, ozonolysis, reduction with zinc and propionic acid, chlorination with thionyl chloride, and treatment with triphenylphosphine, transformed 130 into 132 with the trichloroethyl carbonate group remaining intact.

An alcohol was formed on removal of the trichloroethyl carbonate group by reduction with zinc and acetic acid. Oxidation of this alcohol with dimethyl sulfoxide and acetic anhydride afforded oxalyl ester which spontaneously cyclized, giving 133 exclusively with a six-membered 2-oxo-1-oxacephem skeleton. Transformations of 133 into 134 and 135 were carried out. In accord with the instability of 2-oxocephalosporins reported by Ernest (1980), they were found very labile and accordingly devoid of antibacterial activity.

4. *Syntheses via Intramolecular Acetalization:*
   Nonstereocontrolled Syntheses

   a. General Remarks. Syntheses belonging to this category effectively utilize the valine moiety derived from penicillin (or cephalosporin) for formation of the dihydrooxazine ring. Although various hydroxylated valine residues could be used in the intramolecular acetalization, all syntheses discussed in this section employ functionalized α,β-dehydro-valine systems. The stereoselective functionalization has proven difficult, especially when the more desirable bis-hydroxylation of the α,β-dehy-drovaline moiety is attempted (see, e.g., Campbell and Rawson, 1979). Although difficulties in producing the correct C-6 stereochemistry by applying intramolecular acetalization reduced the utility of this approach, the high, albeit wrong, stereospecificity involved in these conversions afforded useful mechanistic information.

   b. Wolfe's Synthesis. Wolfe *et al.* (1974) reported the first synthesis of the 1-oxacephem skeleton starting from anhydropenicillin (136). This compound was chlorinated to give chloroacid chloride which, upon treatment with methanol, was converted to an epimeric mixture of 137. Both epimers were separated, and each epimer was independently subjected to further similar transformations. Azobisisobutyronitrile initiated the bromination of 137 with *N*-bromosuccinimide, which afforded a mixture of geometrical isomers of 138. Substitution with tetramethylguanidinium

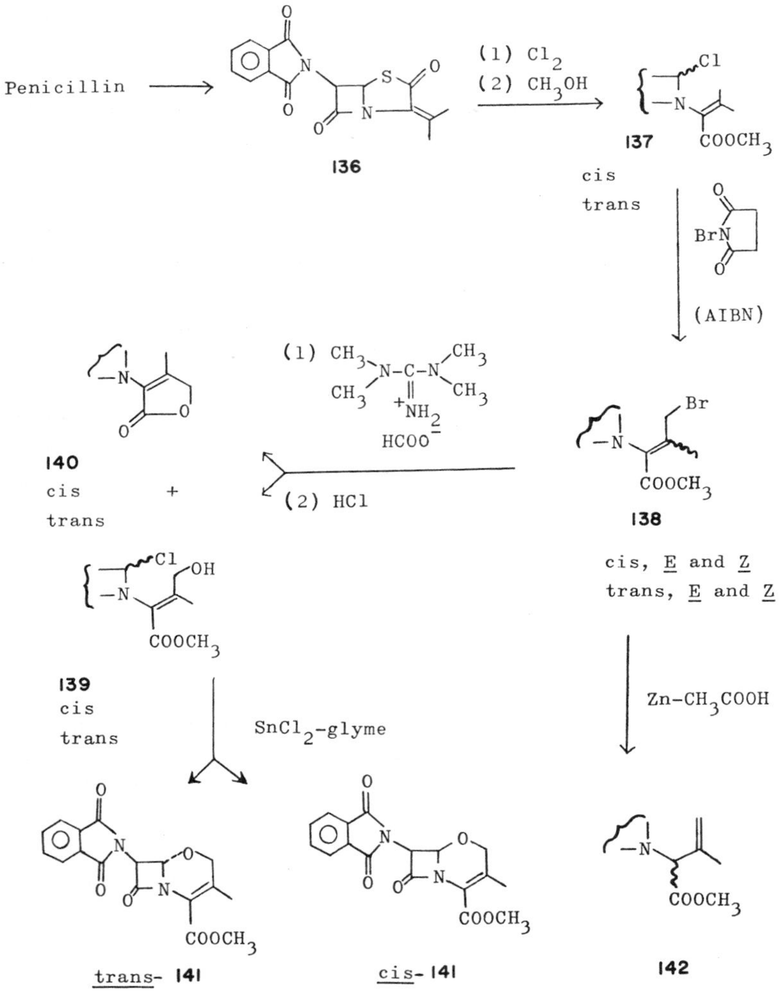

formate and subsequent deformylation yielded the desired allyl alcohol
139 and lactone **140**. These workers reported that the cyclization proceeded smoothly to give the same mixture of *trans*-**141** and *cis*-**141** from
either epimer of **139** and that treatment of *cis*-**139** with 1.38 molar equivalents of stannous chloride in dimethoxyethane yielded only *trans*-
141, whereas 1.67 molar equivalents of the reagent in a doubly diluted
solution afforded a 1:1 mixture of *trans*-**141** and the desired *cis*-**141**. The
cis structure was assigned on the basis of nuclear magnetic resonance
(NMR) data. Reduction of **138** with zinc and acetic produced an epimeric
mixture of β,γ-dehydrovaline derivatives (**142**).

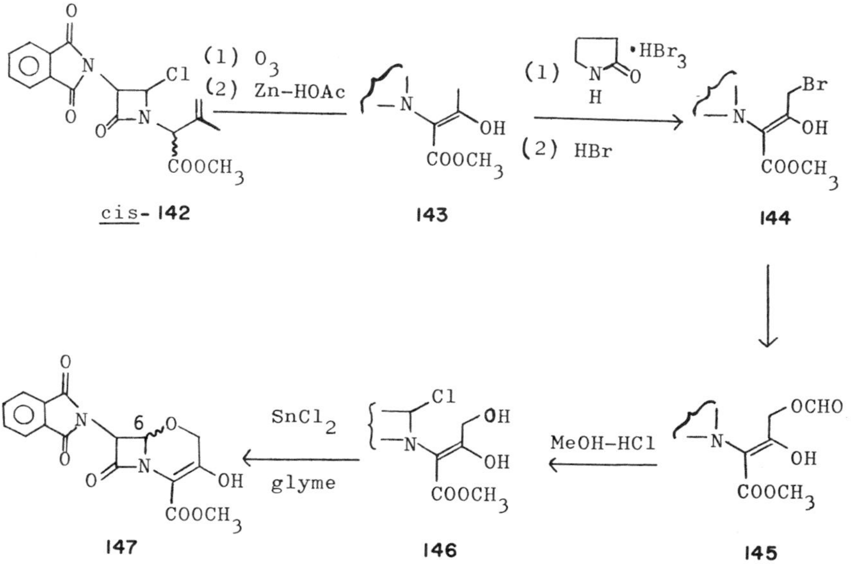

Starting from **142**, synthesis of 3-hydroxy-1-oxacephem (**147**) was accomplished (Japanese Kokai, 1976). Ozonolysis of *cis*-**142** and subsequent reduction with zinc and acetic acid produced enol **143**. Bromination with pyrrolidone hydroperbromide gave an α-bromide, and subsequent rearrangement by prolonged treatment with hydrogen bromide yielded the desired γ-bromide (**144**). Conversion of **144** to **145**, hydrolysis to **146**, and cyclization proceeded smoothly to afford 3-hydroxy-1-oxacephem (**147**) with unidentified C-6 stereochemistry.

Compounds *cis*-**141** and **147** were not transformed into their free acid with 7β-amide functionality, therefore no information about their antibacterial activity is available.

c. Bristol's Synthesis. Bristol chemists reported a stereospecific synthesis of 6-epimeric 3-methyl-1-oxacephem starting from 3-methylcephem (**148**) (Kim and McGregor, 1978). Chlorination at the C-2 position of **148** with *N*-chlorosuccinimide in methanol produced 2α-methoxycephem (**149**). Further chlorination with chlorine cleaved the cephem ring system to give aldehyde **150**, which was reduced with sodium borohydride to give **151** with a hydroxydehydrovaline function of correct geometry. Intramolecular acetalization mediated with silver tetrafluoroborate and silver oxide proceeded stereospecifically from the α side to give 6-epi-1-oxacephem (**152**). Carboxylic acid (**153**), obtained by deprotection of the ester group, was reported to exhibit substantially diminished antibacterial activity.

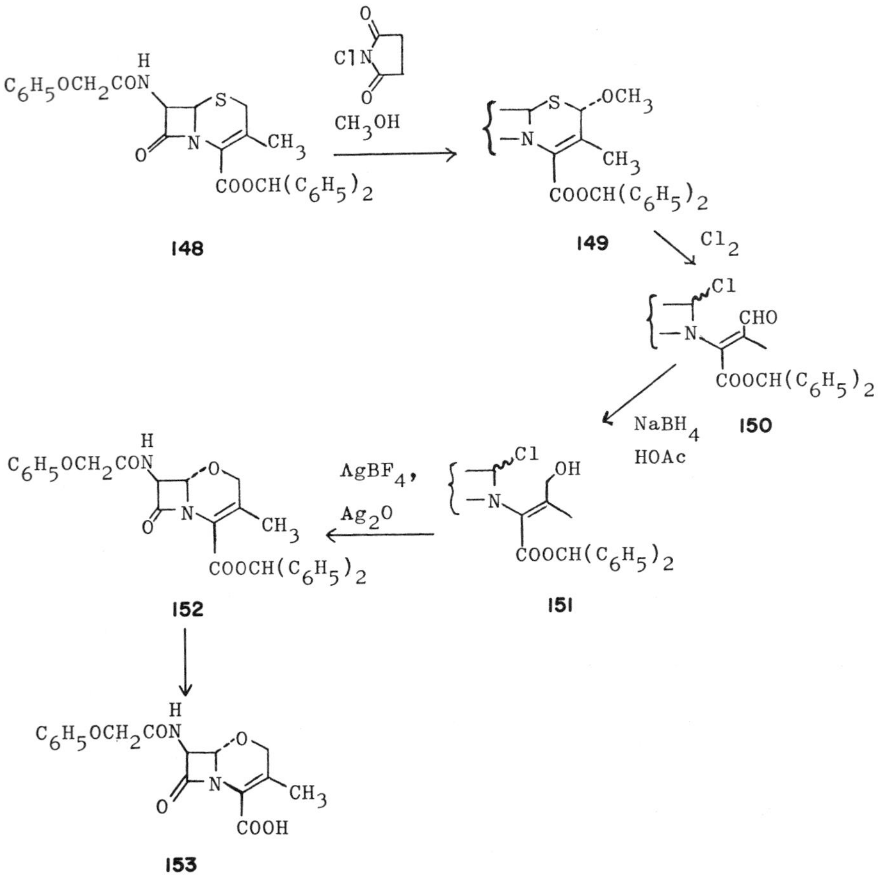

5. Syntheses via Intramolecular Acetalization— Stereocontrolled Syntheses

a. General Remarks. Substantial improvement could be obtained if the preceding syntheses via intramolecular acetalization were performed in a stereocontrolled manner. The problem was solved by applying the previously described method for the intermolecular stereospecific trans-acetalization to *enantio*-oxazolinoazetidinones (Section II,A,3,a). Formation of the allylic alcohol moiety necessary for this intramolecular acetalization could take place most effectively by terminal methyl functionalization of the β,γ-dehydrovaline moiety derived from penicillin.

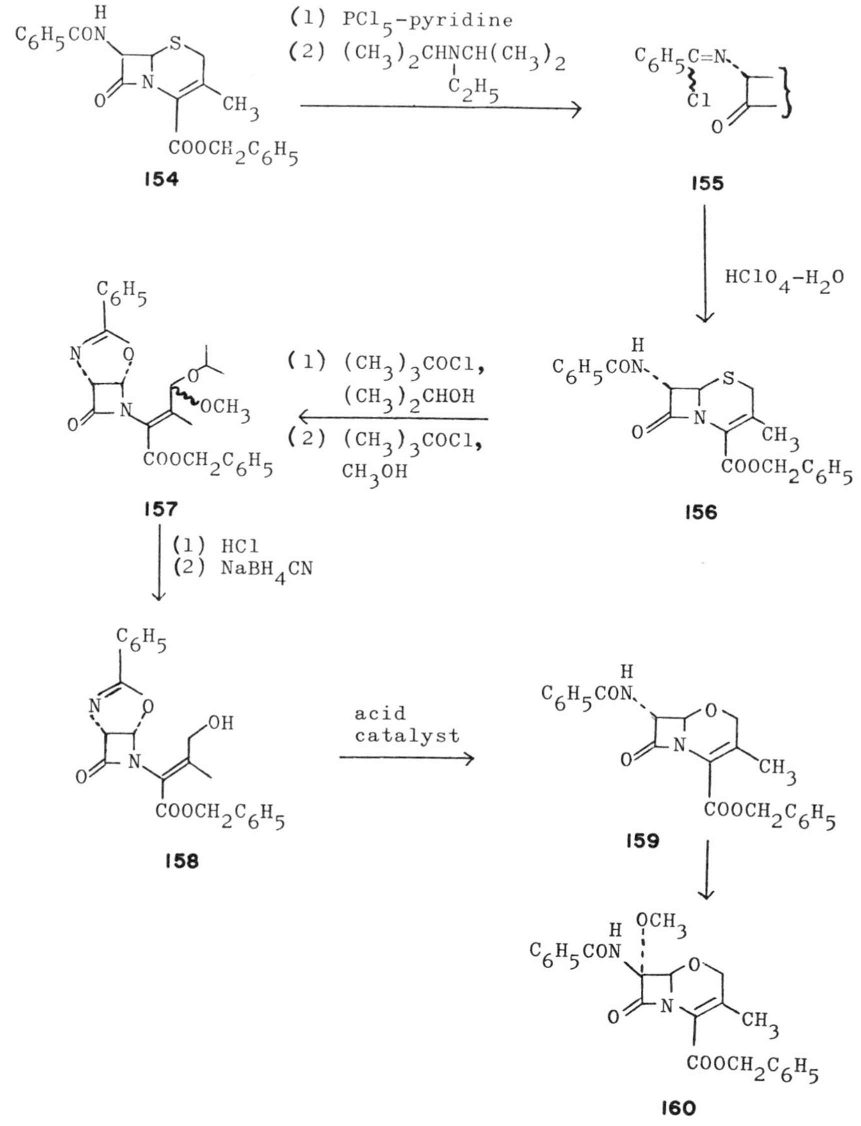

b. Synthesis by the Shionogi Group (VII). By using 7-epi-3-methyl-cephem as the starting material, stereocontrolled synthesis of 7α-methoxy-3-methyl-1-oxacephem was performed (Hamashima *et al.*, 1979a). Epimerization of the C-7 side chain of cephem **154** was carried out by way of the imide chloride (**155**), and the desired 7-epicephem (**156**) was obtained in moderate yield. Sankyo chemists had developed a method similar to that of Bristol (Section II,A,4,c) for cleaving the dihydrothiazine ring with formation of a regioselectively functionalized isopropylidene group (Yoshida *et al.*, 1976, 1977). This method was applied to the 7-epi-isomer (**156**) with a slight modification. Thus by repeated treatments with tertiary butylhypochlorite in isopropanol and then in methanol, *enantio*-oxazolines (**157**) were obtained. Acid hydrolysis of the acetal group followed by hydride reduction gave the hydroxy compound (**158**) which was cyclized with an acid catalyst to yield exclusively 7-epi-3-methyl-1-oxacephem (**159**). On methoxylation with *tert*-butyl hypochlorite and lithium methoxide (Koppel and Koehler, 1973), 7α-methoxy-3-methyl-1-oxacephem (**160**) was prepared with the desired C-7 stereochemistry.

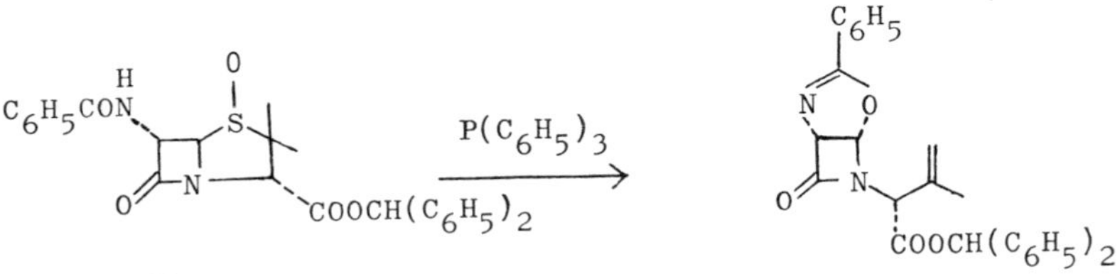

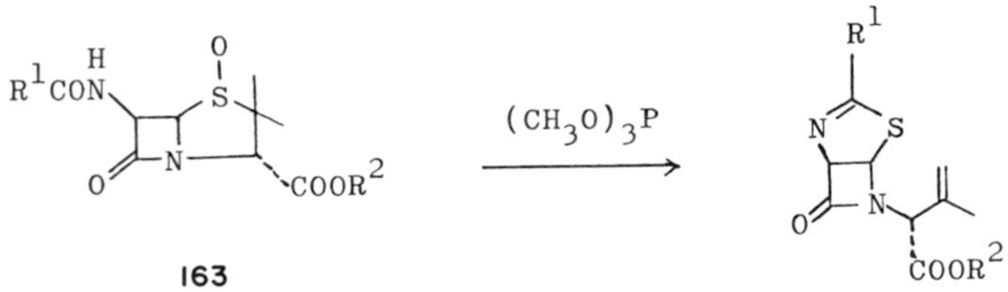

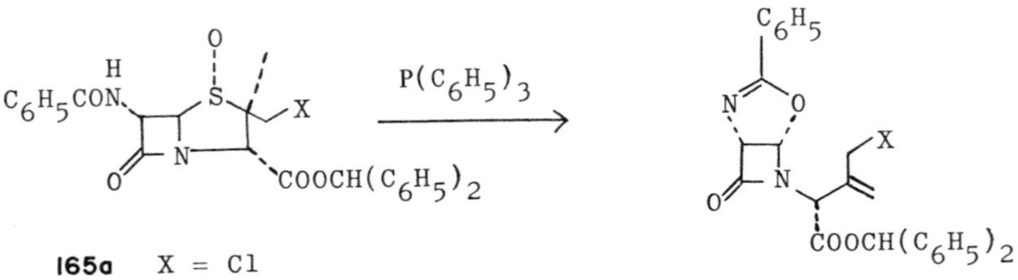

c. Synthesis by the Shionogi Group (VIII). A new method that could directly provide an *enantio*-oxazolinoazetidinone (**162**) with the β,γ-

161 **162**

163 **164**

165a X = Cl
165b X = OCHO
165c X = $OCOCH_2Cl$

166a–c
167 X = OH

dehydrovaline moiety was sought. Although this functional group could be prepared from the isomeric α,β-dehydrovaline derivatives by γ-bromination followed by zinc reduction as described previously (Section II,B,4,b), this procedure was too lengthy. However, this conversion was realized when two research groups independently found a method for the preparation of enantiomeric oxazolines such as **162** by heating 6-epipenicillin sulfoxides (**161**) with triphenylphosphine or trialkyl phosphite (Hamashima *et al.*, 1979c; Busson *et al.*, 1978). In contrast, the conversion of penicillin ester *S*-oxide (**163**) is well known to give thiazolinoazetidinone (**164**) with the β,γ-dehydrovaline moiety (Cooper and Jose, 1970). The new method was also proven to be applicable to 6-epipenicillin sulfoxides with a 2'-substituted methyl group (**165a–c**) obtained by the method of Kamiya *et al.* (1973). The enantiomeric oxazolines with the correspondingly functionalized isopropenyl group (**166a–c**) were obtained.

Although conversion of **166b,c** gave only low yields of **167**, a more direct procedure for its preparation starting from **162** was found by way of **166a**. This achievement provided an excellent synthetic route to 7α-methoxy-1-oxacephems (Yoshioka *et al.*, 1980). Oxazoline (**162**) was converted in good yield to allylic chloride (**166a**) by reaction with molecular chlorine and subsequent treatment with sodium bicarbonate. An "ene-type reaction" was suggested as the mechanism of this interesting allylic chlorination. Cooper (1980) suggested a chlorinium ion mechanism in addition to the ene-type reaction in the case of chlorination of a similar type of thiazoline derivative (Volume 1, Chapter 1).

The allylic chloride (**166a**) could be transformed into allylic alcohol (**167**) in various ways. Although the allylic chloride (**166a**) was not reactive enough to effect direct hydrolysis, displacement with phenylmercaptide proceeded to give sulfide **168**. This was oxidized with peracid to a mixture of sulfoxides and then rearranged by heating with triphenylphosphine in the presence of methanol to give the desired **167** in good yield. Substitution of an iodine atom for the chlorine atom of **166a** improved its reactivity; thus the resulting iodide (**169**) was smoothly hydrolyzed either with silver perchlorate in aqueous acetone or with cuprous oxide in hot aqueous dimethyl sulfoxide to produce **167**. Alternatively, **169** was first transformed into nitrate **170**, either by treatment with silver nitrate or by heating with sodium nitrate in the presence of methyl methanesulfonate as the iodide ion scavenger. The resulting nitrate (**170**) was reduced qualitatively with zinc and acetic acid to the allylic alcohol (**167**). The most efficient and practical transformation is considered to be that performed with cuprous oxide. Stereospecific intramolecular acetalization of **167** proceeded well, as expected, in the presence of a catalytic amount of boron trifluoride etherate, exomethylene 1-oxace-pham (171) with 6R stereochemistry being obtained in high yield.

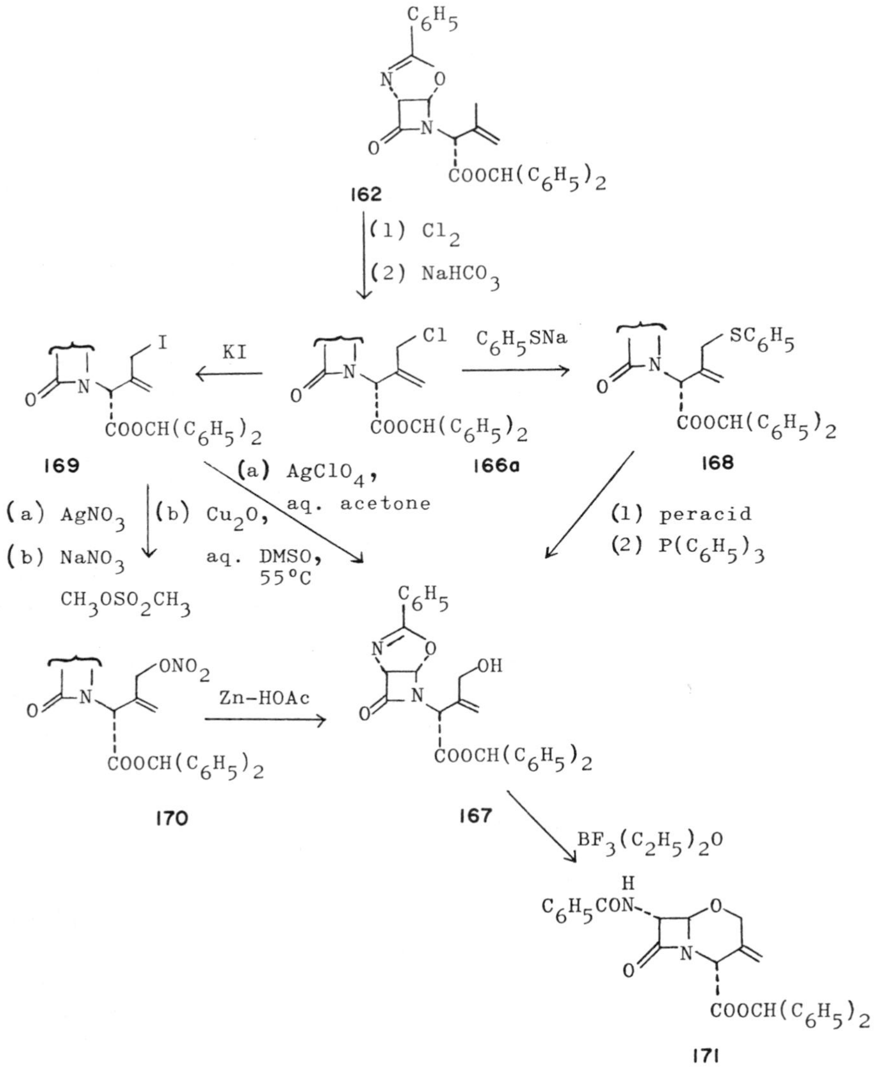

Although the chlorine addition to 171, when performed in a manner similar to that described for 3-methylene cepham (Koppel *et al.*, 1977), was unsatisfactory, it proceeded quite well under irradiation. Subsequent treatment with 1,7-diazabicyclo[4.5.0]undec-6-ene (DBU) produced 3-chloromethyl 7-*epi*-1-oxacephem (172) in high overall yield. Methoxylation of **172** according to the known method (Koppel and Koehler, 1973) yielded 3-chloromethyl-7α-methoxy-1-oxacephem (**173**) which was converted to **174** by a replacement reaction with N-methyltetrazolyl thiolate.

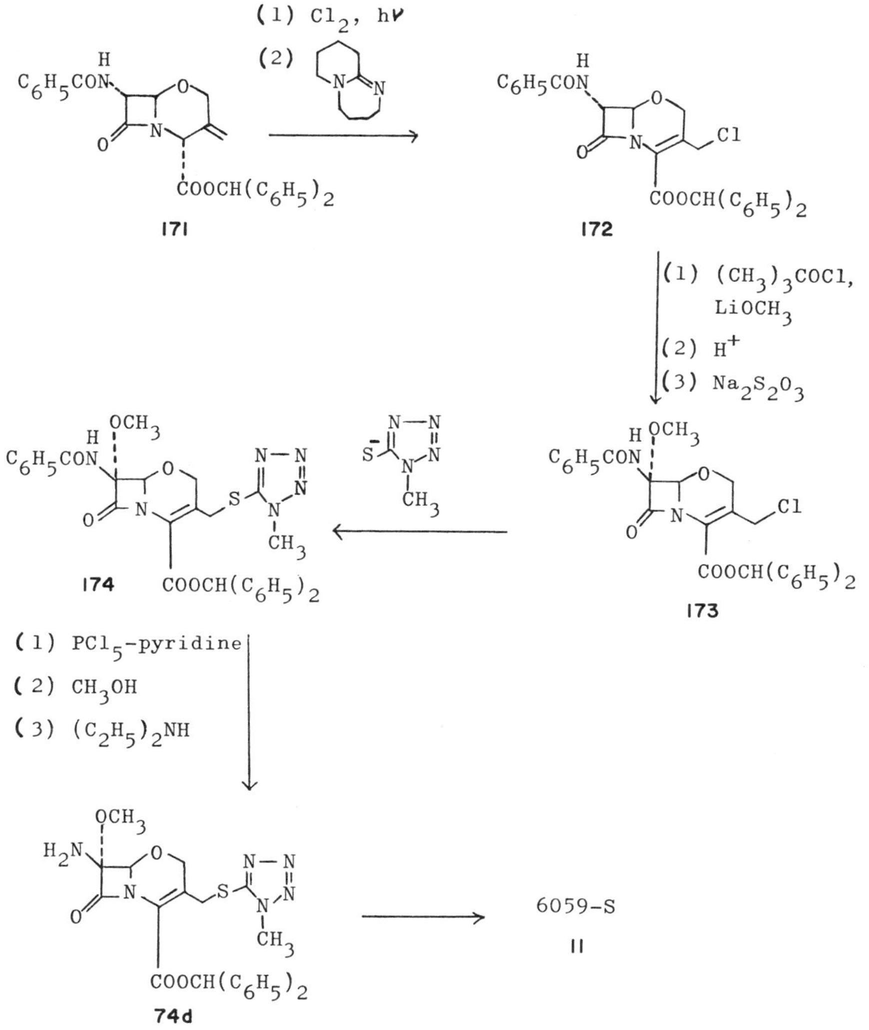

Cleavage of the benzamide side chain by successive treatments with phosphorus pentachloride, methanol, and diethylamine proceeded smoothly to give the methoxyamine (**74d**), the key intermediate for this type of antibiotic, in a satisfactory yield. The latter was also converted to 6059-S (**11**) in high yield.

d. Synthesis by the Shionogi Group (IX). Synthesis by way of glycol or halohydrin derivatives was also investigated at Shionogi (Aoki *et al.*,

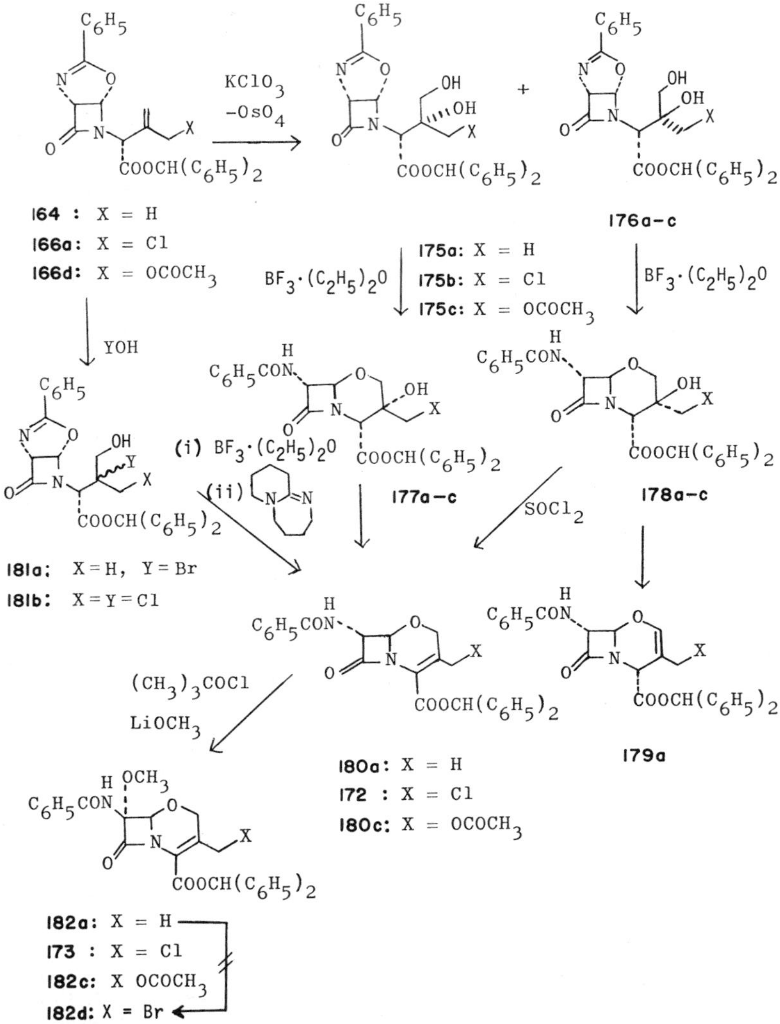

C_6H_5

KClO$_3$
$-OsO_4$

C_6H_5

OH
$_{\text{,,}}$OH
X

COOCH(C$_6$H$_5$)$_2$

+

C_6H_5

OH
OH
X

COOCH(C$_6$H$_5$)$_2$

COOCH(C$_6$H$_5$)$_2$

164 : X = H
166a: X = Cl
166d: X = OCOCH$_3$

176a–c

BF$_3 \cdot$(C$_2$H$_5$)$_2$O

175a: X = H
175b: X = Cl
175c: X = OCOCH$_3$

BF$_3 \cdot$(C$_2$H$_5$)$_2$O

YOH

C_6H_5

OH
Y
X

COOCH(C$_6$H$_5$)$_2$

C_6H_5CON

O
OH
X

COOCH(C$_6$H$_5$)$_2$

(i) BF$_3 \cdot$(C$_2$H$_5$)$_2$O
(ii)

177a–c

C_6H_5CON

O
OH
X

COOCH(C$_6$H$_5$)$_2$

178a–c

181a: X = H, Y = Br
181b: X = Y = Cl

SOCl$_2$

(CH$_3$)$_3$COCl
LiOCH$_3$

C_6H_5CON

O
X

COOCH(C$_6$H$_5$)$_2$

180a: X = H
172 : X = Cl
180c: X = OCOCH$_3$

C_6H_5CON

O
X

COOCH(C$_6$H$_5$)$_2$

179a

C_6H_5CON

H OCH$_3$
O
X

COOCH(C$_6$H$_5$)$_2$

182a: X = H
173 : X = Cl
182c: X OCOCH$_3$
182d: X = Br

1979, 1981). Compounds **164**, **166a**, and **166d** were used as the starting material for this synthesis. The last compound (**166d**) was prepared either by acetylation of **167** or by the treatment of **169** with silver tetrafluoroborate in dimethylacetamide, followed by hydrolysis. Glycolation was effected by treatment with potassium chlorate and a catalytic amount of osmium tetroxide, giving after chromatographic separation the glycols

(175a–c) and their corresponding epimers (176a–c). On treatment with boron trifluoride etherate, the former (175a–c) were cyclized exclusively to 3α-hydroxy-1-oxacephams (177a–c) and the latter (176a–c) to 3β-hydroxy-1-oxacephams (178a–c). The configuration and the conformation of 177a–c and 178a–c were determined by means of NMR spectroscopy. The structural determination of 177a will be discussed in detail later (Section III,B,3). On dehydration with thionyl chloride and pyridine, 178a mainly gave Δ^2-oxacephem (179a), whereas 178b,c and 177a–c afforded the corresponding Δ^3-1-oxacephems 180a, 172, and 180c, respectively. Similarly, halohydrin formation was also investigated. Treatment of 164 with N-bromosuccinimide yielded 181a, whereas that of 166a with trichloroisocyanuric acid afforded 181b. It is noteworthy that the addition reaction proceeded in an anti-Markownikoff manner in both cases. Both 181a and 181b were cyclized with boron trifluoride etherate, and the subsequent dehydrohalogenation of the resulting cyclized products gave 180a and 172, respectively. The 7-epi-1-oxacephems 180a, 172, and 180c obtained by the above two alternative routes were methoxylated (Koppel and Koehler, 1973) to afford 182a, 173, and 182c, respectively. Yields of 182a and 173 do not exceed those obtained by the previous method; however, this method is the best one for the preparation of 182c. Attempts to brominate 3-methyl-1-oxacephem (182a) to give 182d failed.

6. *Other Approaches*

Cyclization by bond formation between O-1 and C-2, i.e., intramolecular etherification of 183 to give 171, could provide another possible approach to 1-oxacephems. Syntheses utilizing this approach have been carried out in cephalosporin chemistry. For example, in the synthesis of 3-hydroxycephems (Hamashima et al., 1977), thiazoline (184) underwent acid hydrolysis, giving mercaptoazetidinone (185) as an intermediate (Volume 1, Chapter 2). The stability of this intermediate in acid medium is well documented (Narisada et al., 1978), and intramolecular alkylation of this intermediate proceeds well even in strong acid medium because of the high nucleophilicity of the thiol group and also because of the potent alkylating ability of the α-bromoketo group.

Such a route to 1-oxacephems was investigated by Shionogi chemists (Kamata et al., 1979). Since acid hydrolysis of oxazolinoazetidinone is known to give an amino ester derivative such as 130 (Wolfe et al., 1975) (Section II,A,3,d), other methods are necessary to obtain the presumably unstable hydroxyazetidinone (183) from an oxazolinoazetidinone. Thus trans cleavage of oxazoline (166a) with hydrogen peroxide in the presence of sodium tungstate afforded a stable hydroperoxide (187) with 6R stereochemistry. Although the desired 183 was formed by reduction of 187

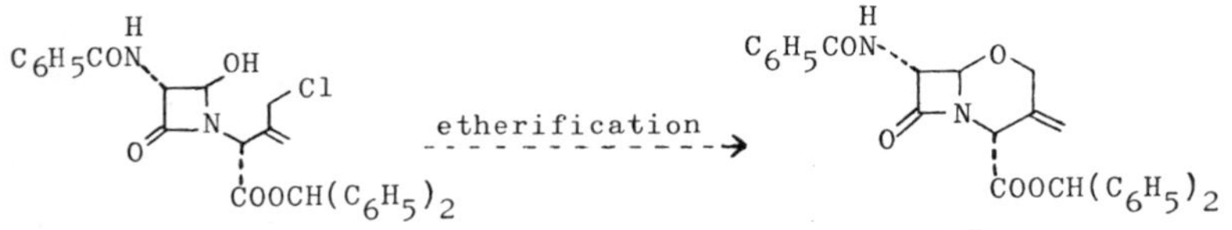

C_6H_5CON ... OH Cl

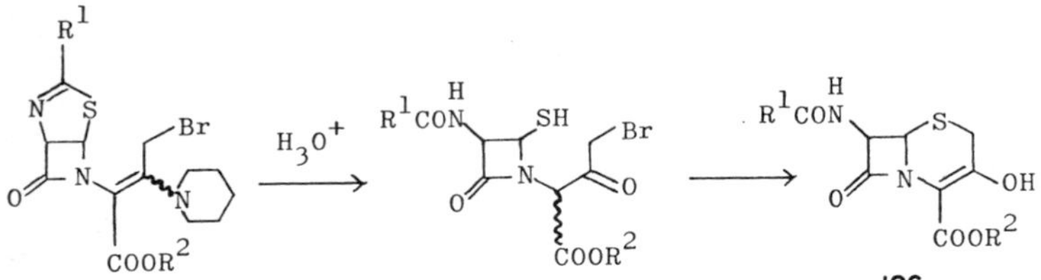

183

etherification
- - - - - - - - - ->

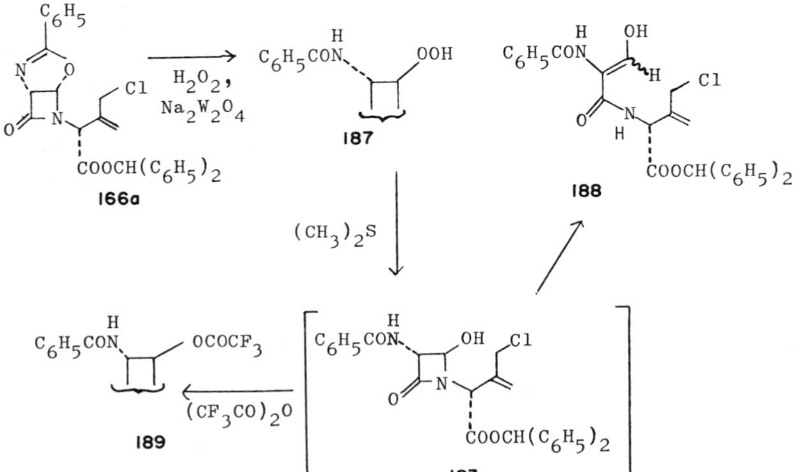

C_6H_5CON ...

$COOCH(C_6H_5)_2$

171

184   H_3O^+ ->   185   ->   186

C_6H_5

166a $\xrightarrow{H_2O_2, Na_2W_2O_4}$ C_6H_5CON ... OOH   187

C_6H_5CON ... OH H Cl

$COOCH(C_6H_5)_2$

188

$(CH_3)_2S$

C_6H_5CON ... $OCOCF_3$

189

$\xleftarrow{(CF_3CO)_2O}$

$\left[\begin{array}{c} C_6H_5CON \cdots OH\ Cl \\ COOCH(C_6H_5)_2 \\ 183 \end{array} \right]$

with dimethyl sulfide, it was too unstable to be isolated. The formation of **183** was proven only by NMR measurements at low temperature. It quickly decomposed to yield **188** but could be isolated as its trifluoroacetate (**189**) which was prone to recyclize to oxazoline (**166a**). Thus it was concluded that this approach was not promising.

B. Other Nuclear Analogs

1. *Introduction*

Only a few examples of the synthesis of 1-cephem analogs other than 1-oxacephems are known. The synthesis of 1-azacephem analogs starting from penicillin has been reported. The other interesting analog is 1-carbacephem, the synthesis of which was carried out by a total synthesis; it is discussed in Chapter 2 of this volume.

2. Syntheses of 1-Azacephems

a. Wolfe's Synthesis. Wolfe *et al.* (1972a,b) synthesized 6-epi-1-azacephem (**192**). Bromide **138**, described previously (Section II,A,4,b), was

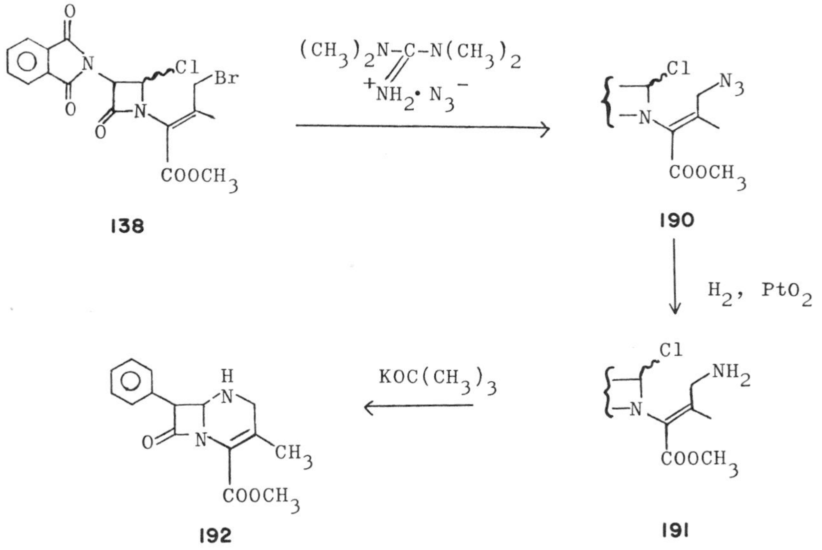

treated with tetramethylguanidinium azide to give **190**. Hydrogenation of the azide group using platinum oxide afforded amine **191**. Cyclization was effected by treatment with potassium tertiary butoxide, giving 6-epi-1-azacephem (**192**). No information about the antibacterial activity of this kind of compounds is available.

b. Synthesis by the Beecham Group. Beecham chemists achieved the first synthesis of a biologically active 1-azacephem compound (Japanese Kokai, 1979c). Azetidinone **193** was successively treated with lithium hexamethylsilazane and 3-butyn-2-one to give **194**, which underwent an intramolecular 1,3-dipolar addition reaction giving **195**. Dehydration of this compound with thionyl chloride afforded 1-azacephem **196** with a fused triazolo ring system. Removal of the trityl group, acylation, and subsequent deprotection of the *tert*-butyl ester group on **196** furnished several acylamino carboxylic acids (**197**). These were reported to show moderate antibacterial activity against gram-positive bacteria.

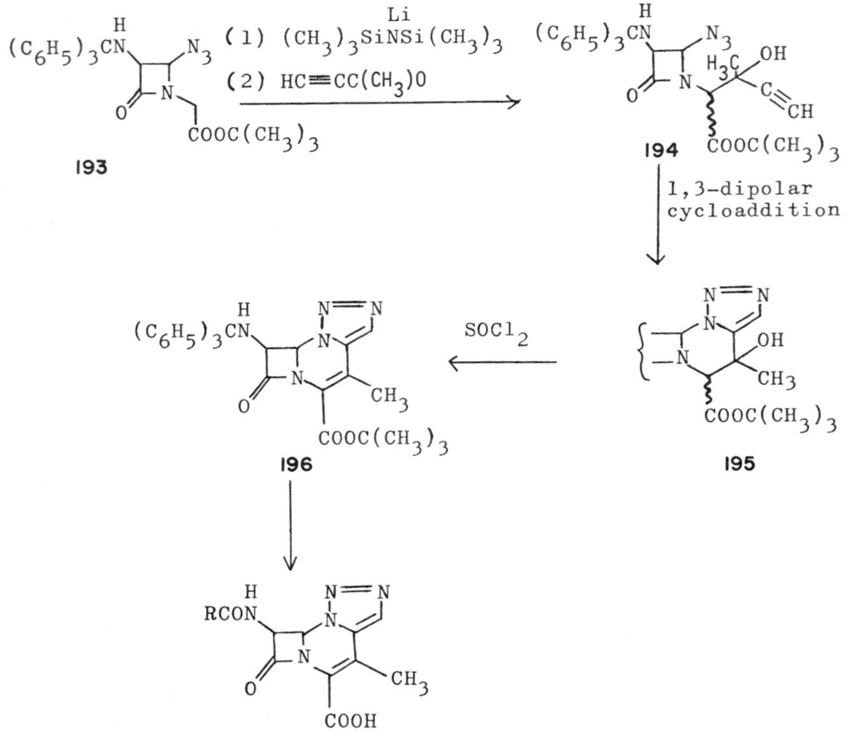

III. Chemical and Physicochemical Properties of 1-Oxacephems

A. Introduction

Contributions of recently developed physicochemical methods to structure elucidation studies on penicillins and cephalosporins have been described in an earlier β-lactam monograph (Sweet, 1972; Demarco and Nagarajan, 1972). These methods have furnished knowledge of the conformations of the antibiotics, as well as information regarding the correlation between the structure of the β-lactam moiety and the biological activity. It will be interesting to examine how the conclusions obtained for cephalosporins can be extended to 1-oxacephems, especially to 7α-methoxy-1-oxacephems.

In this section applications of physicochemical methods to structure elucidation of 1-oxacephems and to investigation of the relationship between chemical reactivity of the β-lactam ring and antibacterial activity are discussed. In order to understand the significant difference in anti-bacterial activity among cephem nuclear analogs, discussions are concentrated mainly on comparison of the physicochemical properties of 1-oxacephems with those of cephalosporins and racemic 1-carbacephems.

B. X-Ray Crystallography

X-Ray crystallographic analyses of 1-oxacephem esters **198** and **199** have been carried out by Shiro et al. (1981a,b), providing some information on the molecular structure of 1-oxacephems. Bond distances and angles for **198** and **199** are compared with those reported recently for cephapirin (**200**) (Declercq et al., 1977) (Table I), and perspective views of these molecules are shown in Figs. 1 and 2.

Figure 3 shows a comparison of the geometries of the skeletons of the 1-oxacephem ester (**198**), the 7α-methoxy-1-oxacephem ester (**199**), and cephapirin (**200**). The interatomic distances of the C-8—O-9 and N-5—C-8 bonds of **198** and **199** are slightly different from those of cephapirin (**200**) (1.195 and 1.201 Å compared with 1.211 Å for C-8—O-9 and 1.391 and 1.393 Å compared with 1.377 Å for N-5—C-8). This suggests a weaker amide resonance in the β-lactam rings of both **198**, and **199**, even though the differences are not statistically significant. Significant differences in the bond angles of N-5—C-4—C-10 and C-4—N-5—C-6 between **198** (119.4 and 119.3°, respectively) or **199** (117.3 and 119.7°, respectively) and cephapirin (**200**) (110.5 and 125.4°, respectively) are recorded. The latter difference may arise from distortion in the C-2—O-1—C-6 triangle caused by replacement of the sulfur atom in the C-2—S-1—C-6 triangle by the oxygen atom. The carboxyl group in **198** and **199** is less twisted out of the C-3—C-4—N-5 plane (~5 and ~6°) than that of cephapirin (**200**) (~35°); this fact may indicate a stronger contribution of the carboxyl resonance to the C-3—C-4 double bond in 1-oxacephems, although no evidence for this view has been obtained from the spectral data of 1-oxacephems measured in solution.

The displacement of the β-lactam nitrogen atom out of the plane of its three substituents has been pointed out by Sweet (1972) as an indication of the decrease in the amide resonance in the β-lactam ring. The values of the displacement out of the plane in the 1-oxacephem ester (**198**) (0.30 Å) and in the 7α-methoxy-1-oxacephem ester (**199**) (0.22 Å) are obviously greater than the corresponding values for cephapirin (**200**) (0.22 Å) and a 7α-methoxycephem (0.15 Å), respectively (Applegate et al., 1974), again suggesting a weaker amide resonance in 1-oxacephems.

In summary, X-ray crystallographic studies reveal that the O-1 substitution results in a geometry modification that suggests weaker β-lactam

TABLE I Molecular Parameters for Some 1-Oxacephem and Cephalosporin Derivatives[a]

Bond	Bond length (Å)		
	1-Oxacephem (198)[b,c]	7α-Methoxy- 1-oxacephem (199)[d,e]	Cephapirin sulfate (200)[f]
O-1—C-2	1.428	1.439	1.813
O-1—C-6	1.407	1.397	1.798
C-2—C-3	1.518	1.515	1.514
C-3—C-4	1.344	1.333	1.331
C-3—C-13	1.489	1.510	1.500
C-4—N-5	1.415	1.419	1.415
C-4—C-10	1.482	1.488	1.489
N-5—C-6	1.469	1.463	1.478
N-5—C-8	1.391	1.393	1.377
C-6—C-7	1.536	1.547	1.545
C-7—C-8	1.546	1.550	1.557
C-7—N-21	1.437	1.430	1.453
C-7—O-31	—	1.395	—
C-8—O-9	1.195	1.201	1.211
C-10—O-11	1.213	1.209	1.178
C-10—O-12	1.333	1.322	1.315
O-12—C-33	1.473	1.469	—
N-21—C-22	1.352	1.367	1.333
C-22—O-23	1.227	1.221	1.228
C-22—C-24	1.514	1.511	1.524
O-31—C-32	—	1.437	—

Bond	Bond angle (deg)		
	1-Oxacephem (198)[b,c]	7α-Methoxy- 1-oxacephem (199)[d,e]	Cephapirin sulfate (200)[f]
C-2—O-1—C-6	109.6	108.9	93.2
O-1—C-2—C-3	114.5	113.9	115.8
C-2—C-3—C-4	120.2	121.3	123.4
C-2—C-3—C-13	114.2	113.9	112.9
C-4—C-3—C-13	125.6	124.7	123.5
C-3—C-4—N-5	117.4	116.3	120.1
C-3—C-4—C-10	123.2	126.2	129.2
N-5—C-4—C-10	119.4	117.3	110.5
C-4—N-5—C-6	119.3	119.7	125.4
C-4—N-5—C-8	133.6	138.0	132.4
C-6—N-5—C-8	93.4	94.6	94.3
O-1—C-6—N-5	109.4	109.6	110.1
O-1—C-6—C-7	111.4	115.5	117.3
N-5—C-6—C-7	88.5	88.5	88.0
C-6—C-7—C-8	85.0	85.3	84.9
C-6—C-7—N-21	119.1	118.9	118.3
C-6—C-7—O-31	—	108.4	—
C-8—C-7—N-21	116.2	111.2	115.2

TABLE I (*continued*)

	Bond angle (deg)		
Bond	1-Oxacephem (**198**)[b,c]	7α-Methoxy- 1-oxacephem (**199**)[d,e]	Cephapirin sulfate (**200**)[f]
C-8—C-7—O-31	—	114.9	—
N-21—C-7—O-31	—	114.9	—
N-5—C-8—C-7	91.0	90.9	91.2
N-5—C-8—O-9	132.9	133.8	132.3
C-7—C-8—O-9	136.1	135.3	136.5
C-4—C-10—O-11	123.6	123.3	122.3
C-4—C-10—O-12	112.1	110.9	114.1
O-11—C-10—O-12	124.3	125.8	123.6
C-10—O-12—C-33	115.2	119.9	—
C-7—N-21—C-22	121.7	120.9	116.6
N-21—C-22—O-23	122.1	122.2	121.6
N-21—C-22—C-24	115.1	114.6	116.4
O-23—C-22—C-24	122.7	123.2	122.0

[a] Structures:

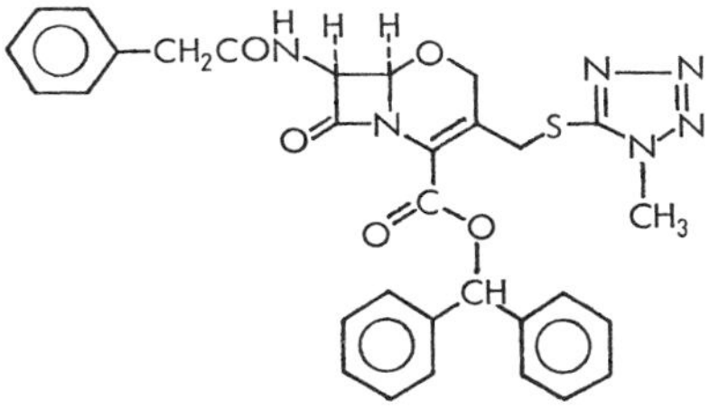

198

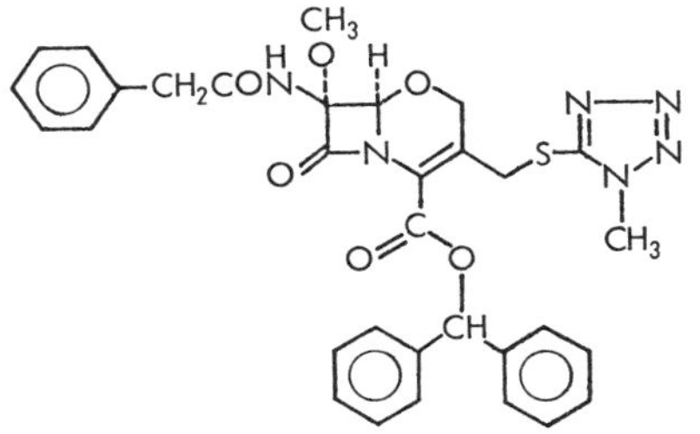

199

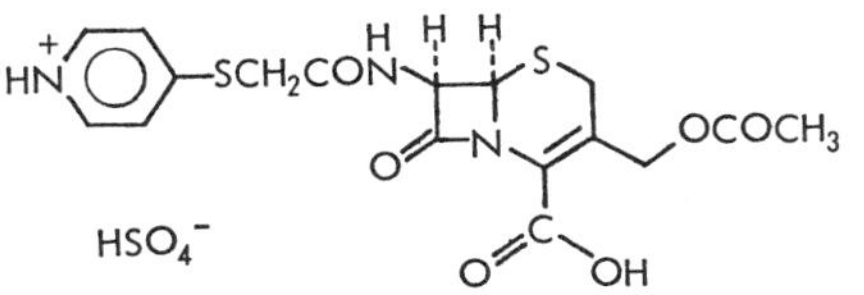

200

[b] Shiro *et al.* (1981a,b).

[c] The mean estimated standard deviations are 0.004 Å for bond lengths and 0.3° for angles.

[d] Shiro *et al.* (1981a,b). The atomic numbering is consistent with (**199**).

[e] The mean estimated standard deviations are 0.003 Å for bond lengths and 0.3° for angles.

[f] Declercq *et al.* (1977).

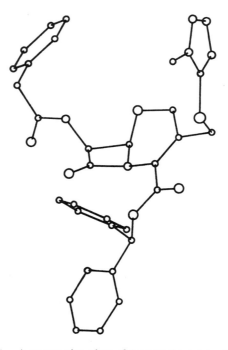

Fig. 1. A perspective view of 1-oxacephem ester (**198**).

amide resonance. That is, 1-oxacephems show (1) slightly shortened carbonyl and lengthened amide bonds and (2) a greater displacement of the amide nitrogen out of the C-4—C-6—C-8 plane. These features may correlate with enhanced reactivity of the β-lactam ring and accordingly with the increased biological activity of 1-oxacephems.

Introduction of the 7α-methoxy group results in a more planar β-lactam moiety for both cephem analogs. Accordingly, the β-lactam carbonyl bond is weakened through enhanced amide resonance. The reason for a more planar structure on introduction of the 7α-methoxy group is not known.

C. Nuclear Magnetic Resonance Spectroscopy

In addition to ¹H-NMR spectra and the nuclear Overhauser effect (NOE) (Demarco and Nagarajan, 1972), ¹³C-NMR spectroscopy has afforded a useful method for determining the electronic structure of the β-lactam moiety in cephalosporins (Mondelli and Ventura, 1977; Paschal *et al.,* 1978; Dereppe *et al.,* 1978; Schanck *et al.,* 1979).

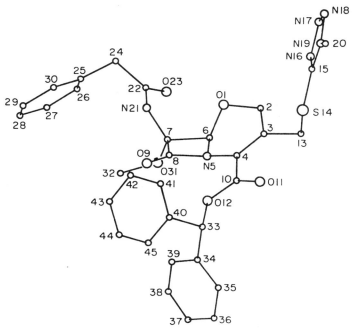

Fig. 2. A perspective view of 7α-methoxy-1-oxacephem ester (**199**).

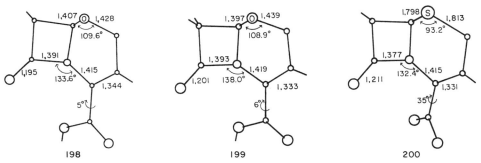

Fig. 3. Comparison of 1-oxacephem, 7α-methoxy-1-oxacephem, and cephem skeletons of **198**, **199**, and **200**.

1. ¹H-NMR Spectra

In Table II, ¹H-NMR data for 1-oxacephem esters **198**, **199**, **201**, and **202** (Tori *et al.*, 1980) are compared with those for the corresponding cephalosporins **203–206**. Most 1-oxacephem signals are assigned as described for cephalosporins (Demarco and Nagarajan, 1972). Assignments of the H-2 and H-3′ signals of **199** are confirmed by their selective

TABLE II ^{1}H-NMR Data for Some 1-Oxacephems and Corresponding Cephalosporins[a,b]

Resonance	(198)	(203)	(199)	(204)
H-2	4.68 (4.56) s	3.74 (3.60) s	4.58 (4.58) s	3.60 (3.52) s
H-3′	4.23 (4.23) s	4.22 (4.22), 4.28 (4.28)	4.22 (4.23) s	4.16 (4.20), 4.37 (4.42)
H-6	5.18 (4.99) d, $J = 4.0$	5.12 (4.89) d, $J = 5.0$	5.14 (5.01) s	5.13 (4.98) s
H-7	5.65 (5.72) dd, $J = 4.0$, $J = 9.5$	5.78 (5.84) dd, $J = 5.0$, $J = 8.5^c$	—	—
7-OCH$_3$	—	—	3.40 (3.44) s	3.38 (3.41) s
CONH	8.97 (6.19) d, $J = 9.5$	9.18 (6.39) d, $J = 8.5^c$	9.23 (6.36) s	9.50 (6.52) s
C$_6$H$_5$CH_2	3.54 (3.61) s	3.54 (3.62) s	3.57 (3.63) s	3.60 (3.63) s
(C$_6$H$_5$)$_2$CH	6.90 (6.88) s	6.92 (6.90) s	6.78 (6.89) s	6.89 (6.88) s
NCH$_3$	3.86 (3.80) s	3.86 (3.77) s	3.85 (3.78) s	3.84 (3.78) s

Resonance	(201)	(205)	(202)[d]	(206)
H-2	4.66 (4.63) s	3.70 (3.68) s	4.63 (4.65) s	3.55 (3.57) 3.67
H-3′	4.23 (4.26) s	4.13 (4.19), 4.32 (4.34)	4.22 (4.25) s	4.13 (4.23), 4.36 (4.45)
H-6	5.03 (4.96) d, $J = 4.0$	5.00 (4.90) AB, $J = 5.0$	4.99 (4.84) s	4.94 (4.81) s
H-7	4.60 (4.48) d, $J = 4.0$	4.84 (4.74) AB, $J = 5.0$	—	—
7-OCH$_3$	—	—	3.36 (3.49) s	3.34 (3.47) s
NH$_2$	3.41 (1.88) s	2.79 (1.84) s	2.90 (2.05) s (br s)	3.14 (2.23) s (br s)
(C$_6$H$_5$)$_2$CH	6.87 (6.91) s	6.89 (6.93) s	6.87 (6.92) s	6.87 (6.92) s
NCH$_3$	3.85 (3.80) s	3.84 (3.78) s	3.86 (3.80) s	3.84 (3.78) s

[a] Measured at 60 MHz using about 0.1 mmol/cm^3 solutions (unless otherwise noted) in CD$_3$SOCD$_3$ and in CDCl$_3$ (values in parentheses). Accuracies of δ_H and J values are ± 0.02 ppm and ± 0.5 Hz, respectively.

[b] Structures:

	A	Y	R
(198)	O	H	C$_6$H$_5$CH$_2$CO
(203)*	S	H	C$_6$H$_5$CH$_2$CO
(199)	O	OCH$_3$	C$_6$H$_5$CH$_2$CO
(204)*	S	OCH$_3$	C$_6$H$_5$CH$_2$CO
(201)	O	H	H
(205)*	S	H	H
(202)	O	OCH$_3$	H
(206)*	S	OCH$_3$	H
(207)†	CH$_2$	H	C$_6$H$_5$CH$_2$CO

* Narisada *et al.* (1980, 1981).

† Uyeo and Ona (1980). Only ^{13}C-NMR chemical shifts for the benzyl ester derivative are reported in Table III.

[c] All J values are identical for both solvents, except where J values are reported as 9.0 Hz.

[d] Measured for a saturated CDCl$_3$ solution.

decoupling in the unambiguously assigned ^{13}C-NMR spectra of the compound (Section III,C,2). Experiments using Eu(fod)$_3$ as a shift reagent resolved the ambiguity in assigning the H-6 and H-7 signals in **205**.

In contrast to the large downfield shifts in the H-2 signals of 1-oxacephems as compared with those of cephalosporins, the H-6 chemical shift differences are unexpectedly small. This anomaly may be ascribed to the unusual low-field chemical shifts for the axially oriented H-6α in cephalosporins. This is attributed to a deshielding effect of the sulfur atom similar to that postulated by Eliel *et al.* (1975) in the interpretation of such an anomaly observed in the axial H-2 of 1,3-dithiane.

Strong solvent effects on the chemical shifts of the amide protons are seen.

Boucherot and Pilgrim (1979) have pointed out that the $^3J_{\mathrm{H,H}}$ coupling constants on the β-lactam ring in 1-oxacephems are smaller than those in cephalosporins by ~1.0 Hz. The demonstrated $^3J_{\mathrm{H,H}}$ coupling constants of the indicated compounds are in agreement with these findings.

2. ^{13}C-NMR Spectra

The ^{13}C chemical shifts for the 1-oxacephem (**198, 199, 201, 202**), cephem (**203–206**), and 1-carbacephem (**207**) esters, reported by Tori *et al.* (1980), are listed in Tables III and IV. Table III shows the resonances of carbon atoms chracteristic of each compound. In Table IV, chemical shifts are given as their mean values, with standard deviations for carbon atoms common to **198, 199, 201–206**.

The chemical shifts for C-2 and C-6 in 1-oxacephems reflect the expected large α effect (Stothers, 1972) of the O-1. Replacement of the sulfur atom with the O-1 causes a ~2-ppm downfield shift in the resonance of the carbonyl carbon (C-8) in the β-lactam ring. It has been reported that the carbonyl carbon atom of the β-lactam ring in 7β-acylaminocephalosporins and in a Δ^2-cephem compound resonates over a narrow range. In penicillins the signals occur at a + 10-ppm lower field (Mondelli and Ventura, 1977). The small but significant downfield shifts of ~2 ppm might correlate with enhanced chemical reactivity of the β-lactam ring in 1-oxacephems (Section III,E).

The C-3 signals of 1-oxacephems appear at about +3 to +6 ppm lower fields, whereas those for C-4 are at −3 ppm higher fields. Although a relationship between antibacterial activity and chemical shift differences between C-4 and C-3 has been reported by Paschal *et al.* (1978) for several cephalosporin carboxylates with a different C-3' substituent, further investigations are needed to conclude whether the relationship is applicable to the substitution of oxygen at C-1, since the chemical shifts for C-3 and C-4 are reversed in the ester series.

The chemical shifts of C-8, C-4, and C-3 of the 1-carbacephem ester

TABLE III [13]C Chemical Shift for Some 1-Oxacephems and Corresponding Cephalosporins[a]

Carbon	(198)	(203)	(207)	(199)	(204)
C-1	—	—	19.9 (20.5)	—	—
C-2	65.3 (66.2)	27.3 (28.4)	25.5 (26.8)	65.5 (66.5)	27.8 (29.3)
C-3[b]	134.5 (134.9)	128.2 (130.2)	130.3 (132.2)	134.2 (134.3[c])	131.4 (135.2)
C-4[b]	121.9 (123.0)	124.6 (125.2)	123.7 (124.4)	122.2 (123.5)	124.6 (125.9)
C-6	78.2 (78.0)	57.7 (57.3)	52.1 (52.8)	82.9 (83.2)	63.4 (64.7)
C-7	58.5 (58.8)	58.9 (59.1)	58.1 (58.8)	94.4 (94.5)	95.3 (95.7)
C-8	168.5 (168.0)	165.1 (164.9)	166.2 (165.6)	162.5 (162.0)	160.7 (160.5)
C-3'	30.6 (30.4)	35.2 (35.2)	35.2 (35.0)	30.3 (30.4)	34.6 (34.7)
COO	159.7 (160.3)	160.5 (161.0)	161.5 (161.7)	159.3 (159.9)	160.1 (160.8)
CONH	170.5 (170.8)	170.9 (171.2)	170.5 (171.5)	170.7 (171.1)	171.4 (171.7)
OCH₃	—	—	—	52.3 (53.3)	52.5 (53.6)

Carbon	(201)	(205)	(202)[d]	(206)
C-2	65.2 (66.2)	27.0 (28.1)	65.5 (66.6)	27.8 (29.0)
C-3[b]	134.0 (134.0)	128.4 (128.5)	133.0 (132.9)	130.4 (134.7)
C-4[b]	122.2 (123.5)	124.8 (125.8)	122.6 (124.0)	125.1 (126.2)
C-6	78.7 (79.2)	59.2 (58.9)	82.5 (83.1)	63.9 (64.4)
C-7	62.9 (63.7)	63.6 (63.7)	97.4 (97.2)	98.5 (98.2)
C-8	172.0 (171.6)	170.3 (169.0)	165.9 (165.5)	164.0 (164.3)
C-3'	30.6 (30.7)	35.3 (35.5)	30.4 (30.5)	34.9 (34.9)
COO	160.0 (160.6)	161.4 (161.3)	159.5 (160.2)	160.5 (160.9)
OCH₃	—	—	50.5 (51.9)	51.1 (52.4)

[a] Measured at 15.087 MHz using about 0.1 mmol/ml solutions (unless otherwise noted) in CD_3SOCD_3 and $CDCl_3$ (values in parentheses). Accuracies of δ_C (TMS) are ±0.1 ppm. See formulas depicted in Table II, footnote a.

[b] Assigned by comparing the signal intensities which should be almost proportional to the reciprocal relaxation times (l/T) (see Dereppe et al., 1978).

[c] Interchangeable with a signal at δ_C 134.1 (See Table IV.)

[d] Measured for a saturated $CDCl_3$ solution.

(207) are intermediate between those of the 1-oxacephem ester (198) and those of the cephalosporin ester (203). These values parallel the increased rate of alkaline hydrolysis of a 1-carbacephem compound as compared with that of the corresponding cephalosporin (Section III,E). Ring strain in the 1-carbacephem skeleton similar to that in 1-oxacephems may modify the electronic structure of the β-lactam ring moiety, resulting in the observed chemical shifts and the increased chemical reactivity.

Introduction of a methoxy group at the 7α position of 1-oxacephems causes large downfield shifts in the resonances of C-7 and C-6 as well as an upfield shift in the C-8 signal. A similar downfield shift has been observed in a 7α-methoxycephalosporin (Paschal et al., 1978) and ascribed to the α and β effects (Stothers, 1972), respectively. An upfield shift in the C-8 signal of the same compound has also been interpreted

TABLE IV   Mean ^{13}C Chemical Shifts for Carbons in Common Substituents of Cephem Analogs **198, 199, 201,** and **206**[a]

Substituent	Carbon	δ_C
1-Methyl-1*H*-tetrazol-5-yl-thiol	C-5	153.0 ± 0.1 (154.1 ± 0.1)
	CH_3	33.6 ± 0.0 (33.4 ± 0.0)
1,1-Diphenylmethyl	C-2	78.9 ± 0.1 (79.8 ± 0.2)
	Ipso	139.8 ± 0.2 (139.3 ± 0.1)
	Ortho	126.5 ± 0.2 (127.2 ± 0.2)
	Meta	128.4 ± 0.0 (128.6 ± 0.1)
	Para	127.7 ± 0.1 (128.2 ± 0.1)
2-Phenylacetyl	C-1	41.6 ± 0.1 (43.5 ± 0.3)
	Ipso	135.6 ± 0.1 (133.9 ± 0.2)
	Ortho	129.0 ± 0.1 (129.4 ± 0.1)
	Meta	128.2 ± 0.1 (127.6 ± 0.1)
	Para	126.4 ± 0.1 (127.6 ± 0.1)

[a] See Table II, footnote *a*. Mean values and standard deviations (σ_{n-1}) are reported. See formulas depicted in Table II.

as being due to decreased carbonyl polarization (Paschal *et al.,* 1978). Contrary to this intrepretation, the infrared (IR) frequencies of the β-lactam carbonyl are lowered by the introduction of a 7α-methoxy group (Section III,E), indicating rather that polarization of the carbonyl is enhanced. Enhanced polarization of the β-lactam carbonyl is also supported by X-ray crystallographic data (Section III,B).

3. *Nuclear Overhauser Effects and Conformation of a 1-Oxacephem*

On the basis of interproton NOE measurements, the tetrahydrooxazine ring in a 1-oxacephem compound (**177a**) (Section II,A,5,d) is thought to adopt conformation A in Fig. 4 (Aoki *et al.,* 1981), similar to that of the

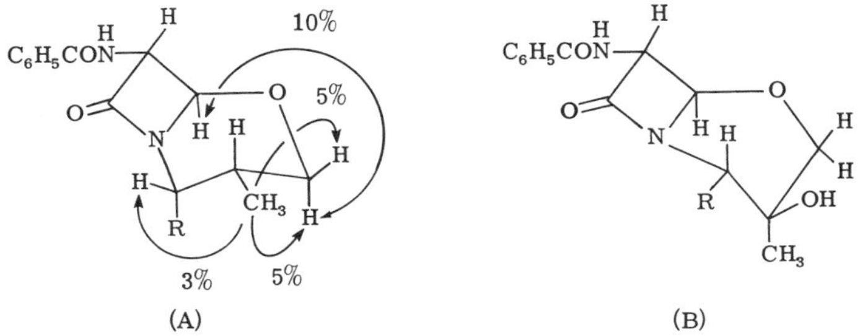

R = COOCH(C_6H_5)$_2$

Fig. 4.   Possible tetrahydroxazine ring conformations and NOEs in 1-oxacepham ester (**177a**).

TABLE V Proton–Proton Coupling Constants of 1-Oxacepham (**177a**)^a

^2J(H-2α, H-2β)	=	-12.2 Hz
^3J(H-6, H-7)	=	$+0.5$ Hz
^3J(H-7, NH)	=	$+7.4$ Hz
$|^4J$(H-2β, H-4)$|$	=	1.0 Hz

^{a} J values ± 0.1 Hz.

tetrahydrothiazine ring in saturated cephalosporins (Demarco and Nagarajan, 1972).

Of conformations A and B in Fig. 4, only A can account for the small but significant NOE of 3% observed between the 3-CH$_3$ and H-4 signals as well as a ^4J(H-4, H-2β) value of 1.0 Hz. Other NOEs observed are indicated in Fig. 4, and the coupling constants are summarized in Table V.

D. Mass Spectrometry

Electron impact mass spectrometry of 1-oxacephems (Nakagawa and Ikenishi, 1980) has proven its usefulness in elucidating the relative configurations at C-7 and C-6 in the 1-oxacephem skeleton. In synthesizing the 1-oxacephem skeleton, the stereochemistry at C-6 and C-7 must be established. Although the relative configurations of H-6 and H-7 have been confirmed by the ^{1}H-NMR coupling constant, this method cannot be applied to 7-methoxy-1-oxacephems. Although X-ray analysis of compound **199** has solved the problem (Section III,B), mass spectrometry furnishes a more direct method for determining the configuration.

In general, 1-oxacephems produce a fragmentation pattern similar to that reported by Demarco and Nagarajan (1972) for cephalosporins. The course of principal fragmentation for cephem analogs is depicted in Fig. 5. The relative abundance of ions A, B, C, D, etc., derived from the cephem analogs with natural and unnatural configurations is shown in Tables VI and VII, respectively.

Major cleavage across the β-lactam ring gives ions A, A′, B, and B′. Ion A (Y = OCH$_3$), derived from 7-methoxy-7-acylamino derivatives **199**, **204**, and **211** appears to lose a hydrogen atom easily from the nethoxy group, giving ion A″. The presence of the amide hydrogen in A″ was confirmed by experiments using deuterated amide compounds. This cleavage in 7-acylamino-1-oxacephems depends strictly upon the relative configuration of C-7 and C-6. In compounds with the natural configuration, peak B′ is more intense than peak B; in the corresponding epimers, peak A is more intense than peak A′. However, this rule is not

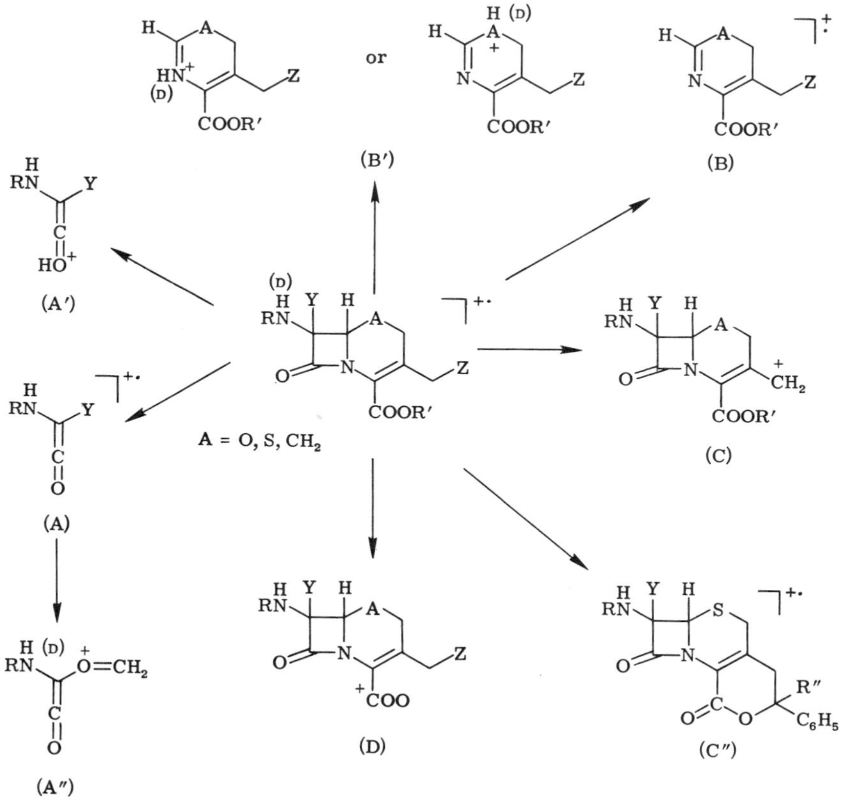

Fig. 5. A general scheme for the mass fragmentation pattern of cephem analogs.

applicable to sulfur cephalosporins; differentiation of C-6 stereochemistry is difficult. The hydrogen attached to ion B′ of 7β-acylamino-1-oxacephems arises from the amide group based on deuteration experiments: ion B′ derived from deuterated 1-oxacephem compounds shifts 1 mass unit higher. Although two structures are possible for the protonated ion B′ (Fig. 5), the observed difficulty in forming ion B′ in the fragmentation of 1-carbacephem **207** suggests that rearrangement occurs during the cleavage to yield the ion protonated at the 1-heteroatom. The amide hydrogen rearranges stereospecifically to the cis-oriented O-1, giving ion B′. No interpretation exists for the poor stereochemical dependency of the hydrogen transfer in cephalosporins.

A lactone structure is tentatively assigned to the ion C″ selectively formed in cephalosporin benzhydryl and benzyl esters. The peak is not formed from methyl esters or 3-methyl compounds.

TABLE VI Relative Abundances in the Mass Spectra of Cephem Analogs with the Natural Configuration

Compound[a]	Ion peak[b]							
	A″	A	A′	B	B′	C″	C	D
(198)	—	175 (2.8)	176 (3.5)	421 ([c])	422 (9.2)	—	481 (1.5)	429 (5.4)
(202)	86 (2.1)	87 (1.0)	88 (2.8)	421 (0.9)	422 (1.5)	—	393 (0.3)	—
(199)	204 (2.1)	205 (3.0)	206 (1.3)	—	422 (9.3)	—	511 (1.2)	459 (3.7)
(208)	—	181 (1.5)	182 (1.3)	—	382 (25.4)	502 (1.2)	503 (0.4)	395 (3.7)
(203)	—	175 (2.2)	176 (5.2)	—	438 (22.1)	496 (0.9)	497 (0.5)	445 (8.5)
(204)	204 (1.5)	205 (1.5)	206 (0.5)	437 (0.3)	438 (6.3)	526 (2.1)	527 (1.2)	475 (0.5)
(207)	—	175 (4.7)	176 (8.8)	343 (0.1)	344 (0.7)	—	403 (40.8)	427 (2.7)

[a] Structures:

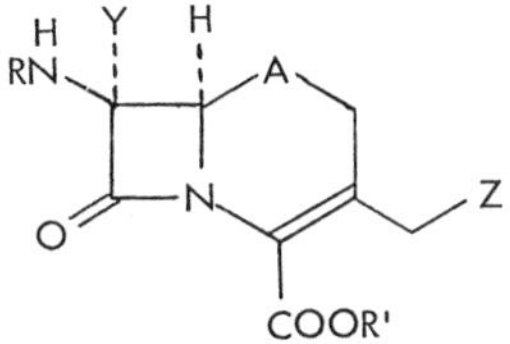

Compound	A	Y	R	R′	Z
(198)	O	H	$C_6H_5CH_2CO$	$CH(C_6H_5)_2$	$S(C_2H_3N_4)$§
(202)	O	OCH_3	H	$CH(C_6H_5)_2$	$S(C_2H_3N_4)$§
(199)	O	OCH_3	$C_6H_5CH_2CO$	$CH(C_6H_5)_2$	$S(C_2H_3N_4)$§
(208)*	S	H	$C_6H_5SCH_2CO$‡	$CH(C_6H_5)_2$	$OCOCH_3$
(203)*	S	H	$C_6H_5CH_2CO$	$CH(C_6H_5)_2$	$S(C_2H_3N_4)$§
(204)*	S	OCH_3	$C_6H_5CH_2CO$	$CH(C_6H_5)_2$	$S(C_2H_3N_4)$§
(207)†	CH_2	H	$C_6H_5CH_2CO$	$CH_2C_6H_5$	$S(C_2H_3N_4)$§

* Narisada et al. (1980).   ‡ 2-Thienylacetyl.
† Uyeo and Ona (1980).   § (1-Methyl-1H-tetrazol-5-yl)thio.

[b] Values are for mass numbers; relative abundances are given in parentheses. The base peak corresponding to $(R')^+$ is observed in each compound except for **202** which gives $(CH_3OH)^+$ instead.

[c] A weak peak with an abundance below 0.1 is detected.

TABLE VII Relative Abundances in the Mass Spectra of Cephem Analogs with the Unnatural Configuration

Compound[a]					Ion peak[b]				
	A″	A	A′	B	B′	C″	C	D
(209)	—	175 (20.6)	176 (4.5)	421 (2.5)	—	—	481 (0.2)	429 (0.1)
(210)	86 (0.1)	87 (1.2)	88 (1.0)	421 (0.7)	422 (0.6)	—	393 (^{c})	—
(211)	204 (7.5)	205 (3.8)	206 (0.7)	421 (1.3)	422 (0.4)	—	511 (0.1)	—
(212)	—	161 (12.2)	162 (15.8)	247 (30.6)	248 (80.2)	—	—	317 (5.3)
(213)	—	161 (47.0)	162 (18.0)	305 (9.5)	306 (77.6)	406 (10.3)	407 (4.1)	375 (1.2)

[a] Structures:

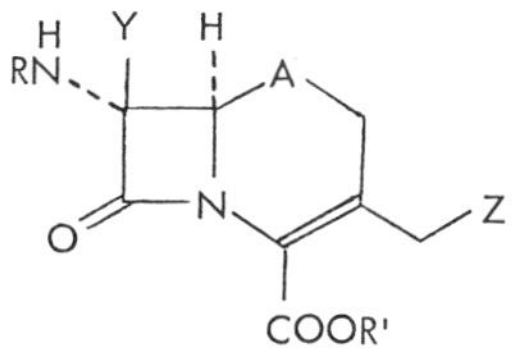

Compound	A	Y	R	R′	Z
(209)	O	H	C$_6$H$_5$CH$_2$CO	CH(C$_6$H$_5$)$_2$	S(C$_2$H$_3$N$_4$)†
(210)	O	OCH$_3$	H	CH(C$_6$H$_5$)$_2$	S(C$_2$H$_3$N$_4$)†
(211)	O	OCH$_3$	C$_6$H$_5$CH$_2$CO	CH(C$_6$H$_5$)$_2$	S(C$_2$H$_3$N$_4$)†
(212)*	S	H	C$_6$H$_5$CO	CH$_2$C$_6$H$_5$	H
(213)*	S	H	C$_6$H$_5$CO	CH$_2$C$_6$H$_5$	OCOCH$_3$

* Hamashima *et al.* (1980a).

† (1-Methyl-1H-tetrazol-5-yl)thio.

[b] See Table V, footnote a. The base peak corresponding to (R′)$^{+\cdot}$ is observed in each compound except for **210** which gives (CH$_3$OH)$^{+\cdot}$ instead.

^{c} See Table VI, footnote c.

E. Infrared Spectroscopy, Alkaline Hydrolysis Rates,
    and Antibacterial Activity

Some investigations have been reported on the interrelations between the antibacterial activity and the acylating ability of β-lactams. Morin *et al.* (1969) have pointed out that the potency of the antibacterial activity of penicillins, Δ^2- and Δ^3-cephems, and cephams is correlated qualitatively with the IR frequencies of the β-lactam carbonyl of their methyl esters. Indelicato *et al.* (1974) have found that the logarithms of the pseudo-first-order rate constant of alkaline hydrolysis of the β-lactam ring at pH 10 and 35°C correlate linearly with the above-described frequencies and that modification of the amide side chain does not significantly affect the reactivity of the β-lactam ring. Yamana and Tsuji (1976) have shown that increased rates of hydroxide ion-catalyzed hydrolysis observed in 3-substituted methylcephalosporins may be correlated with their enhanced antibacterial activity.

Relationships between antibacterial activity and chemical reactivity of the β-lactam carbonyl, which may parallel either IR absorption frequency of the β-lactam carbonyl or alkaline hydrolysis rate, have been studied for some cephem analogs (Narisada *et al.*, 1980). The relevant data are shown in Table VIII.

Comparison of carbonyl frequencies of 1-oxacephems **214**, **11**, **219**, and **221** with those of the corresponding cephems **215**, **216**, **220**, and **222**, respectively, indicates that replacement of the sulfur atom by an oxygen atom results in a higher frequency shift in the β-lactam carbonyl frequencies, whereas the amide carbonyl bands are affected little. The effect of substitution of the methylene group is clearly indicated by a remarkably lower shift in the β-lactam carbonyl frequency of **217**. Also, comparison of the carbonyl frequencies of 7-unsubstituted compounds **214**, **215**, **219**, and **220** with those of 7α-methoxy derivatives **11**, **216**, **221**, and **222**, respectively, indicates a lower shift of the β-lactam carbonyl frequencies and a higher shift of the amide carbonyl freqencies due to introduction of the methoxy group. Introduction of the 7α-methyl group is shown, by comparison of **214** with **218**, to have a small effect. The higher frequency shift of the β-lactam carbonyl band observed in 1-oxacephems may be ascribed to an inductive effect of the O-1 through the lactam nitrogen atom. The higher shift correlates well with enhancement of the pseudo-first-order rate of alkaline hydrolysis, measured at pH 9.2 and 35°C, shown in Table VIII for 1-oxacephems as compared with those of 1-thia congeners.

It should be pointed out that the pseudo-first-order rates of 1-oxa- and 1-thiacephem analogs correlate fairly well with geometrical mean values of the minimum inhibitory concentration (MIC) for susceptible strains

TABLE VIII Infrared Absorption Frequencies, Hydrolysis Rates, and Mean MIC Values of Cephem Analogs

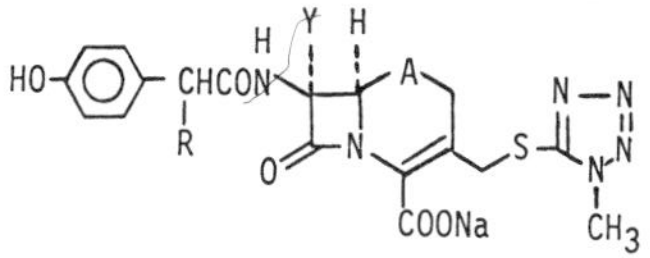

Compound	A	Y	R	V_{max} (C=O) in CH_3SOCH_3 [a]		Alkaline hydrolysis rate ($\times 10^4$ min^{-1}) [b]	Mean MIC ($\times 10^7$ mmol/ml) [c]
				β-Lactam (cm^{-1})	Amide (cm^{-1})		
(214)	O	H	COONa	1779.2	1665.4	21.2	5.02
(215)	S	H	COONa	1770.0	1669.0	3.99	33.7
(11)	O	OCH$_3$	COONa	1771.8	1686.6	29.6	1.30
(216)	S	OCH$_3$	COONa	1767.8	1682.3	3.98	7.77
(217) [d]	CH$_2$	OCH$_3$	COONa	1757.0	1684.5	11.6	78.6 [e]
(218)	O	CH$_3$	COONa	1774.5	1666.2	2.46	228
(219)	O	H	H	1778.2	1674.5	23.2	6.93
(220)	S	H	H	1773.1	1676.3	3.79	26.8
(221)	O	OCH$_3$	H	1772.9	1694.5	38.0	1.79
(222)	S	OCH$_3$	H	1768.1	1690.6	5.85	15.7

[a] V_{max} were measured in dry dimethyl sulfoxide and calibrated for the rotational fine structure of water vapor. Accuracies of V_{max} are ± 0.5 cm^{-1}.

[b] Hydrolysis rates were measured at 35°C in a buffer solution of pH 9.2 prepared from glycine and sodium hydroxide and adjusted to $\mu = 0.5$ with potassium chloride.

[c] Geometrical means of MICs for Es. coli JC-2 and K. pneumoniae SRL-1 measured by a gradient plate technique are indicated.

[d] Uyeo and Ona (1980).

[e] A value of the racemic mixture is indicated.

of *Escherichia coli* JC-2 and *Klebsiella pneumoniae* SRL-1 and that the MIC values of 1-carbacephem (**217**) and 7α-methyl-1-oxacephem (**218**) deviate markedly from the relationship. The lower frequency shift of the β-lactam carbonyl bands caused by the 7α-methoxy group does not parallel the antibacterial activity. However, this may correlate with the possible increase in the amide resonance in the β-lactam ring suggested by X-ray crystallographic analysis (Section III,B) and probably with the higher ^{13}C chemical shift of the β-lactam carbonyl carbon. Similar structure–carbonyl frequency relationships are also valid in a number of the corresponding benzhydryl esters as shown in Table IX.

TABLE IX Mean Values of Absorption Frequencies of Cephem Analog Esters[a]

			V_{max} in CHCl$_3$ (cm^{-1})		
Compound	A	Y	β-Lactam carbonyl	Amide carbonyl	Ester carbonyl
(**223**)	O	H	1799 ± 2 (17)	1684 ± 4 (16)	1721 ± 3 (17)
(**224**)	S	H	1793 ± 2 (2)	1687 ± 3 (2)	1727 ± 0 (2)
(**225**)	O	OCH$_3$	1791 ± 2 (12)	1700 ± 5 (12)[b]	1725 ± 4 (12)
(**226**)	S	OCH$_3$	1787 ± 5 (14)	1703 ± 4 (14)[b]	1727 ± 4 (14)

[a] Mean values and standard deviations (σ_{n-1}) are indicated. Values in parentheses indicate the number of compounds measured. R = H or COOR'. Values are not calibrated.
[b] Usually observed as an inflection.

Murakami *et al.* (1981) have also investigated the effect of replacement of the sulfur atom by oxygen on biological activity and physicochemical properties of cephems with various 7β-actylamino side chains. The stability to β-lactamase is reduced, while IR frequencies of the β-lactam carbonyl bond and intrinsic antibacterial activity against susceptible bacteria strains are invariably enhanced.

F. Ultraviolet and Circular Dichroism Spectra

The 3-cephem chromophore of cephalosporins exhibits two absorption bands in the ultraviolet (UV) region at about 260 and 230 nm. Comparison of many different cephalosporins (Nagarajan and Spry, 1971) and a theoretical treatment by Boyd (1972) led to the proposal that the 260-nm band was due to excitation of an electron from an enamine π-MO to one with both C=O π* and C=C π* character and that the 230-nm band

CEPHALOSPORIN NUCLEAR ANALOGS: PARTIAL SYNTHESIS

arises from the transition of an amide lone pair MO to the C=O, C=C π^* MO.

Table X shows the UV absorption maxima of 1-oxacephems compared with those of cephalosporins and 1-carbacephems. A significant bathochromic shift of about 10 nm is noted on substitution of the 3'-(1-methyl-1H-tetrazol-5-yl)thio group for the corresponding hydrogen. Introduction of the 7α-methoxy group causes a slight bathochromic shift of about 6 nm in the 3'-(1-methyl-1H-tetrazol-5-yl)thiomethyl series, whereas replacement of the sulfur atom by the oxygen atom appears to result in a hypochromic shift of about 3–5 nm.

Circular dichroism (CD) results (Kuriyama and Iwata, 1980) are given in Table XI. The CD curves of 1-oxacephems, as well as cephalosporins,

TABLE X Ultraviolet Absorption Spectra of Cephem Analog Carboxylates[a]

Z	Y	λ_{max} (nm) A = O	A = S	A = CH$_2$[b]
(N–N / S, N,N, CH$_3$)	H	269 (6,930)[c]	272 (10,500)[c]	—
		267 (6,350)[d]	274 (9,910)[d]	—
		265 (8,100)[e]	272 (9,400)[e]	—
	OCH$_3$	273 (11,100)[c]	274 (10,500)[c]	275 (14,200)[c]
		273 (10,800)[d]	276 (9,500)[d]	—
		271 (10,500)[e]	274 (10,000)[e]	—
	CH$_3$	269 (10,300)[c]		
H	H	259 (7,000)[e,g]	264 (7,000)[e,g]	260 (8,200)[e,g]
		259 (6,300)[f,g]	264 (6,200)[f,g]	—
	OCH$_3$	259 (6,700)[e]	265 (7,400)[e]	—
		262 (6,900)[f]	265 (6,300)[f]	—

[a] Spectra were measured in methanol. The molecular extinction coefficient is shown in parentheses.

[b] Uyeo and Ona (1980).

[c] R = HO–⟨O⟩–CH– COONa

[d] R = HO–⟨O⟩–CH$_2$–

[e] R = ⟨O⟩–CH$_2$–

[f] R = CH$_3$.

[g] The corresponding acid is measured.

TABLE XI Circular Dichroism Spectra of Cephem Analogs and Their 7-Epimers

Structure (general formula for compounds): cephem/oxacephem nucleus with substituents R, Y at the 7-position, A at the ring position, COOM ester, and a 1-methyltetrazol-5-ylthiomethyl side chain.

Compound	A	R	Y	M	Solvent	Band I	Band II	Band III	Band IV
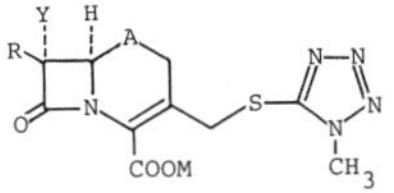						\(\lambda_{max}\) (nm)[a]			
(227)	O	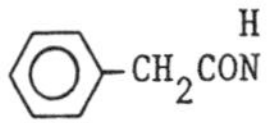 $-\text{CH}_2\text{CON}(\text{H})-\text{C}_6\text{H}_5$	H	Na	Methanol	—	229 (−21.64)	259 (+4.85)	302 (+0.66)
(228)	O	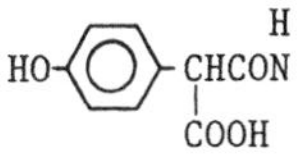 $\text{HO}-\text{C}_6\text{H}_4-\text{CH(COOH)CON(H)}-$	H	H	1% NaHCO$_3$	—	231 (−11.21)	257.5 (+2.21)	284 (−0.61)
(229)	O	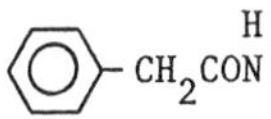 $-\text{CH}_2\text{CON}(\text{H})-\text{C}_6\text{H}_5$	OCH$_3$	Na	Methanol	—	236 (−25.88)	268 (+9.24)	310 (+0.16)
(230)[b]	O	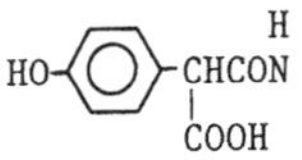 $\text{HO}-\text{C}_6\text{H}_4-\text{CH(COOH)CON(H)}-$	OCH$_3$	H	Methanol	210 (+3.85)	240.5 (−30.1)	170.5 (+8.12)	309 (−0.02)
(202)	O	NH$_2$	OCH$_3$	CH(C$_6$H$_5$)$_2$	Dioxane	220 (+6.42)	250.5 (−32.67)	285 (+3.30)	315 (−0.06)
(231)	S	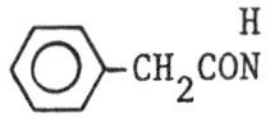 $-\text{CH}_2\text{CON}(\text{H})-\text{C}_6\text{H}_5$	H	Na	Methanol	—	232 (−15.03)	226 (+7.33)	—
(232)	S	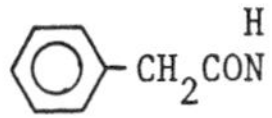 $-\text{CH}_2\text{CON}(\text{H})-\text{C}_6\text{H}_5$	OCH$_3$	Na	Methanol	217 (+2.00)	240.5 (−18.45)	270 (+10.21)	322 (+0.19)
(233)	O	OCH$_3$	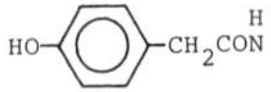 $\text{HO}-\text{C}_6\text{H}_4-\text{CH}_2\text{CON}(\text{H})-$	H	Methanol	210 (−12.5)	243 (−37.1)	271.5 (+14.15)	—
(234)	O	OCH$_3$	NH$_2$	CH(C$_6$H$_5$)$_2$	Dioxane	210 (−5.67)	248 (−32.21)	285 (+5.15)	—

[a] The molecular extinction coefficient is given in parentheses.
[b] Free acid of 6059-S.

exhibit two Cotton effects, a positive maximum near 260 nm and a negative one near 230 nm. In accord with the UV spectra, a bathochromic shift of about 7 nm for both CD maxima is revealed on introduction of the 7α-methoxy group. Intensification of the 230-nm band is seen. The CD curves of the 7-epimers **233** and **234** show a negative 210-nm band and no significant changes in the 230- and 260-nm bands.

On the basis of these observations, it has been suggested that the chiral chromophore indicated in Fig. 6 leads to a positive Cotton effect associated with the 260-nm π–π* transition and to a negative Cotton effect associated with the 230-nm n–π* transition.

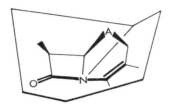

Fig. 6. Conformation of O=C—N—C=C chromophore of (6R)-cephems and (6R)-1-oxacephems.

IV. Structure–Activity Relationships of 1-Oxacephems

A. Evaluation Procedure

In addition to describing structure–activity relationships among 1-oxacephem derivatives, we also will show the shift in biological responses caused by the S → O replacement in the cephem nucleus. For this purpose, we will use data obtained from our own tests rather than comparing literature data which tend to vary among different laboratories.

In vitro tests for antibacterial activity were performed by the agar dilution technique and results expressed as the MIC. One loopful of a bacterial suspension of approximately 10^6 cells/ml was inoculated onto the agar medium containing the compound at twofold serial dilutions. The minimum numbers of test organisms are presented in the tables to define the activity and spectrum for the particular structure. For gram-positive organisms, *Staphylococcus aureus* 209P JC-1 and *Streptococcus pyogenes* were used. Both strains are very sensitive to penicillin G. Gram-negative activity is represented by the following strains: *E. coli* NIHJ JC-2, *E. coli* 73 (produced class III β-lactamase), *K. pneumoniae* SRL-1, *Klebsiella* sp. 363 (produced class IV β-lactamase), *Proteus vulgaris* CN-329, *Enterobacter cloacae* 233, Serratia marcescens ATCC

13880, *Pseudomonas aeruginosa* ATCC 25619 (very sensitive to car-benicillin), and *P. aeruginosa* PS-24. In the tables, the strain number is not given, except for *P. aeruginosa* PS-24, and the β-lactamase-producing strains are distinguished by (R). *In vivo* antibacterial activity, expressed as the 50% effective dose (ED_{50}), was evaluated by a protection test in mice against a lethal systemic infection produced by an intraperitoneal challenge of the organism. Mice were treated by subcutaneous dosings at 1 and 5 hr after infection. The experimental procedure is described by Yoshida *et al.* (1980).

Pharmacological evaluation was performed in rodents. The concentration of the compounds in plasma was determined every 15 min after parenteral administration. The area under the curve (AUC) for the plasma level versus time was calculated on the basis of a trapezoidal method. Excretion of the compound was estimated by its recovery from urine and bile. In mice, bile was collected from washings of whole intestine together with the gallbladder. Urine was collected from the urinary bladder as described previously (Wheeler *et al.*, 1977). In rats, the bile and urine were collected by cannulation of the common bile duct and urinary bladder, respectively.

Serum protein binding was determined by ultrafiltration through Visking tubing. The test compounds were added to 2 ml of human serum albumin solution (50 mg/ml) at a concentration of 10 μg/ml (*C*). Centrifugation of the reaction mixture at 1000 *g* for 15 min at 4°C gave about 0.3 ml of clear ultrafiltrate in which the concentration of the compound (C_f) was determined by bioassay. The binding percentage (*B*) was calculated as $B = (1 - C_f/C) \times 100$.

Measurement of permeability through the outer membrane of gram-negative bacteria was performed according to the procedure of Zimmermann and Rosselet (1977) with a modification. Exponentially growing bacteria were harvested by centrifugation and suspended in 0.05 *M* Na_2HPO_4–KH_2PO_4 buffer (pH 7.0). A portion of the cell suspension was sonicated. β-Lactamase activity of the intact cell suspension and the sonicated cell suspension was measured by spectrophotometric assay (O'Callaghan *et al.*, 1969). Determination of permeability (*C*) is based on the assumptions that β-lactam compounds penetrate through the outer membrane by passive diffusion and that the diffusion rate equals the hydrolysis rate by β-lactamase in the periplasm of the cells at a steady state (Zimmermann and Rosselet, 1977). The penetration index (*P*) (min^{-1} $cell^{-1}$ ml) is calculated as $P = C/n$, where *n* is the number of viable bacteria cells used because the value of *C* depends upon the number of intact cells in the reaction mixture of the β-lactamase assay. Details of this method will be published by Murakami and Yoshida (1982).

The kinetic parameters V_{max} and K_m for the β-lactamases were calculated from double reciprocal plots of V_{max} against substrate concentration, and K_i was determined from plots of apparent K_m against concentrations of an inhibitor. The assay and the purification of β-lactamase were carried out as described previously (Yoshida *et al.*, 1980).

B. Biological Effects of Oxygen Substitution for Sulfur in Cephalosporins

The effect of the substitution of an oxygen atom for the sulfur in the cephalosporin nucleus upon the reactivity of the β-lactam ring has already been discussed (Section III,E). In this section, the change in the biological response caused by a S → O replacement in the cephem nucleus is discussed. The side chains of cephalosporin derivatives at positions 3 and 7 have pronounced effects upon both susceptibility to β-lactamases and antibacterial activity (Richmond and Sykes, 1973; Webber and Ott, 1977). In order to eliminate side-chain effects, comparisons are made between 1-oxacefamandole and cefamandole, the latter having been well characterized by Moellering (1977). In Table XII, some of the biological parameters of the two antibiotics and the S → O effect are summarized.

1. *Antibacterial Activity*

The *in vitro* antibacterial activity of both antibiotics against two gram-positive and seven gram-negative bacteria are shown in Table XIV as compounds **9** and **256**. 1-Oxacefamandole (**9**) has fourfold and eightfold lower MIC values for sensitive strains of gram-positive and gram-negative bacteria, respectively, than cefamandole (**256**). The effect of S → O replacement on *in vitro* activity is always greater for gram-negative than for gram-positive bacteria and tends to be influenced by the side-chain structure at the 7-position (Murakami *et al.*, 1981). The effect of S → O substitution on *in vivo* activity parallels that of *in vitro* activity and is exemplified by ED_{50} values against *E. coli* in infected mice.

2. *β-Lactamase Stability*

The susceptibility of cefamandole and its 1-oxa congener to four typical β-lactamases of gram-negative bacteria was examined. The relative hydrolysis rate was increased by the 1-oxa conversion regardless of the enzyme class tested. The reduction in stability to β-lactamases may be related to the chemical reactivity of the β-lactam carbonyl and is unfavorable to antibacterial activity against bacterial strains which are resistant to either penicillins or cephalosporins as a result of the production of β-lactamases either constitutively or inducibly (Murakami *et al.*, 1981).

TABLE XII Biological Effects of S→O Substitution in Cefamandole and 1-Oxa-1-Dethiacefamandole

System	Cefamandole (256)	1-Oxacefamandole (9)	Change caused by S→O substitution
In vitro activity (MIC, μg/ml)[a]			
Gram-positive bacteria	0.05–0.1	0.012–0.025	4
Gram-negative bacteria	0.4–50	0.05–6.25	8
In vivo activity (ED_{50}, mg/kg)[b]			
Escherichia coli EC-14	3.0	0.87	3.5
β-Lactamase hydrolysis[c]			
Escherichia coli W3110 RTEM (III)	55	371	6.7
Enterobacter cloacae 53 (IV)	20	104	5.2
Escherichia coli 6 (Ib)	14	39	2.8
Proteus vulgaris 31 (Ic)	201	304	1.5
Permeability of outer membrane[d]			
Escherichia coli 6	1.3×10^{-11}	3.3×10^{-11}	2.5
Serum protein binding (%)[e]	79	41	0.52
Mouse plasma level[f]			
Peak (μg/ml)	39.5 ± 7.5	37.0 ± 3.4	0.94
AUC (μg min/ml)	1140	1028	0.90
Mouse excretion (% of dose)[f]			
Recovery in urine, 0–2 hr	41.9 ± 7.8	58.3 ± 11.1	1.4
Recovery in bile, 0–2 hr	30.1 ± 7.5	9.3 ± 5.3	0.3
Total	72.1 ± 1.9	67.5 ± 11.1	0.94

[a] Agar dilution MIC against laboratory strains listed in Table XIV except *P. aeruginosa*.
[b] Protective effect against intraperitoneal infection in mice.
[c] Hydrolysis rate (%) relative to that of cephaloridine.
[d] Permeability index (min^{-1} $cell^{-1}$ ml) (Murakami and Yoshida, 1982).
[e] Ultrafiltration method using human serum albumin (50 mg/ml).
[f] A dose of 20 mg/kg was subcutaneously injected. AUC, Area under curve.

3. Penetrability of the Bacterial Outer Membrane

Since the outer membrane functions as a barrier to the access of β-lactam antibiotics to their target enzyme in gram-negative microorganisms, penetrability through this outer layer of the bacterial envelope is an important factor in controlling the antibacterial activity of β-lactam compounds. The penetration index (P) was measured with *E. coli* 6 which produced a constitutive cephalosporinase. 1-Oxacefamandole exhibited a two- to threefold increase in penetrability over that of cefamandole. Murakami and Yoshida (1982) demonstrated the effect of S → O substitution on the penetrability of three pairs of cephalosporins and their 1-oxa congeners in *E. coli* 6 and *Proteus morganii* 7 using the principle of the method of Zimmermann and Rosselet (1977). They found that the 1-oxa conversion increased not only the penetrability but also the concentrations in the periplasm despite the higher susceptibility of 1-oxa congeners to the β-lactamase of the tested strains. The effect of S → O substitution on penetrability may contribute to the increase in antibacterial activity by 1-oxa conversion. When both antibiotics are compared for their hydrophobicity [determined by reversed-phase thin-layer chromatography according to the method of Biagi *et al.* (1969)], 1-oxacephalosporins have greater hydrophilicity (a lower R_m value) than the corresponding cephalosporins (Murakami and Yoshida, 1982). It is likely that the hydrophilic character of the compound favors penetrability through the bacterial outer membrane. Sawai *et al.* (1979) have reported that β-lactam antibiotics with higher hydrophilicity tend to penetrate more rapidly. This is also supported by the findings of Biagi *et al.* (1970) who demonstrated a good correlation between the hydrophilicity of penicillins and cephalosporins and their antibacterial activity against *E. coli.*

4. *Serum Protein Binding*

Binding to human serum albumin is greatly reduced in the 1-oxa analog of cefamandole. Since only the free drug appears to be bactericidal, the decrease in the degree of protein binding for the 1-oxa congener portends greater antibacterial activity in body fluids. Furthermore, the influence of renal excretion must be taken into account. When a portion of the administered antibiotic is eliminated by glomerular filtration, the recovery rate is accelerated. The effect of S → O replacement on serum protein binding is species-specific and is negligible in mouse plasma.

5. *Pharmacokinetics*

When a dose of 20 mg/kg was subcutaneously administered, no significant effect of S → O replacement was observed in either the peak plasma level or the AUC. However, the excretion pattern was significantly changed. The amount of administered cefamandole recovered was 42% in urine and 30% in bile. Biliary recovery is decreased in the 1-oxa analog, and 1-oxacefamandole is excreted primarily in the urine, although the total recovery of both congeners is the same.

C. Antibacterial Activity of 1-Oxacephem Derivatives

1. *3-Methyl-1-oxacephems*

1-Oxa congeners of 3-methylcephalosporins were prepared with a variety of side-chain structures at the 7β position (Narisada *et al.,* 1977). Table XIII presents a comparison of the *in vitro* antibacterial activity of 3-methylcephalosporin derivatives and their 1-oxa congeners.

TABLE XIII In Vitro Activity of 3-Methylcephalosporins and 1-Oxa Congeners

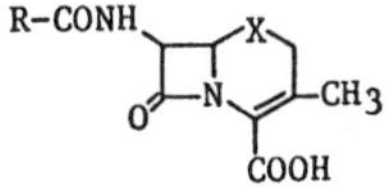

R-CONH — cephalosporin nucleus (X, CH₃, COOH)

Compound	R	X	MIC (µg/ml)									Ref.
			S. aureus	S. pyo-genes	E. coli	K. pneumo-niae	P. mirabilis	P. vulgaris	E. cloacae	S. marces-cens	P. aeruginosa	
(235)	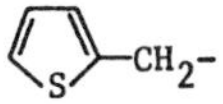 thiophene-CH₂-	S	0.4	0.8	100	25	25	>100	>100	>100	>100	a
(236)		O	0.4	0.2	6.3	3.1	6.3	100	>100	>100	>100	b
(237)	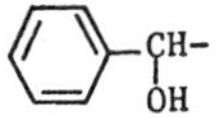 CH(OH)-phenyl	S	1.6	0.8	12.5	6.3	12.5	50	100	>100	>100	a
(10d)		O	0.8	0.2	1.6	1.6	3.1	>100	12.5	>100	>100	b, c
(238)	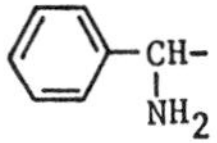 CH(NH₂)-phenyl	S	1.6	0.8	6.3	3.1	6.3	25	>100	>100	>100	d
(10e)		O	25	>3.1	100	50	>100	>100	>100	>100	>100	b, c, e
(239)	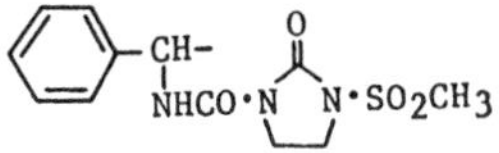 CH-NHCO·N⌐N·SO₂CH₃	S	0.8	0.4	6.3	12.5	25	25	—	>100	>100	a
(10f)		O	1.6	0.1	1.6	0.8	3.1	6.3	12.5	50	>100	f
(240)	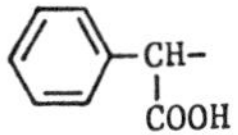 CH(COOH)-phenyl	S	100	>3.1	100	100	>100	100	100	>100	100	a
(10c)		O	50	>3.1	6.3	6.3	12.5	25	6.3	25	6.3	g
(241)	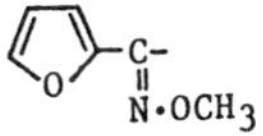 furan-C(=N·OCH₃)	S	12.5	0.4	>100	50	50	50	—	>100	>100	a
(242)		O	3.1	0.2	12.5	6.3	6.3	>100	—	>100	>100	a
(243)	CF₃·S·CH₂-	S	1.6	3.1	50	50	50	>100	>100	>100	>100	h
(244)		O	1.6	0.4	6.3	6.3	25	>100	>100	>100	>100	a

[a] Shionogi Research Laboratories (unpublished work).
[b] Narisada et al. (1977).
[c] Branch and Pearson (1979).
[d] Cephalexin.
[e] Measured as its trifluoroacetate in medium adjusted to pH 6.
[f] Matsumura et al. (1980).
[g] Hamashima et al. (1980b).
[h] Japanese Kokai (1973).

The effect of S → O substitution on the activity against streptococci and gram-negative bacteria is greater by 4- to 16-fold. There is one exception: A phenylglycyl-1-oxacephem derivative shows a reversed effect with diminished *in vitro* activity. This exceptional decrease in the antibacterial activity may be caused by nucleophilic attack by the α-amino group on the β-lactam ring activated by the presence of the oxygen atom in the cephem nucleus. Intramolecular aminolysis of ampicillin was reported to be retarded by steric hindrance generated in the transition state between the amino group of the side chain and H-3β in the penicillin nucleus (Indelicato *et al.*, 1974).

The magnitude of the S → O effect on the MIC values appears to depend on the side-chain structure. A phenylmalonyl derivative manifests the greatest shift (an almost 16-fold increase) with 1-oxa conversion and exhibits a widely expanded antibacterial spectrum which includes antipseudomonal activity. In general, the increase in antibacterial activity seems to be more pronounced against gram-negative bacteria than against gram-positive bacteria.

2. *3-Substituted Methyl-1-oxacephems*

It is well known in the literature that the incorporation of heterocyclic thio groups onto the 3-methyl group of cephems with different 7-acylamido groups produces a favorable effect on the antibacterial activity (Gorman and Ryan, 1972; Webber and Ott, 1977). Table XIV exemplifies trends similar to those observed in the cephalosporin family (Boyd and Lunn, 1979) for 1-oxacephalosporins with three different 7-acylamido side chains including the phenylmalonyl moiety.

The 3-methylene substituents included are methoxy, acetoxy, methyl-1,3,4-thiadiazolylthio, and 1-methyltetrazolylthio. The superiority of the thio-substituted compounds is evident in each of the three series. The tetrazolylthiomethyl analog with the phenylmalonyl side chain [Table XIV (254)] is the most effective in activity and breadth of spectrum against gram-negative bacteria. The activity is approximately 100 times greater than that of the nonsubstituted (3-methyl) congeners [Table XIII (10c)]. The gram-positive activity of the phenylmalonyl derivatives tends to appear better than their inherent activity because of contamination with variable amounts of the decarboxylated congener (G-type side chain).

Table XV lists a number of 3-heterocyclic thiomethylcephalosporins having various 7-acylamido side chains including several which are well documented in the literature. The effects of S → O replacement in individual derivatives are also examined for *in vitro* and *in vivo* activity. It is observed that the effect of S → O substitution is greatly affected

TABLE XIV In Vitro Activity of 3-Substituted Methyl-1-oxacephalosporins

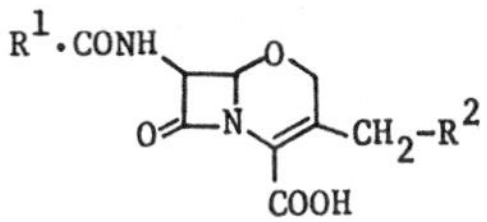

Structure: R¹·CONH— / —CH₂-R² / COOH

R² = A (-OCH₃) R² = B (-OCOCH₃) R² = C $\left(-S-\!\!\!\begin{array}{c}N\!-\!N\\S\end{array}\!\!\!CH_3\right)$ R² = D $\left(-S-\!\!\!\begin{array}{c}N\!-\!N\\N\\CH_3\end{array}\right)$

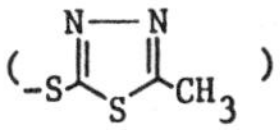

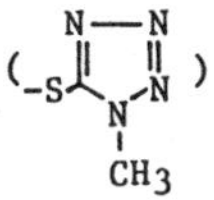

Compound	R¹	R²	MIC (µg/ml) S. aureus	S. pyogenes	E. coli	K. pneumoniae	P. mirabilis	P. vulgaris	E. cloacae	S. marcescens	P. aeruginosa	Ref.
(8)	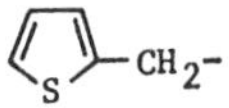 thiophene-CH₂-	B[a]	≦0.01	0.02	0.8	0.2	0.4	50	100	>100	>100	b, c
(246)		C	≦0.01	≦0.01	0.4	0.4	0.8	1.6	50	>100	>100	d
(247)		D	0.02	≦0.01	0.1	0.1	0.4	0.8	3.1	100	>100	d
(248)	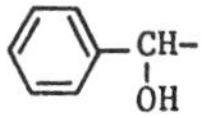 CH-OH phenyl	A	0.2	≦0.01	1.6	1.6	3.1	50	>100	>100	>100	d
(249)		B	0.05	0.02	0.4	0.2	0.4	12.5	12.5	>100	>100	d
(250)		C	0.02	≦0.01	0.1	0.2	0.2	0.4	3.1	25	>100	d
(9)		D[e]	0.02	≦0.01	0.05	0.05	0.1	0.1	0.4	6.3	>100	c, f
(251)	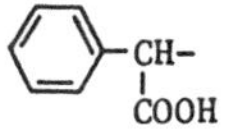 CH-COOH phenyl	A	3.1	3.1	1.6	1.6	3.1	3.1	1.6	3.1	6.3	g
(252)		B	1.6	3.1	0.8	0.8	1.6	1.6	0.8	1.6	3.1	g
(253)		C	0.8	0.8	0.2	0.2	0.2	0.1	0.2	0.4	3.1	g
(254)		D	0.8	0.4	0.05	0.1	0.2	0.1	0.1	0.2	1.6	g
(255)	Cephalothin		0.1	0.1	6.3	1.6	3.1	100	>100	>100	>100	—
(256)	Cefamandole		0.1	0.05	0.4	0.4	0.8	0.8	3.1	50	>100	—

[a] 1-Oxacephalothin.
[b] Cama and Christensen (1974).
[c] Narisada et al. (1979).
[d] Shionogi Laboratories (unpublished work).
[e] 1-Oxacefamandole.
[f] Firestone et al. (1977).
[g] Narisada et al. (1980).

by the nature of the 7-acylamido side chain, showing both a negative and a positive effect as indicated by typical examples for both extremes, e.g., the aminothiazole side chain [Table XV (**265, 266**)] and the phenylmalonyl group [Table XV (**254, 262**)], respectively. As a consequence of the negative shift in resistance to β-lactamase caused by 1-oxa substitution discussed previously, the antibacterial activity of 1-oxa congeners against β-lactamase-producing *E. coli* tends to decrease.

The phenylmalonylamido side chain confers a maximal S → O shift of as much as an 8- to 64-fold increase in both *in vitro* and *in vivo* activity, and the 1-oxa congener (**254**) exhibits an excellent antibacterial activity having a broad spectrum against gram-negative bacteria with the exception of penicillinase-producing *E. coli*. Introduction of a sulfonyl group in the side chain also results in a profound S → O effect (a 16- to 32-fold increase in gram-negative activity), but the activity, both *in vitro* and *in vivo,* of the 1-oxa congener (**261**) is not as great as that of the malonyl derivative (**254**).

Analogs bearing an α-acylureido (**263**) and an α-hydroxy (**256**) group on the phenylacetylamido side chain exhibit a four- to eightfold increase in gram-negative activity after 1-oxa conversion. Compound **268** has an expanded antibacterial spectrum, although an unfavorable S → O effect for antipseudomonal activity is seen. The S → O effect is rather modest in compounds **257** and **258** with the side chains of cephalothin and cefazolin, respectively.

From the available data, significant variations in the S → O effect are seen. These variations may be explained by the enhanced reactivity of the β-lactam ring due to 1-oxa conversion (Murakami *et al.,* 1981). It has been suggested that both transpeptidase inhibition and β-lactamase hydrolysis of β-lactam compounds are similarly mediated by an acylation reaction (Georgopapadakou *et al.,* 1977; Knott-Hunziker *et al.,* 1979). Both effects relate to the activity of the β-lactam ring, the former being favorable, whereas the latter is unfavorable. In addition, outer membrane permeability and chemical stability of a compound also influence the antibacterial activity. The relative importance of all these factors probably varies with side-chain structures and must be taken into account for prediction of the variation in the effect of S → O replacement.

3. *C-3′ Demethyl-1-Oxacephems*

Table XVI provides activity data for C-3′ demethyl-1-oxacephems. Phenylmalonylamino and α-methoxyimino-2-aminothiazole-5-ylacetyl-lamino groups were selected as the side chains because they showed opposite effects of S → O substitution. The 3-chloro-1-oxa compound (**271**) exhibits the best *in vitro* activity in this series, being 2–16 times

TABLE XV Antibacterial Activity of 3-Heterocyclic Thioether Cephalosporins and 1-Oxa Congeners

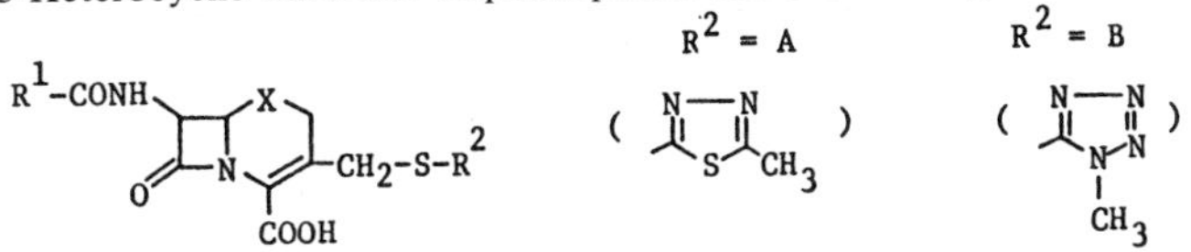

Compound	R¹	R²	X	MIC (μg/ml)									ED₅₀ E. coli EC-14 (mg/kg)	Ref.
				S. aureus	S. pyogenes	E. coli	E. coli (R)	K. pneumoniae	P. vulgaris	E. cloacae	S. marcescens	P. aerugi-nasa		
(257)	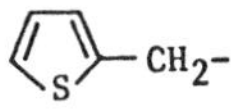 thiophene-CH₂–	A	S	0.02	0.02	1.6	50	0.8	12.5	50	>100	>100	—	a
(246)			O	<0.01	<0.01	0.4	>100	0.4	1.6	50	>100	>100	7.6	b
(258)	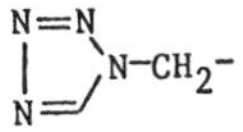 tetrazolyl-CH₂–	A	S	0.1	0.1	1.6	25	1.6	100	>100	>100	>100	5.5	c
(259)			O	0.1	0.02	0.8	>100	1.6	25	100	>100	>100	3.4	b
(256)	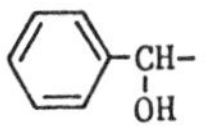 CH– OH	B	S	0.1	0.05	0.4	50	0.4	0.8	3.1	50	>100	3.0	d
(9)			O	0.02	≦0.01	0.05	100	0.05	0.1	0.4	6.3	>100	0.87	e
(260)	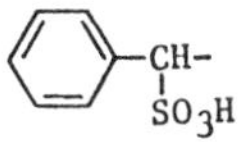 CH– SO₃H	B	S	12.5	12.5	6.3	100	12.5	12.5	12.5	50	50	>50	f
(261)			O	1.6	3.1	0.4	>100	0.8	0.8	0.8	1.6	1.6	8.6	g
(262)	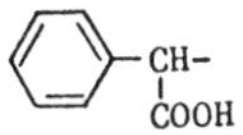 CH– COOH	B	S	6.3	12.5	3.1	25	1.6	0.8	3.1	12.5	25	11	b
(254)			O	0.8	0.4	0.05	12.5	0.1	0.1	0.1	0.2	1.6	0.32	h

(263) HO–⟨phenyl⟩–CH(NHCO–N⟨pyrrolidinone⟩N–SO$_2$CH$_3$)–	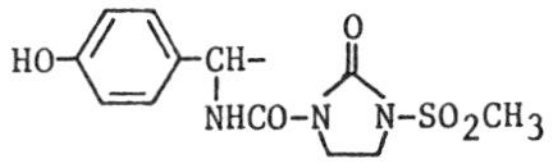 B	S	0.4	0.05	0.2	25	0.2	1.6	1.6	3.1	3.1	0.57	b
(264)		O	0.4	0.02	0.05	25	0.02	0.4	0.4	0.4	6.3	0.17	i
(265) H$_2$N⟨thiazole⟩–CH$_2$–	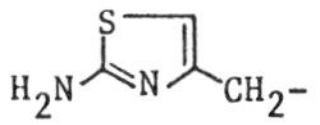 B	S	0.1	0.05	0.1	1.6	0.1	0.8	1.6	6.3	>100	0.58	j
(266)		O	0.05	0.02	0.2	>100	0.2	0.8	12.5	50	>100	0.48	k
(267) H$_2$N⟨thiazole⟩–C(=N–OCH$_3$)–	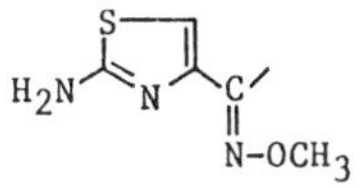 B	S	0.4	0.02	0.02	0.4	0.05	0.05	0.4	0.4	1.6	0.14	l
(268)		O	0.2	<0.01	0.02	6.3	0.02	0.05	0.2	0.2	6.3	0.10	k

[a] Netherlands Patent (1968).
[b] Shionogi Laboratories (unpublished work).
[c] Cefazolin.
[d] Cefamandole
[e] Narisada et al. (1979).
[f] Nomura et al. (1975).
[g] Hayashi et al. (1980).
[h] Narisada et al. (1980).
[i] Matsumura et al. (1980).
[j] Cefotiam.
[k] Hamashima et al. (1980c).
[l] Goto et al. (1980).

TABLE XVI In Vitro Activity of 3'-Demethyl-1-Oxacephem Derivatives

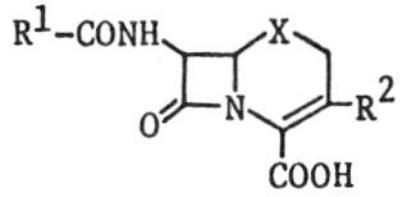

$R^1\text{-CONH}$, X, R^2, COOH bicyclic structure

Compound	R^1	R^2	X	MIC (μg/ml)								Ref.
				S. aureus	E. coli	E. coli (R)	K. pneumoniae	P. vulgaris	E. cloacae	S. marcescens	P. aerugi-nosa	
(269)	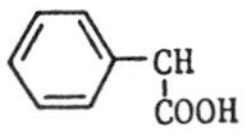 phenyl-CH-COOH	H	O	12.5	6.3	25	6.3	12.5	6.3	12.5	6.3	a
(270)		Cl	S	3.1	6.3	50	6.3	12.5	—	25	6.3	b
(271)		Cl	O	12.5	0.4	12.5	0.4	0.8	0.8	1.6	3.1	a
(272)		OCH_3	O	25	3.1	50	6.3	12.5	3.1	12.5	12.5	a
(273)		OSO_2CH_3	O	12.5	0.8	100	1.6	1.6	1.6	3.1	12.5	a
(274)		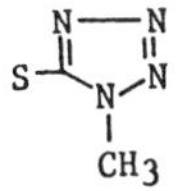 S-tetrazolyl (N-CH_3)	O	6.3	0.8	>100	3.1	6.3	12.5	—	25	a
(109a)	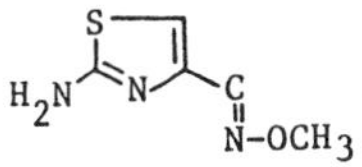 aminothiazole-C(=N-OCH$_3$)	H	S	6.3	0.02	0.1	$\leqq$0.01	$\leqq$0.01	0.2	0.1	1.6	c
(108a)		H	O	3.1	0.1	0.4	0.2	0.1	0.8	0.2	100	d

[a] Japanese Kokai (1978a).
[b] Japanese Kokai (1974).
[c] Ceftizoxime.
[d] Japanese Kokai (1979d).

as active as its 1-thia congener (270). However, none of the C-3'-demethyl substituents inprove the activity of phenylmalonyl-1-oxacephem compared with the 3-heterocyclic thiomethyl substituents. Compound 109a is known to be a very active β-lactam antibiotic as reported by Kamimura *et al.* (1979); however, the S → O shift migrates in the negative direction.

4. *7α-Methoxy-1-oxacephems*

Since 1-oxacephalosporins are unstable toward β-lactamase hydrolysis, they are less active against β-lactamase-producing strains. This disadvantage can be avoided by introducing substituents that protect compounds from β-lactamase hydrolysis. 7α-Methoxycephalosporins (cephamycins) have been shown to be resistant to β-lactamase hydrolysis (Nagarajan *et al.*, 1971; Stapley *et al.*, 1972). Table XVII reveals that introduction of the 7α-methoxy group into 1-oxacephems having various types of 7β-acylamido side chains is quite efficient in restoring activity against a β-lactamase-producing strain of *E. coli* (R).

The preferred side chain structures are again the arylmalonylamido (277, 278) and acylureidophenylacetylamido (279) groups with respect to *in vitro* and *in vivo* activity and broadness of spectrum against gram-negative bacteria including *P. aeruginosa*. However, the phenylglycyl-acetamido group yielded a compound with virtually no activity (282), as already mentioned for the 7α-hydrogen series [Table XIII (10e)].

In order to explore the influence of 7α-methoxy incorporation into 1-oxacephems and their 1-thia counterparts, three different types of side-chain structures were chosen. Table XVIII presents a direct comparison of *in vitro* and *in vivo* activity.

In each pair of 7α-methoxy and nonsubstituted cephem analogs, the methoxy group strikingly increases the activity against *E. coli* (R) over that of the nonsubstituted compound but tends to decrease antistaphylococcal activity. The change in antibacterial activity against gram-negative organisms other than the resistant strain of *E. coli* varies according to the type of 7-acylamido side chain. Only the analog bearing the phenylmalonyl group (230) shows better activity relative to its 7-hydrogen counterpart (228). Moreover, the enhancement of antipseudomonal activity by methoxylation was noteworthy in this pair of compounds. In mice the protective activity of 230 markedly improves and is almost 10 times greater than that of the 1-thia congener (228) as evidenced by the ED_{50} values. Similar trends for the effect of methoxylation are observed in 1-thiacephalosporins (256, 285–289). The introduction of a 6α-methoxy group into carbenicillin is also associated with enhanced gram-negative activity against bacteria (Bentley and Clayton, 1977). A similar dramatic effect of methoxylation has been reported for phenylmalonyl cephalosporins by Webber and Ott (1977).

TABLE XVII Antibacterial Activity of 7α-Methoxy-1-Oxacephem Derivatives

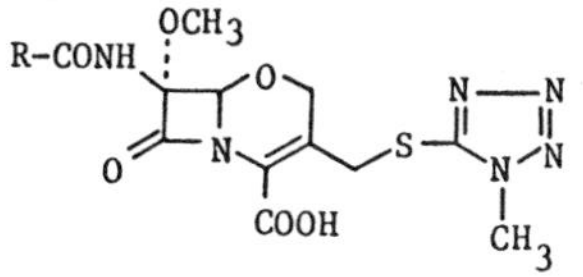

Compound	R	MIC (µg/ml)									ED_{50} E. coli, EC-14 (mg/kg)	Ref.
		S. aureus	E. coli	E. coli (R)	K. pneumo-niae	K. sp. (R)	P. vulgaris	E. cloacae	S. marces-cens	P. aerugi-nosa		
(275)	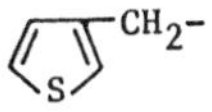 CH₂– (thiophene)	0.1	0.1	0.8	0.2	0.2	0.4	12.5	3.1	>100	1.1	a
(276)	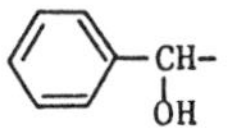 CH–OH (phenyl)	0.4	0.05	0.8	0.1	0.1	0.2	3.1	3.1	>100	0.62	a, b
(277)	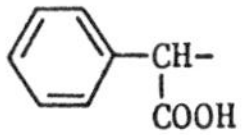 CH–COOH (phenyl)	3.1	0.05	0.2	0.02	0.02	0.05	0.05	0.1	3.1	0.12	c
(278)	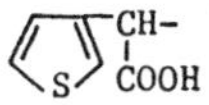 CH–COOH (thiophene)	1.6	0.05	0.1	0.05	0.02	0.1	0.05	0.1	3.1	0.12	c, d
(279)	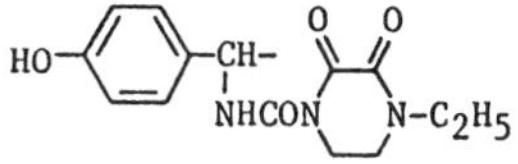 CH–NHCON... N-C₂H₅ (HO-phenyl)	0.8	0.05	0.1	0.01	0.05	0.1	0.2	0.05	1.6	0.07	e, f
(280)	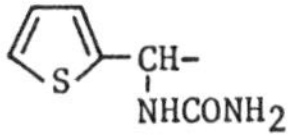 CH–NHCONH₂ (thiophene)	0.4	0.1	0.2	0.05	0.05	0.2	12.5	0.4	100	0.09	a
(281)	NCCH₂S–CH₂–	0.2	0.2	0.2	0.2	0.2	0.8	50	1.6	>100	0.17	a

74

(282)	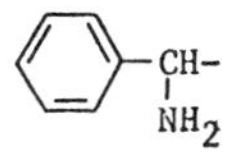 phenyl–CH(NH_2)–	50	>100	>100	100	50	100	>100	>100	>100	—	[a]
(283)	H_2N–C(S)=N ring–CH_2– (2-aminothiazolyl)	6.3	0.2	0.4	0.4	0.2	0.8	50	6.3	>100	0.87	[g]
(284)	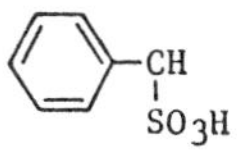 phenyl–CH(SO_3H)–	6.3	0.4	1.6	0.2	0.2	0.4	0.4	0.8	12.5	0.62	[h]

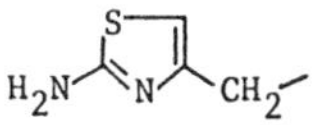

[a] Shionogi Laboratories (unpublished work).
[b] Measured as its O-formate.
[c] United States Patent (1979).
[d] Japanese Kokai (1977c).
[e] Japanese Kokai (1978c).
[f] Austrian Patent (1979).
[g] Hamashima et al. (1980c).
[h] Hayashi et al. (1980).

75

TABLE XVIII Effect of the 7α-Methoxy Substituent on Antibacterial Activity of Three Types of Cephalosporins and 1-Oxa Congeners

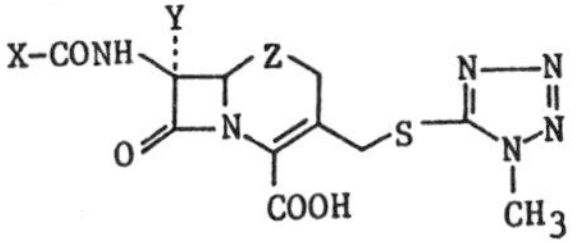

Compound	X	Y	Z	MIC (μg/ml) S. aureus	E. coli	E. coli (R)	P. vulgaris	E. cloacae	S. marcescens	P. aeruginosa	P. aeruginosa PS-24	ED$_{50}$ (mg/kg) E. coli EC-14	Ref.
(285)	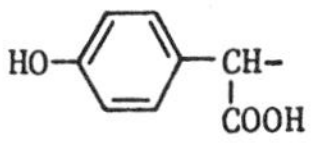 HO–⬡–CH(COOH)–	H	S	12.5	3.1	50	1.6	6.3	12.5	12.5	>100	4.6	a
(286)		OCH₃	S	12.5	0.8	3.1	0.4	0.8	1.6	1.6	25	0.7	a
(228)		H	O	3.1	0.2	50	0.4	0.4	0.8	3.1	>100	1.0	b
(230)		OCH₃	O	6.3	0.2	0.4	0.2	0.1	0.4	6.3	25	0.12	b,c,d,e
(256)	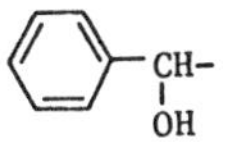 ⬡–CH(OH)–	H	S	0.05	0.2	50	1.6	3.1	25	>100	>100	3.2	f
(287)		OCH₃	S	0.8	1.6	12.5	0.8	12.5	12.5	50	>100	4.0	a,g
(9)		H	O	0.02	0.05	>100	0.1	0.4	6.3	>100	>100	0.87	h
(276)		OCH₃	O	0.4	0.05	0.8	0.2	3.1	3.1	>100	>100	0.62	a,g
(288)	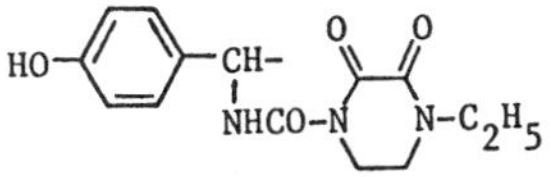 HO–⬡–CH(NHCO–N(ketopiperazine)–N–C₂H₅)–	H	S	0.4	0.1	25	0.8	0.8	0.8	0.8	6.3	0.11	i,j
(289)		OCH₃	S	1.6	0.2	0.8	0.8	1.6	0.4	3.1	12.5	0.4	k
(290)		H	O	0.4	≦0.01	12.5	0.2	0.1	0.05	0.8	3.1	0.04	l,m
(279)		OCH₃	O	0.8	0.05	0.1	0.1	0.2	0.05	1.6	12.5	0.07	l,m

[a] Shionogi Laboratories (unpublished work).
[b] United States Patent (1979).
[c] Free acid of 6059-S (**11**).
[d] Narisada et al. (1979).
[e] Japanese Kokai (1977c).
[f] Cefamandole.
[g] Measured as its O-formate.
[h] Firestone et al. (1977).
[i] Cefoperazone.
[j] Japanese Kokai (1977a).
[k] Australian Patent (1980).
[l] Matsumura et al. (1980).
[m] Japanese Kokai (1978c).

Substitution of the methoxy group at the 7-position was found to be optimal, as evidenced by data in Table XIX. This group is incorporated with the α configuration. The selective effect of methoxylation is also shown in cefmetazole (Nakao *et al.*, 1979).

Among the modifications in the side chain structure of 7α-methoxy-1-oxacephem derivatives, the substitution of carboxyl and acylureido functions at the α position of the 7β-hydroxyphenylacetamide side chain conferred an excellent activity against a wide variety of gram-negative organisms including *P. aeruginosa* as indicated by compounds **230** and **279** in Table XVIII, respectively. These two derivatives were given further evaluation, and a direct comparison of biological properties is shown in Table XX. Based on an examination of these important factors of therapeutic effectiveness, the advantage of the malonyl derivative over the acylureido derivative was verified as follows: (1) high peak plasma level and long half-life as evidenced by the higher AUC values, (2) higher stability in body fluids, and (3) quantitative excretion of the dose injected, which presumably implies metabolic stability. As expected, these properties correlate well with the greater protective activity against infection with a wide variety of gram-negative bacteria. A summary of the results led us to conclude that the phenylmalonyl derivative called 6059-S is superior to the acylureido derivative in therapeutic activity against infectious diseases.

V. Biology of 6059-S

One of the 7β-arylmalonylamino-7α-methoxy-1-oxacephem derivatives (**230**), as the disodium salt, was selected to be a clinical candidate (Yoshida *et al.*, 1978; Matsuura *et al.*, 1978) and was designated 6059-S by the Shionogi Company, Ltd. (Narisada *et al.*, 1979), and LY127935 by the Eli Lilly and Company (Brier *et al.*, 1979). The generic names "moxalactam" (USAN) and "latamoxef" (INN) have been assigned to this new oxa-β-lactam.

A. Pharmacokinetic Properties

In humans, 6059-S has good pharmacokinetic properties (Kurihara *et al.*, 1980; Parsons *et al.*, 1980). Prolonged serum half-life with high serum levels similar to those of cefazolin after parenteral dosing and almost complete excretion of the activity suggesting metabolic stability have been shown.

The *p*-hydroxy function on the phenyl ring in the side chain of 6059-S

TABLE XIX Effect of the 7-Substituent and Its Configuration on the Activity of Arylmalonyl-1-oxacephem Derivatives

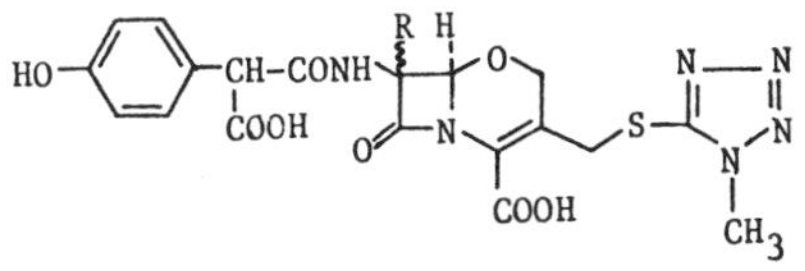

Compound	R	Config-uration	S. aureus	E. coli	E. coli (R)	P. vulgaris	E. cloacae	S. marcescens	P. aeruginosa	P. aeruginosa PS-24	Ref.
							MIC (μg/ml)				
(228)	H	α	3.1	0.2	50	0.4	0.4	0.8	3.1	>100	a
(230)	OCH_3	α	6.3	0.2	0.4	0.2	0.1	0.4	6.3	25	a, b
(291)	OC_2H_5	α	100	3.1	6.3	3.1	6.3	12.5	6.3	50	c
(292)	$OCH_2CH(CH_3)_2$	α	>100	100	100	100	50	>100	100	>100	c
(293)	SCH_3	α	>100	100	>100	100	100	100	>100	>100	c
(294)	$SCOCH_3$	α	>100	25	>100	50	25	100	>100	>100	c
(295)	CH_3	α	>100	12.5	50	12.5	12.5	25	50	>100	c
(296)	H	β	>100	>100	>100	>100	>100	>100	>100	>100	c
(297)	OCH_3	β	>100	50	>100	50	50	100	>100	>100	c
(298)	SCH_3	β	>100	>100	>100	>100	>100	>100	>100	>100	c

[a] United States Patent (1979).

[b] Japanese Kokai (1977c).

[c] Shionogi Laboratories (unpublished work).

TABLE XX Biological Properties of Arylmalonyl and Ureido-Acetyl-Type 7α-Methoxy-1-oxacephems

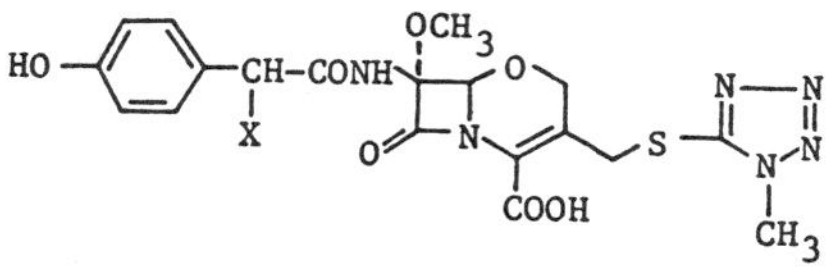

System	X = COOH 230	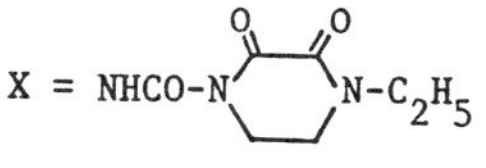 X = NHCO-N⟨⟩N-C$_2$H$_5$ 279
Mouse plasma level[a]		
Peak (μg/ml)	39.6 ± 5.6	13.0 ± 1.4
AUC (μg min/ml)	1240	245
Rat plasma level[b]		
Peak (μg/ml)	16.0 ± 1.3	6.9 ± 1.6
AUC (μg min/ml)	969	261
Rat excretion (% of dose)[b]		
Recovery in urine, 0–24 hr	73.3 ± 4.3	5.2 ± 2.7
Recovery in bile, 0–24 hr	21.7 ± 3.6	79.3 ± 5.3
Serum protein binding (%)[c]	45	24
Stability in human plasma (%)[d]	92	67
In vivo activity (ED$_{50}$, mg/kg)[e]		
Staphylococcus aureus Smith	8.3	4.3
Escherichia coli EC-14	0.12	0.07
Proteus mirabilis PR-4	0.22	1.5
Proteus vulgaris CN-329	0.81	3.5
Enterobacter cloacae CL-1	0.18	0.30
Serratia marcescens 13880	2.0	>10
Pseudomonas aeruginosa PS-24	8.4	47

[a] A dose of 20 mg/kg was subcutaneously injected. AUC, Area under the curve.
[b] A dose of 10 mg/kg was subcutaneously injected.
[c] Ultrafiltration method by using human serum albumin (50 mg/ml).
[d] Remained activity after incubation for 3 hr at 37°C.
[e] Protective effect against intraperitoneal infection.

appears to be associated with the above-mentioned characteristics. The results shown in Table XXI clearly demonstrate that addition of the *p*-hydroxy group brings about an increased peak plasma level and longer duration relative to the unsubstituted derivatives (**277, 278**). When the hydroxy group is placed at the meta or ortho position, the total plasma levels are decreased. Methylation of the *p*-hydroxy group also diminishes the *p*-hydroxy effect. The addition of the hydroxy group somewhat decreased *in vitro* activity, but it resulted in better ED$_{50}$ values against mouse infections similar to those of the unsubstituted analogs. The effect

TABLE XXI Modification of the C-7 Side Chain of 7α-Methoxy-1-oxacephem

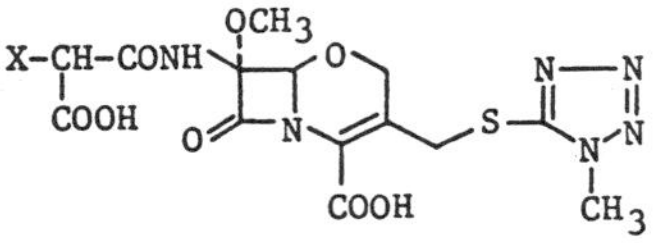

Compound	X	Plasma level[a]		Activity on *E. coli*		Ref.
		Peak (μg/ml)[b]	AUC (μg min/ml)	ED_{50} (mg/kg)	MIC (μg/ml)	
(278)	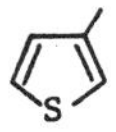	27.8 ± 7.7	590	0.12	0.02	c
(277)	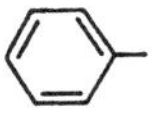	22.6 ± 3.0	506	0.12	0.05	c, d
(230)	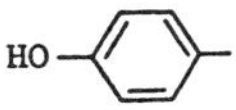 HO—	39.6 ± 5.6	1240	0.12	0.1	c
(299)	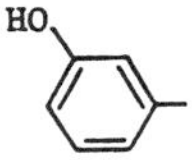	28.2 ± 3.5	761	0.14	0.1	d
(300)	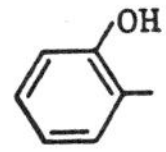	15.9 ± 2.8	387	0.67	0.1	d
(301)	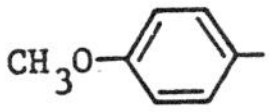 CH_3O—	28.6 ± 1.9	670	0.57	0.4	d

[a] A dose of 20 mg/kg was subcutaneously injected into the mouse.

[b] Mean of results for five mice $\pm$ SD.

[c] United States Patent (1979).

[d] Hamashima *et al.* (1980a).

of aromatic substitution with respect to functional groups and substitution sites has been fully discussed by Hamashima *et al.* (1980b).

Similar effects of aromatic substitution were observed with cephalosporins having a phenylglycyl side chain (Dunn *et al.*, 1976; Webber and Ott, 1977), although these examples were limited to orally absorbable cephalosporins. Pfeffer *et al.* (1977) compared the pharmacokinetic parameters of cephalexin and cefadroxil after oral administration in humans and found higher blood levels and longer duration in the *p*-hydroxy compound. Cefadroxil's longer duration in the blood is attributed to its more rapid saturation of the tubular mechanism (Hartstein *et al.*, 1977)

TABLE XXII Modification of the 3-Substituent of 7α-Methoxy-1-oxacephems

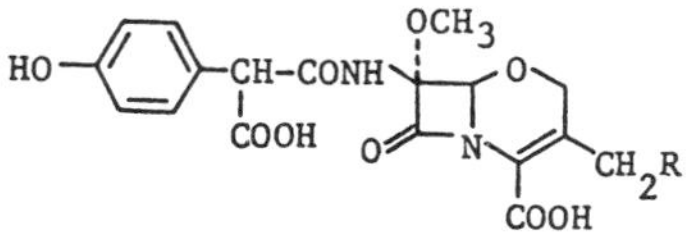

Compound	R	Plasma level[a]		Activity on E. coli		Ref.
		Peak (μg/ml)[b]	AUC (μg min/ml)	ED_{50} (mg/kg)	MIC (μg/ml)	
(302)	$-OCOCH_3$	17.6 ± 3.5	716	0.86	0.4	c
(230)	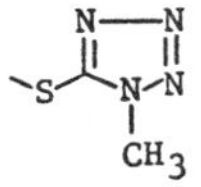	39.6 ± 5.6	1240	0.12	0.1	d, e
(303)	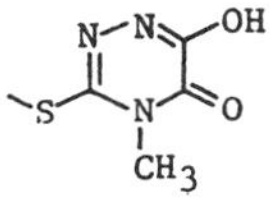	41.6 ± 3.4	1244	0.18	0.4	f, g

[a] A dose of 20 mg/kg was subcutaneously injected into the mouse.
[b] Mean of results for five mice ± SD.
[c] Shionogi Laboratories (unpublished work).
[d] United States Patent (1979).
[e] Japanese Kokai (1977c).
[f] West German Patent (1979).
[g] Japanese Kokai (1979a).

rather than to delayed absorption. Shimada *et al.* (1980) demonstrated in stop-flow studies on dogs that renal excretion of 6059-S took place mainly through glomerular filtration and that there was little tubular excretion. Their experiments in humans indicated that the concomitant administration of probenecid had little influence on the serum levels of 6059-S. The *p*-hydroxy function in 6059-S may be responsible for such renal excretion behavior. When a triazine substituent (**303**) is used instead of the 3-position tetrazole in 6059-S, the pharmacokinetic properties remain unchanged. The decreased plasma levels of the 3-acetoxymethyl compound may be due to metabolic instability caused by deacetylation.

Matsuura *et al.* (1978) found that 6059-S and cefazolin behaved in a similar pharmacokinetic manner in various experimental animals, e.g., plasma levels, half-life, and the ratio between urinary and biliary excretion, as indicated in Table XXIII. The same plasma levels are observed in these structurally unrelated antibiotics, although cefazolin is 74% bound to human serum proteins (Nishida *et al.*, 1970), significantly higher

TABLE XXIII Pharmacokinetic Properties of 6059-S and Cefazolin after Intravenous Administration[a]

Species	Antibiotic	Plasma level at 1 hr (μg/ml)	Half-life (min)	Excretion into[b] Urine (%)	Excretion into[b] Bile (%)
Human	6059-S	59.3	131	94.1	NT[c]
	CEZ	71.5	100	97.9	NT
Monkey	6059-S	47.8	55	77.2	1.4
	CEZ	52.8	49	81.3	NT
Dog	6059-S	35.2	75	89.9	6.0[d]
	CEZ	29.7	60	94.0	6.6[d]
Rabbit	6059-S	19.7	53	107	2.1
	CEZ	19.4	45	102	1.0
Rat	6059-S	8.2	18	81.9	25.3
	CEZ	10.0	26	73.8	26.8
Mouse	6059-S	2.7	17	60.9	13.4
	CEZ	2.9	16	54.1	19.6

[a] Dosage: 20 mg/kg in all animals; 1 g im human.

[b] Collection period: 0–24 hr in human, monkeys, and dogs; 0–6 hr in rabbits and rats; 0–2 hr in mice.

[c] NT, Not tested.

[d] Dosage: 40 mg/kg.

than 6059-S (Table XX). Tubular secretion in renal elimination is evidenced for cefazolin by probenecid administration (Kirby and Regamey, 1973) but not for 6059-S as mentioned above. This may explain the similar half life of both antibiotics.

B. β-Lactamase Stability and Mode of Action Mechanism

Yoshida (1980) has explained the roles of the 7α-methoxy and the side chain α-carboxyl groups in the 6059-S molecule in its stability toward β-lactamases. Data in Table XXIV give a summary of the structural requirements of 6059-S and its 1-sulfur counterpart (Murakami and Yoshida, 1981) for β-lactamase stability. An unsubstituted 1-oxa compound (**304**) was readily hydrolyzed by a variety of β-lactamases including the species-specific cephalosporinases, e.g., class I, and penicillinases, e.g., classes V (RGN 238), III (TEM), and IV (Richmond and Sykes, 1973). It has very poor activity against β-lactamase-producing bacteria.

A 7α-methoxy substitution brought about resistance to hydrolysis by penicillinase-type enzymes but had little effect on the stability toward cephalosporinases. Consequently, the 7α-methoxy compound (**306**) dramatically increased antibacterial activity against penicillinase-producing

TABLE XXIV Effect of Substituents of 1-Oxacephem on Antibacterial Activity and β-Lactamase Stability

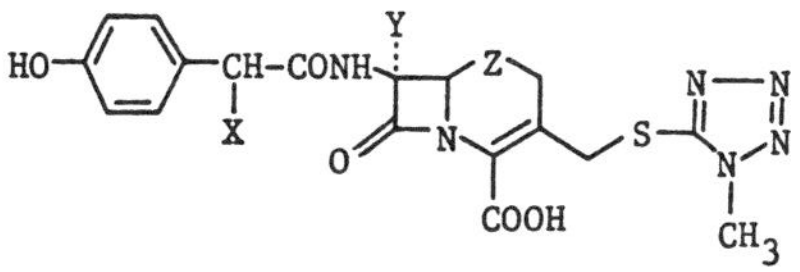

Compound	X	Y	Z	MIC (μg/ml)[a]				Stability toward[b]		Ref.
				E. coli JC-2	E. coli 73 (P)	Klebsiella sp. 363 (P)	E. cloacae 233 (C)	Penicillinase	Cephalosporinase	
(304)	H	H	O	0.8	>100	>100	>100	−	−	c
(305)	H	H	S	3.1	25	100	>100	±	−	c
(306)	H	OCH$_3$	O	0.1	0.8	0.2	100	++	±	c
(307)	H	OCH$_3$	S	3.1	12.5	3.1	>100	++	+	c
(228)	COOH	H	O	0.2	50	100	0.4	−	++	d
(285)	COOH	H	S	3.1	50	50	6.3	±	++	c
(230)	COOH	OCH$_3$	O	0.2	0.4	0.1	0.2	++	++	d, e
(286)	COOH	OCH$_3$	S	0.8	3.1	0.4	0.8	++	++	c

[a] Type of β-lactamase produced by tested strains: P, penicillinase; C, cephalosporinase.
[b] Hydrolysis rate relative to cephaloridin (100): ++, no hydrolysis; +, <10; ±, <100; −, >100.
[c] Shionogi Laboratories (unpublished work).
[d] United States Patent (1979).
[e] Japanese Kokai (1977c).

E. coli and *Klebsiella* sp. but bacteria such as *Enterobacter* sp. 233 with inducible cephalosporinases retained resistance.

The inability of the 7α-methoxy function to protect cephalosporins from β-lactamase hydrolysis has been reported by Onishi *et al.* (1974). They demonstrated that cephamycin C and cefoxitin were hydrolyzable by 28 and 7 out of 91 β-lactamase preparations, respectively, although the correlation between the ability of β-lactamase to hydrolyze 7α-methoxycephalosporins and the type of enzyme was not mentioned. The value of K_m or K_i indicated that the 7α-methoxy group had little effect on affinity for β-lactamases except for the *P. vulgaris* enzyme (Murakami and Yoshida, 1981). Thus the 7α-methoxy group does not affect the interaction between the compound and β-lactamase. Indelicato and Wilham (1974) showed that the 6α substituent in penicillins provided steric hindrance to nucleophilic attack on β-lactams in solution and that, in contrast, the 7α-methoxy substituent in cephalosporins did not have such steric effects. It can be considered that the nucleophilic attack by amino acid residues at the active site of the enzyme is sterically more restricted.

On the basis of three-dimensional structures of β-lactam compounds, Boyd (1977) conversely suggested that the β-lactam ring was attacked on the α face at the active site of the enzyme. Therefore it seems likely that, at the active site of β-lactamase, the 7α-methoxy function in cephalosporins provides steric hindrance to penicillinases and, though to a lesser extent, to cephalosporinases.

Substituents at the α position of the acylamino side chain of penicillins and cephalosporins are known to be of considerable importance in changing the spectrum of antibacterial activity against gram-positive and gram-negative bacteria (Price, 1977; Webber and Ott, 1977). O'Callaghan and Muggleton (1972) have indicated changes in enzyme stability by introducing a substituent in the side chain α-carbon atom. As shown in Table XIII, the carboxyl function of the phenylmalonylamino moiety stabilizes the β-lactam bond toward hydrolysis by cephalosporinase-type enzymes; but there is only a negligible protecting effect against penicillinases (Yoshida, 1980). Compounds having a carboxyl group in the C-7 side chain [Table XXIV (**228, 285**)] show a very high affinity for cephalosporinases (low K_i values) except the *P. vulgaris* enzyme (Murakami and Yoshida, 1981). The negatively charged α-carboxyl substituent may exert a protective effect by strong interaction with the active site of cephalosporinases. On the contrary, the affinity of these compounds for penicillinases and the *P. vulgaris* enzyme is decreased by introduction of the carboxyl group, indicating the absence of a stabilizing effect against these enzymes.

These stabilizing effects produced by either the 7α-methoxy group or the carboxy group are always more pronounced in 1-oxacephem derivatives than in the 1-sulfur congeners, since the former are consistently more sensitive to β-lactamase than the latter (Table XII). When both functional groups reside in a compound, they work together for complete protection against β-lactamase attack and contribute to extensive improvement of the antibacterial activity against β-lactamase-producing bacteria [Table XXIV (230, 286)]. The 1-oxa compound (6059-S) has much higher potency toward all bacteria than its 1-sulfur counterpart. Thus, a main problem causing bacterial resistance to cephalosporins, e.g., production of β-lactamase, was solved by the concomitant introduction of a methoxy group at the 7α position and a carboxyl group in the side-chain α-carbon atom. Consequently, 6059-S possesses an exceptionally expanded antibacterial spectrum.

To elucidate the mechanism of the bactericidal activity of 6059-S against gram-negative bacteria, its binding affinity to the penicillin-binding proteins (PBPs) of *E. coli* K12 was measured (Komatsu and Nishikawa, 1980). In a competition experiment using [^{14}C]penicillin G, the binding affinity of 6059-S to the inner membrane proteins was highest for PBPs 3 and 7/8. Also, 6059-S showed a higher affinity than benzylpenicillin for PBPs 1A, 1Bs, 4, and 5/6. The affinity of 6059-S for PBP-2 was low. These results were confirmed by direct binding studies using ^{14}C-labeled 6059-S, although some other minor proteins bound by ^{14}C-labeled 6059-S but not by [^{14}C]penicillin G were noted. A correlation between the binding features of β-lactams and the selectivity of morphological effects had been elucidated earlier (Spratt, 1975). The preferential binding to PBP-3 of 6059-S was paralleled by the presence of filamentous cells at concentrations lower than its MIC (Yoshida *et al.*, 1980). 6059-S shows a strong bactericidal effect caused by cell lysis at concentrations near the MIC (Yoshida *et al.*, 1980). This is consistent with the high affinity for PBPs 1A and 1Bs.

The effects of the S → O replacement in the nucleus of 6059-S was also examined (Komatsu and Nishikawa, 1980). The 1-sulfur congener of 6059-S showed binding properties similar to those of PBPs 1A, 1Bs, 3, and 4, but a much lower affinity for PBPs 5/6 and 7/8 than did 6059-S. However, 6059-S was 15 times more active against *E. coli* K12 than its 1-sulfur congener. PBP-5 is identified with D-alanine carboxypeptidase 1A (Spratt and Strominger, 1976; Matsuhashi *et al.*, 1978), which is assumed to be nonessential for normal peptidoglycan synthesis (Matsuhashi *et al.*, 1977). However, Tamaki *et al.* (1978) recently reported an important role of PBP-5 in sensitizing cells to β-lactam antibiotics. The 7α-methoxy substitution greatly enhances the binding of β-lactam antibiotics to PBPs 5/6 (Curtis *et al.*, 1979; Matsuhashi and

Tamaki, 1978), which correlates with their increased inhibitory activity for membrane-bound model transpeptidase activity in *E. coli* K12 (Curtis *et al.*, 1979). Thus it is likely that the higher antibacterial activity of 6059-S as compared with that of the 1-sulfur congener against gram-negative bacteria can be partly ascribed to the enhanced affinity for these particular PBPs.

C. Evaluation of 6059-S

6059-S is highly active against a broad range of gram-negative microorganisms including those resistant to classic cephalosporins. Its expanded spectrum of antibacterial activity includes *Haemophilus influenzae*, indole-positive *Proteus, Enterobacter, S. marcescens, Pseudomonas aeruginosa*, and *Bacteroides fragilis* (Yoshida *et al.*, 1978). Table XXV indicates the *in vitro* and *in vivo* antibacterial activity of 6059-S against the representative bacterial strains compared with that of several cephalosporins including the recently introduced cefotaxime (Hamilton-Miller *et al.*, 1978) and cefoperazone (Matsubara *et al.*, 1979).

The antibacterial activity of 6059-S was compared with that of cefazolin and cefmetazole against the clinically important gram-negative bacilli shown in Table XXVI. The gram-negative activity of 6059-S is superior to that of classic cephalosporins and cephamycin-type antibiotics but is comparable to that of cefotaxime and cefoperazone. The latter two antibiotics and 6059-S have similar activity against *P. aeruginosa*. However, 6059-S has outstanding activity against *B. fragilis*. The therapeutic efficacy of 6059-S in treating experimental infections in mice is excellent against gram-negative bacteria, including strains highly resistant to cefazolin. It should be noted that 6059-S is significantly more effective against pseudomonal infection than piperacillin and sulbenicillin (Yoshida *et al.*, 1980).

Many investigators have examined the antibacterial spectrum of 6059-S. Outbreaks of nosocomial infection due to multiresistant gram-negative bacilli have become more frequent. Among multiresistant strains, 6059-S is notably effective against *Serratia* and *Klebsiella*, and its activity is comparable to that of cefotaxime (Hall *et al.*, 1980). For gentamicin-resistant *Enterobacter* strains, 6059-S was 16-fold more inhibitory than cefotaxime, whereas cefoperazone was ineffective (Trager *et al.*, 1980). In a population of multi-drug-resistant isolates, a concentration of 32 μg or less of 6059-S per milliliter inhibited 100% of Enterobacteriaceae and 40% of *P. aeruginosa* (Fass, 1979). Brier *et al.* (1980) found a synergistic response with 90% of multiple-antibiotic-resistant gram-negative orga-

TABLE XXV Antibacterial Activity of 6059-S Compared with Other Cephalosporins against Laboratory Strains[a]

	6059-S	Cefamandole	Cefoxitin	Cefotaxime	Cefoperazone
MIC (μg/ml)					
Staphylococcus aureus 209P	6.3	0.5	1.6	0.4	0.8
Escherichia coli NIHJ JC-2	0.1	0.2	3.1	0.05	0.1
Escherichia coli 73	0.4	50	12.5	0.2	25
Proteus vulgaris CN329	0.2	1.6	3.1	0.02	0.8
Enterobacter cloacae 233	0.1	3.1	>100	0.4	0.4
Serratia marcescens 13880	0.4	25	12.5	0.4	0.8
Pseudomonas aeruginosa PS-24	12.5	>100	>100	12.5	6.3
Bacteroides fragilis W-1	0.8	12.5	6.3	3.1	>100
ED$_{50}$ in mice (mg/kg)					
Staphylococcus aureus SMITH	10.6	0.25	5.3	2.4	NT
Escherichia coli EC-14	0.12	2.3	7.9	0.77	0.11
Proteus vulgaris CN329	0.37	9.8	11.8	0.09	2.2
Enterobacter cloacae CL-47	0.15	NT	NT	0.47	0.19
Pseudomonas aeruginosa PS-24	11.4	NT	NT	31.9	7.7
Haemophilus influenzae 88562	0.03	3.0	6.2	0.02	NT

[a] NT, Not tested.

TABLE XXVI Antibacterial Activity of 6059-S and Selected Compounds against Clinical Isolates

Organism[a]	MIC for inhibition of 70% of clinical isolates (μg/ml)		
	6059-S	Cefazolin	Cefmetazole
Escherichia coli (114)	0.2	6.3	1.6
Klebsiella sp. (132)	0.2	6.3	1.6
Proteus mirabilis (63)	0.2	12.5	6.3
Proteus sp. indole-positive (210)	0.2	>100	6.3
Enterobacter sp. (85)	0.4	>100	6.3
Serratia marcescens (82)	0.8	>100	25
Citrobacter freundii (47)	0.2	100	50
Pseudomonas aeruginosa (112)[b]	25	—	—
Haemophilus influenzae (23)[c]	0.2	25	—
Bacteroides fragilis subsp. *fragilis* (56)[d]	0.8	—	6.3

[a] Number of strains is shown in parentheses.
[b] Sulbenicillin and piperacillin, 50 and 6.3 μg/ml, respectively.
[c] Ampicillin, 0.8 μg/ml.
[d] Cefoxitin, 12.5 μg/ml.

nisms using 6059-S combined with tobramycin. Combination studies with selected strains of *P. aeruginosa* showed synergy between 6059-S and gentamicin (Trager *et al.*, 1980); this synergistic effect was found to be indifferent to the resistance patterns of the strains. However, several investigators were unable to demonstrate synergy in antipseudomonal activity when 6059-S was combined with either aminoglycosides or antipseudomonal β-lactams (Neu *et al.*, 1979; Yu *et al.*, 1980).

6059-S is inhibitory not only to *Pseudomonas aeruginosa* but also to other nonfermenters such as *P. maltophilia*, *P. putida*, *Achromobacter* sp., and *Acinetobacter* sp., organisms which are becoming important causative agents of nosocomial infections (Jorgensen *et al.*, 1980a; Verbist, 1980). In this regard, 6059-S seems promising for use in single-drug therapy for infectious processes involving these organisms (Jorgensen *et al.*, 1980c). Among anaerobic bacteria, the *Bacteroides* group is the most resistant to antibiotics. Cefoxitin has proven to be a clinically useful β-lactam for abdominal anaerobic sepsis (Wilson *et al.*, 1978). Against *B. fragilis*, 6059-S was four to eight times more active than cefoxitin (Wise *et al.*, 1979; Barza *et al.*, 1979; Borobio *et al.*, 1980) and showed the lowest MIC values of the recently developed cephalosporins, although some variations from laboratory to laboratory were noted. 6059-S and cephamycin-type antibiotics were not hydrolyzed by the β-lactamase produced by *B. fragilis* but competitively inhibited this enzyme

(Sato *et al.*, 1980). This may partly explain the potent activity of 6059-S against *B. fragilis*. Although the anti-anaerobic bacteria spectrum of 6059-S favors gram-negative organisms, the other cephamycin-type antibiotics tend to be most active against gram-positive ones, e.g., *Peptococci* (Yoshida *et al.*, 1980; Borobio *et al.*, 1980).

The antibacterial activity of 6059-S appears to be less affected by β-lactamase than the other clinically applicable β-lactam antibiotics. Kazmierczak *et al.* (1980) demonstrated that the range of MIC values against *P. morganii* was narrow for 6059-S (0.06–0.5 μg/ml) but wide for cefotaxime (0.015–16 μg/ml), and that this difference was due to relatively more efficient hydrolysis of cefotaxime than of 6059-S by either inducible or constitutively produced cephalosporinases. Sanders *et al.* (1980) reported that 6059-S selected resistant mutants with difficulty when compared with cefotaxime. They also interpreted this effect as being due to resistance to β-lactamase inactivation. However, similar cefoxitin-inducible resistance among *Enterobacter* species was demonstrated for both 6059-S and cefotaxime (Lang *et al.*, 1980), although neither was as effective an inducer as cefoxitin (Sanders *et al.*, 1980). 6059-S was highly active against *H. influenzae* irrespective of β-lactamase production (Jorgensen *et al.*, 1980b) and inhibited more than 90% of strains tested at the extremely low concentration of 0.1 μg/ml (Khan *et al.*, 1980; Mason *et al.*, 1980). Landesman *et al.* (1979) reported that cerebrospinal fluid (CSF) levels of 6059-S closely paralleled serum levels and that penetration into the CSF remained high even when meningeal inflammation was minimal. Similar results were obtained with experimental gram-negative meningitis in rats (Cordera and Pekarek, 1980) and in rabbits (Schaad *et al.*, 1980), and 6059-S was found to be superior to ampicillin or netilmicin in sterilizing the CSF.

The pharmacokinetics of 6059-S were studied in normal volunteers (Kurihara *et al.*, 1980; Parsons *et al.*, 1980; Israel *et al.*, 1980). The mean serum half-lives of 6059-S ranged from 1.3 to 2.3 hr for the β phase of intravenous (iv) injection and from 2.3 to 2.8 hr for intramuscular (im) injection. After a 1-g im injection, peak serum levels occurred from 30 min to 1 hr, and the mean serum levels varied from 28.2 μg/ml (Israel *et al.*, 1980) to 52 μg/ml (Parsons *et al.*, 1980). At 8 hr, the mean serum levels were 3.8 and 4.8 μg/ml after iv and im administration, respectively (Parsons *et al.*, 1980). Table XXVII shows a comparison of serum levels after a 0.5-g iv dose for 6059-S and other recently developed cephalosporins cited in a collaborative study by the Japan Society of Chemotherapy. A prolonged duration of effective concentrations of 6059-S in serum was also evident.

The kidney appears to be the primary route of excretion of 6059-S,

TABLE XXVII Plasma Levels of 6059-S Compared with Other Cephalosporins after Intravenous Injection (500 mg) in Humans

Time (hr)	Concentration (μg/ml)			
	6059-S[a]	Cefamandole[b]	Cefotaxime[a]	Cefoperazone[a]
0.25	44.3	56.0	30.0	75.8
0.5	32.6	18.0	14.5	56.3
1	23.0	8.1	6.6	32.0
2	13.7	2.6	2.3	20.4
4	6.1	0	0.7	8.8
Half-life (min)	93	10.3	47.3	115

[a] The collaborative works from New Drug Symposium in Japan Society of Chemotherapy (1979).

[b] The collaborative works from New Drug Symposium in Japan Society of Chemotherapy (1978).

with some excretion in the feces, presumably via the biliary pathway (Israel et al., 1980), which caused changes in fecal flora (Allen et al., 1980). Some volunteers experienced brief periods of diarrhea which resolved spontaneously before treatment was stopped. Neither phlebitis nor any other significant adverse reactions were observed.

Clinical examination of 6059-S was first reported by Matsumoto et al. (1979). 6059-S was given to 54 patients. Most of these patients had respiratory tract infections and received less than 2 g daily, two- to threefold less than the ordinary dose of cefazolin. All causative bacteria were eradicated from 44 patients with clinical cures (Matsumoto et al., 1980).

At a symposium on 6059-S organized by the Japan Society of Chemotherapy in December 1979, case reports for 1289 patients from 90 institutions in Japan were reviewed for safety and efficacy. The daily dosages ranged from 0.5 to 9 g, and 1 (29%) and 2 g (49%) were most commonly administered. Most cases (85%) were intravenously dosed twice a day. Of the 1289 total cases, 1221 were evaluatable. The primary diagnosis and clinical response are listed in Table XXVIII. Overall, 6059-S was found to be satisfactory in 976 patients (80%). The causative bacteria ranged from gram-positive cocci to gram-negative bacilli. Of the 1221 qualified cases in the total treated with 6059-S, only 31 patients (2.5%) had adverse effects including skin rash, pyrexia, etc., that were judged to be drug-related by the investigators. No serious adverse effects were encountered during the 6059-S evaluation. In 29 cases, abnormal laboratory values were noted. Mild elevations of serum transaminases

TABLE XXVIII   Clinical Effectiveness of 6059-S for Various Infections[a]

Diagnosis	No. of cases		Satisfactory clinical response	
	Total	Evaluated	Cases	Percentage
Systemic infections	40	28	19	68
Lower respiratory tract infection	371	346	272	79
Urinary tract infection	484	471	356	76
Genital infection	78	77	71	92
Biliary tract infection	106	103	89	86
Peritonitis	48	45	35	78
Skin and soft tissue infection	68	66	57	86
Other	94	85	80	94
Overall	1289	1221	976	80

[a] The collaborative works from New Drug Symposium in Japan Society of Chemotherapy (1979).

were observed in 13 patients, eosinophilia in 3, and leucopenia in 3. The observed reactions, however, were reversible in every case.

Acknowledgment

We gratefully acknowledge the assistance of Miss Michiko Katayama and Miss Teruyo Matsumoto who typed the manuscript with skill and forbearance.

REFERENCES

Allen, S. D., Siders, J. A., Cromer, M. D., Fischer, J. A., Smith, J. W., and Israel, K. S. (1980). *In* "Current Chemotherapy and Infectious Disease" (J. D. Nelson and C. Grassi, eds.), Vol. 1, pp. 101–103. Am. Soc. Microbiol., Washington, D. C.

Aoki, T., Yoshioka, Sendo, Y., and Nagata, W. (1979). *Tetrahedron Lett.* 4327–4330.

Aoki, T., Yoshioka, M., Kamata, S., Konoike, T., Haga, N., and Nagata, W. (1981). Heterocycles **15**, 409–413.

Applegate, H. E., Dolfini, J. E., Puar, M. S., Slusarchyk, W. A., Toeplitz, B., and Gougoutas, J. Z. (1974). *J. Org. Chem.* **39**, 2794–2796.

Aratani, M., and Hashimoto, M. (1980). *J. Am. Chem. Soc.* **102**, 6171–6172.

Aratani, M., Hagiwara, D., Takeno, H., Hemmi, K., and Hashimoto, M. (1980). *J. Org. Chem.* **45**, 3682–3686.

Australian Patent, (1980). No. 505,773.

Austrian Patent (1979). No. 353,964; *C.A.* **89**, 6330s.

Barza, M., Tally, F. P., Jacobus, N. V., and Gorbach, S. L. (1979). *Antimicrob. Agents Chemother.* **16**, 287–292.

Bentley, P. H., and Clayton, J. P. (1977). *In* "Recent Advances in the Chemistry of β-Lactam Antibiotics" (J. Elks, ed.), Spec. Publ. No. 28, pp. 68–72. Chem. Soc., London.

Biagi, G. L., Barbaro, A. M., Gamba, M. F., and Guerra, M. C. (1969). *J. Chromatogr.* **41,** 371–379.

Biagi, G. L., Guerra, M. C., Barbaro, A. M., and Gamba, M. F. (1970). *J. Med. Chem.* **13,** 511–516.

Borobio, M. V., Aznar, J. Jimenez, R., Garcia, F., and Perea, E. J. (1980). *Antimicrob. Agents Chemother.* **17,** 129–131.

Boucherot, D., and Pilgrim, W. R. (1979). *Tetrahedron Lett.* 5063–5066.

Boyd, D. B. (1972). *J. Am. Chem. Soc.* **94,** 6513–6519.

Boyd, D. B. (1977). *Proc. Natl. Acad. Sci. U.S.A.* **74,** 5239–5243.

Boyd, D. B., and Lunn, W. H. W. (1979). *J. Antibiot.* **32,** 855–856.

Brain, E. G., Branch, C. L., Eglington, A. J., Nayler, J. H. C., Osborne, N. F., Pearson, M. J., Smale, T. C., Southgate, R., and Tolliday, P. (1977). *In* "Recent Advances in the Chemistry of β-Lactam Antibiotics" (J. Elks, ed.), Spec. Publ. No. 28, pp. 204–213. Chem. Soc., London.

Branch, C. L., and Pearson, M. J. (1979). *J. C. S. Perkin I* 2268–2275.

Brier, G. L., Black, H. R., Griffith, R. S., Israel, K. S., and Wolny, J. O. (1979). *Abst. Annu. Meet. Am. Soc. Microbiol.* No. A38.

Brier, G. L., Black, H. R., Griffith, R. S., and Wolny, J. D.-(1980). *In* "Current Chemotherapy and Infectious Disease" (J. D. Nelson and C. Grassi, eds.), Vol. 1, pp. 62–63. Am. Soc. Microbiol. Washington, D. C.

Busson, R., Roets, E., and Vanderhaeghe, H. (1978). *J. Org. Chem.* **43,** 4434–4437.

Cama, L. D., and Christensen, B. G. (1974). *J. Am. Chem. Soc.* **96** 7582–7584.

Cama, L. D., and Christensen, B. G. (1978). *Annu. Rep. Med. Chem.* **13,** 149–158.

Campbell, M. M., and Rawson, D. I. (1979). *Tetrahedron Lett.* 1257–1260.

Cooper, R. D. G. (1979). *Top. Antibiot. Chem.* **3,** 40–203.

Cooper, R. D. G. (1980). *Tetrahedron Lett.,* 781–784.

Cooper, R. D. G., and Jose, F. L. (1970). *J. Am. Chem. Soc.* **92** 2575–2576.

Corbett, D. F., and Stodley, R. J. (1974). *J. C. S., Perkin I* 185–188.

Cordera, C. S., and Pekarek, R. S. (1980). *Antimicrob. Agents Chemother.* **17,** 258–262.

Curtis, N. A. C., Ross, G. W., and Boulton, M. G. (1979). *J. Antimicrob. Chemother.* **5,** 391–398.

Declercq, J. P., Germain, G., Moreaux, C., and Van Meerssche, M. (1977). *Acta Crystallogr., Sect. B* **33,** 3868–3871.

Demarco, P. V., and Nagarajan, R. (1972). *In* "Cephalosporins and Penicillins: Chemistry and Biology" (E. H. Glynn, ed.), pp. 311–369. Academic Press, New York.

Dereppe, J.-M., Schanck, A., Coene, B., Moreau, C., and Van Meerssche, M. (1978). *Org. Magn. Reson.* **11,** 638–640.

Dunn, G. L., Hoover, J. R. E., Berges, D. A., Taggart, J. J., Davis, L. D., Dietz, E. M., Jakas, D. R., Yim, N., Actor, P., Uri, J. V., and Weisbach, J. A. (1976). *J. Antibiot.* **29,** 65–80.

Eliel, E. L. Rao, V. S., Vierhapper, F. W., and Juaristi, G. Z. (1975). *Tetrahedron Lett.* 4339–4342.

Ernest, I. (1980). *Helv. Chim. Acta* **63,** 201–213.

Fass, R. J. (1979). *Antimicrob. Agents Chemother.* **16,** 503–509.

Firestone, R. A., Fahey, J. L., Maciejewicz, N. S., Patel, G. S., and Christensen, B. G. (1977). *J. Med. Chem.* **20,** 551–556.

Georgopapadakou, N., Hammarstrom, S., and Strominger, J. L. (1977). *Proc. Natl. Acad. Sci. U.S.A.* **74**, 1009–1012.

Gorman, M., and Ryan, C. W. (1972). *In* "Cephalosporins and Penicillins: Chemistry and Biology" (E. H. Flynn, ed.), pp. 532–582. Academic Press, New York.

Goto, S., Ogawa, M., Tsuji, A., Kawahara, S., Tsuchiya, K., Kondo, M., and Kida, M. (1980). *In* "Current Chemotherapy and Infectious Disease" (J. D. Nelson and C. Grassi, eds.), Vol. 1, pp. 264–266. Am. Soc. Microbiol. Washington, D. C.

Gunda, E. T., and Jaszberenyi, J. C. (1977). *Prog. Med. Chem.* **14**, 181–248.

Hall, W. H., Opfer, B. J., and Gerding, D. N. (1980). *Antimicrob. Agents Chemother.* **17**, 273–279.

Hamashima, Y., Ishikura, K., Ishitobi, H., Itani, H., Kubota, T., Minami, K., Murakami, M., Nagata, W., Narisada, M., Nishitani, Y., Okada, T., Onoue, H., Satoh, H., Snedo, Y., Tsuji, T., and Yoshioka, M. (1977). *In* "Recent Advances in the Chemistry of β-Lactam Antibiotics" (J. Elks, ed.), Spec. Publ. No. 28, pp. 243–251 Chem. Soc. London.

Hamashima, Y., Kubota, T., Ishitobi, K., and Nagata, W. (1979a). *Tetrahedron Lett.* 4943–4946.

Hamashima, Y., Yamamoto, S., Kubota, T., Tokura, K., Ishikura, K., Minami, K., Matsubara, F., Yamaguchi, M., Kikkawa, I., and Nagata, W. (1979b). *Tetrahedron Lett.* 4947–4950.

Hamashima, Y., Yamamoto, S., Uyeo, S., Yoshioka, M., Murakami, M., Ona, H., Nishitani, Y., and Nagata, W. (1979c). *Tetrahedron Lett.* 2595–2598.

Hamashima, Y., Matsumura, H., Ishikura, K., Yoshida, T., Matsuura, S., and Nagata, W. (1980a). *100th Anniv. Meet. Jpn. Pharm. Soc. Tokyo.* Pap. No. 2F 0-4S (Abstr.).

Hamashima, Y., Matsumua, H., Matsuura, S., Nagata, W., Narisada, M., and Yoshida, T. (1980b). *Int. Symp. Recent Adv. Chem. β-Lactam Antibiot., 2nd, Cambridge, Engl.*

Hamashima, Y., Matsumura, H., Tokura, K., Minami, K., and Kubota, T. (1980c). *100th Anniv. Meet. Jpn. Pharm. Soc., Tokyo.* Pap. No. 2F 10-3S (Abstr.).

Hamilton-Miller, J. M. T., Brumfitt, W., and Reynolds, A. V. (1978). *J. Antimicrob. Chemother.* **4**, 437–444.

Hartstein, A. I., Patrick, K. E., Jones, S. R., Miller, M. J., and Bryant, R. E. (1977). *Antimicrob. Agents Chemother.* **12**, 93–97.

Hayashi, S., Narisada, M., Watanabe, F., and Nagata, W. (1980). *100th Anniv. Meet. Jpn. Pharm. Soc., Tokyo.* Pap. No. 4J 2-4S (Abstr.).

Hemmi, K., Hagiwara, D., Takeno, H., Aratani, M., and Hashimoto, M. (1980). *J. Med. Chem.* **23**, 1108–1113.

Heusler, K. (1972). *In* "Cephalosporins and Penicillins: Chemistry and Biology" (E. H. Flynn, ed.), pp. 265–273. Academic Press, New York.

Indelicato, J. M., and Wilham, W. L. (1974). *J. Med. Chem.* **17**, 528–529.

Indelicato, J. M., Norvillas, T. T., Pfeiffer, R. R., Wheeler, W. J., and Wilham, W. L. (1974). *J. Med. Chem.* **17**, 523–527.

Israel, K. S., Black, H. R., Griffith, R. S., Brier, G. L., and Wolny, J. D. (1980). *In* "Current Chemotherapy and Infectious Disease" (J. D. Nelson and C. Grassi, eds.), Vol. 1, pp. 107–108. Am. Soc. Microbiol., Washington, D.C.

Japanese Kokai Tokkyo Koho (1973). No. 73 43,997.

Japanese Kokai Tokkyo Koho (1974). No. 74 110,689; *C.A.* **82**, 4278.

Japanese Kokai Tokkyo Koho (1976). No. 76 41,385; *C.A.* **84**, 180239.

Japanese Kokai Tokkyo Koho (1977a). No. 77 87,189; *C.A.* **88**, 170160.

Japanese Kokai Tokkyo Koho (1977b). No. 77 122,386; *C.A.* **88**, 22936.

Japanese Kokai Tokkyo Koho (1977c). No. 77 133,997; *C.A.* **88**, 22936.

Japanese Kokai Tokkyo Koho (1978a). No. 78 21,188; *C.A.* **88**, 152636.
Japanese Kokai Tokkyo Koho (1978b). No. 78 21,191; *C.A.* **88**, 170178.
Japanese Kokai Tokkyo Koho (1978c). No. 78 31,690; *C.A.* **89**, 6330.
Japanese Kokai Tokkyo Koho (1978d). No. 78 135,997; *C.A.* **90**, 72212.
Japanese Kokai Tokkyo Koho (1979a). No. 79 19,990; *C.A.* **90**, 186968; **92**, 164007.
Japanese Kokai Tokkyo Koho (1979b). No. 79 36,287; *C.A.* **90**, 72212.
Japanese Kokai Tokkyo Koho (1979c). No. 79 125,698; *C.A.* **92**, 111048.
Japanese Kokai Tokkyo Koho (1979d). No. 79 106,491; *C.A.* **92**, 41967.
Japanese Kokai Tokkyo Koho (1980). No. 80 19,250; *C.A.* **93**, 150262.
Jaszberenyi, J. C., and Gunda, E. T. (1975). *Prog. Med. Chem.* **12**, 395–477.
Jorgensen, J. H., Crawford, S. A., and Alexander, G. A. (1980a). *In* "Current Chemotherapy and Infectious Disease" (J. D. Nelson and C. Grassi, eds.), Vol. 1, pp. 78–79. Am. Soc. Microbiol., Washington, D.C.
Jorgensen, J. H., Crawford, S. A., and Alexander, G. A. (1980b). *Antimicrob. Agents Chemother.* **17**, 516–517.
Jorgensen, J. H., Crawford, S. A., and Alexander, G. A. (1980c). *Antimicrob. Agents Chemother.* **17**, 901–904.
Jung, F. A., Pilgrim, W. R., Poyser, J. P., and Siret, P. J. (1980). *Top. Antibiot, Chem.* **4**, 51–119.
Kamata, S., Yamamoto, S., Haga, N., and Nagata, W. (1979). *J.C.S. Chem. Commun.* 1106–1107.
Kamimura, T., Matsumoto, Y., Okada, N., Mine, Y., Nishida, M., Goto, S., and Kuwahara, S. (1979). *Antimicrob. Agents Chemother.* **16**, 540–548.
Kamiya, T., Teraji, T., Saito, Y., Hashimoto, M., Nakaguchi, O., and Oku, T. (1973). *Tetrahedron Lett.* 3001–3004.
Kazmierczak, A., Bolle, M., Siebor, E., Pothier, P., and Labia, R. (1980). *In* "Current Chemotherapy and Infectious Disease" (J. D. Nelson and C. Grassi, eds.), Vol. 1, pp. 71–72. Am. Soc. Microbiol., Washington, D.C.
Khan, W. N., Willert, B., Ahmad, S., Rodriguez, W. J., and Ross, S. (1980). *In* "Current Chemotherapy and Infectious Disease" (J. D. Nelson and C. Grassi, eds.), Vol. 1, pp. 82–84. Am. Soc. Microbiol., Washington, D.C.
Kim, C. U., and McGregor, D. N. (1978). *Tetrahedron Lett.* 409–412.
Kirby, W. M. M., and Regamey, C. (1973). *J. Infect. Dis.* **128**, Suppl., s341–s346.
Knott-Hunziker, V., Waley, S. G., Orlek, B. S., and Sammes, P. G. (1979). *FEBS Lett.* **99**, 59–61.
Komatsu, Y., and Nishikawa, T. (1980). *Antimicrob. Agents Chemother.* **17**, 316–321.
Koppel, G. A., and Koehler, R. E. (1973). *J. Am. Chem. Soc.* **95**, 2403–2404.
Koppel, G. A., Kinnick, M. D., and Nummy, L. J. (1977). *J. Am. Chem. Soc.* **99**, 2822–2823.
Kurihara, J., Matsumoto, K., Uzuka, Y., Shishido, H., Nagatake, T., Yamada, H., Yoshida, T., Oguma, T., Kimura, Y., and Tochino, Y. (1980). *In* "Current Chemotherapy and Infectious Disease" (J. D. Nelson and C. Grassi, eds.), Vol. 1, pp. 110–111. Am. Soc. Microbiol., Washington, D.C.
Kuriyama, K., and Iwata, T. (1980). Unpublished results.
Landesman, S. H., Cleri, D., Goetz, R., Goldstein, E. J. C., Corrado, M., and Cherubin, C. (1979). *Clin. Res.* **27**, 590A.
Lang, S. D. R., Edwards, D. J., and Durack, D. T. (1980). *Antimicrob. Agents Chemother.* **17**, 488–493.
Lowe, G. (1975). *Chem. Ind. (London)* 459–464.
Lunn, W. H. W., Burchfield, R. W., Elzey, T. K., and Mason, E. V. (1974). *Tetrahedron Lett.* 1307–1310.

Mason, E. O., Jr., Kaplan, S. L., Anderson, D. C., Hinds, D. B., and Feigin, R. D. (1980). *Antimicrob. Agents Chemother.* **17,** 470–473.

Matsubara, N., Minami, S., Muraoka, T., Saikawa, I., and Mitsuhashi, S. (1979). *Antimicrob. Agents Chemother.* **16,** 731–735.

Matsuhashi, M., and Tamaki, S. (1978). *J. Antibiot.* **31,** 1292–1295.

Matsuhashi, M., Takagaki, Y., Maruyama, I. N., Tamaki, S., Nishimura, Y., Suzuki, H., Ogino, U., and Hirota, Y. (1977). *Proc. Natl. Acad. Sci. U.S.A.* **74,** 2976–2979.

Matsuhashi, M., Maruyama, I. N., Takagaki, Y., Tamaki, S., Nishimura, Y., and Hirota, Y. (1978). *Proc. Natl. Acad. Sci. U.S.A.* **75,** 2631–2635.

Matsumoto, K., Uzuka, Y., Nagatake, T., and Shishido, H. (1979). *Intersci. Conf. Antimicrob. Agents Chemother., 19th, Boston, Mass.* Pap. No. 172. (Abstr.)

Matsumoto, K., Uzuka, Y., Nagatake, T., and Shishido, H. (1980). *In* "Current Chemotherapy and Infectious Disease" (J. D. Nelson and C. Grassi, eds.), Vol. 1, pp. 112–113. Am. Soc. Microbiol., Washington, D.C.

Matsumura, H., Narisada, M., Okada, T., Haga, N., Yano, T., and Nagata, W. (1980). *100th Anniv. Meet. Jpn. Pharm. Soc., Tokyo.* Pap. No. 4J 2-3S (Abstr.).

Matsuura, S., Yoshida, T., Sugeno, K., Harada, Y., Harada, M., and Kuwahara, S. (1978). *Intersci. Conf. Antimicrob. Agents Chemother., 18th, Atlanta, Ga.* Pap. No. 152. (Abstr.)

Moellering, R. C., Jr. (1977). *J. Infect. Dis.* **137,** Suppl., s1–s194.

Mondelli, R., and Ventura, P. (1977). *J.C.S. Perkin II* 1749–1752.

Morin, R. B., Jackson, B. G., Mueller, R. A., Lavagnino, E. R., Scanlon, W. B., and Andrews, S. L. (1969). *J. Am. Chem. Soc.* **91,** 1401–1407.

Mukerjee, A. K., and Singh, A. K. (1975). *Synthesis* 547–589.

Murakami, K., and Yoshida, T. (1981). *Antimicrob. Agents Chemother.* **19,** 1–7.

Murakami, K., and Yoshida, T. (1982). *Antimicrob. Agents Chemother.* **21**(2), in press.

Murakami, K., Takasuka, M., Motokawa, K., and Yoshida, T. (1981). *J. Med. Chem.* **24,** 88–93.

Nagarajan, R., and Spry, D. O. (1971). *J. Am. Chem. Soc.* **93,** 2310–2312.

Nagarajan, R., Boeck, L. D., Gorman, M., Hamill, R. L., Higgens, C. E., Hoehn, M. M., Stark, W. M., and Whitney, J. G. (1971). *J. Am. Chem. Soc.* **93,** 2308–2310.

Nakagawa, Y., and Ikenishi, Y. (1980). Unpublished results.

Nakao, H., Yanagisawa, H., Ishihara, S., Nakayama, E., Ando, A., Nakazawa, J., Shimizu, B., Kaneko, M., Nagano, M., and Sugawara, S. (1979). *J. Antibiot.* **32,** 320–329.

Narisada, M., Onoue, H., and Nagata, W. (1977). *Heterocycles* **7,** 839–849.

Narisada, M., Onoue, H., Ohtani, M., Watanabe, F., Okada, T., and Nagata, W. (1978). *Tetrahedron Lett.* 1755–1758.

Narisada, M., Yoshida, T., Onoue, H., Ohtani, M., Okada, T., Tsuji, T., Kikkawa, I., Haga, N., Satoh, H., Itani, H., and Nagata, W. (1979). *J. Med. Chem.* **22,** 757–759.

Narisada, M., Yoshida, T., Matsuura, S., Onoue, H., Ohtani, M., and Nagata, W. (1980). *100th Anniv. Meet. Jpn. Pharm. Soc., Tokyo.* Pap. No. 4J 3-1S (Abstr.).

Narisada, M., Yoshida, T., Ohtani, M., Ezumi, K., and Takasuka, M. (1981). To be published.

Nayler, J. H. C., Pearson, M. J., and Southgate, R. (1973a). *J.C.S. Chem. Commun.* 57–58.

Nayler, J. H. C., Pearson, M. J., and Southgate, R. (1973b). *J.C.S. Chem. Commun.* 58–59.

Nayler, J. H. C., Osborne, N. F., Pearson, M. J., and Southgate, R. (1976). *J.C.S. Perkin I* 1615–1620.

Netherlands Patent (1968). No. 5179.

Neu, H. C., Aswapokee, N., Fu, K. P., and Aswapokee, P. (1979). *Antimicrob. Agents Chemother.* **16**, 141–149.

Nishida, M., Matsubara, T., Murakwa, T., Mine, Y., Yokota, Y., Kuwahara, S., and Goto, S. (1970). *In* "Antimicrobial Agents and Chemotherapy—1969" (G. L. Hobby, ed.), pp. 236–243. Am. Soc. Microbiol., Bethesda, Maryland.

Nomura, H., Fugono, T., Hitaka, T., Minami, I., Azuma, T., Morimoto, S., and Matsuda, T. (1975). *Am. Chem. Soc. Meet., 170th, Chicago, Ill., Med. Chem. Sect.* Pap. No. 2. (Abstr.)

O'Callaghan, C. H., and Muggleton, P. W. (1972). *In* "Cephalosporins and Penicillins: Chemistry and Biology" (E. H. Flynn, ed.), pp. 438–495. Academic Press, New York.

O'Callaghan, C. H., Muggleton, P. W., and Ross, G. W. (1969). *In* "Antimicrobial Agents and Chemotherapy—1968" (G. L. Hobby, ed.), pp. 57–63. Am. Soc. Microbiol., Bethesda, Maryland.

Onishi, H. R., Daoust, D. R., Zimmerman, S. B., Hendlin, D., and Stapley, E. O. (1974). *Antimicrob. Agents Chemother.* **5**, 38–48.

Parsons, J. N., Romano, J. M., and Levison, M. E. (1980). *Antimicrob. Agents Chemother.* **17**, 226–228.

Paschal, J. W., Dorman, D. E., Srinivasan, P. R., and Lichter, R. L. (1978). *J. Org. Chem.* **43**, 2013–2016.

Pfeffer, M., Jackson, A., Ximenes, J., and DeMenezes, J. P. (1977). *Antimicrob. Agents Chemother.* **11**, 331–338.

Price, K. E. (1977). *In* "Structure–Activity Relationships among the Semisynthetic Antibiotics" (D. Perlman, ed.), pp. 1–59. Academic Press, New York.

Richmond, M. H., and Sykes, R. B. (1973). *Adv. Microb. Physiol.* **9**, 31–88.

Sammes, P. G. (1976). *Chem. Rev.* **76**, 113–155.

Sanders, C. C., Sanders, W. E., Jr., Dykstra, M. A., and Preheim, L. C. (1980). *In* "Current Chemotherapy and Infectious Disease" (J. D. Nelson and C. Grassi, eds.), Vol. 1, pp. 69–70. Am. Soc. Microbiol., Washington, D.C.

Sato, K., Inoue, M., and Mitsuhashi, S. (1980). *Antimicrob. Agents Chemother.* **17**, 736–737.

Sawai, T., Matsuba, K., Tamura, A., and Yamagishi, S. (1979). *J. Antibiot.* **32**, 59–65.

Scartazzini, R., and Bickel, H. (1972). *Helv. Chim. Acta* **55**, 423–429.

Scartazzini, R., Peter, H., Bickel, H., Heusler, K., and Woodward, R. B. (1972). *Helv. Chim. Acta* **55**, 408–417.

Schaad, U. B., McCracken, G. H., Jr., Loock, C. A., and Thomas, M. L. (1980). *Antimicrob. Agents Chemother.* **17**, 406–411.

Schanck, A., Coene, B., Van Meerssche, M., and Dereppe, J.-M. (1979). *Org. Magn. Reson.* **12**, 337–338.

Shimada, J., Ueda, Y., Yamaji, T., Abe, Y., and Nakamura, M. (1980). *In* "Current Chemotherapy and Infectious Disease" (J. D. Nelson and C. Grassi, eds.), Vol. 1, pp. 109–110. Am. Soc. Microbiol., Washington, D.C.

Shiro, M., Nakai, H., Onoue, H., and Narisada, M. (1981a). To be submitted to *Acta Cryst.*

Shiro, M., Nakai, H., Onoue, H., and Narisada, M. (1981b). *Acta Cryst.* **B36**, 3137–3139.

Spratt, B. G. (1975). *Proc. Natl. Acad. Sci. U.S.A.* **72**, 2999–3003.

Spratt, B. G., and Strominger, J. L. (1976). *J. Bacteriol.* **127**, 660–663.

Stapley, E. O., Jackson, M., Hernandez, S., Zimmerman, S. B., Curie, S. A., Mochales, S., Mata, J. M., Woodruff, H. B., and Hendlin, D. (1972). *Antimicrob. Agents Chemother.* **2**, 122–131.

Stothers, J. B. (1972). "Carbon-13 NMR Spectroscopy," pp. 128–205. Academic Press, New York.

Sweet, R. M. (1972). *In* "Cephalosporins and Penicillins: Chemistry and Biology" (E. H. Flynn, ed.), pp. 280–309. Academic Press, New York.

Tamaki, S., Nakagawa, J., Maruyama, I. N., and Matsuhashi, M. (1978). *Agric. Biol. Chem.* **42,** 2147–2150.

Tori, K., Nishikawa, J., Onoue, H., and Narisada, M. (1980). Unpublished results.

Trager, G. M., White, G. W., Zimelis, V. M., Bryk, D. A., and Panwalker, A. P. (1980). *In* "Current Chemotherapy and Infectious Disease" (J. D. Nelson and C. Grassi, eds.), Vol. 1, pp. 96–98. Am. Soc. Microbiol., Washington, D.C.

Tsuji, T., Kataoka, T., Yoshioka, M., Sendo, Y., Nishitani, Y., Hirai, S., Maeda, T., and Nagata, W. (1979). *Tetrahedron Lett.* 2793–2796.

United States Patent (1979). No. 4,138,486.

Uyeo, S., and Ona, H. (1980). *Chem. Pharm. Bull.* **28,** 1563–1577.

Uyeo, S., Kikkawa, I., Hamashima, Y., Ona, H., Nishitani, Y., Okada, K., Kubota, T., Ishikura, K., Ide, Y., Nakano, K., and Nagata, W. (1979). *J. Am. Chem. Soc.* **101,** 4403–4404.

Verbist, L. (1980). *In* "Current Chemotherapy and Infectious Disease" (J. D. Nelson and C. Grassi, eds.), Vol. 1, pp. 65–67. Am. Soc. Microbiol., Washington, D.C.

Webber, J. A., and Ott, J. L. (1977). *In* "Structure–Activity Relationships among the Semisynthetic Antibiotics" (D. Perlman, ed.), pp. 161–237. Academic Press, New York.

West German Patent (1979). No. 2,831,092.

Wheeler, W. J., Wright, W. E., Line, V. D., and Frogge, J. A. (1977). *J. Med. Chem.* **20,** 1159–1164.

Wilson, P., Leung, T., and Williams, J. D. (1978). *J. Antimicrob. Chemother.* **4,** Suppl. B, 127–141.

Wise, R., Andrews, J. M., and Bedford, K. A. (1979). *Antimicrob. Agents Chemother.* **16,** 341–345.

Wolfe, S., Ducep, J.-B., Kannengiesser, G., and Lee, W. S. (1972a). *Can. J. Chem.* **50,** 2902–2905.

Wolfe, S., Lee, W. S., Ducep, J.-B., and Kannengiesser, G. (1972b). *Can. J. Chem.* **50,** 2898–2902.

Wolfe, S., Ducep, J.-B., Tin, K. C., and Lee, S.-L. (1974). *Can. J. Chem.* **52,** 3996–3999.

Wolfe, S., Lee, S.-L., Ducep, J.-B., Kannengiesser, G., and Lee, W. S. (1975). *Can. J. Chem.* **53,** 497–512.

Woodward, R. B. (1977). *In* "Recent Advances in the Chemistry of β-Lactam Antibiotics" (J. Elks, ed.), Spec. Publ. No. 28, pp. 167–180. Chem. Soc., London.

Yanamoto, S., Haga, N., Aoki, T., Hayashi, S., Tanida, H., and Nagata, W. (1977). *Heterocycles* **8,** 283–292.

Yamana, T., and Tsuji, A. (1976). *J. Pharm. Sci.* **65,** 1563–1574.

Yanagisawa, H., Fukushima, M., Ando, A., and Nakao, H. (1976). *Tetrahedron Lett.* 259–262.

Yoshida, T. (1980). *Philos. Trans. R. Soc. London, Ser. B* **289,** 231–237.

Yoshida, A., Oida, S., and Ohki, E. (1976). *Chem. Pharm. Bull.* **24,** 362–365.

Yoshida, A., Oida, S., and Ohki, E. (1977). *Chem. Pharm. Bull.* **24,** 2082–2088.

Yoshida, T., Narisada, M., Matsuura, S., Nagata, W., and Kurahara, S. (1978). *Intersci. Conf. Antimicrob. Agents Chemother., 18th, Atlanta, Ga.* Pap. No. 151. (Abstr.)

Yoshida, T., Matsuura, S., Mayama, M., Kameda, Y., and Kuwahara, S. (1980). *Antimicrob. Agents Chemother.* **17,** 302–312.

Yoshioka, M., Kikkawa, I., Tsuji, T., Nishitani, Y., Mori, S., Okada, K., Murakami, M., Matsubara, F., Yamaguchi, M., and Nagata, W. (1979). *Tetrahedron Lett.* 4287–4290.

Yoshioka, M., Tsuji, T., Uyeo, S., Yamamoto, S., Aoki, T., Nishitani, Y., Mori, S., Satoh, H., Hamada, Y., Ishitobi, H., and Nagata, W. (1980). *Tetrahedron Lett.* 351–354.
Yu, V. L., Vickers, R. M., and Zuravleff, J. J. (1980). *Antimicrob. Agents Chemother.* **17,** 96–98.
Zimmermann, W., and Rosselet, A. (1977). *Antimicrob. Agents Chemother.* **12,** 368–372.

2

Total Synthesis of Penicillins, Cephalosporins, and Their Nuclear Analogs

KENNETH G. HOLDEN

I. Introduction

Since the previous review of this topic (Heusler, 1972), very significant advances have been made both in our ability to synthesize β-lactam antibiotics and their nuclear analogs and in our understanding of the

Chemistry and Biology of
β-Lactam Antibiotics, Vol. 2

structural features required for useful antibacterial activity. Although some nuclear analogs were accessible by degradation and resynthesis starting from penicillin (Volume 2, Chapter 1), it became clear that many attractive structures could be made most readily by total synthesis. When most of the work to be described in this chapter was initiated, it was believed that the minimal structural requirements consistent with good antibacterial potency could be represented by structure A (Fig. 1). Evidence supporting this belief came largely from two major sources: (1) the proposed mechanism of action of penicillins and cephalosporins, and (2) structure–activity relationships developed from modified derivatives of these antibiotics.

The proposal (Tipper and Strominger, 1965) that β-lactam antibiotics owe their antibacterial activity to their ability to acylate the active site of an enzyme required for cell wall biosynthesis (Volume 1, Chapter 7) strongly suggested that only a bicyclic β-lactam of type A had sufficient reactivity to function in this manner. The source of this reactivity was postulated (Woodward, 1949) to result fron the inhibition of amide resonance. Consistent with this view, X-ray crystallography shows that, in penicillins and cephalosporins with potent antibacterial activity, the β-lactam nitrogen is significantly distorted from the plane defined by the three other atoms to which it is joined (Sweet, 1972). On the other hand, monocyclic β-lactams and Δ^2-cephalosporins, which are essentially inactive as antibacterial agents, have nearly planar structures. The distortion measured by X-ray diffraction is also reflected in an increased frequency of the β-lactam carbonyl band in the infrared (IR) and an increased rate of reaction with nucleophiles (Morin *et al.*, 1969; Indelicato *et al.*, 1974). Other features suggested by the proposed mechanism of action of penicillins and cephalosporins include the carboxylic acid and amide side chain of structure A, since the antibiotics are presumed to mimic the natural substrate of the transpeptidase enzyme which has a D-alanyl-D-alanine terminus (Fig. 1B).

From structure–activity relationships among modified penicillins and

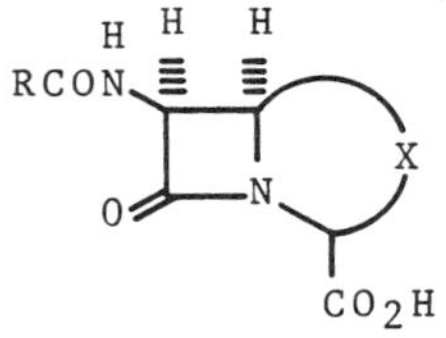

A 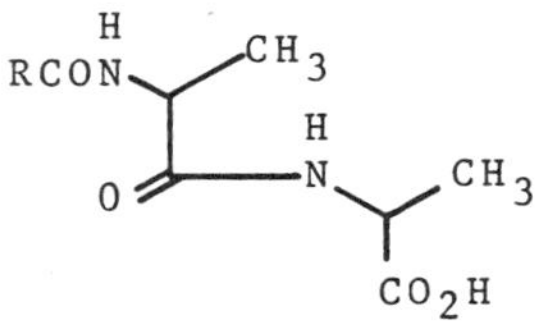   B

Fig. 1. Minimal structural requirements for antibacterial activity (A, R = substituents employed with clinically useful penicillins and cephalosporins, X = two or three atoms) and the D-alanyl-D-alanine terminus of the natural substrate for bacterial transpeptidase enzymes (**B**, R = glycopeptide residue).

cephalosporins (Hoover and Stedman, 1970), it seemed clear that the integrity of both rings of these tricyclic structures was essential for activity. In the case of 4:6-ring systems, it appeared that a Δ^3 double bond was also required, since Δ^2-cephalosporins (Van Heynigen and Ahern, 1968) and saturated analogs (Heusler, 1972) showed only a low order of activity. Furthermore, a cis relationship between the amide side chain and the adjacent ring fusion was required. A carboxylic acid at C-3(4) and an acylated amine at C-6(7) were also apparently essential (Hoover and Stedman, 1970).

Based on these considerations several groups have developed general routes to bicyclic β-lactams of type **A** (Fig. 1). In designing synthetic strategies, one must take into account the inherent instability of these systems. Thus most successful routes postpone formation of the reactive bicyclic structure until late in the synthetic scheme. This has been accomplished in one of two general ways: (1) forming the β-lactam ring late in the synthesis, as exemplified by Sheehan's penicillin synthesis (Sheehan and Henery-Logan, 1962), or (2) generating a monocyclic (unreactive) β-lactam early in the synthetic scheme and closing the second ring late in the synthesis, as exemplified by Woodward's cephalosporin synthesis (Woodward *et al.*, 1966).

II. Synthetic Schemes in Which the β-Lactam Ring Is Formed Late in the Sequence

The general approach of forming the β-lactam ring late in the sequence led to the first demonstrable synthesis of penicillin and was the approach taken by several workers investigating routes to β-lactam nuclear analogs in the late 1960s and early 1970s. As will become apparent as we examine examples of this approach, the major problems encountered were ones of stereochemistry and/or functionality, which required that further reactions be carried out after the strained bicyclic β-lactam ring system had been formed. Since strain and the induced reactivity are almost certainly required for antibacterial activity (Volume 1, Chapter 5), the compounds predicted to display high potency were precisely the ones most likely to lead to side reactions near the end of the synthetic scheme. Nevertheless, some interesting chemistry emerged, and several successes were recorded.

A. Lactam Formation

The now classic synthesis of penicillin (**4a**) (Sheehan and Henery-Logan, 1962) by carbodiimide cyclization of **2a** to **3a** followed by deprotection and acylation has been reviewed previously (Heusler, 1972). Although the synthesis lacks stereospecificity, some degree of selectivity is achieved since only two of four possible isomers of **1a** are formed, and the undesired isomer can be partially converted to the one with the proper stereochemistry by heating in pyridine. In the cyclization reaction it is necessary to use a protecting group such as a trityl, because an amide carbonyl reacts preferentially to give an oxazolone rather than a β-lactam. Although the phthalimido group in **1a** could have served the same purpose as a trityl group, it was not thought possible to remove this group once the bicyclic β-lactam had been formed. Subsequently, Kukolja and Lammert (1975) developed mild reaction conditions compatible with the penicillin nucleus.

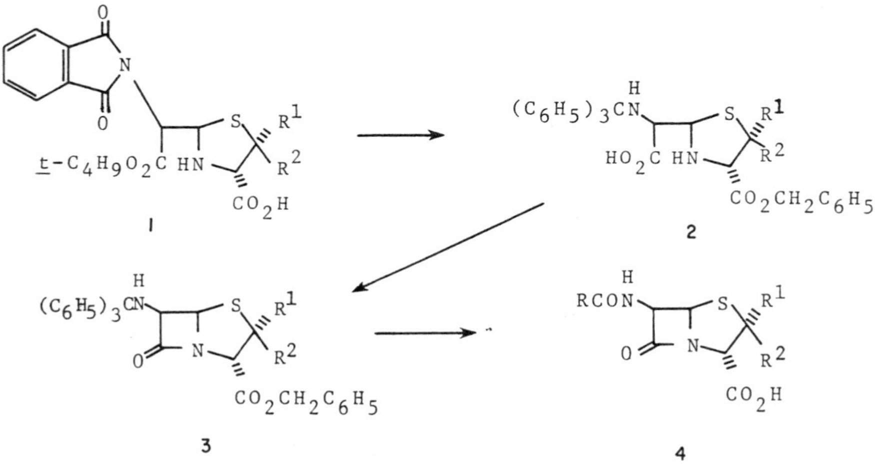

a: R^1 = R^2 = CH_3
b: R^1 = R^2 = H
c: R^1 = CH_3; R^2 = H
d: R^1 = H; R^2 = CH_3
e: R^1 + R^2 = $(CH_2)_n$; n = 3-5

The same general synthetic scheme has been used to prepare bisnor-penicillin (**4b**) (Hoogmartens et al., 1974), the epimeric norpenicillins (**4c,d**) (Claes et al., 1975), and spiro analogs (**4e**) (Leclerco et al., 1978). In the case of bisnorpenicillin synthesis, the instability of some of the intermediates required that reaction conditions be optimized to improve yields. Application of the conditions to the synthesis of penicillin intermediates also improved the efficiency of the original Sheehan route (Hoogmartens et al., 1974).

In the cephalosporin series, Sheehan's carbodiimide cyclization route was successfully pursued by several groups. Most of this work had been summarized previously (Heusler, 1972); however, details of some of the French work appeared subsequently (Heymes *et al.*, 1974, 1977). As in the case of the penicillin route, stereospecificity was not achieved; but, interestingly, the corresponding intermediate mixture was converted essentially quantitatively to the desired threo isomer (**9b**) on acid treatment (Heymes *et al.*, 1974). A new route to intermediate **9** has been described by workers at Merck (Girotra and Wendler, 1972). Starting from **5** and **6** they prepared enamine **7a** which was converted to **7b** in 71% overall yield. Chlorination (*tert*-butyl hypochlorite) followed by elimination (triethylenediamine) gave **8** (90–95% yield), which on treatment with a mild base afforded **9a** stereospecifically (80% yield).

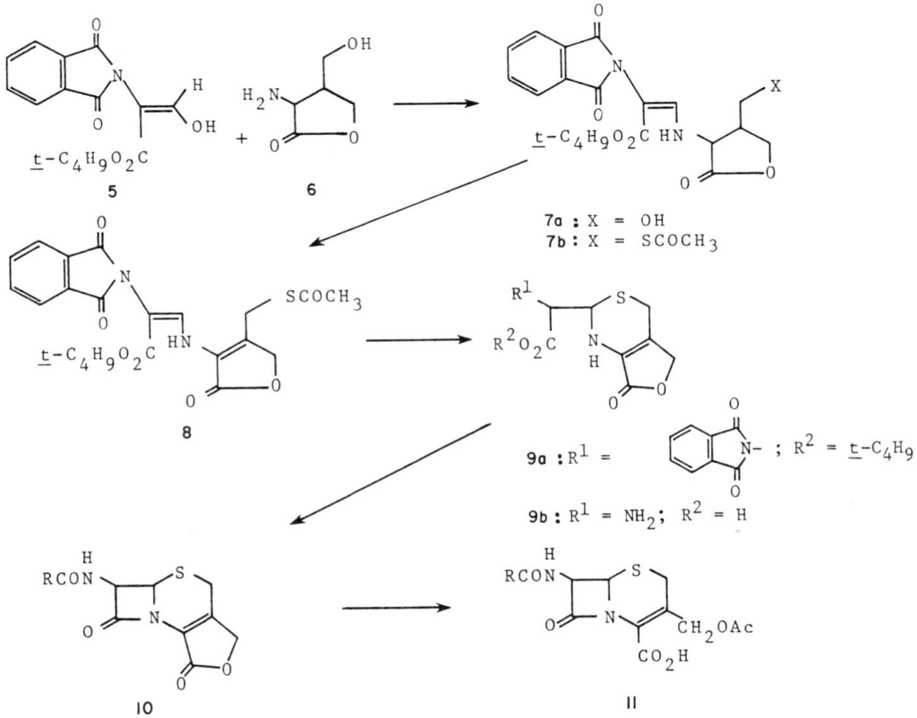

Although **9** can be converted to the cephalosporin nucleus (**10**) in good yield, selective opening of the lactone ring to give a useful cephalosporin such as **11** is achieved only with difficulty (Neidleman *et al.*, 1970). Therefore, although several groups achieved a reasonably efficient total synthesis of lactone (**10**), commercial utilization of the process has not been realized.

B. Cycloaddition

The cycloaddition reaction between a Schiff's base and a ketene to give a β-lactam was first discovered by Staudinger (1907). Bose *et al.* (1968) used this general approach to produce a 6-epipenicillin precursor (**14a**) in very low yield (5–8%) by generating azidoketene from azidoacetyl chloride (**12**) with triethylamine in the presence of thiazoline (**13**). More recently the yield of **14a** was increased somewhat (13%) and, more importantly, a method was devised for converting **14a** to a penicillin with the natural configuration (Firestone *et al.*, 1974a). Although it is possible to partially epimerize 6(7)-α-substituted penicillin and cephalosporin derivatives of type **14b** under equilibrating conditions, the percentage of β- epimer obtained is usually in the range 15–30% (Jackson and Stoodley, 1971). On the other hand, kinetically controlled protonation of the lithium salt of **14b** gives a favorable ratio of isomers (β/α = 2:1) (Firestone *et al.*, 1974a). An explanation of why only the undesired α epimer (**14a**) is formed in the initial cycloaddition, as well as some alternatives to the use of explosive azidoacetyl chloride, will be presented in Section III,B.

14a : R = N_3

14b : R = $p-O_2NC_6H_4CH=N$

The total synthesis of cephalosporins using the cycloaddition approach was achieved by Merck scientists (Ratcliffe and Christensen, 1973a,b,c). Thioformamide (**15**, R = p-$CH_3OC_6H_4CH_2$) was condensed with an α-chloroketone (**16**, R^1 = CH_2OCOCH_3) to give thiazine (**17**) in good yield. Reaction of **17** with azidoacetyl chloride gave 7α-azidocephem (**18**) which, after reduction to the amine, was epimerized via **19** using the kinetically controlled protonation method described above (Firestone *et al.*, 1974a). In this case the epimer ratio was not as favorable (β/α = 45:55). Acylation followed by chromatographic separation of the β isomer and conversion of the ester to the free acid gave (±)-cephalothin (**20a**).

Using this same general approach the Merck group synthesized (±)-cefoxitin (**20b**). In this case the lithium salt of **19** was alkylated with methylsulfenyl chloride to give a 7α-methylthio intermediate which was converted to 7α-methoxy by methanolysis in the presence of thallium

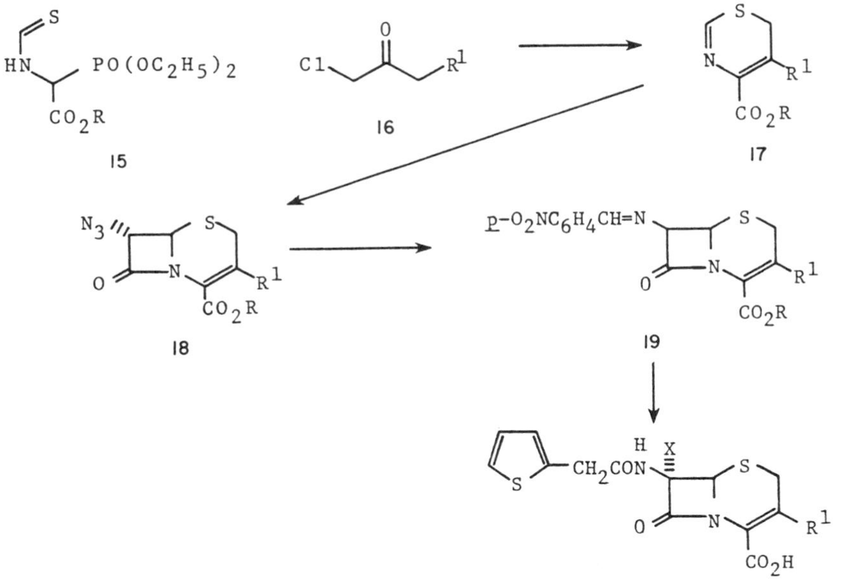

20a: R^1 = CH_2OCOCH_3, X = H
20b: R^1 = $OCONH_2$, X = OCH_3
20c: R^1 = $CH(CH_3)OCOCH_3$, X = H
20d: R^1 = aryl, X = H
20e: R^1 = CF_3, X = H

trinitrate (Ratcliffe and Christensen, 1973c). Subsequently, other 3-sub-stituted cephalosporins (**20c–e**) were prepared in a similar fashion (Stein-berg *et al.*, 1974; Hashimoto *et al.*, 1978).

The synthesis of (±)-6α-methoxycephalothin (**26**) was achieved in a somewhat different manner (Christensen *et al.*, 1977). Alkylation of **21** with 1-acetoxy-3-chloropropan-2-one (**22**) followed by base-catalyzed cyclization afforded dithioimidate **23**. Cycloaddition with azidoacetyl chloride produced **24** which, after mesylation of the hydroxyl group, methanolysis of the methylthio group (thallium trinitrate), and elimination (silica gel), gave **25**. When triethylamine was used for the elimination reaction, a mixture of **25** and the epimeric azide was produced. Similarly, reduction of **25** produced an epimeric mixture of amines. After acylation the epimers were separated and deblocked to give **26** and its 7α epimer.

A novel synthesis of (±)-desacetylcephalothin lactone (**10**, R = thienyl) was achieved by Syntex scientists (Edwards *et al.*, 1974) starting from 4*H*-furo[3,4-*d*]-1,3-thiazine (**27**). Cycloaddition of azidoacetyl chlo-

21 R = p-$O_2NC_6H_4CH_2$ 22 23 24 25 26

ride followed by reduction, epimerization, acylation, and separation gave **28** which was converted to **10** by bromination and *in situ* acetate displacement followed by rearrangement.

27 28 R = (2-thienyl)-CH_2 10

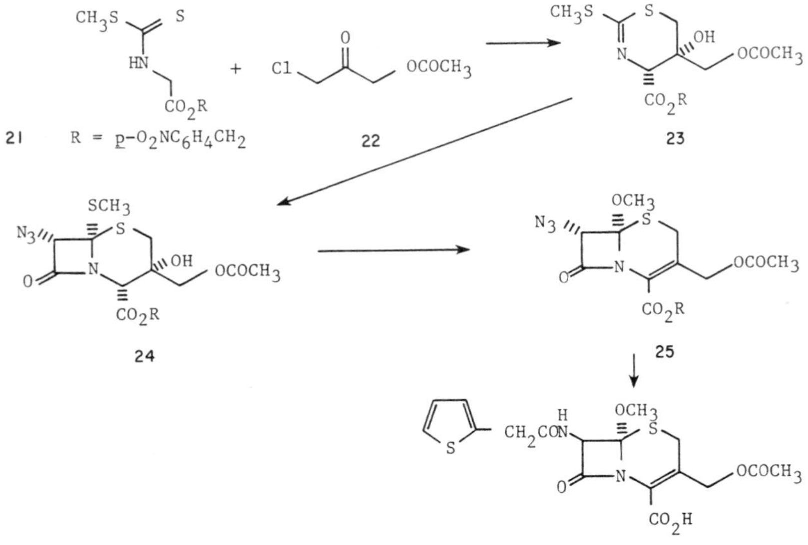

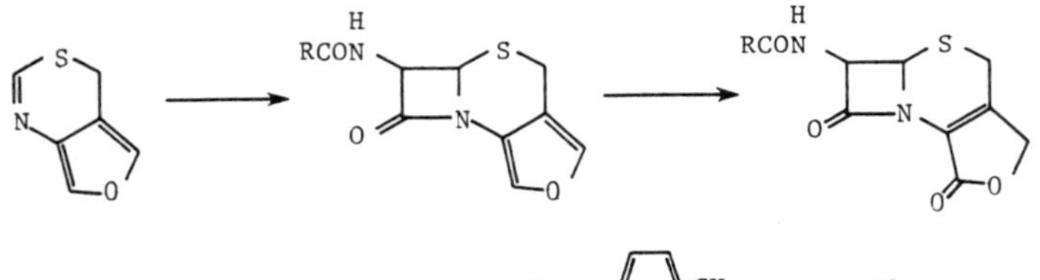

Although the cycloaddition approach usually gives the undesired 6(7)-α-substituted bicyclic β-lactam, which must then be epimerized in a nonstereospecific manner, it affords one of the most direct routes to such systems. Bose and associates (1977, and references cited therein) have produced a large number of bicyclic β-lactams in this way, but in most cases the lack of appropriate functionality detracts from their usefulness. The more efficient epimerization method developed by Firestone *et al.* (1974a) has made it practical to prepare a number of penicillins by the cycloaddition route, which have modified substituents at C-2, C-3, C-5, and C-6 (Vanderhaeghe and Thomis, 1975; Claes and Vanderhaeghe, 1976; Claes *et al.*, 1977; Meyer *et al.*, 1978).

C. Insertion

The successful formation of bicyclic β-lactams by photolysis of α-diazoamides (Corey and Felix, 1965) led Lowe and co-workers at Oxford (Lowe and Parker, 1971) to investigate this route to β-lactam antibiotic nuclear analogs. The initial target was 1-dethiadihydrocephalosporin (33) (Brunwin et al., 1971). The starting material (29) was prepared from pyridine-2-carboxylic acid by catalytic reduction, resolution, and ester formation. Amide formation with the half-ester of malonic acid followed by diazoexchange gave 30. Photolysis of 30 produced a mixture of trans (31) and cis (32a) isomers (trans/cis = 2:1) along with an α-lactone by-product resulting from insertion of the transient carbene intermediate into a C—H bond of the tert-butyl group. Although the reaction was nonstereospecific with regard to the 6,7-substituents, a trans relationship between C-4 and C-6 was obtained exclusively. After chromatographic separation removal of the tert-butyl group from the cis isomer (32a) with trifluoroacetic acid proceeded without epimerization, but attempted formation of the acid azide (32b) by standard methods gave a mixture of epimers. This difficulty was surmounted by carbodiimide coupling of the acid with tert-butyl carbazate followed by removal of the tert-butyl group (trifluoroacetic acid) and diazotization. Curtius rearrangement of the resulting acid azide produced the isocyanate which was trapped with tert-butyl alcohol to yield urethane (32c). The overall yield from 32a to 32c was 20%. Finally, conversion to the amine, followed by acylation and hydrogenolysis of the benzyl ester, afforded the target compound 33.

The Oxford group (Lowe and Ramsay, 1973) also devoted considerable effort aimed at 1-dethia-2-thiacephalosporin, an isomer of the natural

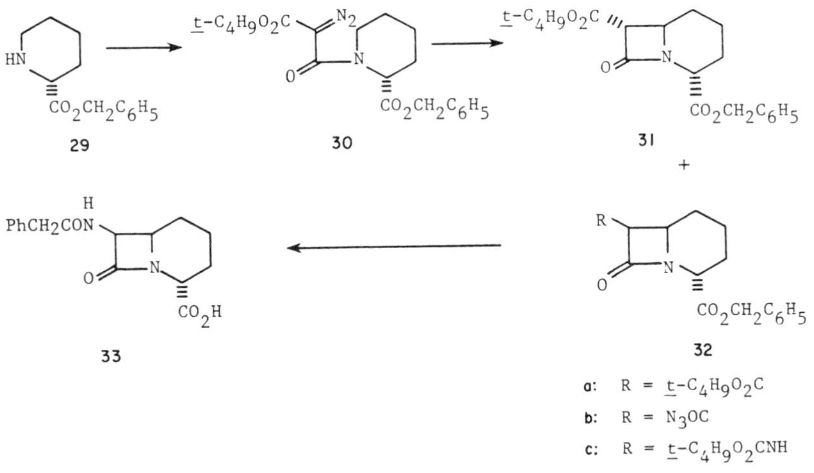

29

30

31

+

33

32

a: R = $\underline{t}$-C$_4$H$_9$O$_2$C

b: R = N$_3$OC

c: R = $\underline{t}$-C$_4$H$_9$O$_2$CNH

product in which the sulfur has been moved one position around the ring. The first attempt aimed at the preparation of a dihydro derivative produced a positional isomer (**38**) of the desired product, because of an ambiguity in the preparation of an early intermediate. Thus reaction of **34** with 2-mercaptoethylamine gave **35** rather than **36**. When **35** was converted to the diazoamide and photolyzed as above, a mixture of all four stereoisomers was obtained. These were separated by chromatography, and each was converted to the target compounds **37–39**; however, one of the 6,7-cis isomers isomerized to the trans intermediate corresponding to **39**, so that only three final products were obtained. The structure of one of the intermediates leading to **37** was established by X-ray crystallography (Vijayan *et al.*, 1973).

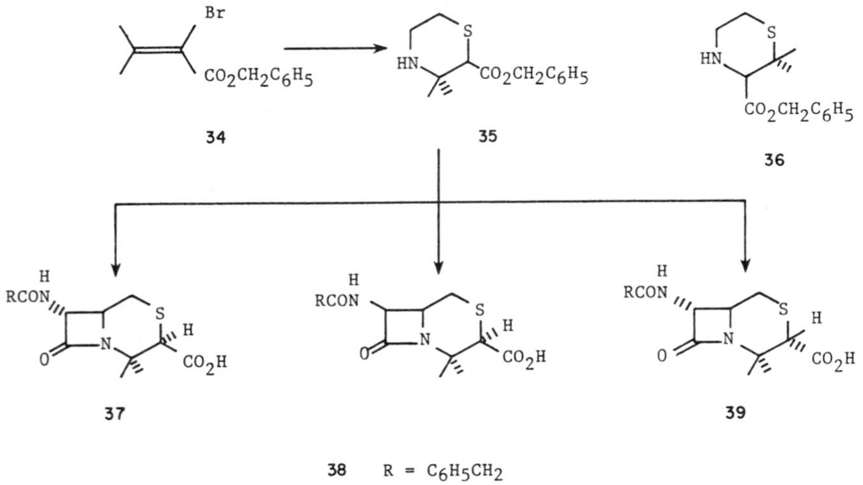

Another approach to the 1-dethia-2-thiacephalosporin system was more successful (Brunwin and Lowe, 1973). Thiomorpholine (**40**) was prepared from *tert*-butyl 1,2-dibromoproprionate and 2-mercaptoethylamine. The structure of **40** was confirmed by formation of a phenylhydantoin with phenyl isocyanate. Conversion to the diazoamide (**41**) followed by photolysis gave **42** and **43** (cis/trans = 7:3). Attempted chromatographic separation on silica gel or neutral alumina resulted in rapid epimerization of **42** to **43**; however, the cis isomer (**42**) could be isolated by fractional crystallization. The trans isomer (**43**) was converted to the final product (**44**) by the route used previously. However, the cis isomer (**42**) epimerized during the Curtius rearrangement step.

In an effort to circumvent the epimerization problem, the trans isomer (**43**) was alkylated (KO*t*-C$_4$H$_9$, CH$_3$I) to give exclusively the desired 7α-methyl derivative (**45**). By the usual route **45** was converted to the dihydro analog (**46**). In addition, the requisite double bond was introduced by chlorination–dehydrochlorination to give 7α-methyl-1-dethia-2-thiacephalosporin (**47**).

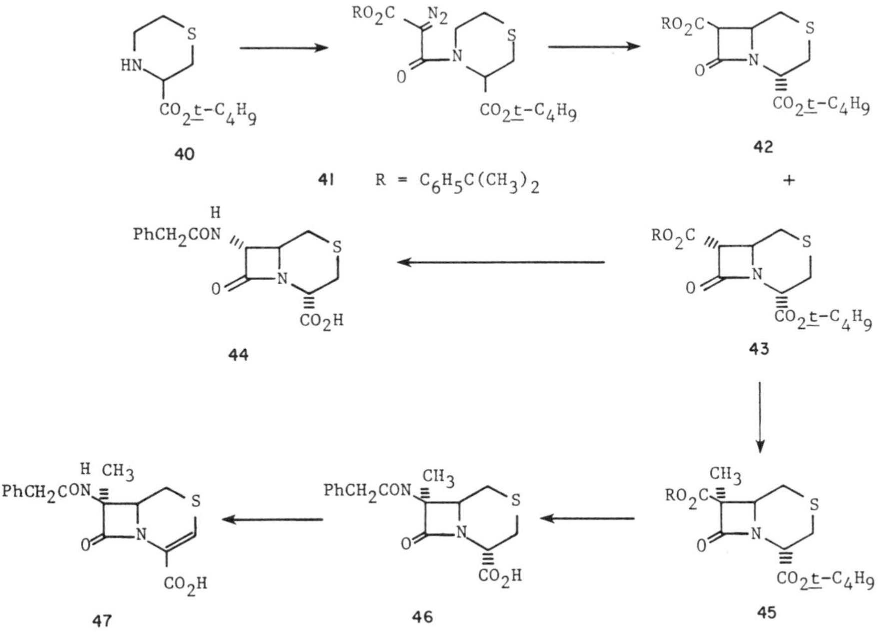

Another method for generating carbenes that will insert to form bicyclic β-lactams involves thermolysis of a dihalomercury intermediate such as **48** in refluxing bromobenzene to give 6α-bromopenam (**49**) in 10% yield (Johansson and Akermark, 1971a). In several subsequent papers from the Swedish group, model compounds of greater stability were studied, and it was found that similar thermolysis of **50** produced 47% **51** along with 14% cis isomer. Displacement with the thallium salt of phthalimide in dimethyl sulfoxide (DMSO) at 150°C afforded 50% cis isomer (**52**) along with 5% trans isomer (Johansson and Akermark, 1971b; Johansson, 1973; Akermark *et al.*, 1974; Lagerlund, 1976). Because of the vigorous reaction conditions it seems unlikely that this approach will prove useful for the synthesis of strained bicyclic systems with the functionality required for antibacterial activity.

Photolysis of α-ketoamides (**53**) affords bicyclic β-lactams (**54**) of uncertain stereochemistry and usually in low yield (Henery-Logan and Chen, 1973; see also Akermark and Johansson, 1969; Johansson *et al.*, 1976).

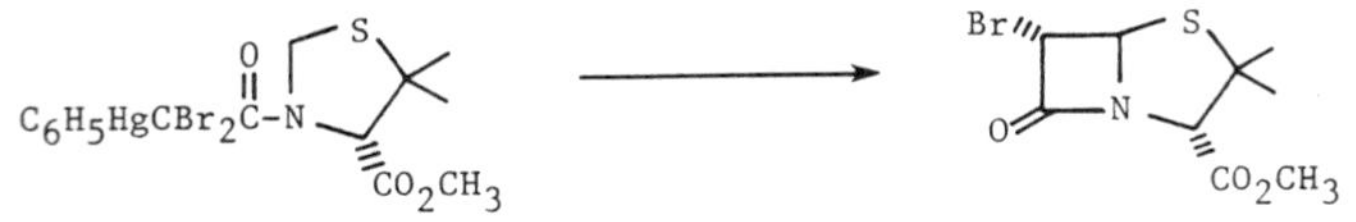

48   **49**

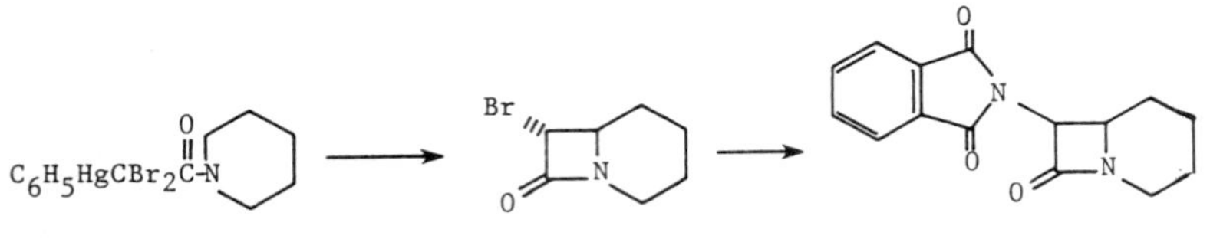

50   **51**   **52**

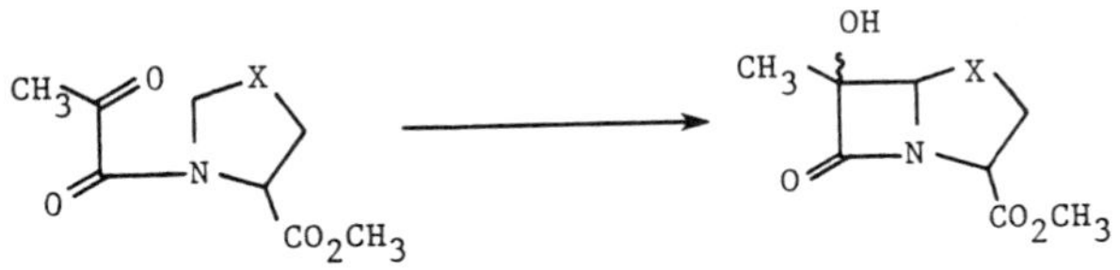

53

54

X = S   (11%),
    SO   (8%),
    SO$_2$ (70%),

D. Ring Contraction

The photolytic Wolff rearrangement has provided an entry into the 6-epi-1-dethiapenam system (**57**) (Lowe and Ridley, 1973). Diekmann cyclization of **55** followed by selective hydrolysis of the *tert*-butyl ester and decarboxylation afforded **56a**. Diazo exchange produced **56b** which on irradiation in the presence of methylphenethyl carbazate at −70°C yielded a solution containing **57**. However, attempts to purify the product led to rapid decomposition, suggesting that the subsequent synthetic manipulations required to convert it to a penicillin nuclear analog would not be feasible.

A more stable model system was investigated by Stork and Szajewski (1974). Irradiation of **58** produced a mixture of isomers (**59**) in 65% yield (cis/trans = 2:5). However, since the cis isomer was found to epimerize very readily, it is not certain that the observed ratio is the one actually formed by the reaction.

The oxidative contraction of α-ketolactams with periodate was studied at Berkeley by Rapoport and associates (Bender *et al.*, 1975a,b). The model system (**60**) reacted smoothly at room temperature to give **62** in

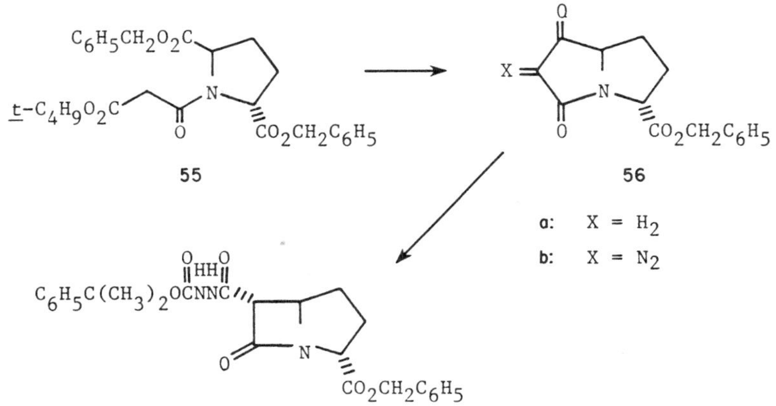

55

56

a: X = H₂
b: X = N₂

57

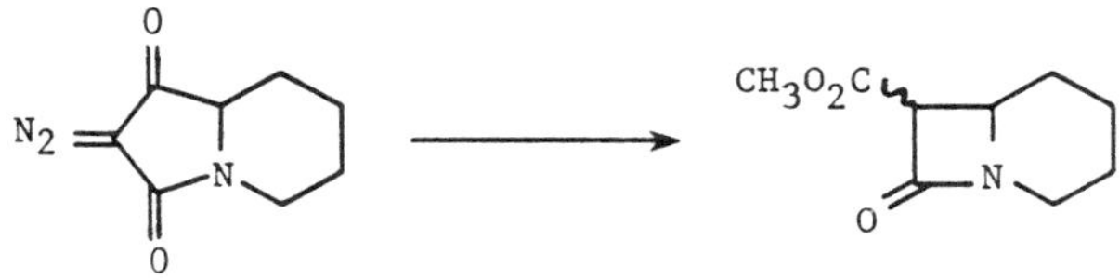

58   59

70% yield. The reaction is postulated to proceed through a cyclopropanone intermediate (61). Application of this method to more complex
systems has not been reported.

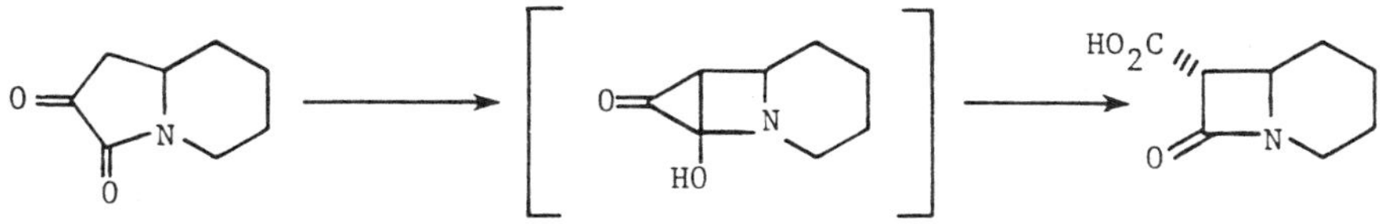

60   61   62

Other contractions of possible utility are photolytic contraction of
mesoionic thiazolones such as 63 to intermediate 63a which yields 64 on
treatment with tributylphosphine (Barton *et al.*, 1977), as well as the
contraction of 65 to 66 (Hirokami *et al.*, 1979).

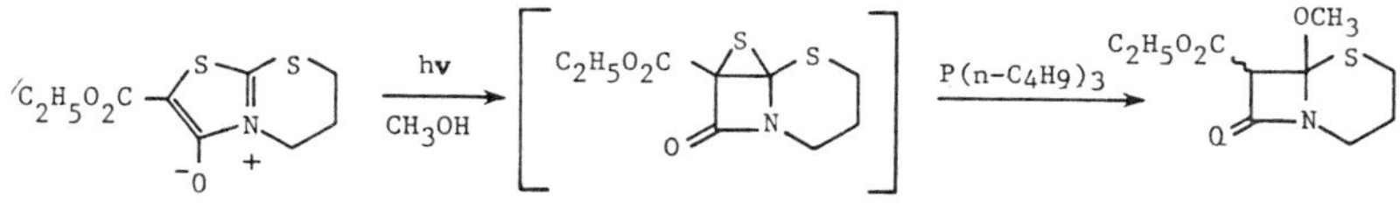

63   63a   64

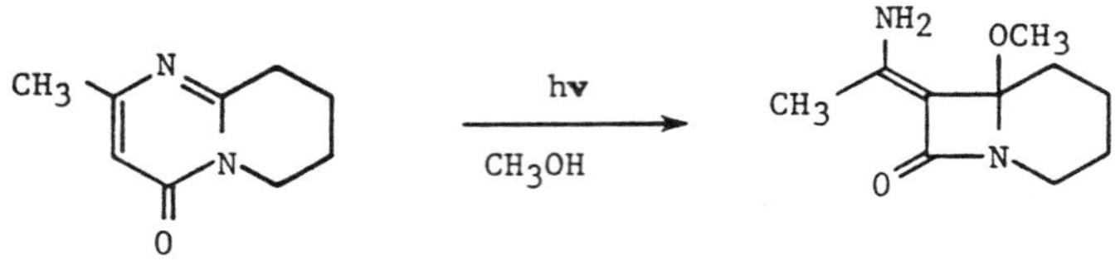

65   66

E. Other Routes

The Ugi reaction has been used to prepare penams in reasonably good yield (Ugi and Wischöffer, 1962). This reaction is a lactam-forming reaction but, in addition, the potential C-3(4) carboxyl function is added simultaneously as an amide. Recently Schutz and Ugi (1979) used this approach to prepare a 3-epipenicillin (68) in high yield (82%) by treatment of the threo isomer of 67 with *tert*-butylisocyanide. However, the conversion of 68 and similar analogs derived from this route to biologically active materials appears formidable.

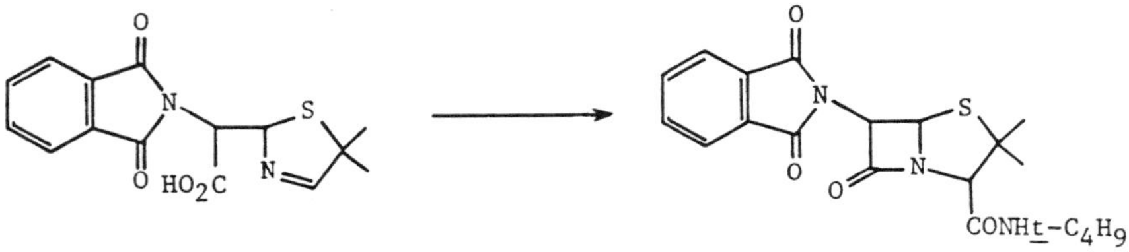

67   68

Just and co-workers (1977) reported an unsuccessful attempt to prepare an oxacepham using the Ugi reaction.

Several groups have attempted the simultaneous formation of both rings of the bicyclic system. Semmelhack and Gilman (1971) investigated the photolysis of dihydrothiazepines (69) but did not obtain the desired transannular ring closure to 70. Similarly transannular nucleophilic displacement in a related system failed (Benn and Mitchell, 1972). An initial report (Hatanaka *et al.*, 1971) that rearrangement of an *o*-quinone oxime benzenesulfonate (71a) produced the highly reactive bicyclic lactam (71c) via a transannular Michael addition of 71b was later corrected when the product was identified as a cyanomethytetronic acid (72) (Fleming *et al.*, 1972).

69   70

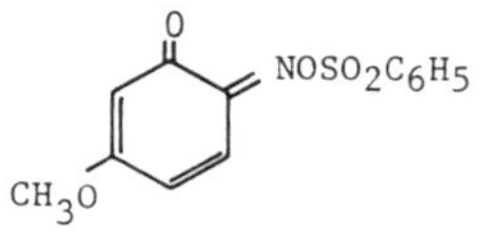

III. Synthetic Schemes in Which the β-Lactam Ring Is Formed Early in the Sequence

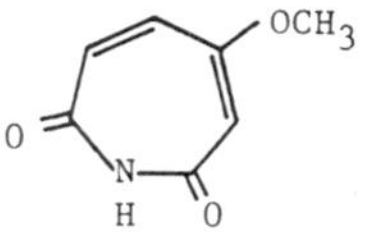

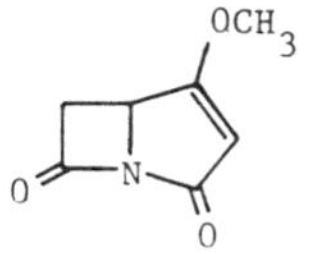

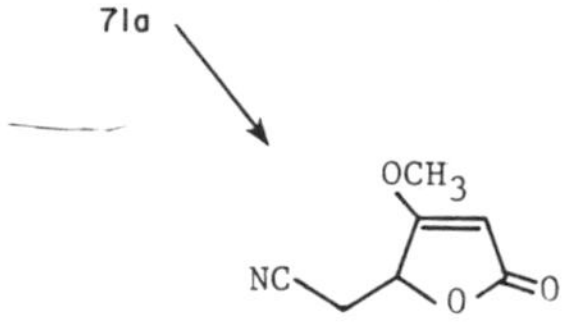

The general approach of forming the β-lactam ring early in the sequence was first effectively employed by Woodward *et al.* (1966) in the synthesis of cephalosporin C. Since that time a number of groups have been successful in applying this strategy to the synthesis of β-lactam antibiotics and their nuclear analogs. There are several reasons why synthetic schemes of this type have been more effective than those in which the β-lactam ring is formed near the end of the sequence. Probably most important is that this approach makes it possible to establish the presence of the amide side chain with cis stereochemistry while the β-lactam is still relatively unreactive. This avoids some of the major problems encountered with the routes described above where epimerization was almost always required to establish the correct stereochemistry and relatively harsh conditions (e.g., Curtius rearrangement) were often needed to obtain proper functionality. Another important advantage of the monocyclic approach is versatility (for example, see also Volume 1, Chapter 1 and this volume, Chapter 1). As will become apparent from the examples described below, a single monocyclic intermediate can be used to generate a wide range of nuclear analogs.

A. Lactam Formation

Woodward's classic synthesis of cephalosporin C has been reviewed previously, as has the application of his key monocyclic intermediate (**77**) to the synthesis of nuclear analogs (Heusler, 1972). In the Woodward synthesis, two of the heteroatoms and three of the carbons of the β-lactam ring were derived from L-cysteine (**74**) which, after conversion to **75,** was functionalized at the methylene group adjacent to sulfur. The initially formed product was the thermodynamically more stable trans isomer which gave the desired cis orientation on displacement with azide. The derived amine **(76)** was cyclized to **77** using triethylaluminum. The β-lactam nitrogen is reasonably nucleophilic and thus provided the first point of attachment of the elements of the dihydrothiazine ring. Subsequent removal of the S- and N-protecting groups followed by cyclization and appropriate acylation and ester hydrolysis provided the first total synthesis of a cephalosporin. Research groups at the Woodward Institute and Ciba–Beigy utilized intermediate **77** for the synthesis of a variety of nuclear analogs of type **78.** Most of these have been summarized previously (Heusler, 1972), but since many of the references were listed as unpublished results the following references to the published work are provided (Scartazzini and Bickel, 1972; Scartazzini *et al.,* 1972a,b; Woodward *et al.,* 1977).

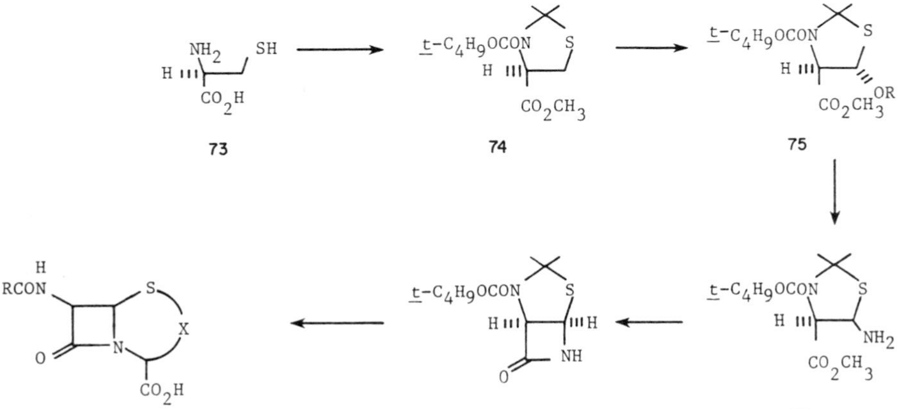

B.   Cycloaddition (N,C-4 → C-2,C-3)

The ketene–imine cycloaddition reaction described in Section II,B has been successfully applied by several groups to the construction of monocyclic β-lactams with appropriate functionality and stereochemistry that can be converted to a variety of β-lactam antibiotic nuclear analogs with potent antibacterial activity. Since the ketene–imine reaction has proved to be so useful, some apsects of its mechanism, stereochemistry, and scope will be discussed.

Although the ketene–imine cycloaddition route to β-lactams has received considerable attention, the exact mechanism and stereochemical consequences of this reaction are still being debated. It is generally agreed that the reaction usually proceeds through a dipolar intermediate of type **C** or **G** (Fig. 2) rather than by a concerted [2 + 2]addition. Evidence for this comes from trapping experiments in which the dipolar species is intercepted. For example, chloroamides corresponding to the protonated form of **E** (Nu = Cl) have been isolated (Duran and Ghosez, 1970; Nelson, 1972), as well as 4-oxo-1,3-thiazolidine 1,2-dioxides resulting from the insertion of sulfur dioxide (Decazes *et al.*, 1972; Bellus, 1975). When the ketene component is generated *in situ*, which is most often the case, it is possible that the dipolar species results from acylation of the imine by the ketene precursor (usually an acid chloride) followed by deprotonation. The most puzzling feature of the ketene–imine reaction has been the stereochemical outcome. Depending on the reaction conditions and the nature of the substituents, the product may be all-cis (**D**), all-trans (**H**), or a variable mixture of the two. Of the various ex-

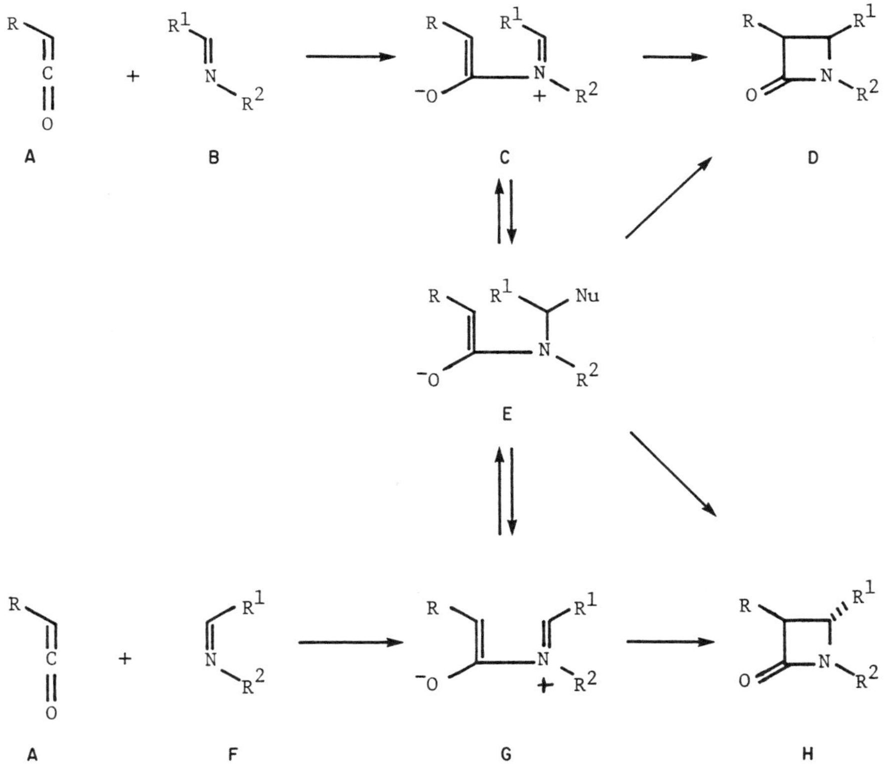

Fig. 2. Possible mechanism of the ketene–imine cycloaddition reaction.

planations offered, the conrotatory ring closure of **C** to **D** and **G** to **H** seems to fit the observed results best (Moore *et al.*, 1978). Thus, when acyclic imine **B** (trans) reacts with ketene **A**, intermediate **C** results and the product resulting from immediate cyclization is the *cis*-β-lactam (**D**). On the other hand, a cyclic imine (**F**) (cis), in which R^1 and R^2 are part of a ring, would produce a *trans*-β-lactam (**H**) via **G**. This appears to be the course followed when R^2 is not an electron-withdrawing group. However, when R^2 is, for example, phenyl, acyclic imines give the trans product (**H**) or a mixture of cis and trans, with trans usually predominating (see, e.g., Zamboni and Just, 1979; Just *et al.*, 1979b). The result could be explained by assuming the formation of intermediate **E** by the addition of a nucleophile (usually chloride) to **C** or **G**. This process is favored in cases where R^2 is an electron-withdrawing group. Direct closure to **D** or **H** could follow, or **E** might serve only as a means of interconverting **C** and **G**. In either case the thermodynamically favored isomer (**H**) (trans) should predominate. Another possibility is that, when R^2 is an electron-withdrawing group, the nucleophilicity of the imine nitrogen is reduced to the point where acylation to give **C** or **G** is not a favorable process, and a [2 + 2]cycloaddition reaction intercedes. A somewhat different explanation is offered by Doyle *et al.* (1977a).

In applying the ketene–imine cyclization to the construction of monocyclic β-lactams suitable for conversion to β-lactam antibiotic nuclear analogs, the stereochemistry of the product and the nature of the substituents are of critical importance. As described in Section II,B, addition of ketenes to cyclic imines invariably gives the undesired trans product. However, addition to acyclic imines can yield exclusively the desired cis isomer as described above. The choice of substituents on the ketene is somewhat limited if the bicyclic target requires a C-6(7) amido function, as in penicillins and cephalosporins. Amides cannot be used because azlactone formation results. Similarly, carbamates usually cannot be employed; however, Bose and associates (1975) have reported some success with benzyloxycarbonylglycine. The most useful substituent has proved to be the azido group which is readily converted to the desired amido function by mild reduction followed by acylation. One drawback in the use of the azido group is that azidoacetyl chloride is explosive and azidoacetic acid and its activated esters can decompose violently under certain conditions (Borowski and Kamholz, 1976). An alternative to the azido group that is safe and thus applicable to large-scale work is phthalamido (see, e.g., Finklestein *et al.*, 1978). Recently, Dane salts have been recommended as suitable alternatives to the azido group (Sharma and Gupta, 1978; Sharma *et al.*, 1979; Bose *et al.*, 1979a,b). Other methods for avoiding the use of azidoacetyl chloride include the use of a mixed anhydride of azidoacetic acid and trifluoroacetic acid (Bose *et al.*, 1973) and the use of activated esters (Manhas *et al.*, 1976a,b; Amin *et al.*, 1979).

The substituents on the imine component are governed by the type of bicyclic β-lactam one desires to construct. The substituent on nitrogen must either be one that is useful in forming the remaining ring or one that can be removed conveniently. Both approaches have been successfully utilized and are exemplified below. There are some limitations with respect to the aldehyde or ketone component of the imine. When the derived imine bears an α carbon with a relatively labile proton, base-catalyzed isomerization to the enamine is often observed. In most successful syntheses this pathway is blocked by using an sp^2-hybridized carbon or a heteroatom in this position.

The first successful application of the ketene–imine approach via a monocyclic precursor was realized by a group at Merck (Cama and Christensen, 1974; Guthikonda *et al.*, 1974). Their two initial targets were cephalosporin analogs in which the sulfur was replaced by oxygen or a methylene group. Treatment of **80** with azidoacetyl chloride (**79**) in the presence of triethylamine gave the *trans*-β-lactam **81**. It appears that obtaining a product with trans stereochemistry is inconsistent with the mechanism of the reaction delineated above. However, thioimidates appear to be a special case with respect to the ketene–imine cycloaddition reaction. Bose and Fahey (1974) noted that thioimidates consistently gave β-lactams in which the sulfur atom was trans to the substituent derived from the ketone. More recently Bachi and Vaya (1979) have found that this type of reaction is not necessarily stereospecific, although the trans isomer is heavily favored. A possible explanation for these observations is that the dipolar intermediate **82**, analogous to C in Fig. 2, can readily equilibrate to the structure analogous to G (Fig. 2) via **83**, or that closure of **83** may give the thermodynamically favored trans isomer directly.

Chlorination of **81** gave a mixture of *cis*- and *trans*-4-chloro isomers (**84a**) which, on reaction with 1-hydroxy-3-acetoxy-2-propanone in the presence of silver tetrafluoroborate and silver oxide produced **84b** as a 1:1 mixture of cis and trans isomers. Ring closure of **84b** with sodium hydride afforded bicyclic β-lactam **85** from which the desired cis isomer was separated by chromatography. Concomitant reduction of the azido function and ester hydrogenolysis, followed by acylation, gave 1-dethia-1-oxacephalosporin (**86**).

The above synthesis suffers from the lack of stereospecificity encountered in the chloride displacement step which then results in a 1:1 mixture of cis and trans isomers of the bicyclic lactam **85**. A stereospecific route to the corresponding carbocyclic cephalosporin (90) was achieved, however. In this case azidoacetyl chloride (79) was reacted with 87 in the presence of triethylamine at $-78°C$ to give 30% cis-β-lactam 88. Other conditions for β-lactam formation failed, presumably because of isomerization of the imine to the corresponding enamine. Deketalization followed by cyclization resulted in a good yield of 89 which was converted to the carbocyclic cephalosporin 90 by standard methods.

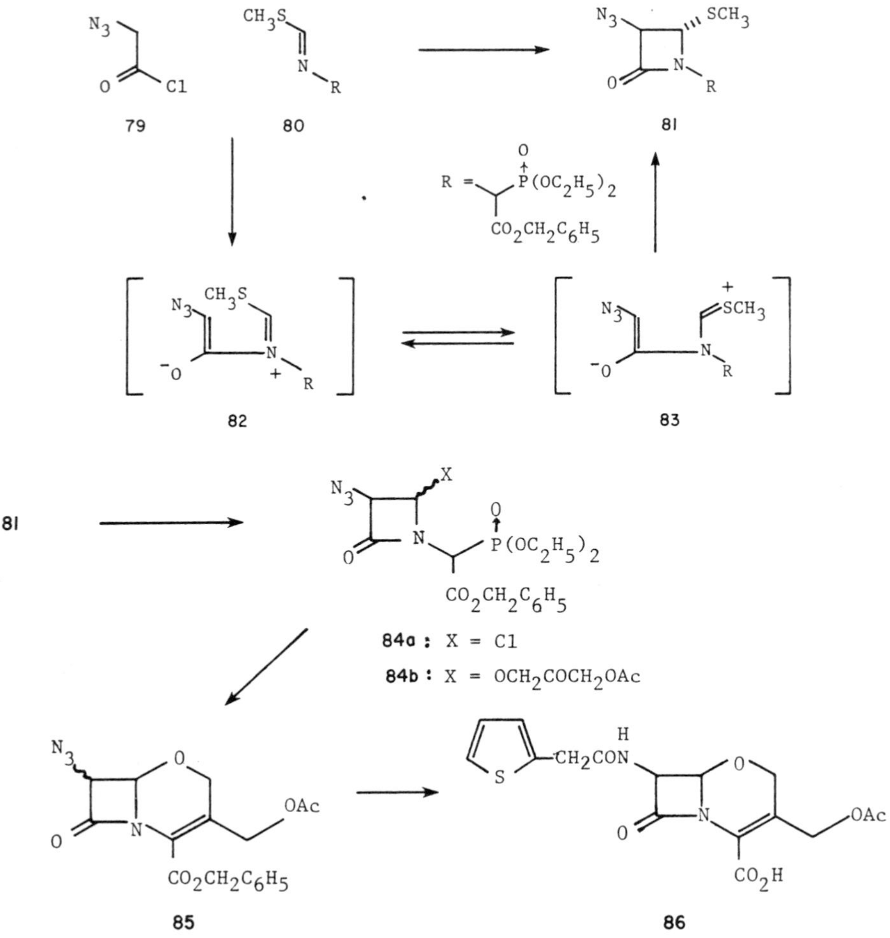

Using the same general approach, the Merck group prepared a number of oxa- and carbacephalosporins analogous to 86 and 90 bearing substituents at C-3 and C-7 designed to optimize antibacterial potency and spectrum (Firestone *et al.*, 1977). Using a route somewhat analogous to the preparation of **86**, they also succeeded in synthesizing a penicillin with sulfur replaced by oxygen (Cama and Christensen, 1978a). In this case azidoacetyl chloride (**79**) was reacted with **91** to give the *trans*-β-lactam **92**. Following the route used previously, **92** was converted to a mixture of *cis*- and *trans*-4-chloro derivatives which were displaced with *N-tert*-butoxycarbonylserine benzyl ester to give **93a**. The substituent on the β-lactam nitrogen was removed by potassium permanganate oxidation, and the desired cis isomer (**93b**) was separated from the resulting mixture. After reducing the azide and acylating the resulting amine, the *tert*-butyl group was removed and the amine was diazotized to yield **94**.

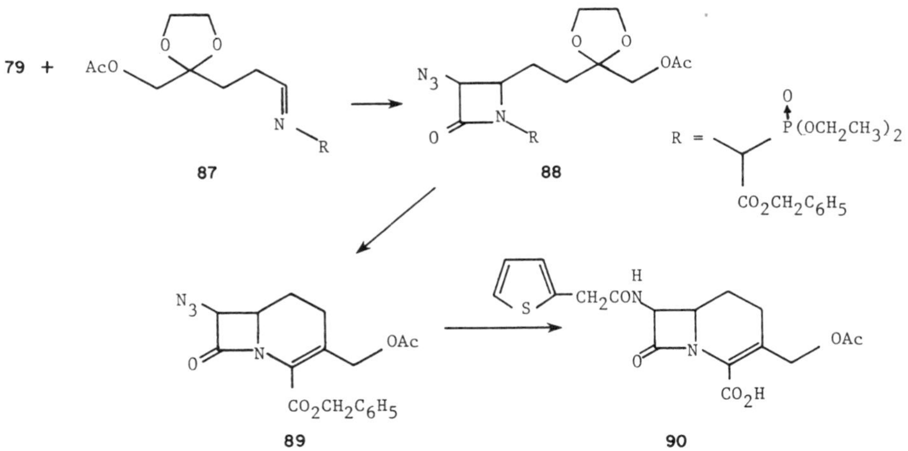

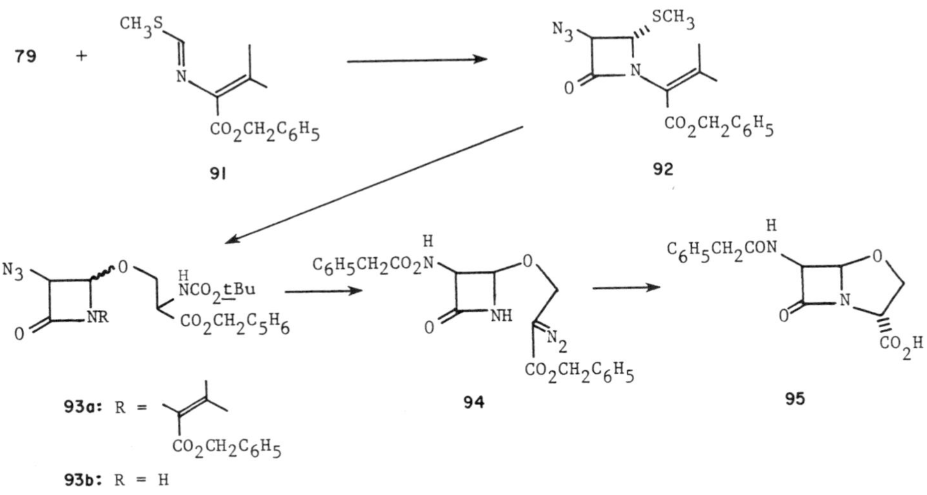

Cyclization was achieved by intramolecular insertion of the carbene derived from **94** into the N—H bond of the β-lactam, using rhodium acetate as the catalyst. After hydrogenolysis of the benzyl ester, 1-dethia-1-oxabisnorpenicillin (**95**) was obtained, the stereochemistry at C-3 being assigned on the basis of nuclear magnetic resonance (NMR).

At Smith Kline & French a somewhat different strategy was adopted for the synthesis of β-lactam antibiotic nuclear analogs, in that a single monocyclic precursor served as the key intermediate for a number of target molecules (Holden *et al.*, 1979). The mixed anhydride of azidoacetic acid (**96a**) (Bose *et al.*, 1973), generated *in situ*, was reacted with imine **96b** in the presence of triethylamine to give exclusively the *cis*-β-lactam **96c** in 58% yield. At this point the dimethoxybenzyl group could be removed by a novel oxidative procedure ($K_2S_2O_8$, CH_3CN–H_2O, pH 5–6.5, Δ). Alternatively, this step could be postponed until the azido group was converted to an amide by reduction followed by acylation or until further modification of the carbomethoxy group was achieved. For the preparation of a 1-dethia-2-azapenam (**98b**), monocyclic β-lactam **96c** was reduced, acylated, and deblocked to give **97a** in 52% overall yield. Selective ester reduction was achieved with sodium borohydride, and the resulting alcohol (**97b**) was converted to the iodide **97d** via tosylate **97c**. Displacement with azide followed by reduction produced amine **97e** which was condensed with benzyl glyoxylate to afford imine **97f**. On treatment with acetyl chloride, acylative cyclization occurred to give the desired bicyclic β-lactam **98a** which was a 3:1 mixture of carboxylate epimers. Hydrogenolysis of the benzyl ester produced the desired acid (**98b**) (Huffman *et al.*, 1977).

For the synthesis of a penicillin analog in which the sulfur has been moved one position around the ring (**101**), the thienyl amide (**99**) corresponding to **97d** was reacted with benzyl glyoxylate to give **100a** as a mixture of carboxylate isomers. Treatment of this mixture with thionyl chloride followed by displacement with potassium thioacetate afforded **100b**. Unexpectedly, selective hydrolysis of the benzyl ester occurred to give **100c** when **100b** was treated with potassium carbonate. Cleavage of the thioacetate with concomitant cyclization was achieved when **100c** was treated with cyclohexylamine in methylene chloride. The desired penicillin analog (**101**) was isolated directly from the reaction mixture as its cyclohexylamine salt (Huffman *et al.*, 1978).

The corresponding cephalosporin analog (**103b**) was prepared from iodide **99** in the following way. Displacement with trityl mercaptan followed by deblocking to the thiol and reaction with benzhydryl β-bromopyruvate gave bicyclic β-lactam **102** directly. Dehydration to the cephem analog (**103a**) was achieved with difficulty. Cleavage of the

96a **96b** **96c**

97a: X = CO_2CH_3
97b: X = CH_2OH
97c: X = CH_2OTs
97d: X = CH_2I
97e: X = CH_2N_2
97f: X = $CH_2N{=}CHCO_2CH_2C_6H_5$

98a: R = $CH_2C_6H_5$
98b: R = H

99

100a: X = OH, R = $CH_2C_6H_5$
100b: X = $SCOCH_3$, R = $CH_2C_6H_5$
100c: X = $SCOCH_3$, R = H

101

benzhydryl ester (CF_3CO_2H, 0°C) gave the free acid (**103b**). In order to introduce functionality at C-3, as is present in the more biologically potent cephalosporins, the synthetic scheme was repeated starting from iodide **99d** and utilizing *tert*-butyl 3-bromo-2-oxobutyrate to yield **104a.**

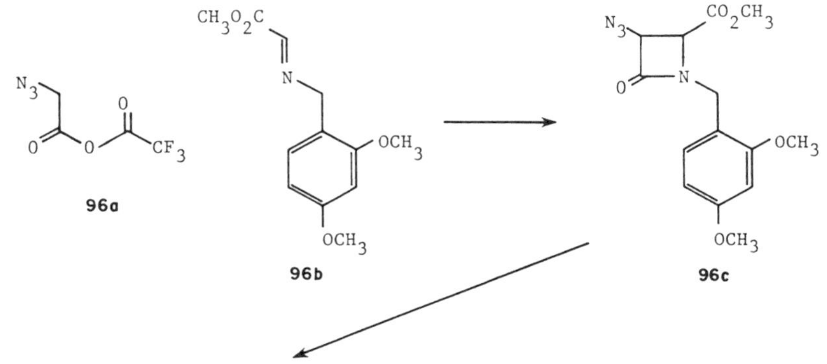

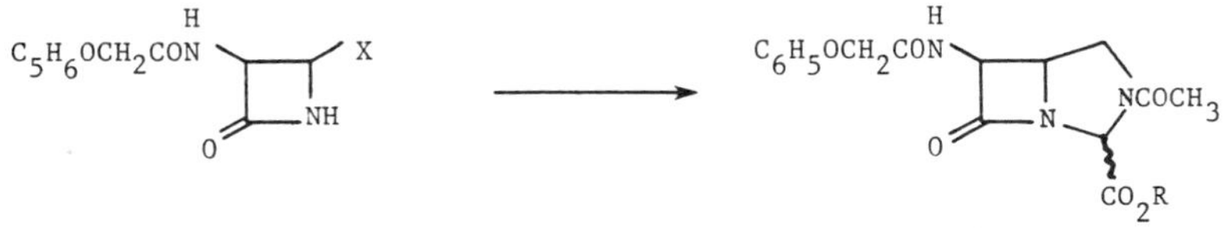

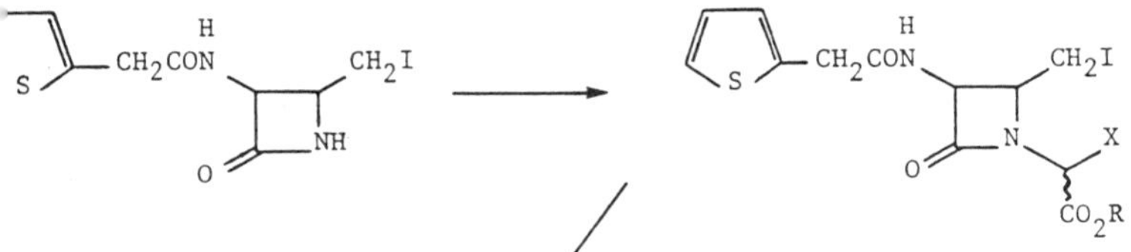

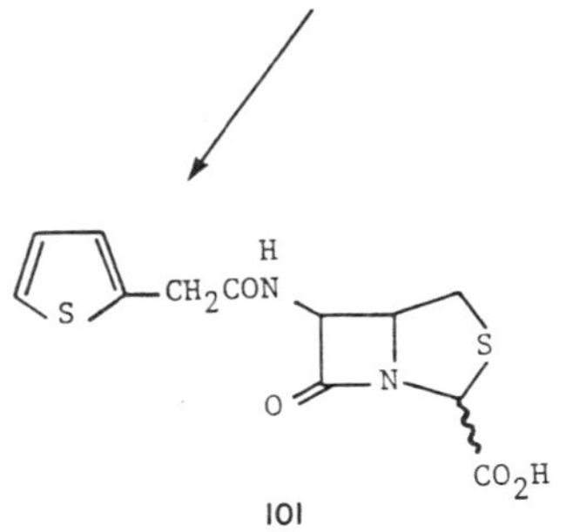

The methyl group was successfully functionalized by bromination followed by displacement with potassium acetate in the presence of crown ether, and the *tert*-butyl ester was cleaved with trifluoroacetic acid to yield **104b** (Bryan *et al.*, 1977).

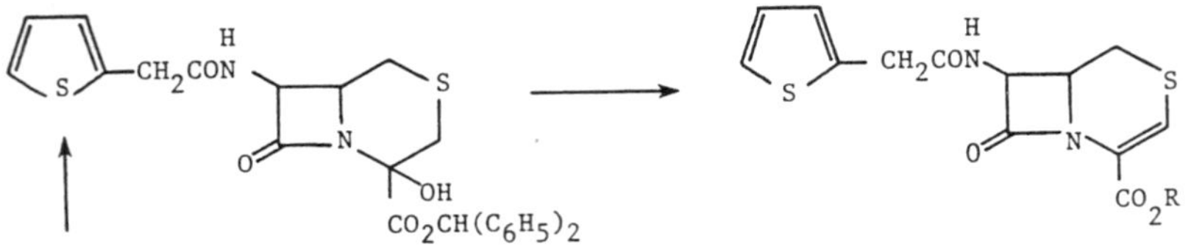

99

102

103a: R = CH(C$_6$H$_5$)$_2$
103b: R = H

97d ⟶

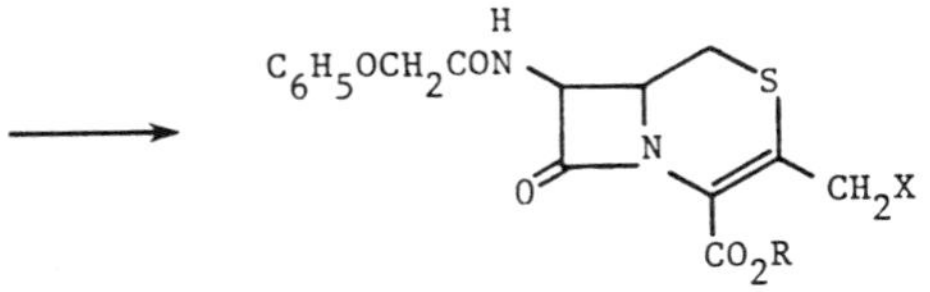

104a: X = H, R = $\underline{t}$-C$_4$H$_9$
104b: X = OAc, R = H

The synthesis of 1-dethia-2,3-diazacephams (**106**) was achieved efficiently by hydrolysis of **99a** to the free acid followed by carbodimide coupling with hydrazines to give **105**. Condensation of **105** with benzyl glyoxylate produced the desired bi- and tricyclic β-lactams as a mixture of epimers which were converted to the free acids (**106**) (Finkelstein *et al.*, 1977).

99a ⟶

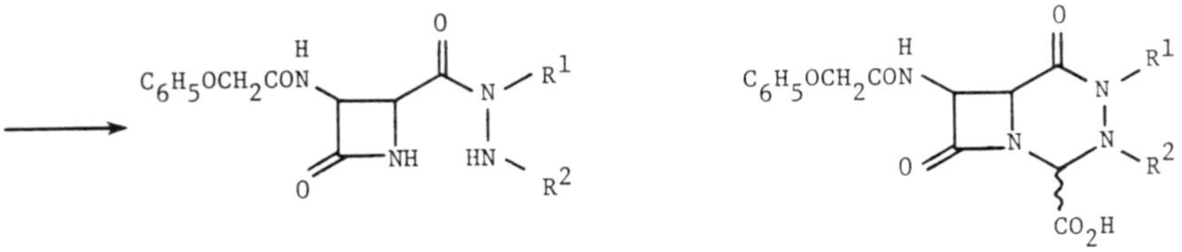

105a: R^1 + R^2 = (CH$_2$)$_4$
105b: R^1 + R^2 = (CH$_2$)$_3$
105c: R^1 + R^2 = CH$_2$CH$_2$CO
105d: R^1 = H, R^2 = CO$_2$CH$_3$

106

To synthesize cephams with a heteroatom at the 3-position it was necessary to homologate intermediate **98**. This was achieved by selective reduction of the ester (NaBH$_4$) followed by oxidation to the aldehyde (**107a**). Condensation with nitromethane followed by dehydration of the intermediate nitroalcohol, and reduction of the resulting nitroolefin gave **107b**. A modified Nef reaction on **107b** produced dimethyl acetal **107c** which could be oxidatively deblocked to yield **108a.** Condensation of **108a** with benzyl glyoxylate afforded **108b** as a separable mixture of diasteromers. One isomer was cyclized to **109** on treatment with *p*-toluenesulfonic acid and 4-Å sieves, whereas the other isomer yielded a mixture of α- and β-methoxy epimers (**110**). The stereochemical assignments made by NMR were confirmed by an X-ray crystallographic study of **109.** Finally, reduction of the azide function to the amine, acylation, and subsequent hydrogenolysis of the ester provided acids **111** and **112** (Gleason *et al.*, 1979).

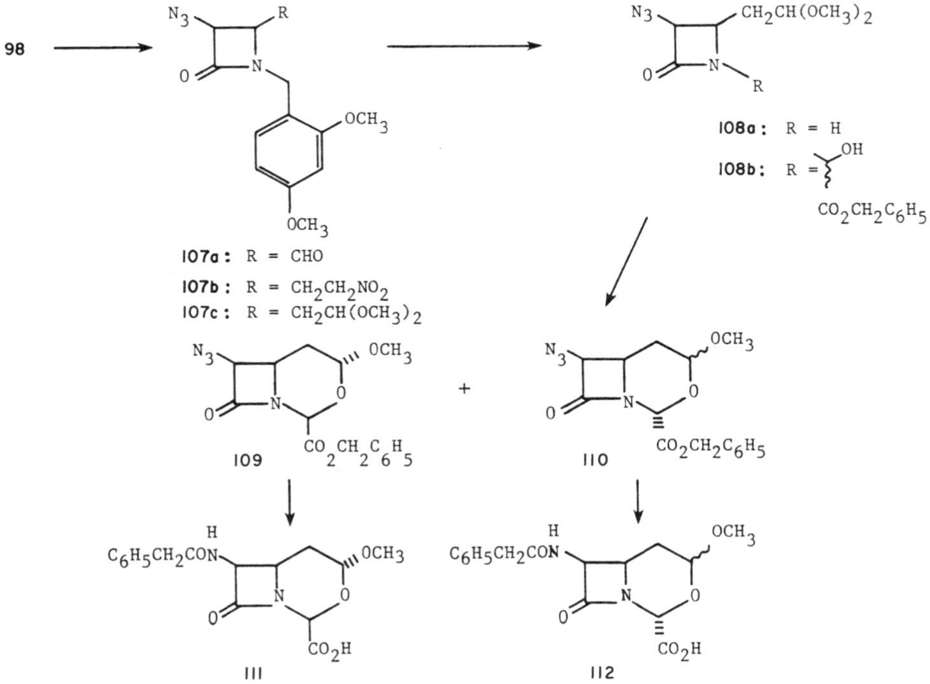

107a : R = CHO
107b : R = CH₂CH₂NO₂
107c : R = CH₂CH(OCH₃)₂

108a : R = H
108b : R =

109

110

111

112

A different monocyclic intermediate was required for the synthesis of 1-dethia-1,2-benzocephem (**116b**). Thus **114a** could be prepared in either of two ways: (1) The mixed anhydride of azidoacetic acid (**96**) was reacted with imine **113,** and the resulting *cis*-β-lactam (49%) was oxidatively deblocked, reduced, and acylated to give **114a,** or (2) phthaloylglycyl chloride (**115**) was reacted with **113** to give a *cis*-β-lactam (64%). Removal of the phthaloyl group (methylhydrazine) followed by reduction, acylation, and oxidative deblocking resulted in a higher overall yield of **114a.** Condensation of **114a** with benzyl glyoxylate afforded **114b** which, on reaction with thionyl chloride followed by triphenylphosphine, gave ylide

114c. Hydrolysis of the acetal resulted in direct cyclization to the tricyclic analog **(116a)**, which was converted to the free acid **(116b)** by hydrogenolysis (Finkelstein *et al.*, 1978).

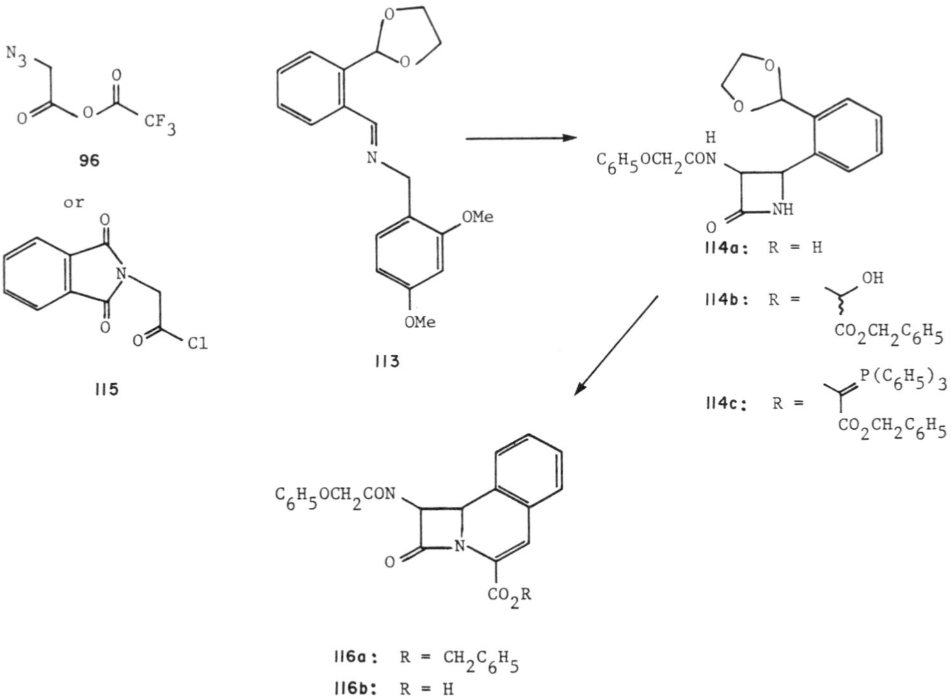

At Bristol Laboratories in Canada a similar general approach to β-lactam nuclear analogs was developed (Doyle *et al.*, 1980). However, in contrast to the Smith Kline & French approach, the substituent on the β-lactam nitrogen of the monocyclic precursor was not removed but was used in construction of the second ring. While this approach is more efficient, it limits the utility of any one intermediate. A group of common intermediates **(119)** was prepared by the addition of azidoacetyl chloride **(79)** to imine **117** in the presence of triethylamine to give *cis*-β-lactam **118a** exclusively. Ozonolysis to the aldehyde **(118b)** followed by reduction to the alcohol **(118c)** and subsequent mesylation gave **118d** which was hydrolyzed to **119**. Base-catalyzed cyclization of **119** followed by conversion of the azide function to an amide and deblocking of the ester in the usual manner gave a series of 1-dethia-2-oxacephems **(120)** (Doyle *et al.*, 1977a,b).

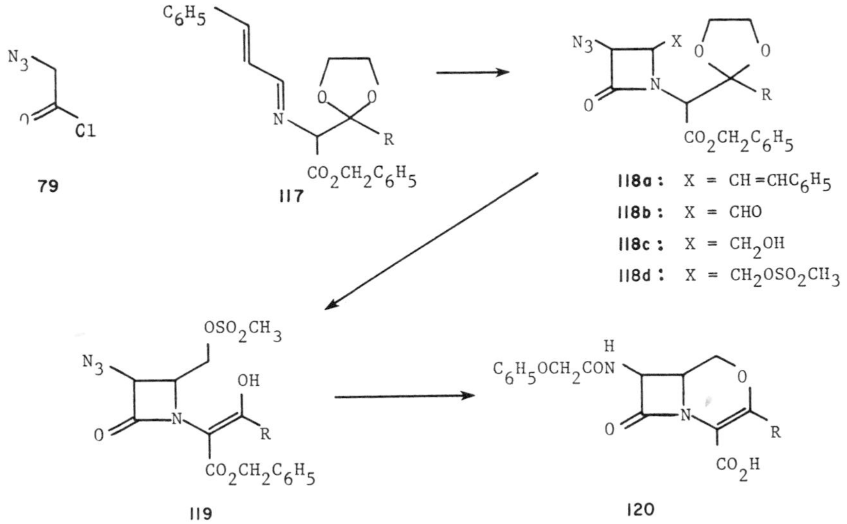

118a : X = CH=CHC$_6$H$_5$

118b : X = CHO

118c : X = CH$_2$OH

118d : X = CH$_2$OSO$_2$CH$_3$

R = H, CH$_3$, C$_2$H$_5$,
CH$_2$C$_6$H$_5$, CH$_2$CH$_2$C$_6$H$_5$

Attempts to introduce an acetoxymethyl group at C-3 were at first unsuccessful. However, it was subsequently found that, when the di-mesylate (121a) or mesylate triflate (121b) derived from 119 was treated with base, elimination occurred to give allene 122. Bromination of 122 produced 123 in good yield, and this could be converted directly to 124a on treatment with potassium acetate. Displacement of acetate by thiols did not take place as it does in the cephalosporin series. Instead displacement was carried out on intermediate 123. Alternatively, formate 124b was prepared, hydrolyzed to alcohol 124c, and converted to mesylate 124d. Displacement of the mesyl group proceeded readily with most thiols to give 3-thiomethyl derivatives (124e). Intermediates 124 were converted to a variety of 1-dethia-2-oxacephems of type 125 (Conway et al., 1978).

Disulfonate 121 and closely related structures also proved to be useful intermediates for the preparation of 1-dethia-2-thiacephems (127), 1-de-thia-2-azacephems (129), and 1-dethiacephems (136). Reaction of 121 with hydrogen sulfide–triethylamine gave the 1-dethia-2-thiacephem (126) which was converted to the final product (127) by standard procedures (Doyle et al., 1977f). Similarly, treatment of 121 with methylamine or ammonia followed by ethyl chloroformate gave 1-dethia-2-azacephems (128) which were also converted to final products (129) in the usual

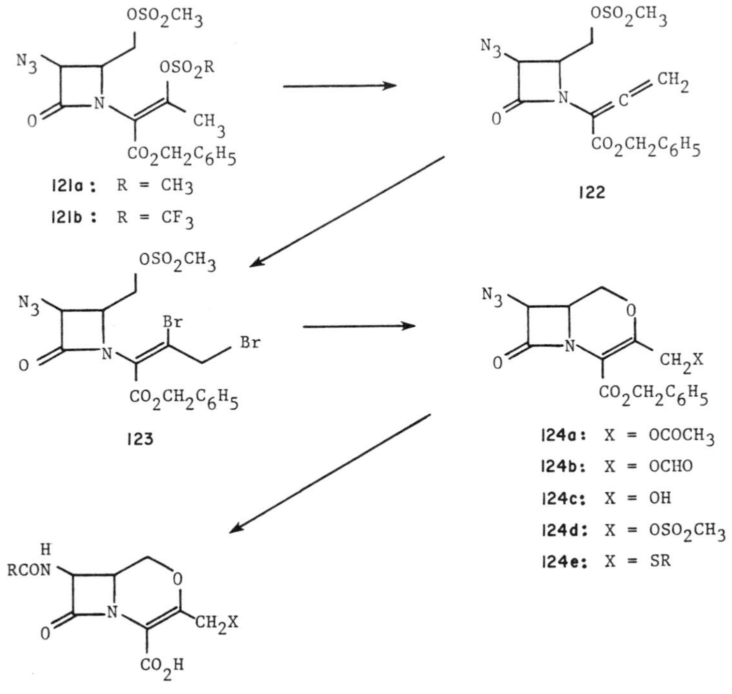

OSO_2CH_3

OSO_2R

N_3

CH_3

$CO_2CH_2C_6H_5$

121a : R = CH₃
121b : R = CF₃

OSO_2CH_3

N_3

CH_2

$CO_2CH_2C_6H_5$

122

OSO_2CH_3

N_3

Br

Br

$CO_2CH_2C_6H_5$

123

N_3

CH_2X

$CO_2CH_2C_6H_5$

124a: X = OCOCH₃
124b: X = OCHO
124c: X = OH
124d: X = OSO₂CH₃
124e: X = SR

RCON

H

O

CH_2X

CO_2H

125

fashion (Doyle *et al.*, 1977e). Finally, dimesylate **121** could also be condensed with malonates to give 1-dethiacephems (**130**). Hydrolysis of the di-*tert*-butyl ester with trifluoroacetic acid followed by decarboxylation in refluxing toluene produced **131** along with some of the Δ^2 isomer (Doyle *et al.*, 1979a). Further decarboxylation of **131** catalyzed by triethylamine afforded **132** which rearranged to **133** in the presence of 1,5-diazabicyclo[4.3.0]-5-nonene (DBN) (Doyle *et al.*, 1979b). Functionalization at C-2 was achieved most readily by epoxidation of **132** to yield **134**. Base-catalyzed (DBN) opening of epoxide **134** gave allylic alcohol **135a** which could be oxidized to the corresponding ketone (**135b**). Reduction of ketone **135b** produced the isomeric allylic alcohol (**135c**) (Martel *et al.*, 1979). Many of the 1-dethiacephem intermediates described above were converted to final products (**136a–i**) for evaluation as antibacterial agents.

1-Dethia-2-oxacephems substituted at C-1 (**138**) were prepared by a variation of the original scheme. Condensation of azidoacetyl chloride with imines derived from methacrylaldehyde or furfural gave *cis*-β-lac-

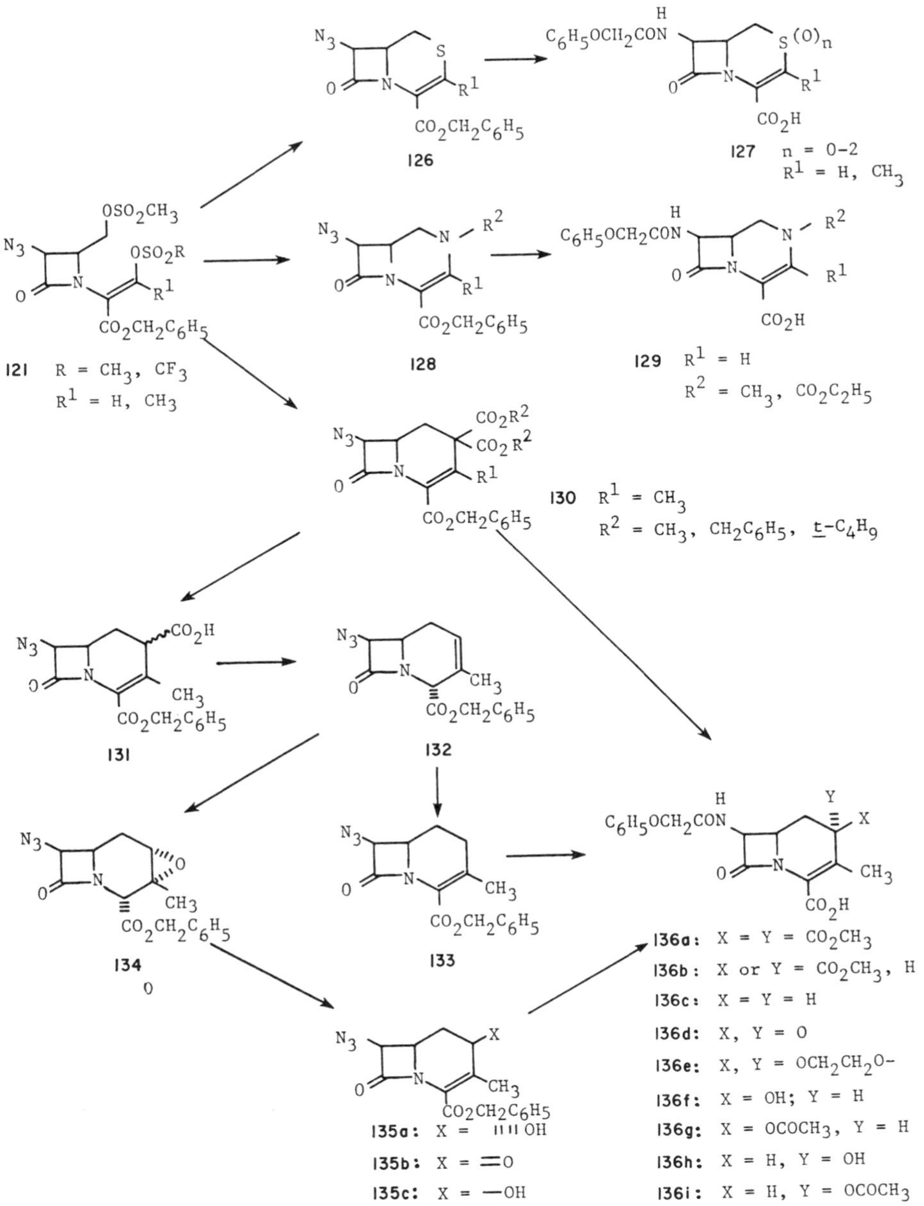

$$121 \quad R = CH_3, \; CF_3$$
$$R^1 = H, \; CH_3$$

$$126$$

$$127 \quad n = 0\text{-}2$$
$$R^1 = H, \; CH_3$$

$$128$$

$$129 \quad R^1 = H$$
$$R^2 = CH_3, \; CO_2C_2H_5$$

$$130 \quad R^1 = CH_3$$
$$R^2 = CH_3, \; CH_2C_6H_5, \; \underline{t}\text{-}C_4H_9$$

$$131$$

$$132$$

$$134$$

$$133$$

136a: X = Y = CO_2CH_3

136b: X or Y = CO_2CH_3, H

136c: X = Y = H

136d: X, Y = O

136e: X, Y = OCH_2CH_2O-

136f: X = OH; Y = H

136g: X = OCOCH_3, Y = H

136h: X = H, Y = OH

136i: X = H, Y = OCOCH_3

135a: X = ıııı OH

135b: X = =O

135c: X = —OH

tams **137a,b.** Ozonolysis of **137a** followed by sodium borohydride reduction gave alcohols **137c,d.** Ozonolysis of **137b** gave **137e.** These compounds were carried through procedures analogous to those used above to yield final products **138a–c** (Doyle *et al.*, 1977c,d). Another variation in the nature of the imine component led to the preparation of a 3,4-benzo-fused analog **(139)** (Doyle, 1977).

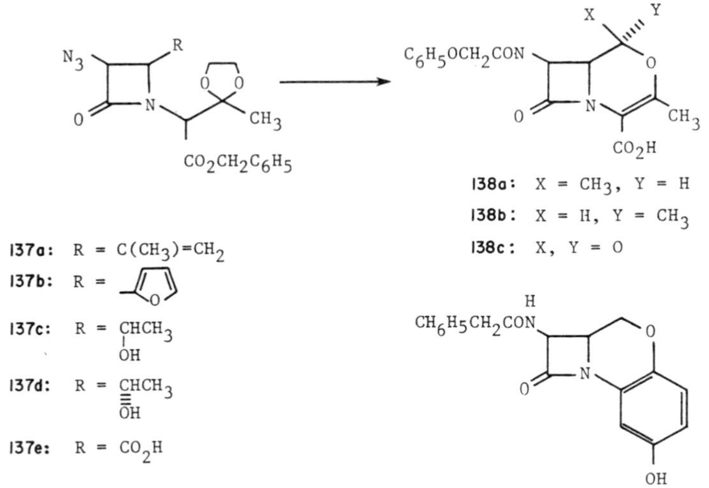

138a: X = CH_3, Y = H
138b: X = H, Y = CH_3
138c: X, Y = O

137a: R = C(CH_3)=CH_2

137b: R =

137c: R = CHCH_3
           OH

137d: R = CHCH_3
           OH

137e: R = CO_2H

139

The major thrust of the total synthesis work carried out at Farbwerke Hoechst used an approach different from the ketene–imine cycloaddition route (Section III,C). However, early work by this group provided access to some potentially useful monocyclic intermediates (Lattrell, 1973, 1974; Lattrell and Lohaus, 1974a,b). Of particular note was the addition of sulfonate esters (Fig. 3) to thioimidates **B** to give *trans*-β-lactams **C** which could be displaced with azide to afford a monocyclic intermediate **D** with the correct cis configuration.

Using this approach Lattrell and Lohaus (1974c) prepared isomeric cephems **142** and **143** by cyclization of **141** which was, in turn, prepared from **140** by ozonization, ketalization, azide displacement, reduction, acylation, and deketalization.

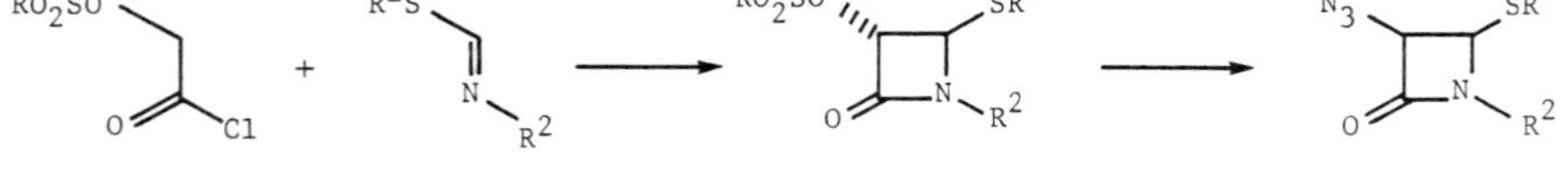

A   B   C   D

Fig. 3. Synthesis of cis monocyclic β-lactams.

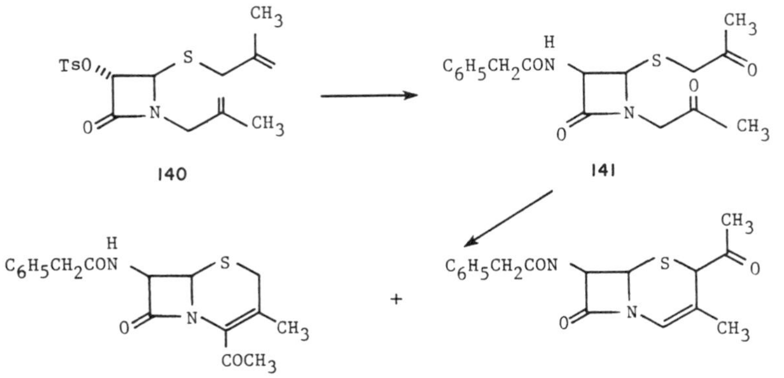

140

141

142

+

143

More recently Bachi and co-workers at the Weizmann Institute have successfully applied a similar approach to the total synthesis of penicillin and cephalosporin analogs (Bachi and Ross-Petersen, 1975; Bachi and Vaya, 1976, 1977, 1979; Bachi *et al.*, 1977; Bachi and Sasson, 1977). Cycloaddition of phthaloylglycyl chloride (**115**) to imine **144** produced the *trans*-β-lactam **145a** as a 1:1 mixture of carboxylate diastereomers in 74% yield. The methylthio group was converted to iodide **145c** by way of sulfonium salt **145b**. Detritylation followed by intramolecular alkylation gave **146** which, however, was not elaborated further.

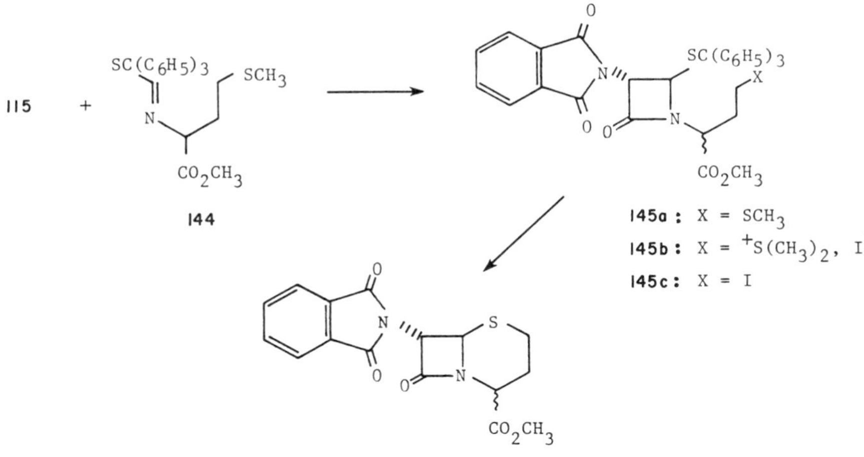

115 +

144

145a : X = SCH₃
145b : X = ⁺S(CH₃)₂, I⁻
145c : X = I

146

Cycloaddition of azidoacetyl chloride (**79**) to imine **147** gave *trans*-β-lactam **148** as a separable mixture of carboxylate diastereomers (55% yield). Chlorinolysis of each isomer resulted in preferential cleavage of the sulfide bonds to give **149** and **150**. Cyclization of **149** with stannous chloride in dioxane produced **151** (2%) and **152** (25%), whereas similar treatment of **150** gave **153** (24%). Although the products were not converted further, procedures for doing so have been described in the literature. Intermediates corresponding to **151–153** were also prepared in the natural penicillin series.

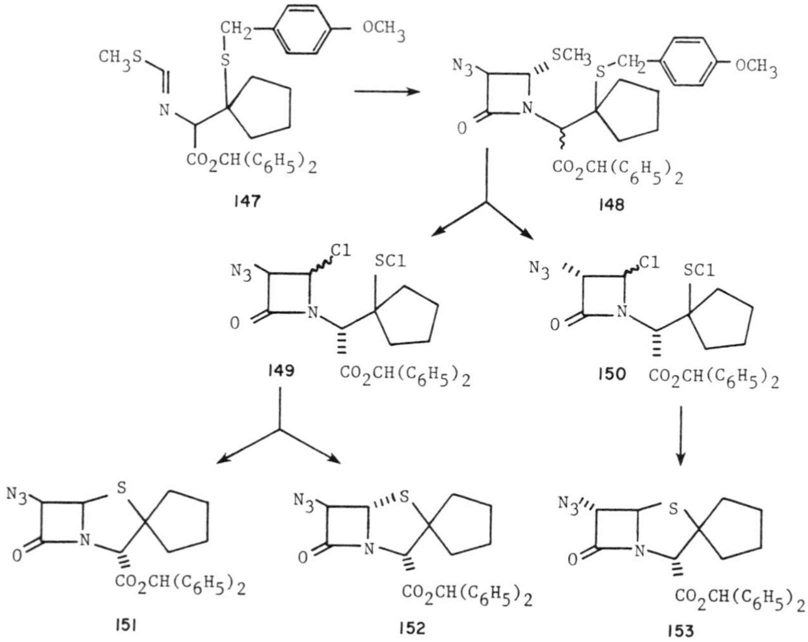

Just and co-workers at McGill have described the synthesis of β-lactam antibiotic nuclear analogs using the approach developed by the Bristol group (Just and Zamboni, 1978a,b; Just *et al.*, 1979a,b; Hakimelahi and Just, 1979; Zamboni and Just, 1979). Of the analogs prepared, perhaps the most interesting are of type **156** which can be regarded as cyclized derivatives of nocardicin. The monocyclic β-lactam **154a** was prepared by the Bristol approach. After conversion to alcohol **154b**, cyclization to **155** was achieved with thionyl chloride–pyridine in refluxing benzene. Conversion to the final product (**156**) was carried out in the usual manner.

Finally, Kametani and co-workers in Japan have adopted the strategies of the Smith Kline & French and Bristol groups in preparing β-lactam antibiotic nuclear analogs (Kametani *et al.*, 1979a,b,c,d). For example, they were able to prepare **158** by oxidative deblocking of the β-lactam nitrogen of **157** followed by reaction with glyoxylate, cyclization, and ester hydrolysis.

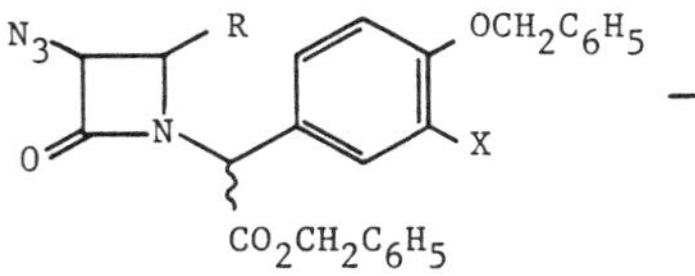

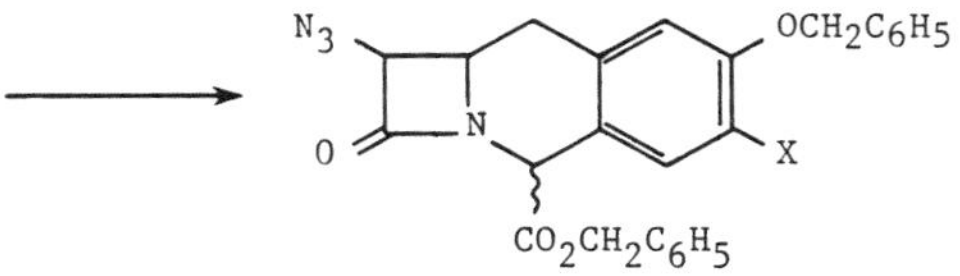

154a R = CH=CHC$_6$H$_5$
154b R = CH$_2$OH
X = H, OCH$_2$C$_6$H$_5$

155 X = H, OCH$_2$C$_6$H$_5$

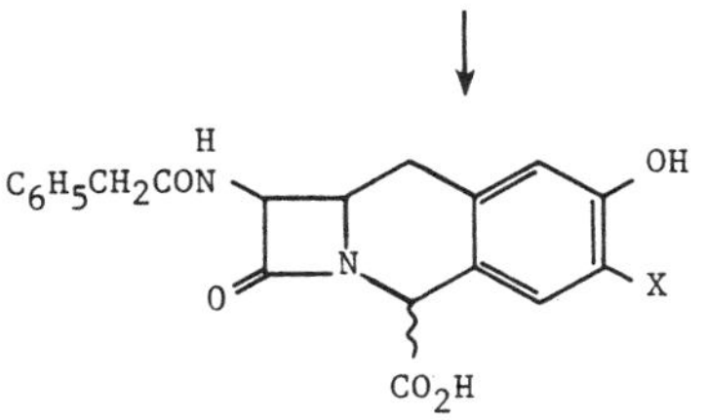

156 X = H, OH

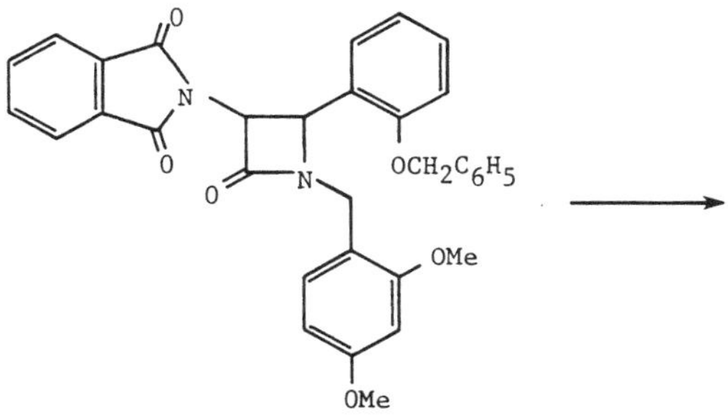

157

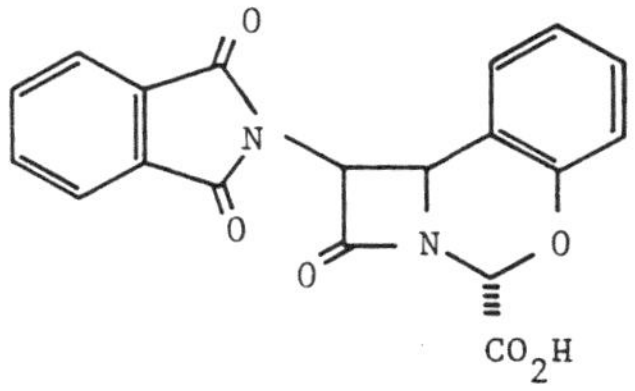

158

C. Cycloaddition (N,C-2 → C-3,C-4)

The second approach used by the Hoechst group utilized the addition of chlorosulfonyl isocyanate (159) to vinyl acetate (160) to give, after mild hydrolysis of the sulfonyl group, the monosubstituted β-lactam 161. Since the acetate group could be displaced by a number of nucleophiles, 161 could be a valuable intermediate provided the amide substituent needed at C-6(7) in the bicyclic target compounds could be introduced (Clauss *et al.,* 1974). Methods for accomplishing this in both the monocyclic and bicyclic series were developed utilizing either addition to a C-3 (monocyclic) or C-6(7) (bicyclic) carbanion or bromination followed by azide displacement (Kuhlein and Jensen, 1974). Several bicyclic analogs were prepared from 161 (Kuhlein and Jensen, 1974; Schnabel *et al.,* 1974; Bormann, 1974) using two similar approaches. Reaction of 161 with mercaptan (162) gave 163a directly, which could be dehydrated to cephem 164. However, to achieve functionality at C-7, 163b was brominated to afford the 7α-bromo epimer which, on displacement with azide, produced the desired 7β-azide (165). An alternative method of ring closure is exemplified by reaction of 161 with mercaptoacetone to give 166 which on addition of glyoxylate to the β-lactam nitrogen afforded 167. Treatment of 167 with thionyl chloride followed by triphenylphosphine and then base generated an ylide which was cyclized to give the cephem 168.

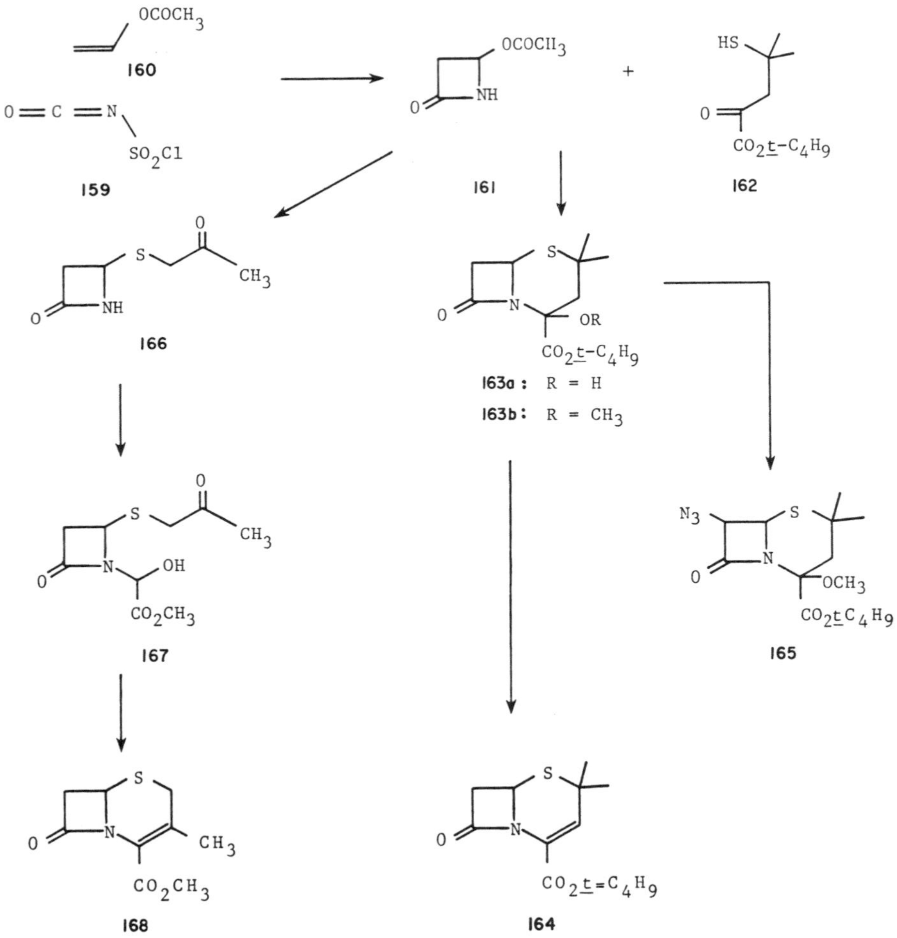

More recently others have used the Hoechst intermediate (161) for the synthesis of nuclear analogs related to clavulanic acid and penems (cf. Volume 2, Chapters 5 and 6) which have no substituent at C-6(7) (Petrzilka *et al.*, 1977; Brown *et al.*, 1977; Branch *et al.*, 1978; Campbell *et al.*, 1979; Shibuya and Kubota, 1979).

D. Biogenetic-Type Closure (N → C-4)

Kishi and co-workers devised two routes to 6(7)-substituted penicillins and cephalosporins based on proposed biosynthetic pathways (Nakatsuka *et al.*, 1975a,b). One route utilized double cyclization of thioamide **169** to give *cis*-β-lactam **170** in low yield. Allylic bromination followed by treatment with zinc in acetic acid gave the deconjugated olefin **171** as a mixture of isomers at the carboxyl position along with some recovered **170**. The product with the natural configuration was oxidized with *m*-chloroperbenzoic acid in benzene containing a catalytic amount of trifluoroacetic acid to yield a complex mixture which, after treatment with phosphorous trichloride, afforded low yields of cephalosporin (**172**) (5%) and penicillin (**173**) (1%). Alternatively one of the isomeric allylic bromide precursors of **171** could be converted to **172** in considerably higher yield (40%) by allowing a thin film of the material to stand at room temperature for 3 days.

The second route employed bromination of thiazoline (**174a**) to give a 1:1 mixture of epimeric bromides (**174b**) only one of which cyclized to β-lactam **175** on treatment with potassium hydride in tetrahydrofuran. The overall yield from **174a** to **175** was 15%. Bromination followed by elimination produced **176** (70%). Although **176** was not converted to a bicyclic β-lactam, the deconjugated olefin corresponding to **171** could presumably yield 6(7)-α-methylpenicillins and cephalosporins by the first method described above. Subsequently, Kishi and co-workers (Tanino *et al.*, 1976) found that thiazoline sulfoxide (**177**), derived by degradation of penicillin, could be converted to penicillin β-sulfoxide (**178**) in high yield, suggesting a more efficient total synthesis route.

Baldwin and co-workers (Baldwin *et al.*, 1975, 1976) used a similar approach, but they achieved a completely stereospecific synthesis by their route. Starting from ethyl 2-nitromethylacrylate, D-isodehydrovaline methyl ester (**179**) was prepared in good yield. This was coupled with a thiazolidine acid (**180**) to give **181a**. Stereospecific functionalization was achieved with benzoyl peroxide, and the benzoate (**181b**) was converted to chloride **181c** by treatment with hydrogen chloride in methylene chloride. Cyclization to *cis*-β-lactam **182** occurred smoothly on treatment with sodium hydride (82% yield). The corresponding sulfoxide was rearranged to **183a** by heating under acidic conditions. Epoxide formation (diazomethane) gave **183b** which was rearranged (boron trifluoride etherate) to aldehyde **183c**. The corresponding sulfoxide underwent thermal syn-elimination of methacraldehyde to generate an intermediate sulfenic acid which afforded penicillin sulfoxide (**184**) directly in 21% overall yield from epoxide **183b.** Deoxygenation to the corresponding penicillin (phosphorous tribromide, dimethylformamide) proceeded readily.

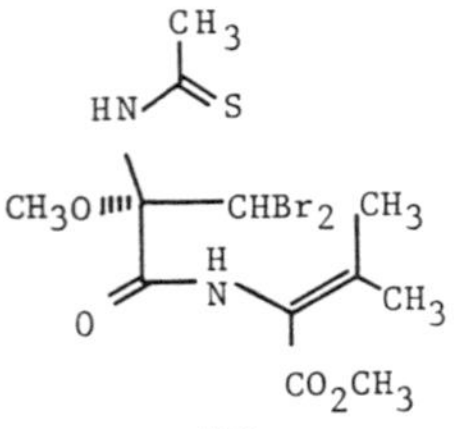

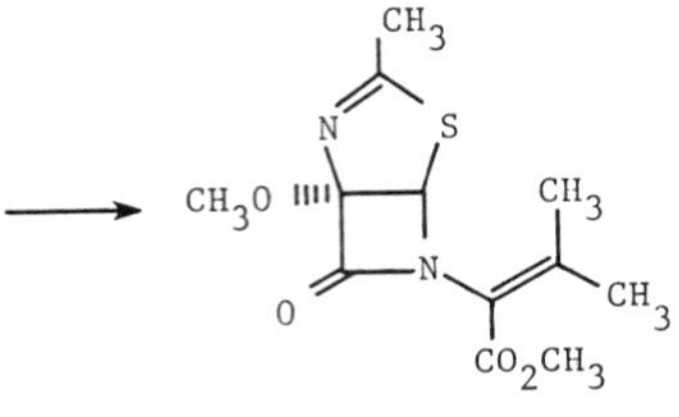

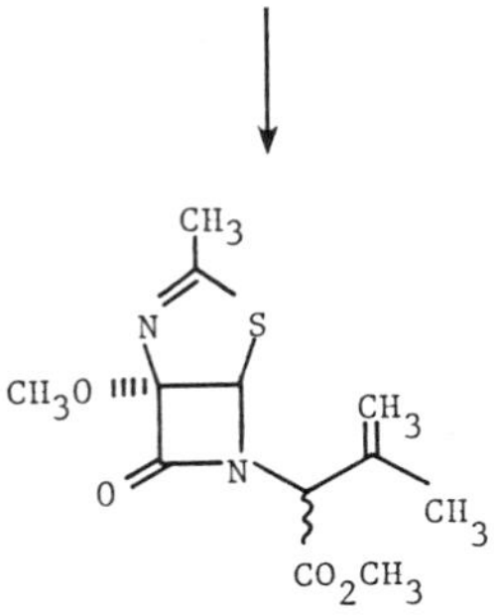

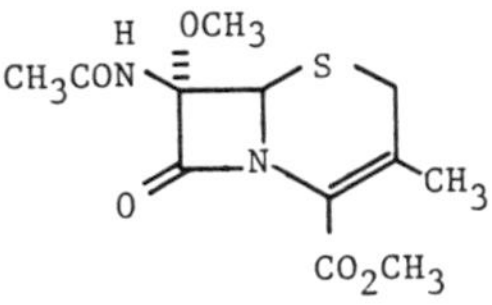

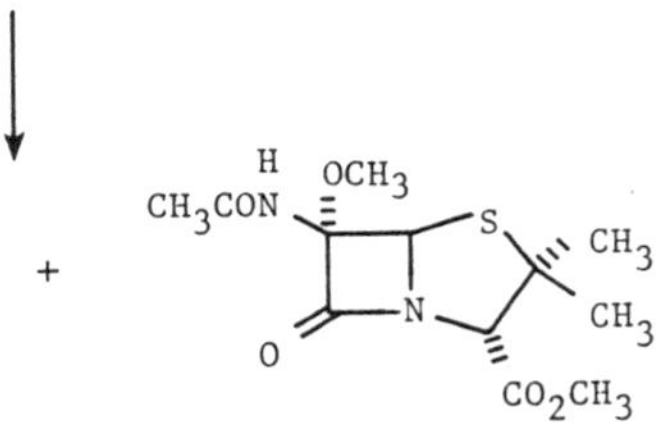

More recently other groups have used the general approach of cyclizing β-haloamides (Koppel *et al.,* 1978; Fletcher and Kay, 1978; Wasserman *et al.,* 1979); however, these investigations were aimed at simpler monocyclic β-lactams related to nocardicins (Chapter 3). One of these routes (Mattingly *et al.,* 1979) utilizes *N*-alkoxy amides which are deprotonated more readily than simple amides. This allowed the direct synthesis of β-lactams **186** from serine derivatives (**185**) without the necessity of forming the β-chloroamide. Reaction of **185** with diethyl azodicaroxylate

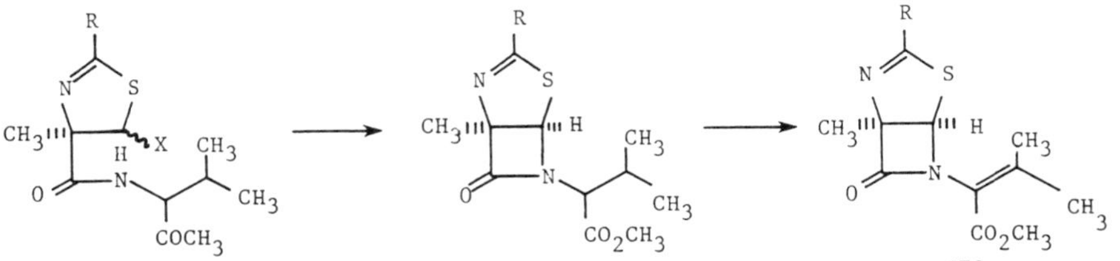

174a X = H
174b X = Br
175
176

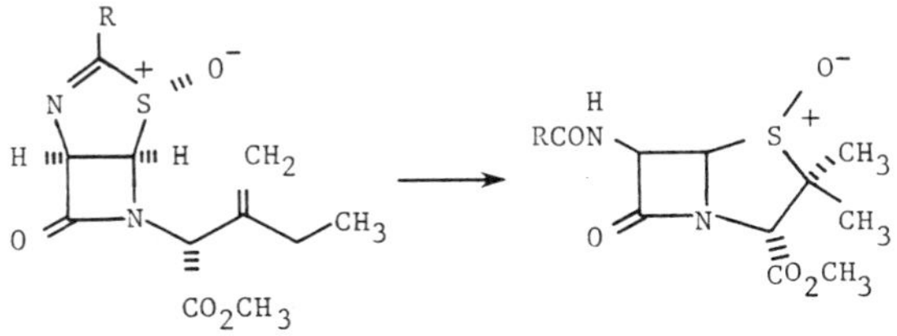

177
178

R = p-CH₃OC₆H₄

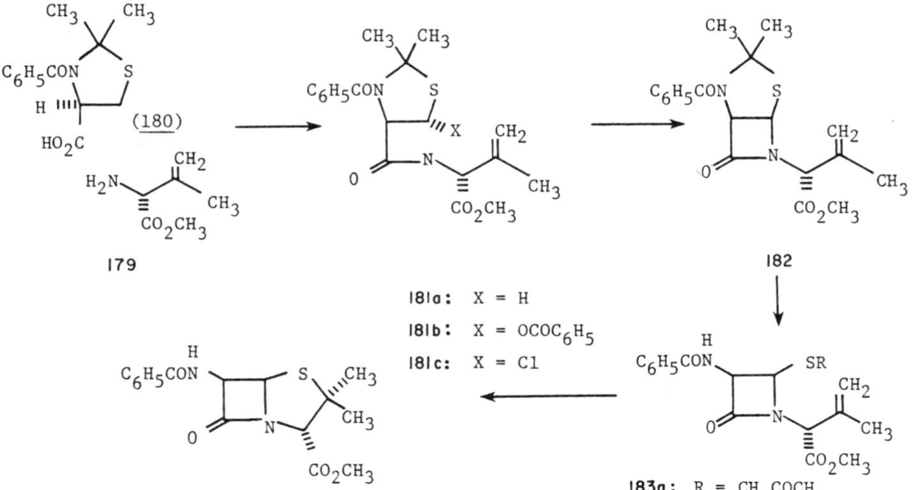

(180)
179

181a: X = H
181b: X = OCOC₆H₅
181c: X = Cl

182

184

183a: R = CH₂COCH₃
183b: R = CH-C-CH₃
183c: R = CH₂CHCH₃

and triphenyphosphine in tetrahydrofuran gave **186** in 54–90% yield with no elimination and complete retention of optical activity.

The reverse approach, displacement of a group from nitrogen by an anion at C-4, has also been reported (Scott *et al.*, 1976). Thus, on treatment of **187** with potassium *tert*-butoxide in tetrahydrofuran, **188** is produced in 50% yield.

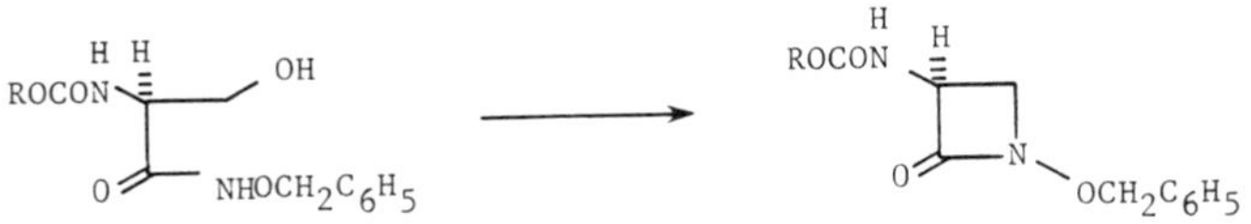

185   R = *t*-C₄H₉, CH₂C₆H₅

186

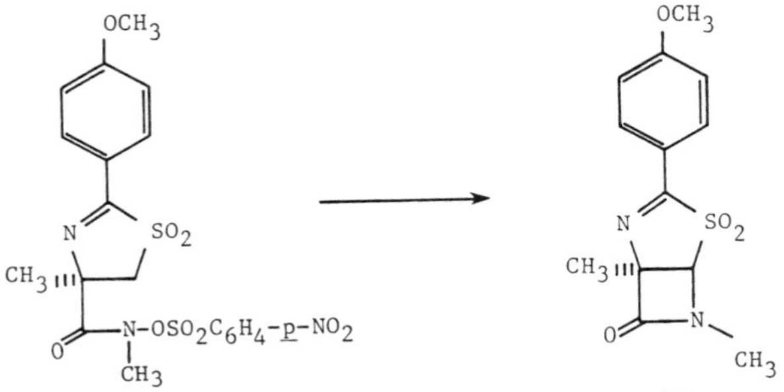

187

188

E.   Other Routes

Over the last several years many novel β-lactam syntheses have been developed. Since most have been reviewed previously (see, e.g., Mukerjee and Srivastava, 1973; Mukerjee and Singh, 1978), only selected examples which may have application in the construction of β-lactam antibiotic nuclear analogs will be discussed in this section.

Of the several reported methods involving ring contraction, only the photolytic Wolff rearrangement used by Lowe and co-workers (Lowe and Yeung, 1973; Hlubucek and Lowe, 1974) produced a monocyclic intermediate that was eventually converted to a bicyclic β-lactam antibiotic nuclear analog (Corrie *et al.*, 1977). Diazoketone **189** gave an approximately equal mixture of *cis-* and *trans-*β-lactams (**190a**) on photolysis in the presence of *tert*-butyl carbazate. The mixture was carried through the same series of reactions used in the bicyclic examples (Section II,D) to yield monocyclic precursors with the usual amide side chain (**190b**). The cis isomer was separated by fractional crystallization, and, after removal of the benzyl groups with sodium in liquid ammonia, the resulting disodium salt was condensed with 1-acetoxy-3-chloroacetone to afford **191.** Only one of the possible stereoisomers appeared to be formed. Dehydration of the tertiary alcohol (**191**) with thionyl chloride in pyridine gave **192a** which was converted to alcohol **192b** with orange peel acetylesterase. Oxidation to the corresponding carboxylic acid was not achieved, but aldehyde **192c** was obtained by treatment of **192b** with 2,3-dichloro-5,6-dicyano-1,4-benzoquinone.

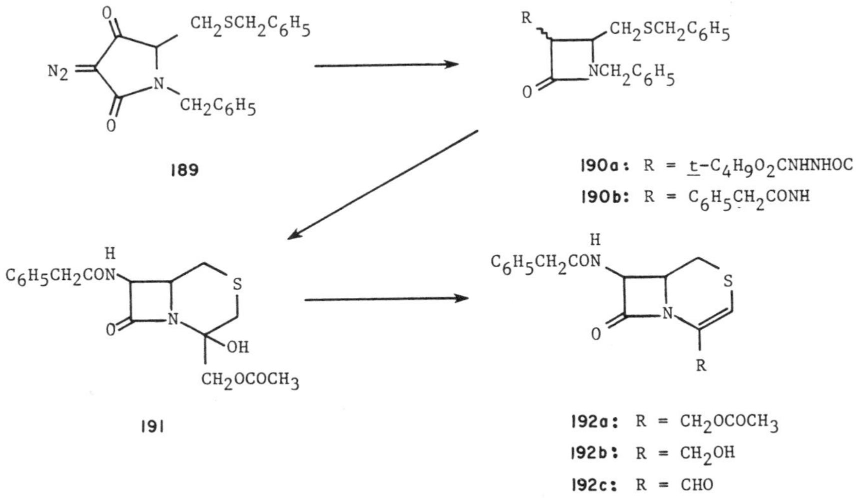

$CH_2SCH_2C_6H_5$
N_2
$CH_2C_6H_5$
R
$NCH_2C_6H_5$
$C_6H_5CH_2CONH$
S
OH
CH_2OCOCH_3
R
189
190a: R = $\underline{t}$-$C_4H_9O_2CNHNHOC$
190b: R = $C_6H_5CH_2CONH$
191
192a: R = CH_2OCOCH_3
192b: R = CH_2OH
192c: R = CHO

Another type of ring contraction that holds considerable promise for the stereospecific formation of *cis*-β-lactams that might be converted to β-lactam antibiotic nuclear analogs is the photolytic contraction of pyridones and pyrazinones (**193**) to give bicyclic β-lactams **194** (Corey and Streith, 1964; DeSelms and Schleigh, 1972; Furrer, 1972). Cleavage of the double bond of **194** affords monocyclic precursors with desirable functionality and stereochemistry (Gleason *et al.*, 1977). An interesting acyclic analog of this ring contraction has been reported (Sen *et al.*, 1977); photolysis of **195** gives **196.**

Other methods of ring contraction that have been reported (Hatch and Johnson, 1974; Johnson and Hatch, 1975a,b; Chasle and Foucaud, 1972; Moore *et al.*, 1976) appear to be less useful for the construction of monocyclic precursors.

Wasserman and co-workers (Wasserman *et al.*, 1971; Wasserman and Glazer, 1975) developed a ring expansion route to β-lactams based on a cyclopropanone intermediate constructed from ketene and diazomethane. The same group (Wasserman and Lipshutz, 1976) also discovered

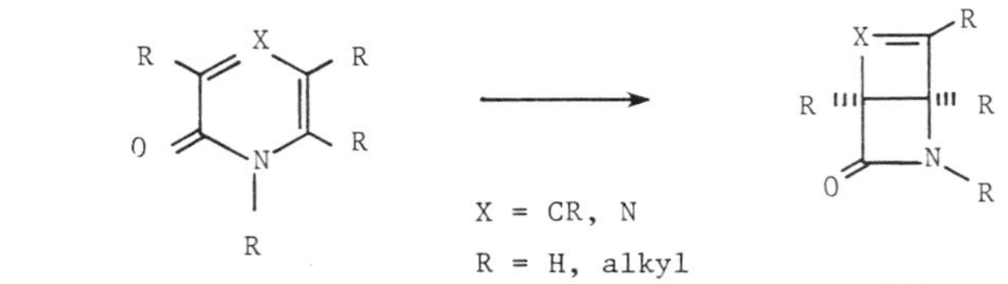

193

194

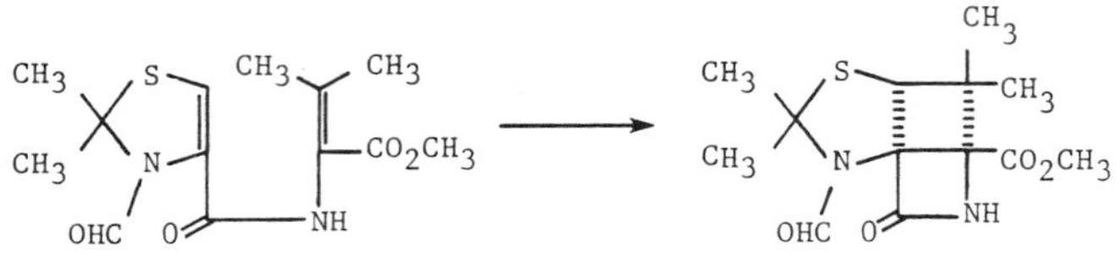

X = CR, N
R = H, alkyl

195

196

that oxygenation of the dianion of N-substituted azetidine-2-carboxylic acids led to the formation of β-lactams in 50–61% yield.

A method for the construction of simple β-lactams involving lactam bond formation (Birkofer and Schramm, 1975), as well as three routes analogous to the ketene–imine cycloaddition, have been reported (De Poortere *et al.*, 1974; Prasad and Petrzilka, 1975; Ojima *et al.*, 1977). The cycloaddition of nitrones with copper acetylides produces mixtures of cis and trans-3,4-disubstituted β-lactams (Ding and Irwin, 1976). Two methods for the construction of β-lactams involving carbon monoxide as the source of the β-lactam carbonyl have been reported (Wong *et al.*, 1977; Mori *et al.*, 1979), as has alkylation of the dianion of amides bearing an α-phenylthio group with methylene diiodide (Hirai and Iwano, 1979). Several reports of the synthesis of monocyclic β-lactams by photolysis of α-ketoamides have appeared (Aoyama *et al.*, 1978, 1979; Shiozaki and Hiraoka, 1979).

IV. Totally Synthetic β-Lactam Antibiotics and Their Nuclear Analogs

A. Summary Tables

Collected in the following tables are selected β-lactam antibiotics and their nuclear analogs that have been produced by total synthesis. A number of structural types are excluded because they were prepared by partial synthesis (Chapter 1) or because they are covered separately in this volume (i.e., thienamycins, clavulanic acids, nocardicins, penems, and their closely related analogs). Also excluded from the tables are a large number of bicyclic β-lactams whose structures are far removed from the natural products and inactive. On the other hand, a few examples of this type are included when they represent novel systems which might indeed display antibacterial activity if proper functionality were present. Totally synthetic β-lactams reviewed previously (Heusler, 1972) are not repeated here.

The tables are organized so that the penicillins (Table I) and cephalosporins (Table II) appear first, followed by analogs in which sulfur has been replaced by oxygen or nitrogen. Analogs in which the heteroatom has been moved one and then two positions around the ring follow. Rings containing two heteroatoms and, finally, carbocyclic analogs complete the entries. Table III lists analogs with rings containing more than six atoms and monocyclic β-lactams of interest as antibacterial agents.

B. Structure–Activity Relationships

When one considers the newly discovered β-lactam antibiotics thienamycin (197) and clavulanic acid (198) (Chapters 4 and 6), it is clear that the structural requirements for good antibacterial activity do not necessarily include an amide side chain at the C-6(7) position oriented cis to the ring fusion as proposed earlier (Fig. 1, structure A). One might also speculate that a bicyclic structure is not even required based on the antibacterial activity of nocardicin (199) (Chapter 5). However, these examples appear to be rather special cases, since penicillins and cephalosporins in which the amide side chain has been replaced by a hydroxyethyl residue corresponding to that in thienamycin (197) are considerably less potent (DiNinno et al., 1977). Similarly, removal of the side chain from penicillin (Evrard et al., 1964) gives a compound (200a) with a very low order of activity. In fact, clavulanic acid (198) is actually a relatively weak antibiotic, its most useful property being the irreversible inhibition of bacterial β-lactamases. Interestingly, sulfone 200b is reported to be a potent β-lactamase inhibitor (English et al., 1978). Nocardicin (199) shows a relatively low order of activity in vitro and prob-

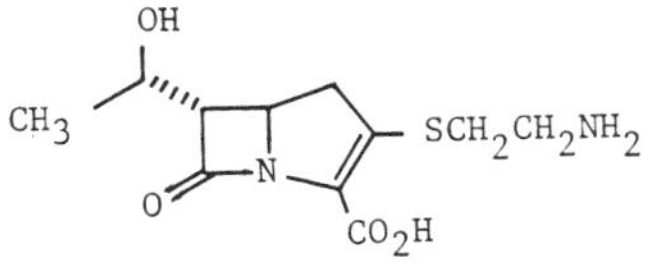

197

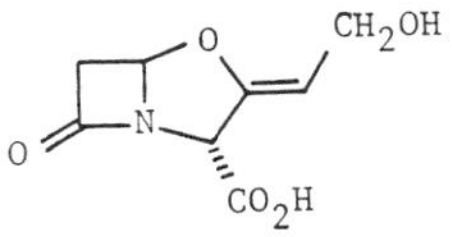

198

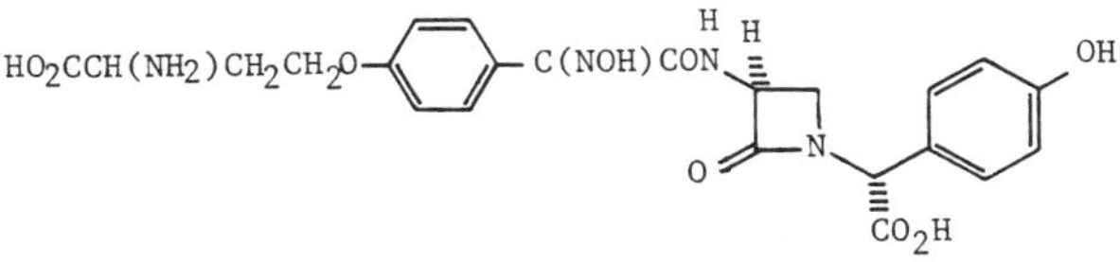

199

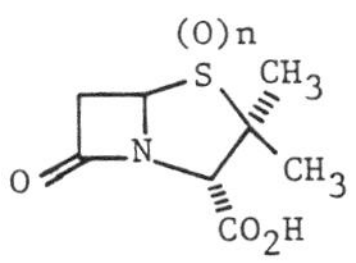

200a: $n = 0$
200b: $n = 2$

TABLE I Penams and Related Ring Systems

Number	Structure	Method of synthesis[a]	Antibacterial activity[b]	Reference
1	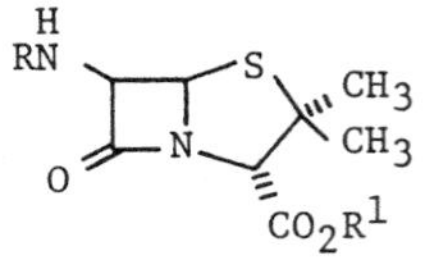 $R = H$; $R^1 = CH_2C_6H_5$	II, B	NR	Firestone et al. (1974a)
2	$R = C_6H_5CO$; $R^1 = CH_3$	III, D	NR	Baldwin et al (1976)
3	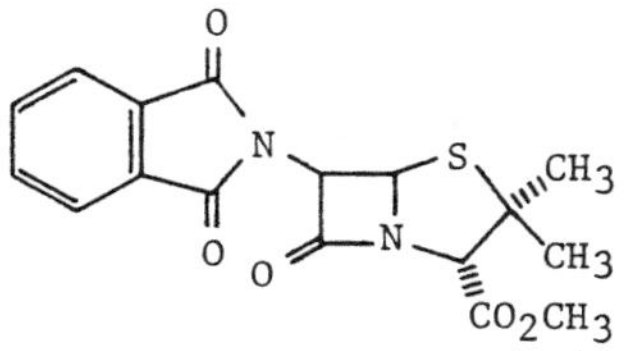 CO_2CH_3	III, B	NR	Bachi et al. (1977)
4	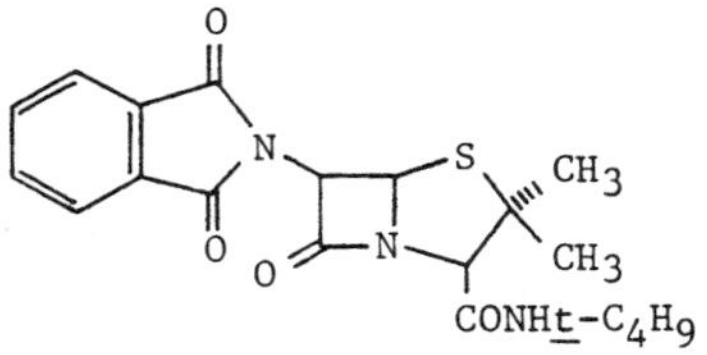 $CONH\underline{t}\text{-}C_4H_9$	II, E	NR	Schutz and Ugi (1979)
5	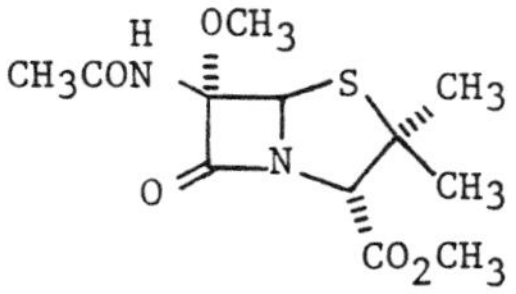 CH_3CON, OCH_3, CO_2CH_3	III, D	NR	Nakatsuka et al. (1975a)
6	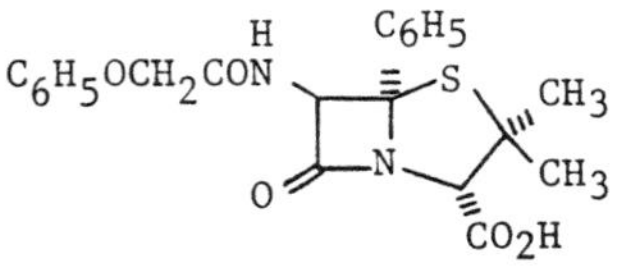 $C_6H_5OCH_2CON$, C_6H_5, CO_2H	II, B	+	Vanderhaeghe and Thomis (1975)
7	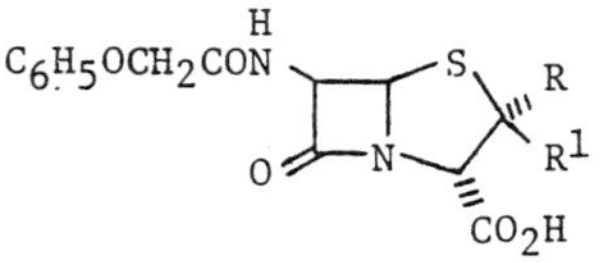 $C_6H_5OCH_2CON$, CO_2H; $R = R^1 = H$	II, A	+ +	Hoogmartens et al. (1974)

TABLE I (Continued)

Number	Structure	Method of synthesis[a]	Antibacterial activity[b]	Reference
8	$R = H;\ R^1 = CH_3$	II, A	+ +	Claes et al. (1975)
9	$R = CH_3;\ R^1 = H$	II, A	+ +	Claes et al. (1975)
10	$R = R^1 = C_2H_5$	II, B	+ +	Claes and Vanderhaeghe (1976)
11	$R + R^1 = (CH_2)_3$	II, B	+ +	Claes et al. (1977)
12	$R + R^1 = (CH_2)_4$	II, B	+ +	Claes et al. (1977); Leclerco et al. (1978)
13	$R + R^1 = (CH_2)_5$	II, B	+ +	Leclerco et al. (1978)
14	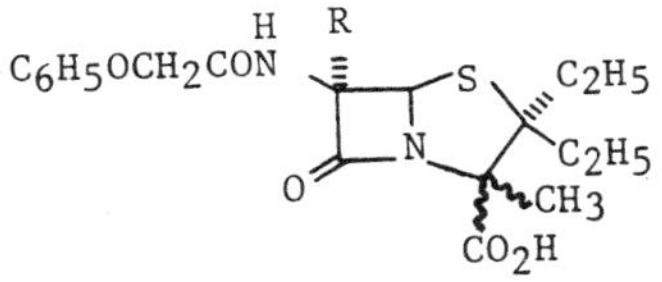 $R = H,\ CH_3$	II, B	0	Meyer et al. (1978)
15	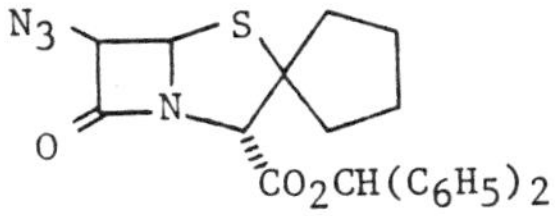	III, B	NR	Bachi and Sasson (1977)
16	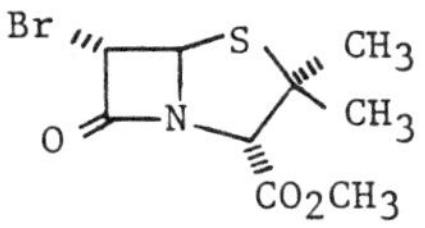	II, C	NR	Johansson and Akermark (1971a)
17	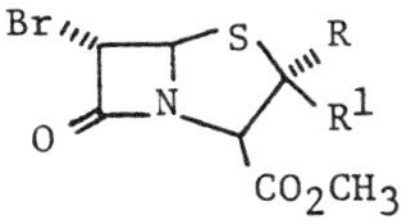 $R = R^1 = H$ or CH_3	II, C	NR	Johansson (1976)

TABLE I (Continued)

Number	Structure	Method of synthesis[a]	Antibacterial activity[b]	Reference
18	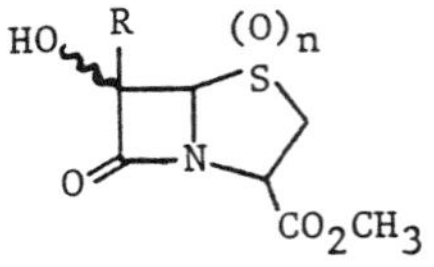 R = CH$_3$, H; n = 0,1,2	II, C	NR	Henery-Logan and Chen (1973)
19	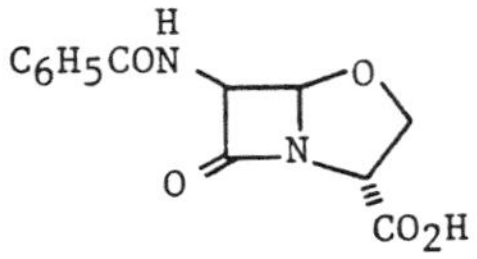	III, B	+	Cama and Christensen (1978a)
20	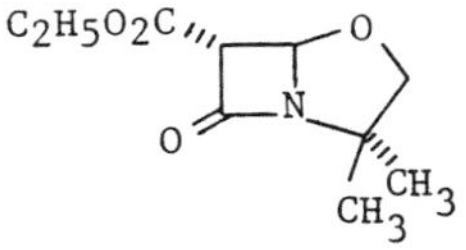	II, C	NR	Golding and Hall (1975)
21	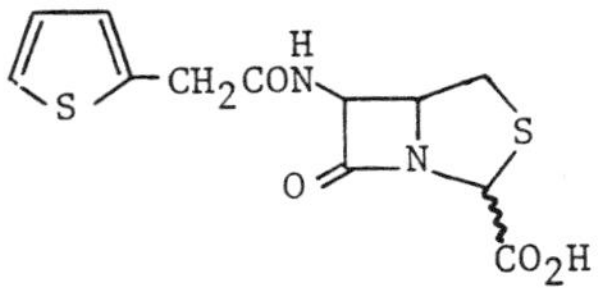	III, B	+ +	Huffman et al. (1978)
22	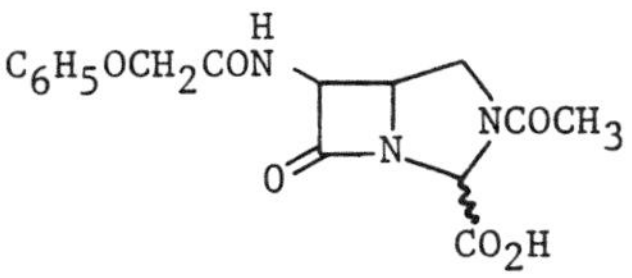	III, B	+	Huffman et al. (1977)
23	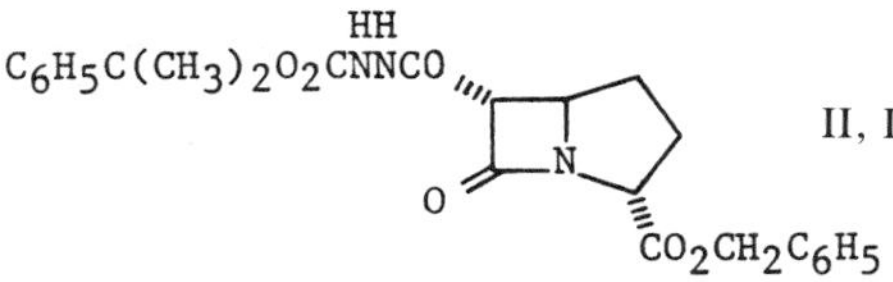	II, D	NR	Lowe and Ridley (1973)

[a] Number of chapter section in which synthesis is described.

[b] + +, Antibacterial potency in the range of clinically useful penicillins and cephalosporins; +, active but of considerably less potency; 0, not active at the highest concentration tested; NR, not reported.

TABLE II Cephams and Related Ring Systems

Number	Structure	Method of synthesis[a]	Antibacterial activity[b]	Reference
1	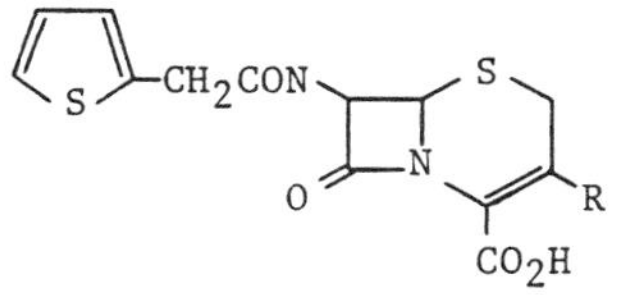 R = CH$_2$OAc	II, B	+ +	Ratcliffe and Christensen (1973b)
2	R = CH(CH$_3$)OAc	II, B	NR	Steinberg *et al.* (1974)
3	R = C$_6$H$_5$, C$_6$H$_4$CO$_2$CH$_3$(p), 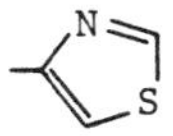 	II, B	NR	Firestone *et al.* (1974b)
4	R = CF$_3$	II, B	NR	Wantanabi *et al.* (1977)
5	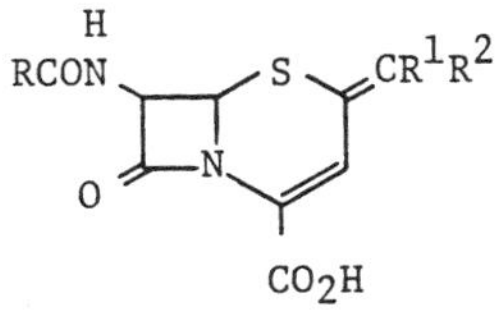 R = C$_6$H$_5$CH$_2$, C$_6$H$_5$OCH$_2$, NCCH$_2$, BrCH$_2$; R^1= H, CH$_3$; R^2= Various alkyl and aryl	III, A	+ +	Woodward *et al.* (1977)
6	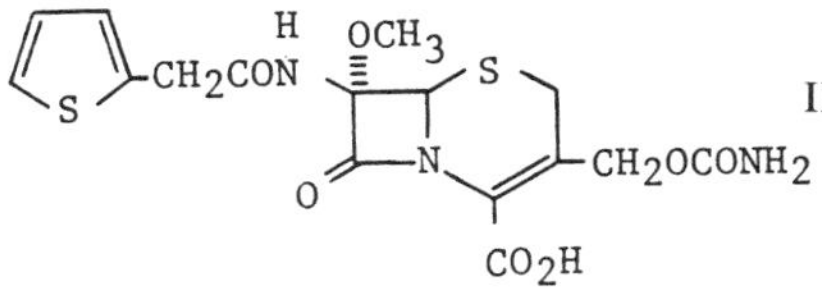	II, B	+ +	Ratcliffe and Christensen (1973c)
7	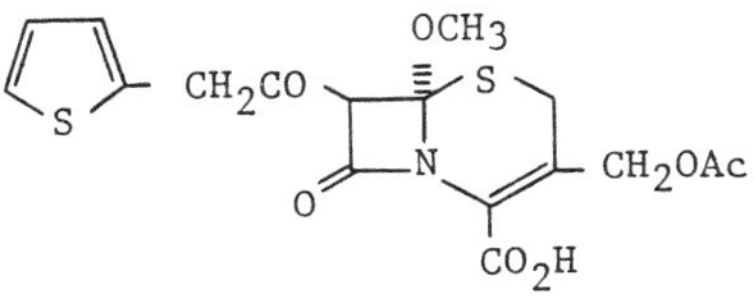	II, B	+	Christensen *et al.* (1977)

(Continued)

TABLE II (Continued)

Number	Structure	Method of synthesis[a]	Antibacterial activity[b]	Reference
8	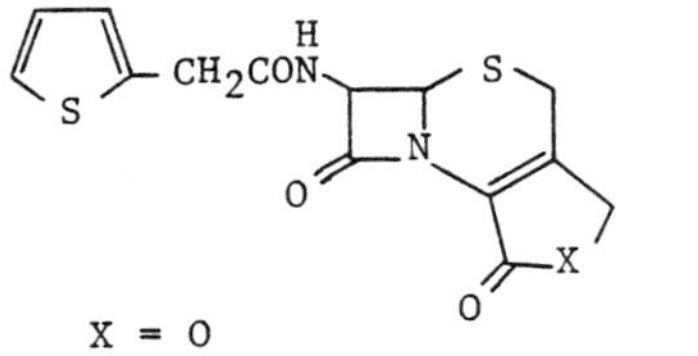 (thiophene)—$CH_2CON\overset{H}{-}$ ... $X = O$	II, A; II, B	NR	Heymes et al. (1974); Edwards et al. (1974)
9	$X = NH$	II, A	NR	Heymes et al. (1977)
10	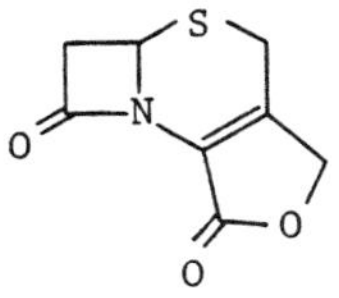 (structure)	III, C	NR	Schmid et al. (1976); Petzilka et al. (1977)
11	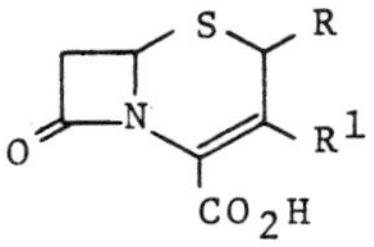 (structure) CO_2H $R = H, CH_3$ $R^1 = CH_3, C_6H_5$	III, C	NR	Bormann (1974)
12	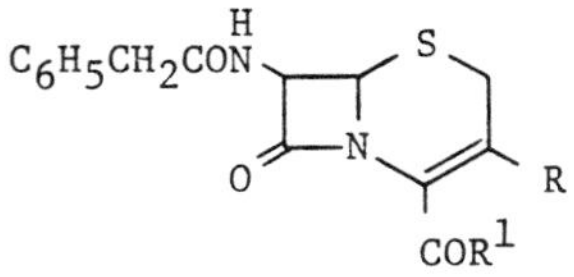 $C_6H_5CH_2CON\overset{H}{-}$ ... COR^1 $R = CH_3, C_6H_5;$ $R^1 = CH_3, C_6H_5, CH_2O_2CCH_3,$ $CH_2CH_2SC_2H_5, CH_2C_6H_5$	III, C	NR	Lattrell and Lohaus (1974c)
13	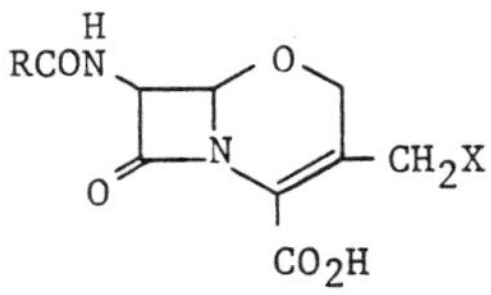 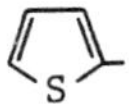 $RCON\overset{H}{-}$ ... CH_2X CO_2H $R =$ (thiophene)—$CH_2;$ $X = OAc$	III, B	+ +	Cama and Christensen (1974)

TABLE II   (Continued)

Number	Structure	Method of synthesis[a]	Antibacterial activity[b]	Reference
14	R = $C_6H_5CH(OH)$; X = S 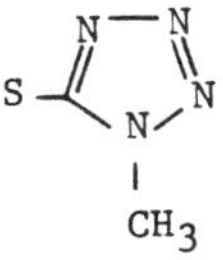	III, B	+ +	Firestone et al. (1977)
15	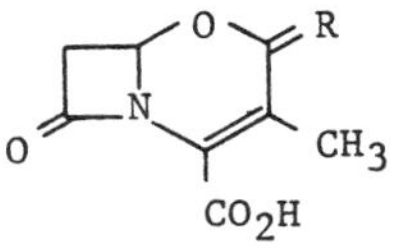 R = H_2, $CHCH_3$	III, C	0	Branch et al. (1978)
16	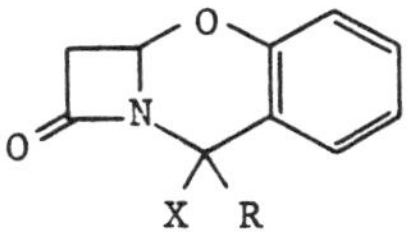 R = H, CH_3; X = OH, $OCOCH_3$, N_3, $CO_2C_2H_5$	III, C	0	Campbell et al. (1979); Shibuya and Kubota (1979)
17	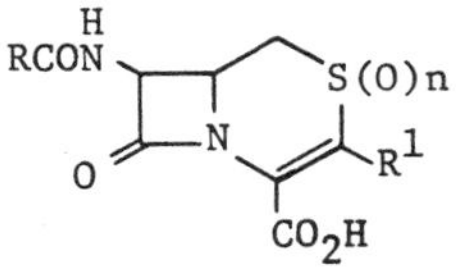 R 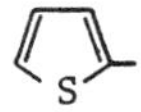 = CH_2, $C_6H_5OCH_2$; R^1 = H, CH_3, CH_2OAc; n = 0, 1, 2	III, B	+ +	Bryan et al. (1977); Doyle et al. (1977f)
18	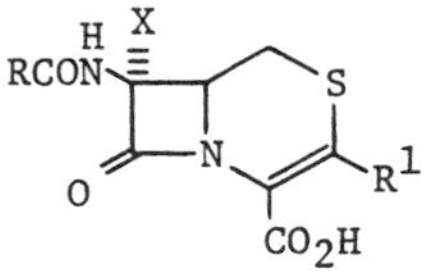 R = $C_6H_5CH_2O$; R^1 = CH_3, X = OCH_3	III, B	0	Douglas et al. (1978)
19	R = $C_6H_5CH_2$; R^1 = H, X = CH_3	II, C	0	Brunwin and Lowe (1973)

(Continued)

TABLE II   (Continued)

Number	Structure	Method of synthesis[a]	Antibacterial activity[b]	Reference
20	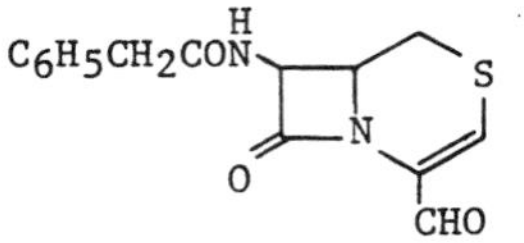	III, E	+	Corrie et al. (1977)
21	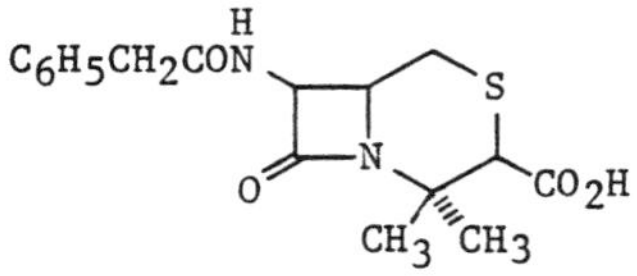	II, C	0	Lowe and Ramsey (1973)
22		III, B	+ +	Doyle et al. (1977b, 1980); Conway et al. (1978)

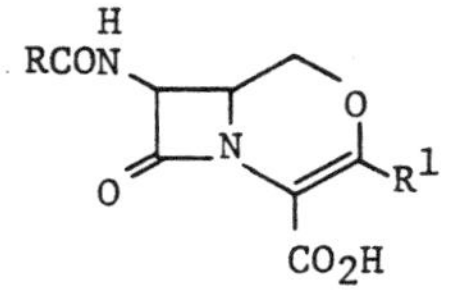

R = $C_6H_5CH_2O$ and many other groups

R^1 = H, CH_3, CH_2X, where X = $OCOCH_3$ and many others groups

| 23 | 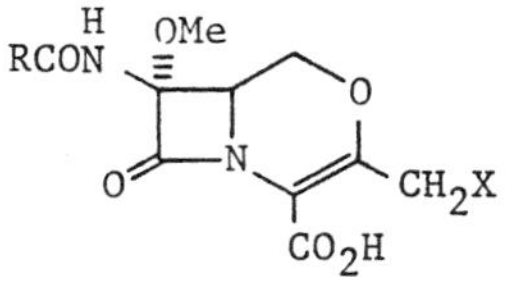 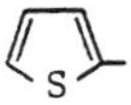 | III, B | + + | Douglas et al. (1978) |

R = CH2; X = OCOCH3

| 24 | R = $C_6H_5OCH_2$; X = H | III, B | 0 | Douglas et al. (1978) |
| 25 | | III, B | + | Doyle et al. (1977c, 1980) |

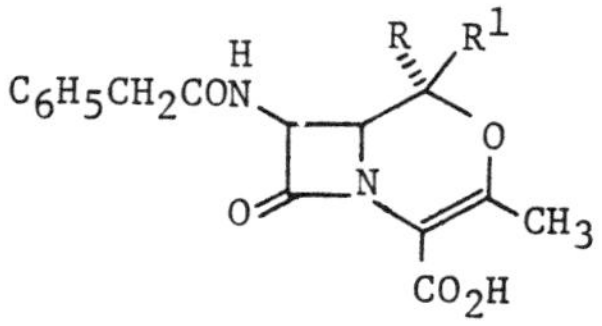

R = H; R^1 = CH_3; R = CH_3, R^1 = H

TABLE II (Continued)

Number	Structure	Method of synthesis[a]	Antibacterial activity[b]	Reference
26	$R + R^1 = O$	III, B	0	Doyle et al. (1977c, 1980)
27	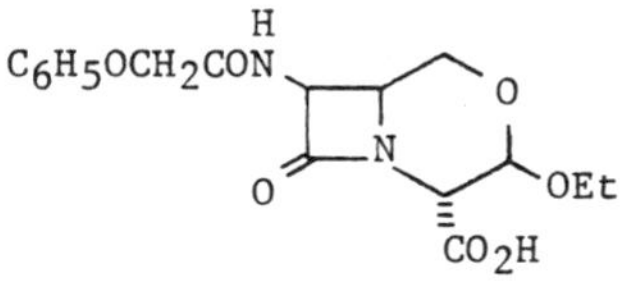	III, B	+	Doyle et al. (1977a,b)
28	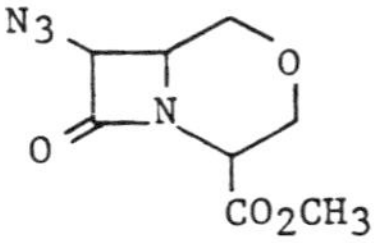	III, B	NR	Just et al. (1979a)
29	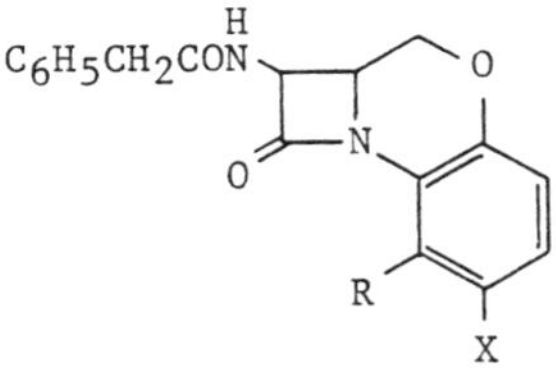 $R = CO_2H; \ X = H$	III, B	0	Just and Zamboni (1978b)
30	$R = H; \ X = OH$	III, B	+	Doyle (1977)
31	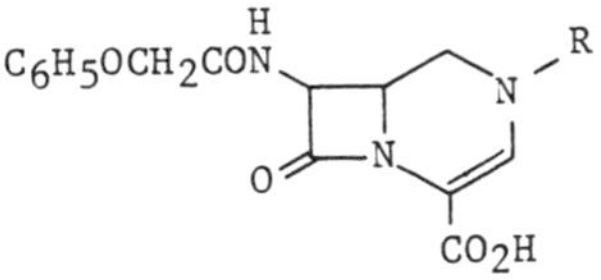 $R = CO_2C_2H_5$	III, B	+	Doyle et al. (1977e, 1980)
32	$R = CH_3$	III, B	0	Doyle et al. (1977e)
33	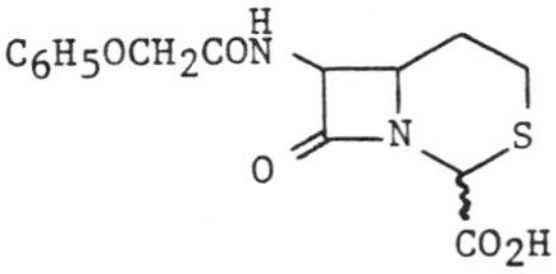	III, B	0	Holden et al. (1979)

(Continued)

TABLE II (Continued)

Number	Structure	Method of synthesis[a]	Antibacterial activity[b]	Reference
34	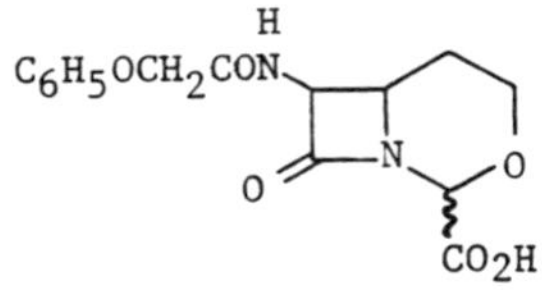	III, B	0	Holden et al. (1979)
35	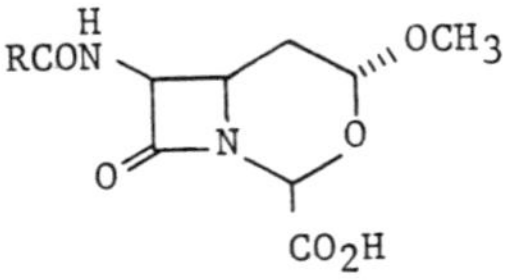 R = $C_6H_5OCH_2$, $C_6H_5CH(OH)$	III, B	+ +	Gleason et al. (1979)
36	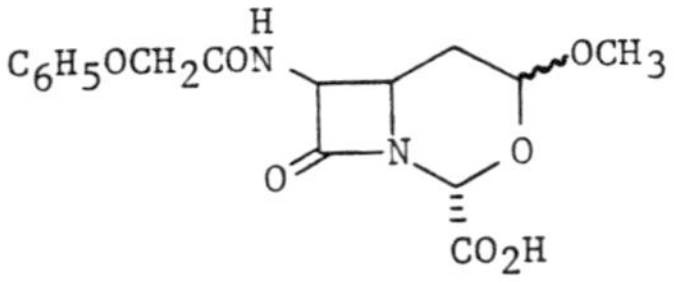	III, B	0	Gleason et al. (1979)
37	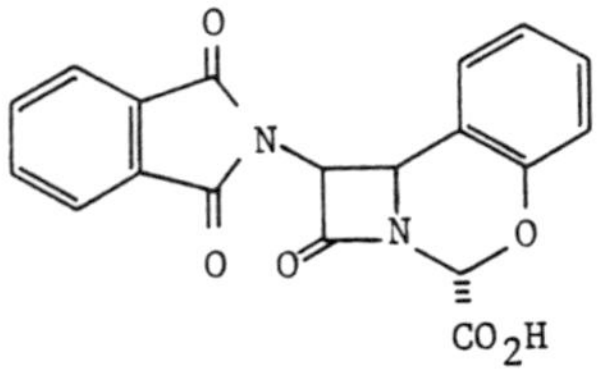	III, B	NR	Kametani et al. (1979d)
38	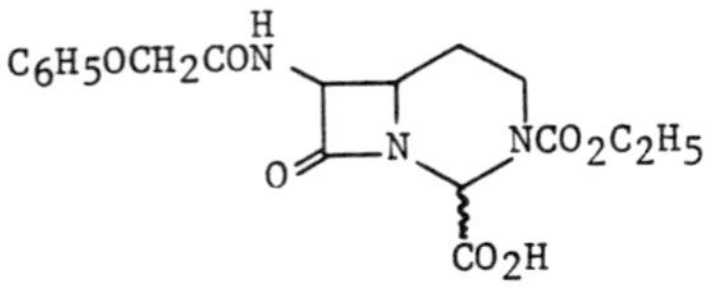	III, B	0	Holden et al. (1979)
39	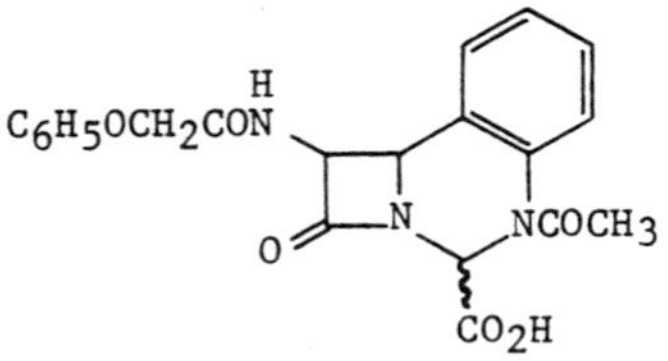	III, B	0	Holden et al. (1979)

TABLE II   (Continued)

Number	Structure	Method of synthesis[a]	Antibacterial activity[b]	Reference
40	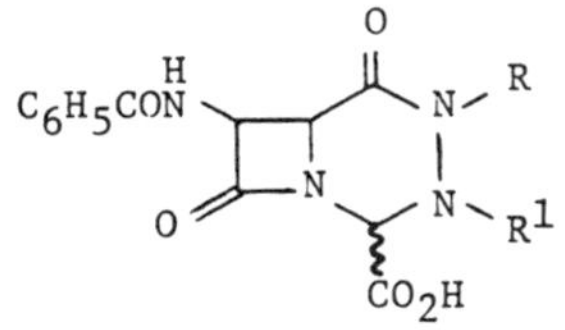 $R + R^1 = (CH_2)_4$, $(CH_2)_3$	III, B	+	Finkelstein et al. (1977)
41	$R + R^1 = CH_2CH_2CO$; $R = H$; $R^1 = CO_2CH_3$		0	Finkelstein et al. (1977)
42	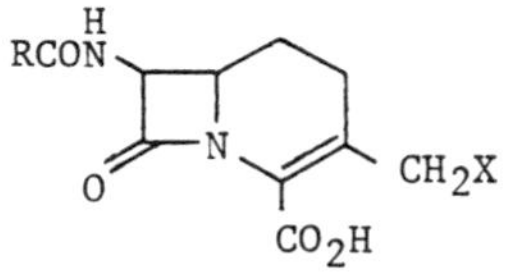 $R = \ce{}$ 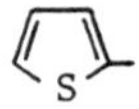 CH_2, $C_6H_5OCH_2$, $C_6H_5CH(OH)$; $X = H$, $OCOCH_3$, 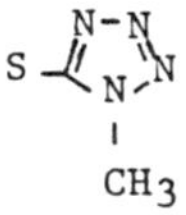	III, B	+ +	Guthikonda et al. (1974); Firestone et al. (1977); Doyle et al. (1979b)
43	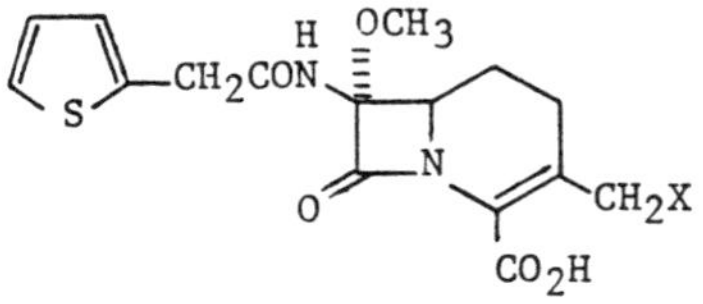 $X = OCONH_2$	III, B	+ +	Firestone et al. (1977)
44	$X = H$	III, B	NR	Firestone et al. (1977)

(Continued)

TABLE II (Continued)

Number	Structure	Method of synthesis[a]	Antibacterial activity[b]	Reference
45	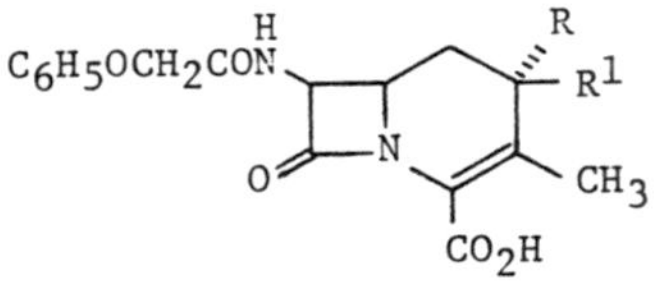 $C_6H_5OCH_2CON$ structure with R, R^1, CH_3, CO_2H R = OH; R^1 = H R = H; R^1 = OH, OAc R + R^1 = O, OCH_2CH_2O R or R^1 = CO_2CH_3 or H R = R^1 = CO_2CH_3	III, B	+ +	Doyle et al. (1979, 1980); Martel et al. (1979)
46	R = OAc, R^1 = H R or R^1 = CO_2H or H	III, B	+	Doyle et al. (1979, 1980); Martel et al. (1979)
47	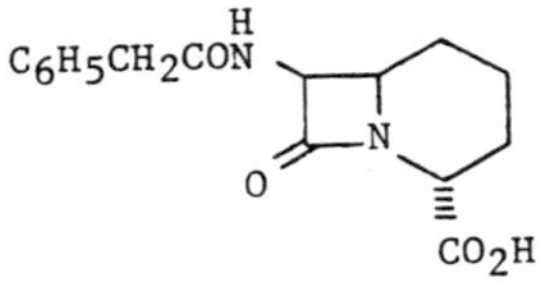 $C_6H_5CH_2CON$ structure with CO_2H	II, C	0	Brunwin et al. (1971)
48	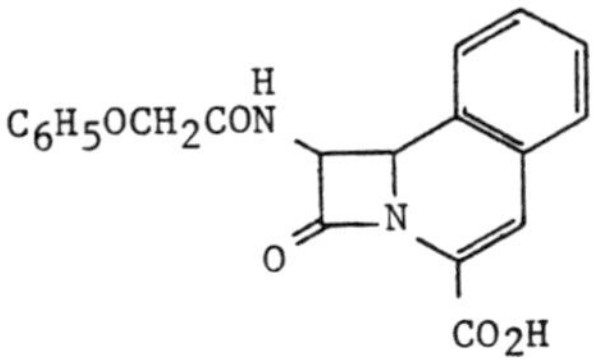 $C_6H_5OCH_2CON$ structure with CO_2H	III, B	+	Finkelstein et al. (1978)
49	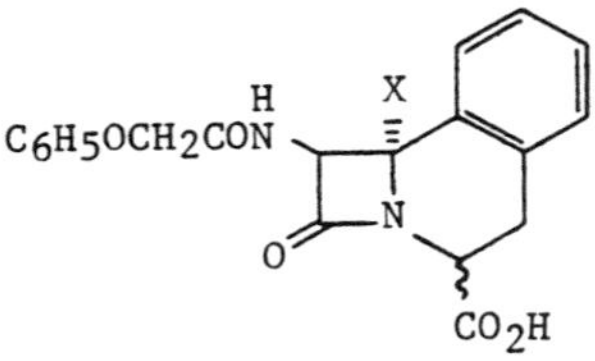 $C_6H_5OCH_2CON$ structure with X, CO_2H X = H, SCH_3	III, B	+	Bose et al. (1979c)

TABLE II (Continued)

Number	Structure	Method of synthesis[a]	Antibacterial activity[b]	Reference
50	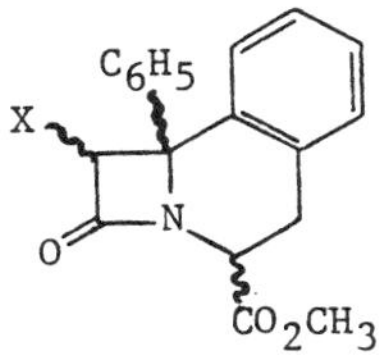 X = C₆H₅O, N₃	III, B	+	Bose et al. (1976)
51	X = C₆H₅OCH₂CONH	III, B	0	Bose et al. (1976)
52	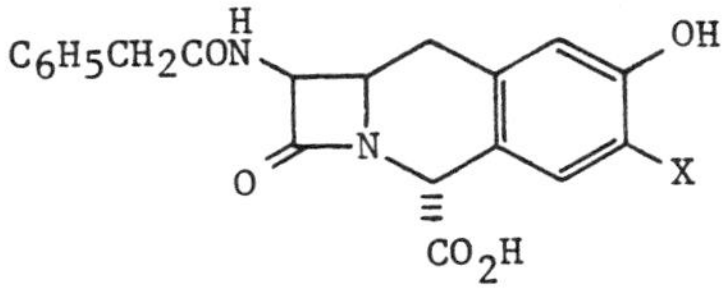 X = H, OH	III, B	0	Hakimelahi and Just (1979)

[a] See Table I, footnote a.
[b] See Table I, footnote b.

ably works by a mechanism different from that of other β-lactam antibiotics. Since acylation of the active site of enzymes involved in bacterial cell wall biosynthesis requires an activated (strained) β-lactam, a monocyclic example such as nocardicin could not be expected to function in this way. Thus, in spite of some apparent exceptions, the structural requirements of **A** in Fig. 1 may still be considered reasonably valid.

The information on antibacterial activity contained in Tables I–III is only a fraction of the information available, since many related structures are covered in other chapters of this book and the previous edition. Accordingly, to facilitate discussion, some information is included from these sources without reference. The general approach to deriving structure–activity relationships from Tables I–III will be to consider the effect of substituents starting at the 1-position and moving around the ring system to C-6(7) for all the analogs related to penams and cephams (Tables I and II). After comparing the various nuclear changes within

TABLE III Other Ring Systems

Number	Structure	Method of synthesis[a]	Antibacterial activity[b]	Reference
1	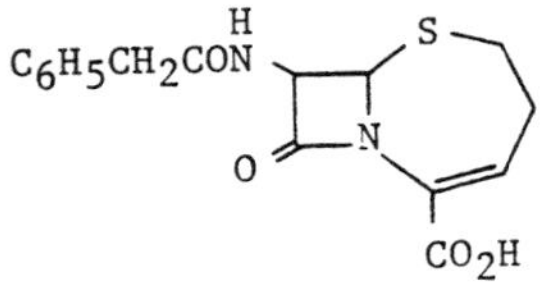	III, A	0	Scartazzini et al. (1972b)
2	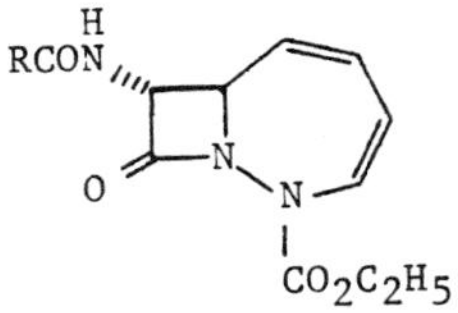 $R = C_6H_5OCH_2, \ C_6H_5CH_2,$ $p\text{-}NO_2C_6H_4CH_2, \ \langle\!\langle{}_S\rangle\!\rangle\text{-}CH_2$ 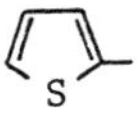	II, B	NR	Streith and Wolff (1976)
3	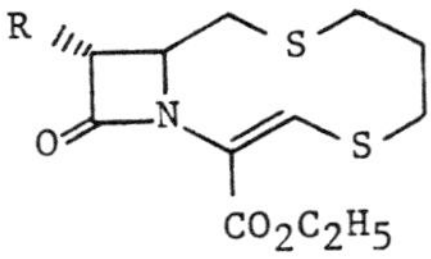 $R = H, \ C_6H_5$	III, B	NR	Kametani et al. (1979b)
4	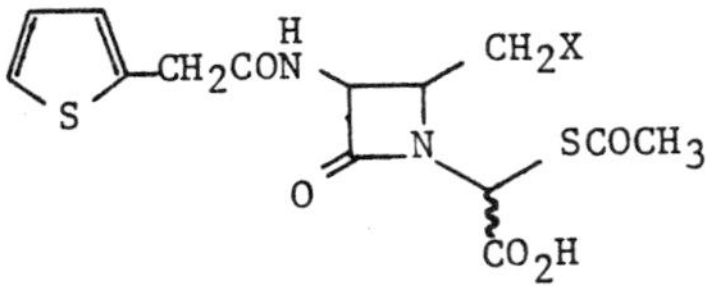 $X = I, \ Br, \ Cl$	III, B	+ +	Huffman et al. (1978); Holden et al. (1979)
5	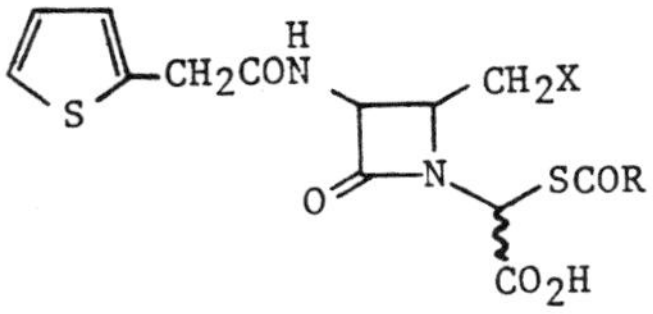 $X = OSO_2C_6H_4CH_3\text{-}p, \ R = CH_3$ $X = I, \ R = C_6H_5$	III, B	+	Holden et al. (1979)

TABLE III (Continued)

Number	Structure	Method of synthesis[a]	Antibac-terial activity[b]	Reference
6	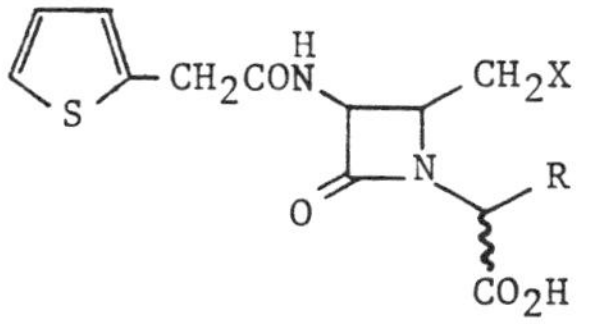 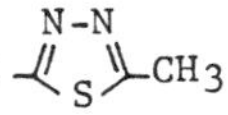	III, B	0	Holden et al. (1979)
7	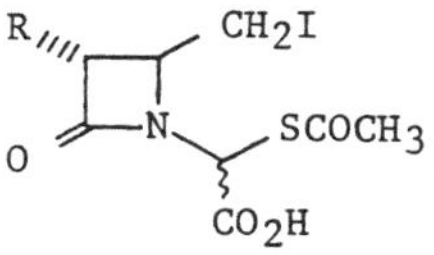	III, B	0	Holden et al. (1979)
8	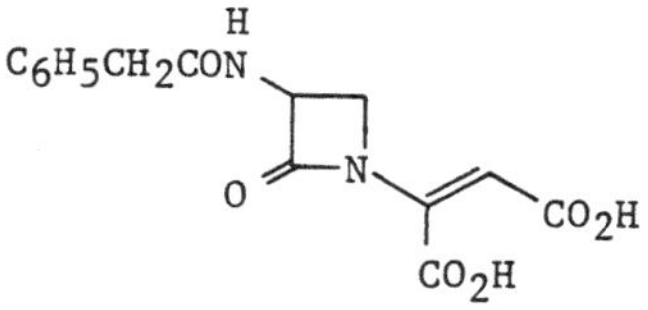	III, E	0	Lowe and Yeung (1973)
9	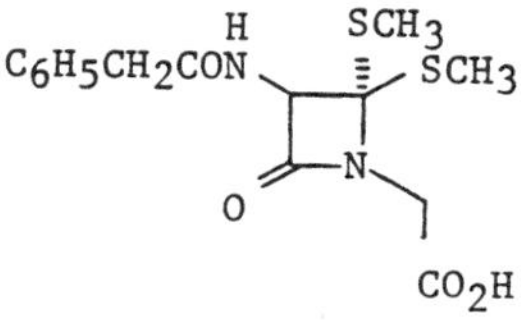	III, B	0	Sullivan et al. (1976)
10	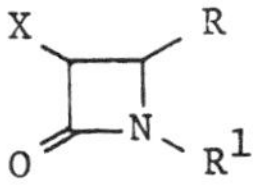	III, B	+	Bose et al. (1974)

For 6:

X = $OCOCH_3$, OH, $SCH_2C_6H_5$, CH_2CH_2I;
R = $SCOCH_3$;

X = I; R = $OCOCH_3$, H, S—[N-N ring with S, CH_3]

For 7:

R = H, $CH_3CH(OH)$

For 10:

X = OCH_3, NH_2, OC_6H_5;
R = aryl;
R^1 = aryl, $CH_2C_6H_5$, $CH(C_6H_5)_2$, C_6H_{11}

(Continued)

TABLE III (Continued)

Number	Structure	Method of synthesis[a]	Antibacterial activity[b]	Reference
11	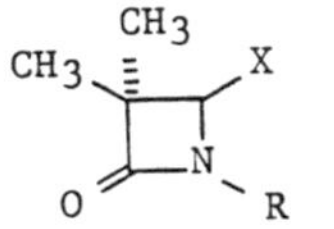 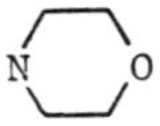 X = N(CH₃)₂, N⟨ ⟩O ; R = substituted phenyl	III, C	+	Abdulla and Fuhr (1975)

[a] See Table I, footnote a.
[b] See Table I, footnote b.

the same two series, larger ring systems and monocyclic β-lactams found in Table III will be discussed.

Substituents on C-1, the position normally occupied by sulfur in the natural series, seem to be detrimental to good antibacterial activity (compare 22 with 25 and 42 with 48 in Table II). Also, penicillin and cephalosporin sulfoxides and sulfones derived from the natrual products often show markedly decreased antibacterial activity.

The change in bulk and lipophilicity introduced by modification of the C-2 methyl groups in penicillin (Table I: 7–16) does not greatly affect antibacterial potency. Similarly, in the cephalosporin series modified substituents at C-2 and C-3 do not appear to decrease activity appreciably (Table II: 5, 17, 22, 45). Unfortunately, antibacterial testing results have not been reported for a number of analogs of this type (Table II: 2–4, 11, 12).

The need for a free carboxyl group at C-3(4) seems to be a universal requirement for good activity. Cephalosporin lactones (Table II: 8) may retain some activity as a result of enzymic hydrolysis *in vitro*. The corresponding amide (Table II: 9) would be expected to be essentially inactive. The cephalosporin bearing a methyl group on the 3-acetoxymethyl substituent (Table II: 2) is reported to lactonize spontaneously ($t_{1/2} = 20$ min at 37°C), which should decrease its activity appreciably. Other structures lacking a C-4 carboxyl in the cephalosporin series have little activity (Table II: 12, 16, 20, 21, 29, 30).

Introduction of a phenyl substituent at the C-5 position of penicillin

(Table I: 6) markedly reduces activity. Similarly, introduction of a methoxy group at the C-6 bridgehead position in a cephalosporin (Table II: 7) is quite detrimental.

Although not apparent from the data presented, introduction of a methoxy or methyl group at C-6 (Table I: 5, 15) is known to diminish greatly or eliminate antibacterial activity in the penicillin series. In the cephalosporin series a methoxy group at C-7 can be tolerated (Table II: 6) and even expands the spectrum of antibacterial activity (see Volume 1, Chapter 3). However, this is not true when the C-3 methyl lacks a good leaving group; for example, in Table II compare 17 with 18 and 23 with 24. A methyl group at C-7 is also deleterious in all known examples (Table II: 19).

It is clear from inspection of the tables that the sulfur atom at C-1 common to both penicillins and cephalosporins is not required for activity. It can be replaced by oxygen or carbon, or the heteroatom may be moved around the ring and good activity still retained. In the case of oxygen substitution in the penicillin series (Table I: 20), the decreased activity is probably due to limited stability. The same is true of the 1-dethia-2-aza analog (Table I: 22), whereas the corresponding thia derivative (Table I: 21) is stable enough to have reasonable antibacterial potency. In the cephalosporin series, the 1-dethia analogs having an oxygen at the 1-position, sulfur or oxygen at the 2-position, or no heteroatom all have antibacterial activity in the range of naturally derived cephalosporins (Table II: 13, 14, 17, 22, 23, 42–45). The 1-dethia-2-aza analog (Table II: 32) is inactive because of instability, whereas the more stable carbamate (Table II: 31) has reduced activity compared to the other analogs.

In the cephalosporin series, the 3,4-double bond has always been considered essential for good antibacterial activity. All the nuclear analogs lacking this feature (Table II: 27, 33, 34, 36, 38, 39, 40, 47, 49–52) have, at best, weak activity. There is, however, one outstanding exception (Table II: 35). X-Ray crystallography indicates that the β-lactam nitrogen of this analog is significantly distorted out of the plane defined by the three other atoms to which it is joined. The degree of deformation is in the range of that of active cephalosporins and considerably greater than in inactive Δ^2-cephalosporins. The observed spatial orientation of the carboxyl group is actually quite close to that of Δ^3-cephalosporins. This suggests that the relationship between the carboxyl group and the β-lactam bond, and not the relative configuration of the carboxyl, may be important for enzyme recognition and antibacterial activity. The lack of activity of closely related structures (Table II: 34, 36) is more difficult to explain. One could assume that the orientation of the carboxyl group is detrimental to enzyme recognition in the isomer (Table II: 36), whereas the necessity for participation of the methoxy group, possibly by concerted elimination during β-lactam cleavage, could explain the inactivity of the desmethoxy derivative (Table II: 34).

Since deformation of the β-lactam nitrogen is a major source of activation, it might be anticipated that the fusion of rings containing more than six atoms would decrease strain to the point where acylating power, hence antibacterial activity, would be eliminated. The best evidence that this is so is provided by a homocephalosporin (Table III: 1). Other examples (Table III: 2, 3) lack proper functionality and stereochemistry. Similarly, monocyclic β-lactams are expected to be inactive because of a lack of reactivity. Two examples of this type (Table III: 8, 9) were indeed inactive. Other monocyclic β-lactams (Table III: 10, 11) showed weak activity probably unrelated to the type of antibacterial activity associated with penicillins and cephalosporins. One series of monocyclic β-lactams (Table III: 4) showed clinically useful levels of antibacterial activity almost surely due to their *in situ* cyclization to 1-dethia-2-thiapenicillins (Table I: 22). Liberation of the thiol by hydrolysis, perhaps by a bacterial enzyme, results in spontaneous cyclization when a good leaving group is present (Table III: 4). However, the presence of a poorer leaving group or a less easily generated thiol gives compounds with weaker activity (Table III: 5). When either no leaving group is present or a thiol cannot be formed, inactive compounds result (Table III: 6). In the case of the homologous iodide (Table III: 6, X = CH_2CH_2I) cyclization can take place, but the product is known to be inactive (Table II: 33). Monocyclic precursors of the 1-dethia-2-thiapenicillin ring system lacking the amide side chain (Table III: 7) are essentially inactive, as are the corresponding penicillins and cephalosporins discussed earlier. It may turn out that the normal amide side chain is required for most β-lactams and that only in cases where a particularly reactive nucleus is present can other groups be substituted.

Since the method of presenting the antibacterial activity in Tables I–III allows only a rough approximation, the original literature should be consulted for more precise information. Relatively small, but perhaps significant, differences in antibacterial potency and spectrum may become apparent on closer inspection. It is hoped that the structure–activity relationships presented here coupled with new information regarding the sites and mechanism of action of β-lactam antibiotics will lead to the design and synthesis of new nuclear analogs with enhanced antibacterial properties.

V. Summary

Since the first compilation of information on the total synthesis of β-lactam antibiotics and their nuclear analogs (Heusler, 1972), a number of reviews have appeared which cover, at least in part, some additional aspects of this subject (Gleason, 1975; Gleason and Dunn, 1977; Gleason and Kingsbury, 1979; Lowe, 1975, 1979; Sammes, 1976; Christensen and Ratcliffe, 1976; Cama and Christensen, 1978b; Mukerjee and Srivastava, 1973; Mukerjee and Singh, 1975, 1978; Jaszberenyi and Gunda, 1975; Gunda and Jaszberenyi, 1977; Holden *et al.*, 1979; Doyle *et al.*, 1980). In this chapter an attempt has been made to compile the most significant work on this subject since 1972 in such a way that the differences in synthetic approach are clearly apparent and the relationship of structure to antibacterial activity can be appreciated.

In terms of synthesis, schemes in which the β-lactam ring is formed early in the sequence have proved most effective in producing bicyclic β-lactams with the proper functionality and stereochemistry for good antibacterial activity. Among routes of this type, the ketene–imine cycloaddition reaction has been used most often for construction of the key monocyclic β-lactam intermediate. This route is particularly effective for the synthesis of 1-dethia-2-hetero nuclear analogs, since the desired cis-substituted β-lactam is obtained stereospecifically. Closure of the second ring can be accomplished in a variety of ways, but for the construction of very strained bicyclic systems mild conditions are required. In addition, a relatively energetic intermediate, such as a carbene, may be most appropriate for difficult closures of this type. Total synthesis of β-lactam antibiotics or their nuclear analogs has not yet evolved to the point where this route can compete with partial synthesis on a commercial scale. However, total synthesis has provided access to nuclear analogs difficult to obtain by partial degradation and resynthesis from the natural products.

The nuclear analogs synthesized over the last several years and the isolation of three new classes of β-lactams of microbial origin have caused considerable revision of some of the long-held tenets of structure–activity relationships based on modified penicillins and cephalosporins. While acylation of the active site of enzymes required for bacterial cell wall biosynthesis appears to be the mechanism by which β-lactam antibiotics and their nuclear analogs kill bacteria, it now appears that there are multiple killing sites and that the relative affinity for these sites varies considerably among β-lactams of different structure. Further complications in understanding the relationship of structure to antibiotic activity are provided by the instability of some of the more strained systems under physiological conditions, degradation by bacterial β-lactamases or the ability to inhibit them irreversibly, and barriers to penetration to the site of action. In spite of these difficulties, it is clear that a reactive β-lactam with a free carboxyl group appropriately positioned with respect to the β-lactam carbonyl is a minimum requirement for activity. Activation is achieved by fusion of a second five or six-membered ring. In six-membered rings a double bond conjugated to the carboxyl is usually required for good activity. In addition, when the β-lactam is not exceedingly reactive, an amide side chain oriented cis to the fused ring seems to be essential. In some cases further fragmentation of the ring system following opening of the β-lactam may be an important feature for antibacterial activity.

Information gained from the diverse ring systems investigated thus far suggests that, to achieve large increases in antibacterial potency and spectrum above those displayed by penicillins and cephalosporins, highly strained (reactive) β-lactams will be the most likely candidates. The lack of stability of such ring systems not only poses a synthetic challenge but also presents a practical problem in delivery of the drug to the site of action. The design of a β-lactam with the proper balance of stability to hydrolysis coupled with the ability to penetrate to the site of action and react rapidly with bacterial enzymes, but having no appreciable effect on the host, remains a challenge for future. research.

References

Abdulla, R. F., and Fuhr, K. H. (1975). *J. Med. Chem.* **18,** 625.
Akermark, B., and Johansson, N. G. (1969). *Tetrahedron Lett.* p. 371.
Akermark, B., Lagerlund, I., and Lewandowska, J. (1974). *Acta Chem. Scand., Sect. B.* **28,** 1238.
Amin, S. G., Glazer, R. D., and Manhas, M. S. (1979). *Synthesis* p. 210.
Aoyama, H., Hasegawa, T., Watabe, M., Shiraishi, H., and Omote, Y. (1978). *J. Org. Chem.* **43,** 419.
Aoyama, H., Hasegawa, T., and Omote, Y. (1979). *J. Am. Chem. Soc.* **101,** 5343.
Bachi, M. D., and Ross-Petersen, K. J. (1975). *J.C.S. Perkin I* p. 2525.
Bachi, M. D., and Sasson, S. (1977). *In* "Recent Advances in the Chemistry of β-Lactam Antibiotics" (J. Elks, ed.), Spec. Publ. No. 28, p. 277. Chem. Soc., London.
Bachi, M. D., and Vaya, J. (1976). *J. Am. Chem. Soc.* **98,** 7825.
Bachi, M. D., and Vaya, J. (1977). *Tetrahedron Lett.* p. 2209.
Bachi, M. D., and Vaya, J. (1979). *J. Org. Chem.* **44,** 4393.
Bachi, M. D., Frydman, N., Sasson, S., Stern, C., and Vaya, J. (1977). *Tetrahedron Lett.* p. 641.
Baldwin, J. E., Au, A., Christie, M., Haber, S. B., and Hesson, D. (1975). *J. Am. Chem. Soc.* **97,** 5957.

Baldwin, J. E., Christie, M. A., Haber, S. B., and Kruse, L. I. (1976). *J. Am. Chem. Soc.* **98**, 3045.

Barton, D. H. R., Buschmann, E., Hausler, J., Holzapfel, C. W., Sheradsky, T., and Taylor, D. A. (1977). *J.C.S. Perkin I* p. 1107.

Bellus, D. (1975). *Helv. Chim. Acta* **58**, 2509.

Bender, D. R., Bjeldanes, L. F., Knapp, D. R., and Rapoport, H. (1975a). *J. Org. Chem.* **40**, 1264.

Bender, D., Rapoport, H., and Bordner, J. (1975b). *J. Org. Chem.* **40**, 3208.

Benn, M. H., and Mitchell, R. E. (1972). *Can. J. Chem.* **50**, 2195.

Birkofer, L., and Schramm, J. (1975). *Justus Liebigs Ann. Chem.* p. 2195.

Bormann, D. (1974). *Justus Liebigs Ann. Chem.* p. 1391.

Borowski, S. J., and Kamholz, K. K. (1976). *Chem. Eng. News* Oct. 25, p. 5.

Bose, A. K., and Fahey, J. L. (1974). *J. Org. Chem.* **39**, 115.

Bose, A. K., Spiegelmann, G., and Manhas, M. D. (1968). *J. Am. Chem. Soc.* **90**, 4506.

Bose, A. K., Sharma, S. D., Kapur, J. C., and Manhas, M. S. (1973). *Tetrahedron Lett.* p. 2319.

Bose, A. K., Manhas, M. S., Kapur, J. C., Sharma, S. D., and Amin, S. G. (1974). *J. Med. Chem.* **17**, 541.

Bose, A. K., Manhas, M. S., Chawla, H. P. S., and Dayal, B. (1975). *J.C.S. Perkin I* p. 1880.

Bose, A. K., Amin, S. G., Kapur, J. C., and Manhas, M. S. (1976). *J.C.S. Perkin I* p. 2193.

Bose, A. K., Hoffmann, W. A., and Manhas, M. S. (1977). *In* "Recent Advances in the Chemistry of β-Lactam Antibiotics" (J. Elks, ed.), Spec. Publ. No. 28, p. 269. Chem. Soc., London.

Bose, A. K., Manhas, M. S., Amin, S. G., Kapur, J. C., Kreder, J., Mukkavilli, L., Ram, B., and Vincent, J. E. (1979a). *Tetrahedron Lett.* p. 2771.

Bose, A. K., Ram, B., Amin, S. G., Mukkavilli, L., Vincent, J. E., and Manhas, M. S. (1979b). *Synthesis* p. 543.

Bose, A. K., Ram, B., Hoffman, W. A., Hutchison, A. J., and Manhas, M. S. (1979c). *J. Heterocycl. Chem.* **16**, 1313.

Branch, C. L., Nayler, J. H. C., and Pearson, M. J. (1978). *J.C.S. Perkin I* p. 1450.

Brown, A. G., Corbett, D. F., and Howarth, T. T. (1977). *Chem. Commun.* p. 359.

Brunwin, D. M., and Lowe, G. (1973). *J.C.S. Perkin I* p. 1321.

Brunwin, D. M., Lowe, G., and Parker, J. (1971). *J. Chem. Soc. C* p. 3756.

Bryan, D. B., Hall, R. F., Holden, K. G., Huffman, W. F., and Gleason, J. G. (1977). *J. Am. Chem. Soc.* **99**, 2353.

Cama, L. D., and Christensen, B. G. (1974). *J. Am. Chem. Soc.* **96**, 7582.

Cama, L. D., and Christensen, B. G. (1978a). *Tetrahedron Lett.* p. 4233.

Cama, L. D., and Christensen, B. G. (1978b). *Ann. Rep. Med. Chem.* **13**, 149.

Campbell, M. M., Nelson, K. H., and Cameron, A. F. (1979). *Chem. Commun.* p. 532.

Chasle, M.-F., and Foucaud, A. (1972). *Bull. Chim. Soc. Fr.* p. 195.

Christensen, B. G., and Ratcliffe, R. W. (1976). *Ann. Rep. Med. Chem.* **11**, 271.

Christensen, B. G., Hoogsteen, K., Plavac, F., and Ratcliffe, R. W. (1977). *In* "Recent Advances in the Chemistry of β-Lactam Antibiotics" (J. Elks, ed.), Spec. Publ. No. 28, Chem. Soc., London.

Claes, P. J., and Vanderhaeghe, H. (1976). *Eur. J. Med. Chem.* **11**, 359.

Claes, P. J., Hoogmartens, J., Janssen, G., and Vanderhaeghe, H. (1975). *Eur. J. Med. Chem.* **10**, 573.

Claes, P. J., Janssen, G., and Vanderhaeghe, H. (1977). *Eur. J. Med. Chem.* **12**, 521.

Clauss, K., Grimm, D., and Prossel, G. (1974). *Justus Liebigs Ann. Chem.* p. 539.
Conway, T. T., Lim, G., Douglass, J. L., Menard, M., Doyle, T. W., Rivest, P., Horning, D., Morris, L. R., and Cimon, D. (1978). *Can. J. Chem.* **56**, 1335.
Corey, E. J., and Felix, A. M. (1965). *J. Am. Chem. Soc.* **87**, 2518.
Corey, E. J., and Streith, J. (1964). *J. Am. Chem. Soc.* **86**, 950.
Corrie, J. E. T., Hlubucek, J. R., and Lowe, G. (1977). *J.C.S. Perkin I* p. 1421.
Decazes, J. M., Luche, J. L., and Kagan, H. B. (1972). *Tetrahedron Lett.* p. 3633.
De Poortere, M., Marchand-Brynaert, J., and Ghosez, L. (1974). *Angew. Chem.* **13**, 267.
DeSelms, R. C., and Schleigh, W. R. (1972). *Tetrahedron Lett.* p. 3563.
Ding, L. K., and Irwin, W. J. (1976). *J.C.S. Perkin I* p. 2382.
DiNinno, F., Beattie, T. R., and Christensen, B. G. (1977). *J. Org. Chem.* **42**, 2960.
Douglas, J. L., Horning, D. E., and Conway, T. T. (1978). *Can. J. Chem.* **56**, 2879.
Doyle, T. W. (1977). *Can. J. Chem.* **55**, 2714.
Doyle, T. W., Belleau, B., Luh, B.-Y., Ferrari, C. F., and Cunningham, M. P. (1977a). *Can. J. Chem.* **55**, 468.
Doyle, T. W., Belleau, B., Luh, B.-Y., Conway, T. T., Menard, M., Douglas, J. L., Chu, D. T.-W., Lim, G., Morris, L. R., Rivest, P., and Casey, M. (1977b). *Can. J. Chem.* **55**, 484.
Doyle, T. W., Luh, B.-Y., and Martel, A. (1977c). *Can. J. Chem.* **55**, 2700.
Doyle, T. W., Martel, A., and Luh, B.-Y. (1977d). *Can. J. Chem.* **55**, 2708.
Doyle, T. W., Luh, B.-Y., Chu, D. T.-W., and Belleau, B. (1977e). *Can. J. Chem.* **55**, 2719.
Doyle, T. W., Douglas, J. L., Belleau, B., Meunier, J., and Luh, B.-Y. (1977f). *Can. J. Chem.* **55**, 2873.
Doyle, T. W., Conway, T. T., Casey, M., and Lim, G. (1979a). *Can. J. Chem.* **57**, 222.
Doyle, T. W., Conway, T. T., Lim, G., and Luh, B.-Y. (1979b). *Can. J. Chem.* **57**, 227.
Doyle, T. W., Douglas, J. L., Belleau, B., Conway, T. T., Ferrari, L., Horning, D. E., Lim, G., Luh, B.-Y., Martel, A., Menard, M., and Morris, L. R. (1980). *Can. J. Chem.* **58**, 2508.
Duran, F., and Ghosez, L. (1970). *Tetrahedron Lett.* p. 245.
Edwards, J. A., Guzman, A., Johnson, R., Beeby, P. J., and Fried, J. H. (1974). *Tetrahedron Lett.* p. 2031.
English, A. R., Retsema, J. A., Girard, A. E., Lynch, J. E., and Barth, W. E. (1978). *Antimicrob. Agents Chemother.* **14**, 414.
Evrard, E., Claesen, M., and Vanderhaeghe, H. (1964). *Nature (London)* **201**, 1124.
Finkelstein, J., Holden, K. G., Sneed, R., and Perchonock, C. D. (1977). *Tetrahedron Lett.* p. 1855.
Finkelstein, J. F., Holden, K. G., and Perchonock, C. D. (1978). *Tetrahedron Lett.* p. 1629.
Firestone, R. A., Maciejewicz, N. S., Ratcliffe, R. W., and Christensen, B. G. (1974a). *J. Org. Chem.* **39**, 437.
Firestone, R. A., Maciejewicz, N. S., and Christensen, B. G. (1974b). *J. Org. Chem.* **39**, 3384.
Firestone, R. A., Fahey, J. L., Maciejewicz, N. S., Patel, G. S., and Christensen, B. G. (1977). *J. Med. Chem.* **20**, 551.
Fleming, I., Hatanka, N., Ohta, H., Simamura, O., and Yoshida, M. (1972). *Chem. Commun.* p. 242.
Fletcher, S. R., and Kay, I. T. (1978). *Chem. Commun.* p. 903.
Furrer, H. (1972). *Chem. Ber.* **105**, 2780.
Girotra, N. N., and Wendler, N. L. (1972). *Tetrahedron Lett.* p. 5301.

Gleason, J. G. (1975). *In* "Organic Compounds of Sulfur, Sellenium, and Tellurium" (D. H. Reid, ed.), Vol. 3, p. 190. Chem. Soc., London.

Gleason, J. G., and Dunn, G. L. (1977). *In* "Organic Compounds of Sulfur, Selenium and Tellurium" (D. R. Hogg, ed.), Vol. 4, p. 466. Chem. Soc., London.

Gleason, J. G., and Kingsbury, W. D. (1979). *In* "Organic Compounds of Sulfur, Selenium and Tellurium" (D. R. Hogg, ed.), Vol. 5, p. 454. Chem. Soc., London.

Gleason, J. G., Hoskins, C. J., and Holden, K. G. (1977). Unpublished results.

Gleason, J. G., Buckley, T. F., Holden, K. G., Bryan, D. B., and Siler, P. (1979). *J. Am. Chem. Soc.* **101**, 4730.

Golding, B. T., and Hall, D. R. (1975). *J.C.S. Perkin I* p. 1517.

Gunda, E. T., and Jaszberenyi, J. C. (1977). *Prog. Med. Chem.* **14**, 181.

Guthikonda, R. N., Cama, L. D., and Christensen, B. G. (1974). *J. Am. Chen. Soc.* **96**, 7584.

Hakimelahi, G. H., and Just, G. (1979). *Can. J. Chem.* **57**, 1939.

Hashimoto, T., Watanabe, T., Kawano, Y., Tanaka, T., and Miyadera, T. (1978). *Heterocycles* **11**, 207.

Hatanaka, N., Ohta, H., Simamura, O., and Yoshida, M. (1971). *Chem. Commun.* p. 1364.

Hatch, C. E., and Johnson, P. Y. (1974). *Tetrahedron Lett.* p. 2719.

Henery-Logan, K. R., and Chen, C. G. (1973). *Tetrahedron Lett.* p. 1103.

Heusler, K. (1972). *In* "Cephalosporins and Penicillins: Chemistry and Biology" (E. H. Flynn, ed.), p. 255. Academic Press, New York.

Heymes, R., Amiard, G., and Nomine, G. (1974). *Bull. Soc. Chim. Fr.* p. 563.

Heymes, R., Martel, J., and Nomine, G. (1977). *Bull. Soc. Ghim. Fr., Part 2* p. 906.

Hirai, K., and Iwano, Y. (1979). *Tetrahedron Lett.* p. 2031.

Hirokami, S.-I., Hirai, Y., Nagata, M., Yamazaki, T., and Date, T. (1979). *J. Org. Chem.* **44**, 2083.

Hlubucek, J. R., and Lowe, G. (1974). *Chem Commun.* p. 419.

Holden, K. G., Gleason, J. G., Huffman, W. F., and Perchonock, C. D. (1979). *In* "Drug Action and Design: Mechanism-Based Enzyme Inhibitors" (T. I. Kalman, ed.), p. 225. Elsevier/North-Holland, New York.

Hoogmartens, J., Claes, P. J., and Vanderhaeghe, H. (1974). *J. Med. Chem.* **17**, 389.

Hoover, J. R. E., and Stedman, R. J. (1970). *In* "Medicinal Chemistry" (A. Burger, ed.), 3rd ed., p. 371. Wiley (Interscience), New York.

Huffman, W. F., Holden, K. G., Buckley, T. F., Gleason, J. G., and Wu, L. (1977). *J. Am. Chem. Soc.* **99**, 2352.

Huffman, W. F., Hall, R. F., Grant, J. A., and Holden, K. G. (1978). *J. Med. Chem.* **21**, 413.

Indelicato, J. M., Norvilas, T. T., Pfeiffer, R. R., Wheeler, W. J., and Wilham, W. L. (1974). *J. Med. Chem.* **17**, 523.

Jackson, J. R., and Stoodley, R. J. (1971). *Chem. Commun.* p. 647.

Jaszberenyi, J. C., and Gunda, T. E. (1975). *Prog. Med. Chem.* **12**, 395.

Johansson, N. G. (1973). *Acta Chem. Scand.* **27**, 1417.

Johansson, N. G. (1976). *Acta Chem. Scand., Sect. B* **30**, 377.

Johansson, N. G., and Akermark, B. (1971a). *Tetrahedron Lett.* p. 4785.

Johansson, N. G., and Akermark, B. (1971b). *Acta Chem. Scand.* **25**, 1927.

Johansson, N. G., Akermark, B., and Sjoberg, B. (1976). *Acta Chem. Scand., Sect. B* **30**, 383.

Johnson, P. Y., and Hatch, C. E. (1975a). *J. Org. Chem.* **40**, 3502.

Johnson, P. Y., and Hatch, C. E. (1975b). *J. Org. Chem.* **40**, 3510.

Just, G., and Zamboni, R. (1978a). *Can. J. Chem.* **56**, 2720.

Just, G., and Zomboni, R. (1978b). *Can. J. Chem.* **56**, 2725.

Just, G., Chung, B. Y., and Grozinger, K. (1977). *Can. J. Chem.* **55**, 274.

Just, G., Hakimelahi, G. H., Ugolini, A., and Zamboni, R. (1979a). *Synth. Commun.* **9**, 113.

Just, G., Ugolini, A., and Zamboni, R. (1979b). *Synth. Commun.* **9**, 117.

Kametani, T., Yokohama, S., Shiratori, Y., Aihara, S., Fukumoto, K., and Satoh, F. (1979a). *Heterocycles* **12**, 405.

Kametani, T., Yokohama, S., Shiratori, Y., Satoh, F., Ihara, M., and Fukumoto, K. (1979b). *Heterocycles* **12**, 669.

Kametani, T., Kigasawa, K., Hiiragi, M., Wakisaka, K., Sugi, H., and Tanigawa, K. (1979c). *Heterocycles* **12**, 735.

Kametani, T., Kigasawa, K., Hiiragi, M., Wakisawa, K., Sugi, H., and Tanigawa, K. (1979d). *Heterocycles* **12**, 795.

Koppel, G. A., McShane, L., Jose, F., and Cooper, R. D. G. (1978). *J. Am. Chen. Soc.* **100**, 3933.

Kuhlein, K., and Jensen, H. (1974). *Justus Liebigs Ann. Chem.* p. 369.

Kukolja, S., and Lammert, S. R. (1975). *J. Am. Chem. Soc.* **97**, 5582.

Lagerlund, I. (1976). *Acta Chem. Scand., Sect. B* **30**, 318.

Lattrell, R. (1973). *Angew. Chem., Int. Ed. Engl.* **12**, 925.

Lattrell, R. (1974). *Justus Liebigs Ann. Chem.* p. 1361.

Lattrell, R., and Lohaus, G. (1974a). *Justus Liebigs Ann. Chem.* p. 870.

Lattrell, R., and Lohaus, G. (1974b). *Justus Liebigs Ann. Chem.* p. 901.

Lattrell, R., and Lohaus, G. (1974c). *Justus Liebigs Ann. Chem.* p. 921.

Leclerco, J., Cossement, E., Boydens, R., Rodriguez, L. A. M., Brouwers, L., De-Laveleye, F., and Walburgis, L. (1978). *Chem. Commun.* p. 46.

Lowe, G. (1975). *Chem. Ind. (London)* p. 459.

Lowe, G. (1979). *In* "Comprehensive Organic Chemistry" (E. Haslam, ed.), Vol. 5, p. 289. Pergamon, Oxford.

Lowe, G., and Parker, J. (1971). *Chem. Commun.* p. 577.

Lowe, G., and Ramsay, M. V. J. (1973). *J.C.S. Perkin I* p. 479.

Lowe, G., and Ridley, D. D. (1973). *J.C.S. Perkin I* p. 2024.

Lowe, G., and Yeung, H. W. (1973). *J.C.S. Perkin I* p. 2907.

Manhas, M. S., Lal, B., Amin, S. G., and Bose, A. K. (1976a). *Synth. Commun.* **6**, 435.

Manhas, M. S., Amin, S. G., Ram, B., and Bose, A. K. (1976b). *Synthesis* p. 689.

Martel, A., Doyle, T. W., and Luh, B.-Y. (1979). *Can. J. Chem.* **57**, 614.

Mattingly, P. G., Kerwin, J. F., and Miller, M. J. (1979). *J. Am. Chem. Soc.* **101**, 3893.

Meyer, R., Schollkopf, U., Madawinata, K., and Stafforst, D. (1978). *Justus Liebigs Ann. Chem.* p. 1982.

Moore, H. W., Hernandez, L., and Sing, A. (1976). *J. Am. Chem. Soc.* **98**, 3728.

Moore, H. W., Hernandez, L., and Chambers, R. (1978). *J. Am. Chem. Soc.* **100**, 2245.

Mori, M., Chiba, K., Okita, M., and Ban, Y. (1979). *Chem. Commun.* p. 698.

Morin, R. B., Jackson, B. G., Mueller, R. A., Lavagnino, E. R., Scanlon, W. B., and Andrews, S. L. (1969). *J. Am. Chem. Soc.* **91**, 1401.

Mukerjee, A. K., and Singh, A. K. (1975). *Synthesis* p. 547.

Mukerjee, A. K., and Singh, A. K. (1978). *Tetrahedron* **34**, 1731.

Mukerjee, A. K., and Srivastava, R. C. (1973). *Synthesis* p. 327.

Nakatsuka, S.-I., Tanino, H., and Kishi, Y. (1975a). *J. Am. Chem. Soc.* **97**, 5008.

Nakasuka, S.-I., Tanino, H., and Kishi, Y. (1975b). *J. Am. Chem. Soc.* **97**, 5010.

Neidleman, S. L., Pan, S. C., Last, J. A., and Dolfini, J. E. (1970). *J. Med. Chem.* **13**, 386.

Nelson, D. A. (1972). *J. Org. Chem.* **37**, 1447.
Ojima, I., Inaba, S.-I., and Yoshida, K. (1977). *Tetrahedron Lett.* p. 3643.
Petrzilka, T., Prasad, K. K., and Schmid, G. (1977). *Helv. Chim. Acta* **60**, 2911.
Prasad, K. K., and Petrzilka, T. (1975). *Helv. Chim. Acta* **58**, 2504.
Ratcliffe, R. W., and Christensen, B. G. (1973a). *Tetrahedron Lett.* p. 4645.
Ratcliffe, R. W., and Christensen, B. G. (1973b). *Tetrahedron Lett.* p. 4649.
Ratcliffe, R. W., and Christensen, B. G. (1973c). *Tetrahedron Lett.* p. 4653.
Sammes, P. G. (1976). *Chem. Rev.* **76**, 113.
Scartazzini, R., and Bickel, H. (1972). *Helv. Chim. Acta* **55**, 423.
Scattazzini, R., Peter, H., Bickel, H., Heusler, K., and Woodward, R. B. (1972a). *Helv. Chim. Acta* **55**, 408.
Scartazzini, R., Gosteli, J., Bickel, H., and Woodward, R. B. (1972b). *Helv. Chim. Acta* **55**, 2567.
Schmid, G., Prasad, K. K., and Petrzilka, T. (1976). *Helv. Chim. Acta* **59**, 2294.
Schnabel, H. W., Grimm, D., and Jensen, H. (1974). *Justus Liebigs Ann. Chem.* p. 477.
Schutz, A., and Ugi, I. (1979). *J. Chem. Res.* p. 2064.
Scott, A. I., Yoo, S. E., Chung, S.-K., and Lacadie, J. A. (1976). *Tetrahedron Lett.* p. 1137.
Semmelhack, M. E., and Gilman, B. F. (1971). *Chem. Commun.* p. 988.
Sen, P. K., Veal, C. J., and Young, D. W. (1977). *Chem. Commun.* p. 678.
Sharma, S. D., and Gupta, P. K. (1978). *Tetrahedron Lett.* p. 4587.
Sharma, S. D., Sunita, M., and Gupta, P. K. (1979). *Tetrahedron Lett.* p. 1265.
Sheehan, J. C., and Henery-Logan, K. R. (1962). *J. Am. Chem. Soc.* **84**, 2983.
Shibuya, M., and Kubota, S. (1979). *Heterocycles* **12**, 947.
Shiozaki, M., and Hiraoka, T. (1979). *Synth. Commun.* **9**, 179.
Staudinger, H. (1907). *Justus Liebigs Ann. Chem.* **356**, 51.
Steinberg, N. G., Ratcliffe, R. W., and Christensen, B. G. (1974). *Tetrahedron Lett.* p. 3567.
Stork, G., and Szajewski, R. P. (1974). *J. Am. Chem. Soc.* **96**, 5787.
Streith, J., and Wolff, G. (1976). *Heterocycles* **5**, 471.
Sullivan, D. F., Scopes, D. I. C., Kluge, A. F., and Edwards, J. A. (1976). *J. Org. Chem.* **41**, 1112.
Sweet, R. M. (1972). *In* "Cephalosporins and Penicillins: Chemistry and Biology" (E. H. Flynn, ed.), p. 280. Academic Press, New York.
Tanino, H., Nakatsuka, S., and Kishi, Y. (1976). *Tetrahedron Lett.* p. 581.
Tipper, D. J., and Strominger, J. L. (1965). *Proc. Natl. Acad. Sci. U.S.A.* **54**, 1133.
Ugi, I., and Wischöffer, E. (1962). *Chem. Ber.* **95**, 136.
Vanderhaeghe, H., and Thomis, J. (1975). *J. Med. Chem.* **18**, 486.
Van Heynigen, E., and Ahern, L. K. (1968). *J. Med. Chem.* **11**, 933.
Vijayan, K., Anderson, B. F., and Hodgkin, D. C. (1973). *J.C.S. Perkin I* p. 484.
Wantanabi, T., Kawando, Y., Tanaka, T., Hashimoto, T., Nagando, M., and Miyadera, T. (1977). *Tetrahedron Lett.* p. 3053.
Wasserman, H. H., and Glazer, E. (1975). *J. Org. Chem.* **40**, 1505.
Wasserman, H. H., and Lipshutz, B. H. (1976). *Tetrahedron Lett.* p. 4613.
Wasserman, H. H., Adickes, H. W., and deOchoa, O. E. (1971). *J. Am. Chem. Soc.* **93**, 5586.
Wasserman, H. H., Hlasta, D. J., Tremper, A. W., and Wu, J. S. (1979). *Tetrahedron Lett.* p. 549.
Wong, P. K., Madhavarao, M., Marten, D. F., and Rosenblum, M. (1977). *J. Am. Chem. Soc.* **99**, 2824.

Woodward, R. B. (1949). *In* "The Chemistry of Penicillin" (H. T. Clarke, J. R. Johnson, and R. Robinson, eds.), p. 440. Princeton Univ. Press, Princeton, New Jersey.

Woodward, R. B., Heusler, K., Gosteli, J., Naegeli, P., Oppolzer, W., Ramage, R., Ranganathan, S., and Vorbruggen, H. (1966). *J. Am. Chem. Soc.* **88,** 852.

Woodward, R. B., Heusler, K., Ernest, I., Burri, K., Friary, R. J., Haviv, F., Oppolzer, W., Paioni, R., Syhora, K., Wenger, R., and Whitesell, J. K. (1977). *Nouv. J. Chim.* **1,** 85.

Zamboni, R., and Just, G. (1979). *Can. J. Chem.* **57,** 1945.

3

Nocardicins

TAKASHI KAMIYA, HATSUO AOKI,
AND YASUHIRO MINE

Chemistry and Biology of
β-Lactam Antibiotics, Vol. 2

I. Introduction

β-Lactam antibiotics are one of the most widely prescribed classes of antibiotics in clinical practice because of their high therapeutic index in humans and the availability of a large number of semisynthetic analogs. Strominger and Tipper (1965) proposed a mechanism of action of β-lactam antibiotics and showed that these antibiotics were cell wall biosynthesis inhibitors. As the remarkable safety of cell wall biosynthesis inhibitors became clear, a massive search for other β-lactam antibiotics was undertaken throughout the world. The search for novel β-lactam antibiotics at the Fujisawa Research Laboratories has resulted in the discovery of new β-lactam antibiotics, nocardicin A and its congeners, from *Nocardia* species (Fig. 1).

Nocardicins are unique in several respects: (1) They are the first monocyclic β-lactam antibiotics possessing a relatively high potency, especially against *Escherichia coli* and *Pseudomonas;* (2) they are biologically and stereochemically related to penicillin and cephalosporin; (3) they contain *p*-hydroxyphenylglycine and oxime functions which are rarely found in nature. This chapter will be devoted to a discussion of these new β-lactam antibiotics.

II. Screening Procedures and Occurrence

A. β-Lactam Antibiotic-Supersensitive Mutants

At the Fujisawa Research Laboratories (Aoki *et al.,* 1976), cells of *E. coli* NIHJ JC-2 were treated with *N*-methyl-*N'*-nitro-*N*-nitrosoguanidine and plated on antibiotic medium no. 3 agar (Difco). Colonies appearing after 24 hr of incubation at 37°C were replicated on agar medium containing graded concentrations of penicillin G. Mutant colonies that showed higher sensitivity to penicillin G than the parent strain were put on agar slants. After single-cell isolation, subisolates were examined for

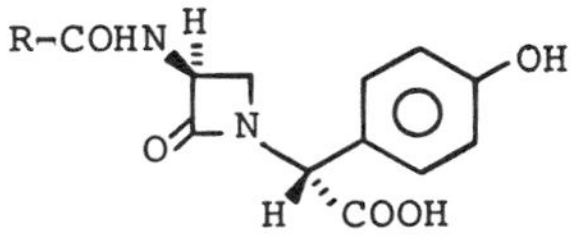

Nocardicins

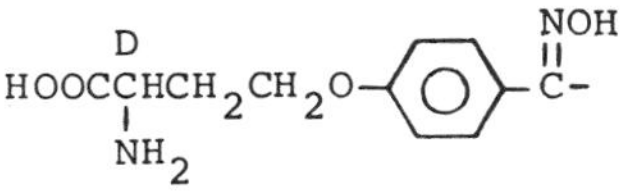

A : 1

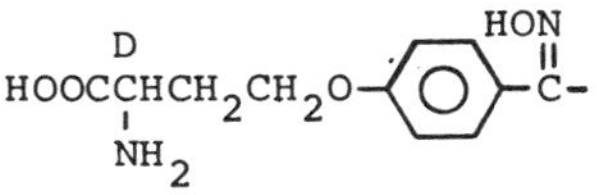

B : 2

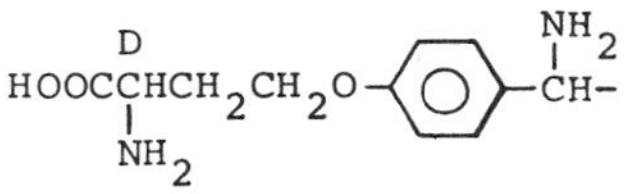

C : 3

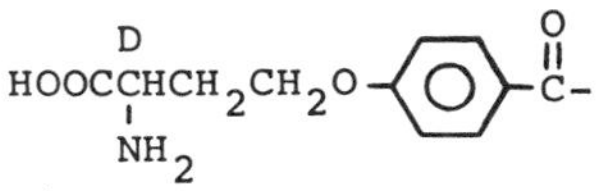

D : 4

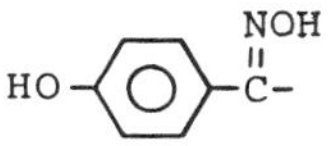

E : 5

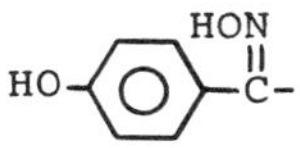

F : 6

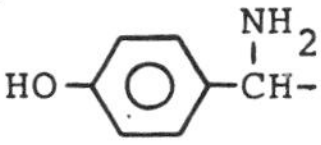

G : 7

Fig. 1. Structures of nocardicins.

their sensitivity to various antibiotics, and those that showed specific supersensitivity to β-lactam antibiotics were selected (Tables I and II). Mutants obtained by this procedure were found to be supersensitive to cephalosporin C (cephem), cephamycin C (7-methoxycephem), and other semisynthetic β-lactam antibiotics, as well as to penicillin G. It is interesting, however, that mecillinam, an amidinopenicillin, did not have any selective activity on these sensitive mutants (Table II).

B. Screening Procedure for β-Lactam Antibiotics

A screening procedure for β-lactam antibiotics carried out at the Fujisawa Research Laboratories (Aoki *et al.*, 1977) is illustrated in Fig. 2. Antibacterial substances with stronger activity on a β-lactam-supersensitive mutant were selected. Characterization of crude samples of the

TABLE I Mutants of *Escherichia coli* Supersensitive to β-Lactam Antibiotics

Strain	MIC (μg/ml)						
	Cephalosporin C	Penicillin G	Cephamycin C	Nocardicin A	Cycloserine	Fosfomycin
Es-11	0.8	3.2	0.8	0.8	25.0	0.8
Es-12	1.6	6.3	3.2	1.6	50.0	1.6
Es-21	6.3	6.3	3.2	1.6	25.0	0.8
Es-22	3.2	1.6	1.6	0.4	50.0	0.8
Es-23	1.6	6.3	1.6	0.4	50.0	1.6
Es-25	3.2	6.3	1.6	0.8	50.0	1.6
Es-26	3.2	0.8	1.6	0.8	25.0	3.2
Es-31	0.8	0.8	1.6	0.8	50.0	1.6
Es-33	1.6	0.8	1.6	1.6	50.0	1.6
Es-36	0.8	3.2	1.6	0.8	50.0	0.8
Es-41	1.6	3.2	1.6	0.8	25.0	1.6
Es-42	100.0	6.3	12.5	25.0	25.0	0.8
NIHJ JC-2	200.0	100.0	25.0	400.0	25.0	1.6

TABLE II MIC of Antibiotics on *Escherichia coli* NIHJ JC-2 and Its Mutant Supersensitive to β-Lactam Antibiotics

Antibiotics	MIC (μg/ml)	
	NIHJ JC-2	Es-114
Penicillin G	100.0	3.2
Cephalosporin C	200.0	0.8
6-APA	200.0	50.0
7-ACA	50.0	12.5
A-16886 A	200.0	3.2
A-16886 B (cephamycin C)	25.0	1.6
Clavulanic acid	200.0	50.0
Thienamycin	2.0	0.125
Aminobenzylpenicillin	6.4	0.8
Carboxybenzylpenicillin	50.0	3.2
Cloxacillin	>800.0	3.2
Mecillinam	0.2	0.2
Cephalothin	6.3	0.4
Cephaloridine	50.0	1.6
Cephalexin	100.0	6.3
Cefazolin	6.3	1.6

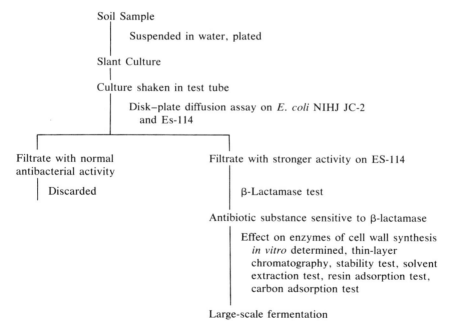

Fig. 2.   A screening procedure for new β-lactam antibiotics.

substances was conducted by examining their sensitivity to various β-lactamases, their effect on *in vitro* peptidoglycan-synthesizing systems, and their R_f value on thin-layer or paper chromatography. Examination of the sensitivity of antibacterial substances to β-lactamases is useful for the differentiation and classification of β-lactam antibiotics (Table III).

TABLE III Sensitivity of β-Lactam Antibiotics to β-Lactamases from Clinical Isolates

Enzyme origin	Sensitivity of antibiotics[a]			
	Penicillin G	Cephalo-sporin C	Cephamycin C	Nocar-dicin A
Escherichia coli 602	+ +	+ +	−	+
Escherichia coli 386	+ +	+ +	+ +	−
Escherichia coli 3032	+ +	+ +	−	+
Staphylococcus aureus 277	+ +	−	−	−

[a] Exposure of a 1000 μg/ml solution of antibiotics to washed bacteria in 1/15 *M* phosphate buffer (10 times the original concentration) of an 18-hr nutrient broth culture (*E. coli*) and to the supernatant of a centrifuged culture (*S. aureus*). + +, >90% degradation; +, 10–90% degradation; −, no degradation.

By the procedure mentioned above, characterization and differentiation of the substances in question from known β-lactam antibiotics can be achieved at an early stage of a screening program.

C.   Nocardicin A

1.   *Characterization of Nocardicin A-Producing Cultures*

The nocardicin A-producing strain WS 1571 was isolated from a soil sample collected in Okayama Prefecture, Japan (Aoki *et al.*, 1976). This organism produces aerial mycelium composed of a network of sympodially branched aerial hyphae which eventually segment into spores. The spores are oblong or cylindrical and have smooth surface. Neither fragmentation of hyphae nor formation of spores occurs in the substrate mycelium. Orange vegetative growth develops moderately on most media tested, and the aerial mass is thin and white. No soluble pigment formation is observed. Whole-cell hydrolysate contains *m*-diaminopimelic acid. Microscopic and culture studies and cell wall components of strain WS 1571 indicated that this strain belonged to the genus *Nocardia*. Comparisons of this organism with the published description of *Nocardia* species showed its close resemblance to *Nocardia uniformis*, although some minor differences were observed. As a result of these investigations strain WS 1571 has been designated *Nocardia uniformis* subsp. *tsuyamanensis*.

Recently, another wild isolate of actinomycetes was found to produce nocardicin A (E. Iguchi *et al.*, unpublished data). This organism produces monopodially branched and flexuous mycelium. Spores forming chains of 20–50 are cylindrical and 0.4–0.7 × 1.0–1.6 μm in length. The surface of the spores is smooth. The aerial mycelium is light gray, and the reverse side of the colony is colorless or pale yellow on most media tested. No melanin-like pigment is produced on media commonly used in taxonomic studies. Whole-cell hydrolysate contains LL-diaminopimelic acid. The most distinct characteristic of this organism is its alkalophilic poperty; the organism grows only in an alkaline pH range (>7.5; the optimum for growth is pH 9.5), and no growth is observed at neutral pH (6–7).

Characteristics of this strain, other than its alkalophilic property, resemble those of *Streptomyces flavovirens*, *S. atroolivaceus*, *S. fluvoviridis*, and *S. flavogriseus*, but distinct differences are observed. Thus this organism is considered a new species and has been designated *Streptomyces alcalophilus*.

2. *Production and Isolation of Nocardicin A from a* Nocardia *Strain*

At the initial stage of investigation, nocardicin A was extracted and purified by the use of activated carbon and an anion-exchange resin such as Duolite A-6 (Aoki *et al.*, 1976). This method was not practical, because it was laborious and expensive. Examination of various extraction and purification methods resulted in a procedure that used macroporous adsorption resins such as Diaion HP-20 and Amberlite XAD-4 as illustrated in Fig. 3 (Kurita *et al.*, 1976). Nocardicin A can be adsorbed onto Diaion HP-20 from the culture filtrate at pH 4 and eluted from the resin with

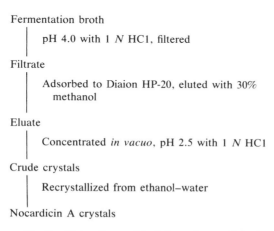

Fig. 3.   Extraction and isolation of nocardicin A.

30% aqueous methanol. The improved extraction and purification method gave an overall purification of about 100-fold in a 70–80% yield of crude nocardicin crystals. Recrystallization from ethanol–water yielded a crystalline sample of more than 95% purity.

3. Biological Activities

   a. Antibacterial Activity. Nocardicin A shows selective activity, having a moderate antibacterial effect on gram-negative bacteria including *Pseudomonas aeruginosa, Serratia marcescens,* and indole-positive and -negative *Proteus.* It has no significant *in vitro* activity against *Staphylococcus, Mycobacterium,* fungi, and yeasts. No cross-resistance was observed between nocardicin A and other β-lactam antibiotics (Aoki *et al.,* 1976).

   b. Toxicity. The acute toxicity of nocardicin A is very low: Its LD_{50} in laboratory animals exceeds 2 g/kg by any route tested (Table IV).

   c. Mode of Action Studies. The antibacterial action of nocardicin A involves interference with bacterial cell wall synthesis as evidenced by the transformation of susceptible cells into spheroplasts when treated with a lethal concentration of nocardicin A. Preliminary examination of the effect of nocardicin A on enzymes involved in the biosynthesis of bacterial cell walls has been published along with a screening procedure (Aoki *et al.,* 1977).

   Recently, M. Matsuhashi and K. Kunugita (personal communication) examined the binding of nocardicin A to penicillin-binding proteins (PBPs) of gram-negative bacteria. The results of their investigations can be summarized as follows: (1) Very weak binding of nocardicin A to PBP-1A of *E. coli* was observed, but no binding to other components of PBP occurred; (2) the concentration needed for 50% inhibition (IC_{50}) of nocardicin A on cross-linking (transpeptidation) by PBP-1B was 80 μg/ml; the antibiotic also inhibited cross-linking by PBP-1A and/or PBP-3; (3) nocardicin A seemed to induce DL-carboxypeptidase, which cleaves D-alanine from a disaccharide–peptide dimer; (4) the binding affinity of

TABLE IV   Acute Toxicity of Nocardicin A

Species	Sex	LD_{50} (mg/kg)[a]			
		iv	ip	sc	po
Mouse	Male	2000	2500	2900	>8000
	Female	2400	2500	3100	>8000
Rat	Male	>2000	2600	3100	>8000
	Female	>2000	2800	5100	>8000

[a] iv, Intravenous; ip, intraperitoneal; sc, subcutaneous; po, oral.

nocardicin A from PBP-1B of *Proteus mirabilis* (susceptible to nocardicin A) was stronger than for *E. coli*.

III.   Isolation and Description of Related Substances

A.   Detection of Minor Components

During structure elucidation studies on nocardicin A, hydrogenation of the antibiotic carried out over 10% palladium–carbon (Pd–C) yielded reduced nocardicin A (nocardicin C) (Hashimoto *et al.*, 1976a,b). This substance had no significant antibacterial activity even against a β-lactam-supersensitive mutant of *E. coli* used for the detection of nocardicin A. Mutant strains were selected from *P. aeruginosa* NCTC 10490 (sensitive to carbenicillin) for their sensitivity to nocardicin C (Aoki *et al.*, 1977). A mutant, Ps-III, was obtained which showed the same degree of sensitivity to nocardicin C as to nocardicin A. This mutant was used to search for minor components in the fermentation broth producing no-cardicin A. The availability of improved mutants of *Nocardia* and large-scale fermentation broth facilitated the search for the minor components. Crude crystalline nocardicin A showed two antibacterial spots on a thin-layer chromatography bioautogram using the mutant Ps-III. Seven active spots were detected on the bioautogram of the concentrated filtrate of the nocardicin culture after development on a cellulose sheet with an appropriate solvent system (Fig. 4) (Hosoda *et al.*, 1977).

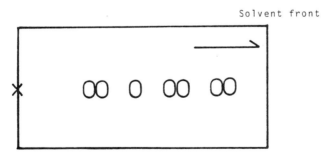

Fig. 4.   Thin layer chromatograph of metabolites in the fermentation Broth of *Nocardia uniformis* subsp. *tsuyamanensis*.

B.   Isolation of New Nocardicins from *Nocardia* Strains

1.   *Isolation Procedures*
a.   Isolation of Nocardicin B. As illustrated in Fig. 5, nocardicin B can be separated from nocardicin A by use of the macroporous nonionic

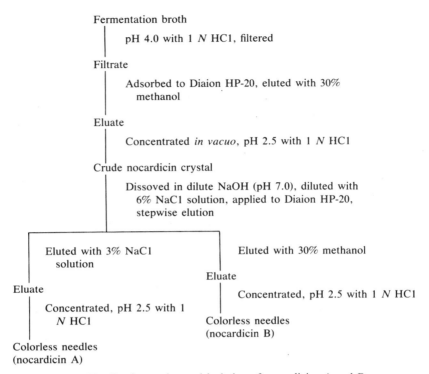

Fig. 5. Separation and isolation of nocardicins A and B.

adsorption resin Diaion HP-20 in the presence of sodium chloride (Kurita *et al.*, 1976). Crude crystalline nocardicin is dissolved in water at pH 7 (6 *N* NaOH), an equal volume of 6% NaCl solution is added, and the mixture is applied to a column of Diaion HP-20. Nocardicin A can be completely washed from the resin with a 3% NaCl solution, whereas nocardicin B is eluted with 30% aqueous methanol. Another procedure for nocardicin B isolation utilizes preparative liquid chromatography under the conditions mentioned in the footnote to Table V.

b. Isolation of Nocardicins C and D. Media used for the production of nocardicins are shown in Table VI. Isolation of nocardicins C and D was achieved as illustrated in Fig. 6 (Hosoda *et al.*, 1977). After 96 hr of fermentation, the mycelium containing most of the antibiotics was separated by filtration and washed with water to remove residual filtrate. The active components were extracted from the washed mycelium with 70% aqueous ethanol. Combined extracts were concentrated by the removal of ethanol under reduced pressure. After adjustment of the pH

TABLE V   Retention Times of Nocardicins A and B on Preparative Liquid Chromatography[a]

Compound	Retention time (min)
Nocardicin A	10.8
Nocardicin B	17.6

[a] The chromatography was performed with Waters liquid chromatography apparatus using a Bondapack C18/Porasil B column ($\frac{3}{8}$ in. × 2 ft) × 2. Mobile phase, 0.01 M Na_2HPO_4–0.01 M KH_2PO_4–methanol (95:95:10 by volume); flow rate, 5.5 ml/min; pressure, 1000 psi; instrument, Model No. M-6000A.

to 3 and extraction of impurities with an organic solvent, the active solution was concentrated, adjusted to pH 4, and applied to a column of macroporous adsorption resin Diaion HP-20. The passed fraction contained nocardicin C, and the eluate with 50% aqueous ethanol contained nocardicins D and A and a small amount of B. The solution containing nocardicin C was adjusted to pH 8 and applied to a column of activated carbon. The column was washed with water and eluted with 80% aqueous methanol. The active eluate was concentrated and freeze-dried. The crude powder of nocardicin C was further purified by the use of column

TABLE VI   Media Used for Production of Nocardicins

Medium component	Concentration (g/liter)			
			Fermentation medium[b]	
	Bennett's agar[a]	Seed medium	A	B
Glucose	10	—	—	—
Peptone	2	—	10	—
Yeast extract	1	—	4	—
Beef extract	1			
Agar	20			
Sucrose	—	20	—	—
Soluble starch	—	20	20	20
Cottonseed meal	—	20	—	20
Dried yeast	—	10	—	20
KH_2PO_4	—	21.8	10	21.8
$Na_2HPO_4 \cdot 12H_2O$	—	14.3	10	14.3
$MgSO_4 \cdot 7H_2O$	—	—	5	5
L-Tyrosine	—	—	1	1
Glycine	—	—	1	1

[a] The pH was adjusted to 6.5 prior to autoclaving.

[b] Medium A was utilized for nocardicins C, D, and F production, and medium B was used for production of nocardicins E and G.

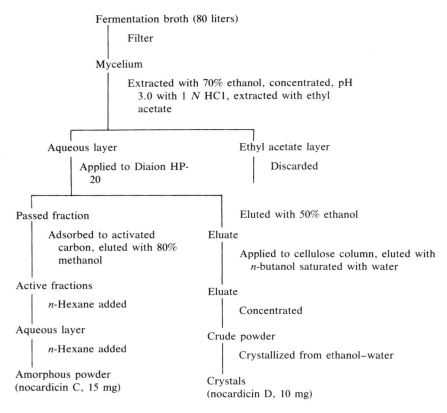

Fig. 6. Isolation of nocardicins C and D.

chromatography on cellulose powder with a developing solvent of *n*-butanol–acetic acid–water (20:6:1). Two volumes of hexane were added to the active fractions, and the antibiotic was recovered in the water layer. Two volumes of acetone were added to the solution to give a precipitate which was then separated by filtration. Crystallization from a water–acetone mixture yielded nocardicin C as crystals.

The eluate from Diaion HP-20 containing nocardicin D was concentrated and freeze-dried. The crude powder was subjected to repeated column chromatography on cellulose powder with developing solvents of *n*-butanol saturated with water and *n*-butanol–ethyl acetate (1:1) saturated with water. The active fractions were collected and concentrated to give a precipitate. The separated precipitate was dissolved in a small volume of water at pH 8 (1 *N* NaOH), adjusted to pH 3 with 1 *N* HCl, and stored at 5°C overnight to give crystalline nocardicin D.

c. Isolation of Nocardicins E and F. Nocardicins E and F were adsorbed onto activated carbon from the culture filtrate and eluted from the carbon with 80% aqueous methanol (Fig. 7) (Hosoda *et al.*, 1977). The extract solution was concentrated under reduced pressure and adjusted to pH 4 with 4 *N* HCl. The precipitate appearing after acidification was filtered off, and the filtrate applied to a column of Diaion HP-20. The antibiotics were eluted with 40% ethanol after washing with water. The active eluate was concentrated and extracted with acetone. The

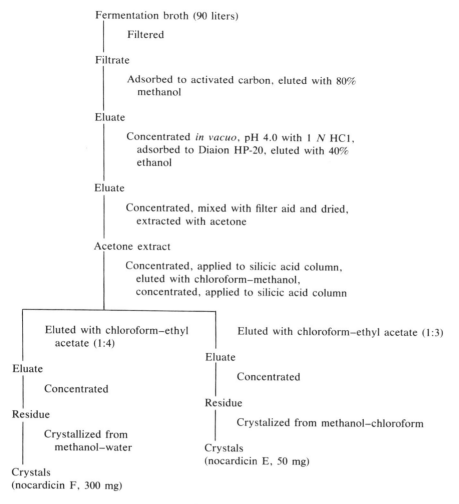

Fig. 7.   Isolation of nocardicins E and F.

acetone extract was evaporated to dryness, and the residue was purified by silica gel column chromatography with a developing solvent of chloroform–methanol (10:1). The active fractions containing nocardicins E and F were collected, concentrated, and further purified by silicic acid column chromatography. Nocardicin F was eluted from the column with a chloroform–ethyl acetate mixture (1:4), dried, and crystallized from methanol–water. Elution of nocardicin E was achieved by a chloroform–ethyl acetate mixture (1:3). Active fractions were collected, and concentrated, and the antibiotic was crystallized from methanol–chloroform.

d. Isolation of Nocardicin G. After 120 hr of fermentation, the culture broth was filtered (Fig. 8) (Hosoda *et al.*, 1977). The filtrate containing most of the antibiotic was concentrated under reduced pressure. Five volumes of methanol were added to the concentrated solution, and the precipitate formed was removed by filtration. The filtrate was concentrated to remove methanol, adjusted to pH 2 with 4 N HCl, and saturated with sodium chloride. The antibiotic was extracted from the solution with n-butanol. Two volumes of n-hexane were added to the butanol extract, and the antibiotic was recovered in the aqueous layer. The water layer was adjusted to pH 7 with a 1 N NaOH solution and concentrated to remove the butanol. The concentrate was adjusted to pH 4 with a 1 N HCl solution and diluted with 10 vol of 1% sodium chloride solution. The solution was passed through a column of Diaion HP-20. The column was washed with 1% KH_2PO_4 solution and eluted with water. The active eluate was added to 2 vol of 3% Na_2HPO_4 solution and adjusted to pH 9 with 1 N NaOH solution. The solution was applied to a column of Diaion HP-20. The column was washed with 1% Na_2HPO_4 solution and eluted with water. The eluate was passed through a column of activated carbon, and the antibiotic was eluted with 80% aqueous methanol. The active fractions were collected, concentrated, and freeze-dried. The crude powder of nocardicin G obtained was further purified by the use of cellulose powder column chromatography with a developing solvent of n-butanol saturated with water. Two volumes of n-hexane were added to the active eluate to recover the antibiotic in the aqueous layer. The antibiotic in the water solution was precipitated by the addition of acetone. The precipitate was collected, dissolved in a small volume of water, and adjusted to pH 5 with a 1 N NaOH solution. After standing overnight at 5 °C, crystals of nocardicin G were obtained and recrystallized from water.

2. *Biological Activities*

The antibacterial activities of nocardicins are compared in Table VII (Aoki *et al.*, 1976; Hosoda *et al.*, 1977). Nocardicins C–E have weak

Fermentation broth (35 liters)
   | Filtered
   |
Filtrate
   | Concentrated and methanol added, precipitate
   | removed
   |
Methanol solution
   | Concentrated, pH 2.0 with 4 N HCl, saturated
   | with NaCl, extracted with n-butanol
   |
Butanol extract
   | N-hexane added
   |
Aqueous layer
   | Concentrated, pH 4.0, diluted with 1% NaCl,
   | adsorbed to Diaion HP-20, eluted with water
   |
Eluate
   | Diluted with 3% Na_2HPO_4 solution, applied to
   | Diaion HP-20, eluted with water
   |
Eluate
   | Adsorbed to activated carbon, eluted with 80%
   | methanol
   |
Eluate
   | Applied to cellulose column, eluted with n-
   | butanol saturated with water
   |
Eluate
   | n-Hexane added
   |
Aqueous layer
   | Acetone added
   |
Precipitate
   | Crystallized from water
   |
Crystals
(nocardicin G, 150 mg)

Fig. 8.   Isolation of nocardicin G.

TABLE VII Antibacterial Activity of Nocardicins

Antibiotic	MIC (µg/ml)					
	E. coli	Es-114	P. aeruginosa NCTC 10490	Ps-III	P. vulgaris IAM 1025	B. subtilis ATCC 6633
Nocardicin A	800	6.3	25.0	0.2	3.1	50.0
Nocardicin B	>800	>100	200	0.8	400	>800
Nocardicin C	>800	>100	200	0.2	400	200
Nocardicin D	200	25.0	100	0.2	12.5	200
Nocardicin E	>800	400	100	0.8	>400	>400
Nocardicin F	>800	>400	100	0.8	>400	>400
Nocardicin G	>800	>400	100	0.4	>400	>400
3-Aminonocardicinic acid	>800	>400	>400	50.0	>400	>400

antibacterial activity compared to that of nocardicin A, whereas nocardicins B, F, and G show no significant *in vitro* activity.

Comparison of the activities of nocardicins A and B with those of nocardicins E and F clearly demonstrates the importance of the stereochemistry of the oxime function on the biological activity of this series of compounds. Contribution of the 3-amino-3-carboxypropoxy moiety to the antibacterial activity is also shown by comparison of nocardicins A and E with nocardicins C and G. It is remarkable, however, that Ps-III, a mutant strain of *P. aeruginosa* NCTC 10490, shows the same degree of sensitivity to all these nocardicins.

Nocardicins are nontoxic substances; no toxic symptoms were observed when 500 mg/kg of these antibiotics was administered intravenously to mice.

IV. Physical and Chemical Properties

The seven nocardicins isolated from *Nocardia* are white, crystalline powders which exhibit a number of common physical and chemical properties. These characteristics are summarized in Tables VIII and IX.

V. Determination of Structure

The structures of nocardicins have been determined by analysis of their spectral data and chemical degradation (Kamiya, 1977, 1978; Hashimoto *et al.*, 1976a,b; Hosoda *et al.*, 1977).

Potentiometric titration of nocardicins revealed the presence of three ionizable moieties identified as amino, carboxyl, and weak acidic hydroxyl groups in the molecules. All nocardicins have a characteristic AMX system in their nuclear magnetic resonance (NMR) spectra originating from the vicinal coupled and adjacent β-lactam protons (see partial structure **I** in Fig. 9 and also Table IX). This partial structure is also supported by an infrared (IR) carbonyl band at 1730–1750 cm^{-1}. Two sets of AB systems in the NMR indicate the presence of two para-substituted aromatic groups (partial structures **III** and **IV** in Fig. 9). These aromatic groups were further characterized as para-alkylated phenols on the basis of ultraviolet (UV) spectra (Table VIII). In addition, the NMR spectra of nocardicins A–D each exhibit two proton methylene multiplets, two proton methylene triplets, and one proton methine triplet, which are derived from the five homoserine protons (partial structure **II** in Fig. 9). Nocardicins E–G do not exhibit the requisite signals for

TABLE VIII   Physical and Chemical Properties of Nocardicins

Property	Nocardicin A	Nocardicin B	Nocardicin C
Molecular formula	$C_{23}H_{24}O_9N_4$	$C_{23}H_{26}O_8N_4$	$C_{23}H_{26}O_8N_4$
Optical rotation, $[\alpha]_D^{24}$	$-135°$ ($c = 1.0$, H_2O)	$-95°C$ ($c = 0.6$, H_2O)	$-95°$ ($c = 0.6$, H_2O)
Melting point	214–216°C (dec.)	220–225°C (dec.)	220–225°C (dec.)
UV absorption	220 (sh), 272 (310) in phosphate buffer (pH 8.0)	223 (507), 271 (181) in phosphate buffer	227 (434), 272 (43), 277 (sh 37) in H_2O
λ_{max} (nm)^a	244 (460), 283 (270) in 0.1 N NaOH		232 (319), 243 (sh 289), 280 (54), 292 (sh 44) in 0.1 N NaOH

^{a} $E_{1\ cm}^{1\%}$ is given in parentheses.

the homoserine protons. These assignments are also supported by the
^{13}C-NMR spectra of nocardicins A and D and their resultant chemical
degradation products (Table X).

The close similarity of the NMR spectra of nocardicins A and B to
those of nocardicins E and F suggests that they are pairs of stereoisomers.
This was further corroborated by results from chemical degradation experiments. Treatment of nocardicins A and B with sodium bisulfite gave
the same oxo derivative which was identical to nocardicin D. Catalytic
hydrogenation of nocardicins A and B gave the same isomeric mixture
of amines, one of which was identified as nocardicin C. This sequence
of reactions conclusively established that both nocardicins A and B contained an oxime function with a different stereochemistry. In addition,
the presence of the oxime group was also established by the fact that
nocardicin A was obtained by treatment of nocardicin D with hydroxylamine. These results also established that the functionalities at C-2'
in nocardicins C and D differed from that in nocardicin A. In a similar
manner, nocardicins E and F were confirmed to be stereoisomers at the
oxime function. The stereochemistry of the oxime group was established
to be *syn-Z* to the acylamino group for nocardicin A and *anti-E* for
nocardicin B. This was determined from the NMR spectrum of nocardicin
A in [D$_6$]DMSO, which showed the amide proton at 9.12 ppm, whereas
in nocardicin B it appeared at 8.81 ppm. This 0.31 ppm downfield shift
suggested that internal hydrogen bonding existed between the oxime
oxygen and the amide proton in nocardicin A. This is only possible with
the oxime in the configuration syn to the amide group. Corresponding
behavior was observed in nocardicins E and F (Table IX). The model
compounds **8** and **9**, in which the oxime is *syn-Z,* show the amide proton

TABLE VIII (Continued)

Nocardicin D	Nocardicin E	Nocardicin F	Nocardicin G
$C_{23}H_{23}O_9N_3$	$C_{19}H_{17}O_7N_3$	$C_{19}H_{17}O_7N_3$	$C_{19}H_{19}O_6N_3 \cdot \frac{1}{2}H_2O$
—	$-192°$ ($c = 1$, H_2O)	$-181°$ ($c = 1$, H_2O)	$-205°$ ($c = 1$, 1% $NaHCO_3$)
230–235°C (dec.)	228–231°C (dec.)	230–231°C (dec.)	200–230°C (dec.)
226 (395), 298 (313) in EtOH–H_2O (1:1)	222 (sh 557), 272 (396), in MeOH	224 (516), 270 (248), in MeOH	228 (454), 273 (52) 278 (sh 45) in 0.1 N HCl
	248 (719), 298 (324) in MeOH–1 N NaOH (9:1)	247 (720), 295 (253) in MeOH–1 N NaOH (9:1)	248 (562), 292 (107) in 0.1 N NaOH

8

9

at 8.30 ppm; whereas in the *anti-E* isomer it appears at 8.00 ppm. This difference in chemical shift (0.3 ppm) is in good agreement with that found in both nocardicins A and B and nocardicins E and F. This conclusion was also supported by the following UV studies. The UV spectra due to the partial structure D of nocardicins A and B were calculated by subtracting the absorbance of *p*-hydroxyphenylglycine from the values of nocardicin A [λ_{EtOH-H_2O} = 270 nm (ε = 14,900) and $\lambda_{EtOH-0.1\ N\ NaOH}$ = 283 nm (ε = 9500)] and nocardicin B [λ_{EtOH-H_2O} = 267 nm (ε = 8900) and $\lambda_{EtOH-0.1\ N\ NaOH}$ = 275 nm (ε = 9400)], respectively. Comparison of these differential spectra showed that the absorption maximum of nocardicin A was at a higher wavelength and had a larger extinction coefficient in both neutral and basic media than the maximum observed for nocardicin B. This was in agreement with the data for model compounds **8** and **9** [λ_{EtOH-H_2O} = 270 nm (ε = 15,800) and $\lambda_{EtOH-0.1\ N\ NaOH}$ = 283 nm (ε = 11,400); λ_{EtOH-H_2O} = 267 nm (ε = 9800) and $\lambda_{EtOH-0.1\ N\ NaOH}$ = 275 nm (ε = 9500)]. This was additional confirmation that the oxime function is *syn-Z* in nocardicins A and E and *anti-E* in nocardicins B and F.

For confirmation of the absolute configuration, the acidic degradation of nocardicin A was carried out. Hydrolysis of nocardicin A in refluxing 6 N HCl gave compounds **10–12**. Compound **12** was further treated with 6 N HCl to give L-α,β-diaminopropionic acid (**13**) and partially racemized *p*-hydroxy-D-phenylglycine (**14**) (optical purity 54). These data confirmed that the absolute configurations at C-3 and C-5 were L and D, respectively.

TABLE IX ^{1}H-NMR Data for Nocardicins

Nocar-dicin	Solvent	H-3	H-4β	H-4α	H-5	H-8 H-7	H-5' H-4'	H-8'	H-9'	H-10'	H-2'	NHCO
A	[D$_6$]DMSO	4.96 m	3.08 dd (5.2)	3.83 t (5)	5.26 s	6.76 d 7.14 d (9)	6.95 d 7.42 d (9)	4.14 t (6)	2.19 m	3.57 t (6)	—	9.12 d (8)
B	[D$_6$]DMSO	4.91 m	3.15 dd (5.2)	3.74 t (5)	5.24 s	6.75 d 7.13 d (9)	6.94 d 7.44 d (9)	4.15 t (6)	2.18 m	3.55 t (6)	—	8.81 d (8)
D	D$_2$O (NAH–CO$_3$)	5.00 dd (5.2)	2.94 dd (6.2)	4.00 dd (6.5)	5.35 s	6.93 d 7.23 d (9)	6.99 d 7.89 d (9)	4.27 t (6)	2.43 m	3.78 t (6)	—	—
E	[D$_6$]DMSO	4.98 m	3.12 dd (5.2)	3.79 t (5)	5.33 s	6.78 d 7.16 d (9)	6.78 d 7.33 d (9)	—	—	—	—	9.06 d (8)
F	[D$_6$]DMSO	4.94 m	3.14 dd (5.2)	3.74 t (5)	5.31 s	6.78 d 7.17 d (9)	6.78 d 7.39 d (9)	—	—	—	—	8.82 d (8)
G	D$_2$O	4.97 dd (5.2)	3.07 dd (5.2)	3.82 t (5)	5.28 s	6.89 d 7.21 d (9)	6.95 d 7.24 d (9)	—	—	—	5.04 s	—

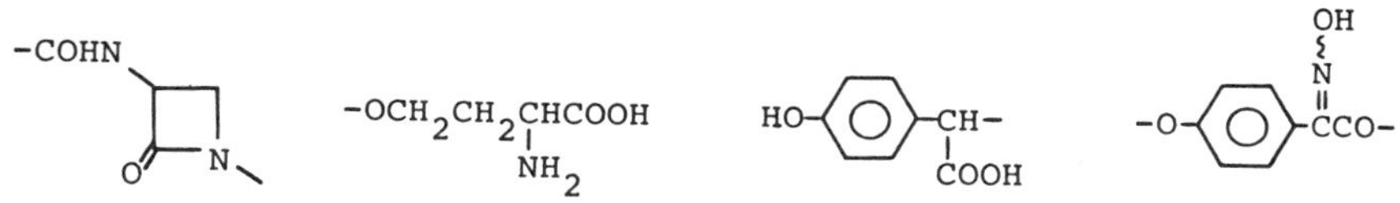

Fig. 9. Partial structures determined from NMR studies.

With regard to the absolute configuration of the remaining homoserine moiety, compound **11** was oxidized with hydrogen peroxide to give the benzoic acid (**15**). Compound **15** was then hydrogenated over Adams catalyst in 3 N HCl to yield D-α-aminobutyrolactone (**16**) and cyclohexane carboxylic acid (**17**). Thus the absolute configuration of the homoserine moiety was confirmed to be D. These chemical data are also in full agreement with the structure of nocardicin A.

The structures of nocardicins have been elucidated by chemical degradation and analysis of their spectral data and finally confirmed by total synthesis (Section VII,B).

TABLE X ^{13}C-NMR Data for Nocardicin A and Its Derivatives[a]

Carbon	(1)[b]	(6)[b]	(11)[c]	(12)[c]
C-9'	30.63	30.63	34.76	—
C-4	47.02	46.77	—	49.44
C-8'	66.01	66.19	66.79	—
C-10'	54.17	53.93	54.42	—
C-5	54.90	54.78	—	55.02
C-3	61.58	61.45	—	67.16
C-6	127.46	127.34	—	129.65
C-7	131.04	131.10	00	129.65
C-8	116.54	116.54	—	117.03
C-9	156.41	156.46	—	158.53
C-3'	123.95	126.01	125.77	—
C-4'	128.68	136.02	133.29	—
C-5'	115.88	115.57	115.94	—
C-6'	160.53	164.47	164.72	—
C-2'	153.74	188.38	196.63	—
C-1 +	166.84	166.17	183.52	—
C-2	168.54	168.36	—	177.70
C-10	176.61	176.61	—	179.76
C-11'	174.73	174.79	174.18	—

[a] Values are given in parts per million δ.
[b] Sodium salt in D$_2$O solution.
[c] In D$_2$O–NaOD solution.

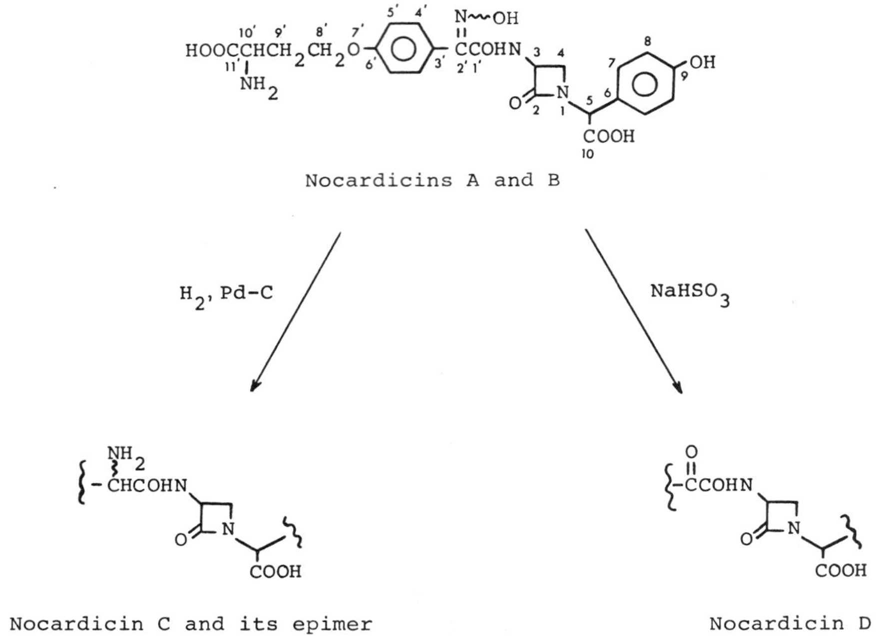
Nocardicins A and B
H2, Pd-C
NaHSO3
Nocardicin C and its epimer
Nocardicin D

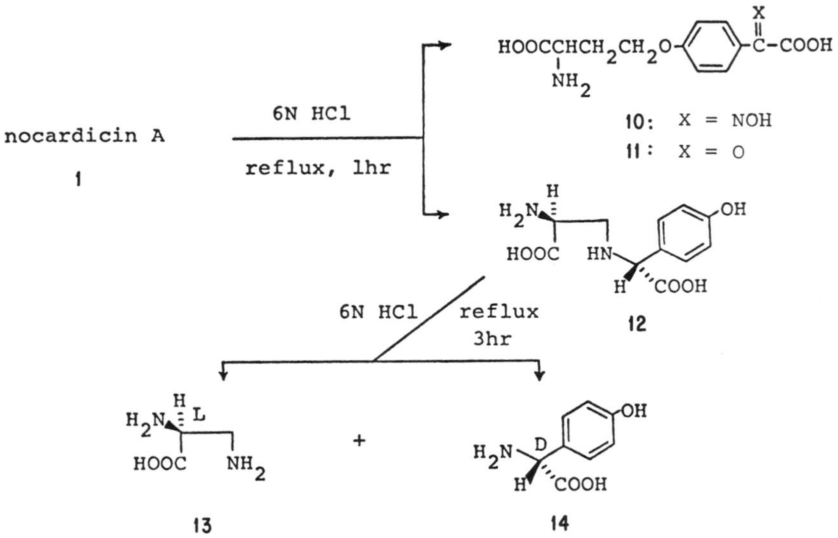
nocardicin A
1
6N HCl
reflux, 1hr
10: X = NOH
11: X = O
12
6N HCl
reflux
3hr
13
14

VI. Side-Chain Cleavage of Nocardicins

Modification of the acyl side chain has affected the potency of both penicillin and cephalosporin antibiotics. Analogously, major differences in activity might result from appropriate changes in the N-acyl side chain of nocardicin. Methods of removing the N-acyl side chain have been investigated as a prerequisite for acyl modifications. This section summarizes the chemical and microbiological methods that have been employed to cleave the side chain amide selectively from nocardicins, giving rise to 3-aminonocardicinic acid (3-ANA) and its derivatives.

A. Chemical Methods

The need for substantial quantities of 3-ANA to be used in preparing new nocardicins necessitated an efficient method of cleaving nocardicin to 3-ANA. Two practical methods have been reported. First, the application of Edman's method to nocardicin has been demonstrated by the Fujisawa group (Kamiya, 1977, 1978). A favored substrate was the N,N-bisthiourea of nocardicin C (18), which was easily obtained from nocardicin C and isothiocyanates. Treatment of bisthiourea (18) with concentrated hydrochloric acid or trifluoroacetic acid in acetic acid at room temperature, followed by adjustment of the pH, gave 3-ANA (19) in 40%

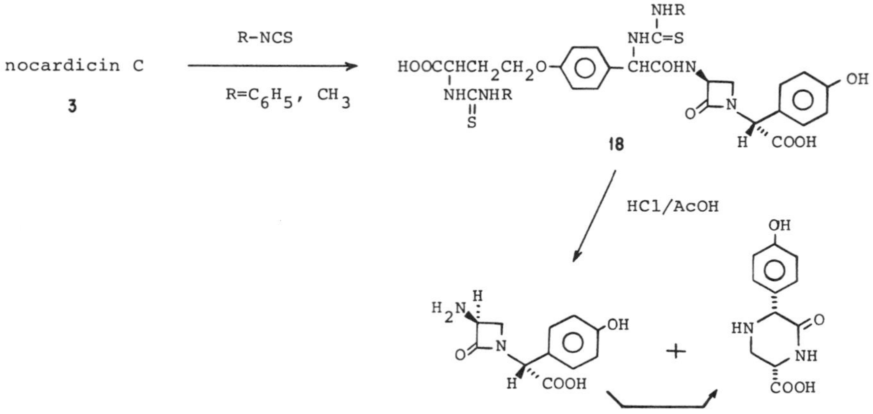

3-aminonocardicinic acid(3-ANA)   **20**

19

yield. Piperidinone (**20**) was also formed as a by-product, since 3-ANA is relatively unstable and is converted to piperidinone under acidic conditions. This method opened the way to the synthesis of a large number of new *N*-acyl derivatives of 3-ANA.

Subsequently, an alternative method for removal of the *N*-acyl side chain from nocardicin A was developed by the Ciba–Geigy group (Japanese Kokai, 1979b). This was a novel and efficient procedure for the preparation of 3-ANA and its derivatives. Treatment of nocardicin A with a large excess of di-*tert*-butyl carbonate in aqueous sodium hydroxide–dioxane at 55°C, followed by treatment with additional di-*tert*-butyl carbonate at 30°C, gave *tert*-butoxycarbonyl (BOC)-protected 3-ANA (**24**) in 80% yield. The reaction is presumed to follow initial formation of the oxime carbonate (**21**) which smoothly eliminated *tert*-butoxycarbonic acid to give the nitrile (**25**) and the isocyanate (**22**). The resulting isocyanate is hydrolyzed to the amine (**23**) which is then converted to product **24** by di-*tert*-butyl carbonate. The use of benzyloxycarbonyl chloride gave the benzyloxycarbonyl derivative (**25**). The *N,O*-BOC-3-ANA (**24**) has proven to be versatile. Treatment of this compound with trifluoroacetic acid gave 3-ANA in 86% yield. Removal of its O-protecting group with aqueous sodium carbonate gave the *N*-BOC-3-ANA (**26**) which was converted to the diphenylmethyl ester (**27**) by treatment with diphenyldiazomethane. Compound **24** was also converted to the corresponding diphenylmethyl ester (**28**). Treatment of **28** with *p*-toluenesulfonic acid gave the *O*-BOC ester (**29**). These products are useful intermediates for the preparation of new derivatives.

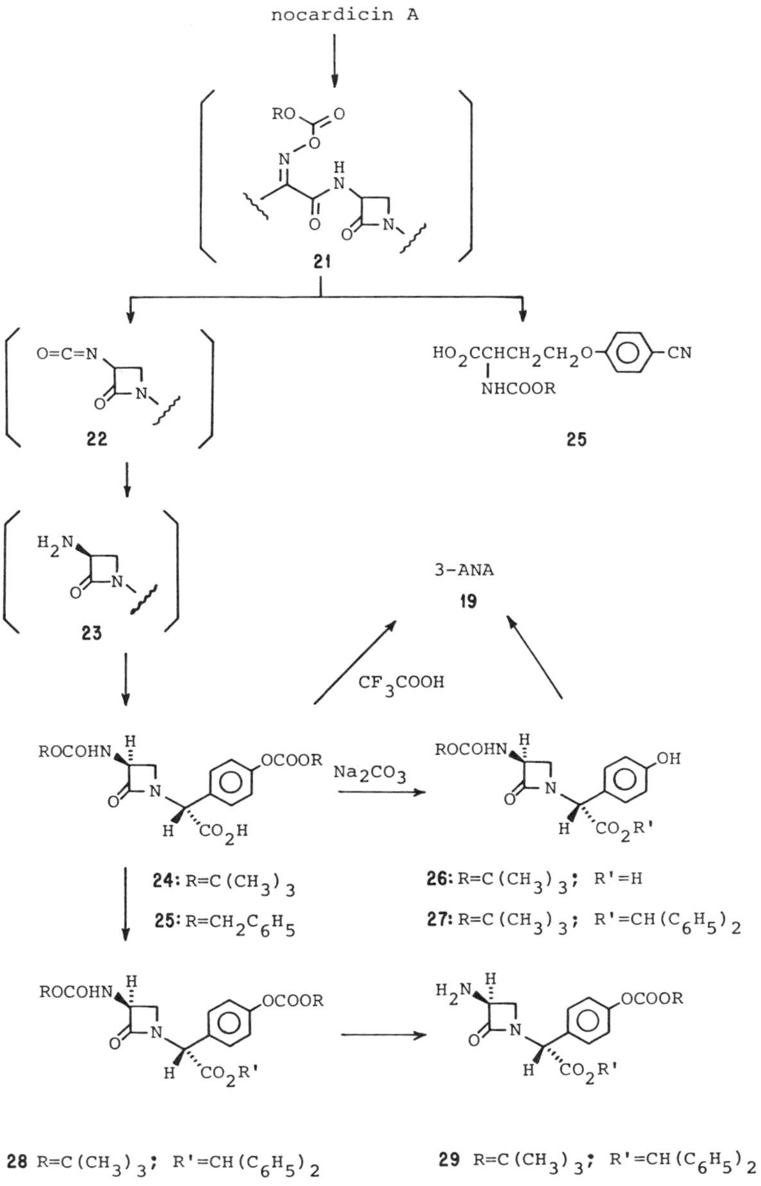

nocardicin A

21

22

23

$HO_2CCHCH_2CH_2O$ —⟨ ⟩— CN
     |
 NHCOOR

25

3-ANA
19

CF_3COOH

Na_2CO_3

24: R=C(CH_3)_3
25: R=CH_2C_6H_5

26: R=C(CH_3)_3; R'=H
27: R=C(CH_3)_3; R'=CH(C_6H_5)_2

28 R=C(CH_3)_3; R'=CH(C_6H_5)_2

29 R=C(CH_3)_3; R'=CH(C_6H_5)_2

B.   Biological Methods

Komori *et al.* (1978) examined approximately 100 bacterial species, 1000 actinomycetes cultures, 20 yeasts, and 100 fungi cultures and found none that cleaved nocardicin A to 3-ANA. Although nocardicin A appears not to be cleaved, nocardicin C and related derivatives have been enzymatically hydrolyzed. Almost all the microorganisms investigated, including bacteria, actinomycetes, and fungi, possess nocardicin C acylase activity.

The purification of nocardicin C acylase of *Pseudomonas schuylkilliensis* IAM 1126 has been reported. Fractionation with ammonium sulfate, followed by column chromatography on DEAE-Sephadex, hydroxylapatite, and Sephadex G-100, gave the pure enzyme. The enzyme appeared as a single component on polyacrylamide gel electrophoresis and had a molecular weight of 5400. The optimal pH (8–9), the optimal temperature (50°C), and the Michaelis constant (K_m 1.1 $\times$ 10^{-2} M, V_{max} 0.211 mmol/min) for the acylase were also reported. However, reversibility (acylation of 3-ANA) of this acylase was not observed.

VII.   Syntheses of 3-ANA and Nocardicins

A total synthesis of nocardicins and their analogs can hardly be expected to be of immediate practical importance. However, much broader variability can be expected once compounds of this type become available by total synthesis. Therefore a more satisfactory answer to the influence of structure on activity relationships can be anticipated from such studies. Partial and total syntheses of nocardicins and their analogs will be described in this section. Syntheses of azetidinones which have not led to nocardicin will not be discussed.

A.   Partial Synthesis from Penicillin

Two approaches have been conceived for the chemical conversion of penicillin to nocardicin, both requiring removal of the thiazolidine ring without any concomitant change in the chemically unstable β-lactam moiety. The first approach is the desulfurization of penicillin followed by removal of the carbon side chain from the β-lactam nitrogen and its replacement with the nocardicin side chain. This approach has been reported by the Fujisawa group (Kamiya, 1977, 1978). Oxidative degradation of the N-substituted side chain in dethiopenicillin (**30**) by lead tetraacetate gave the acetoxy derivative (**31**). Hydrolysis with potassium

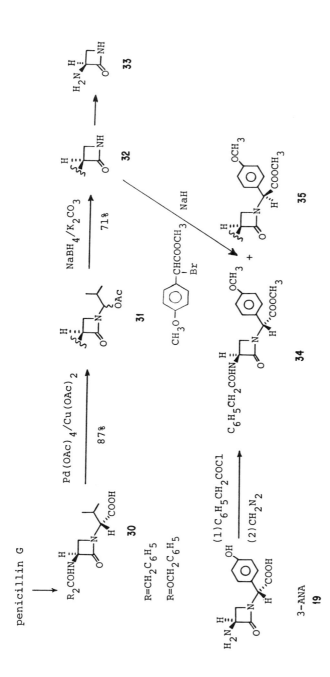

carbonate and sodium borohydride gave azetidinone (32). Catalytic hydrogenation of 32 produced the aminoazetidinone (33) as fine crystals. Alkylation of 32 with methyl α-bromo-p-methoxyphenyl acetate and sodium hydride in dimethylformamide gave a mixture of two isomers, 34 and 35. One of these, 34, which was separated by column chromatography, was identical to the authentic sample prepared from the phenylacetyl derivative of 3-ANA. This result chemically proved that the absolute configuration of the 3-acylamino group in the β-lactam ring of nocardicin was identical to that of penicillin and cephalosporin.

Second, one could open the five-membered ring of the penicillin nucleus and subsequently replace the carbon chain at the β-lactam nitrogen with the nocardicin side chain. Recent progress in penicillin chemistry has led to the development of attractive precursors to be used as starting materials for this purpose. One of these was the fused thiazoline (36) which was prepared from penicillin (Cooper and Jose, 1970; Brain et al., 1976). Alkylation of thiazoline with methyl α-bromophenyl acetate and sodium hydride gave the product 37. Acylation of this produced thiazolidine (38) which was smoothly converted to the fully substituted azetidinone 39 by acidic hydrolysis. Azetidinone 40 was also obtained directly from the thiazoline by treatment with diethyl azodicarboxylate. The desulfurization of both 39 and 40 with Raney nickel afforded nocardicinoid (41) (Foglio et al., 1978). Similarly, the alkylation of methylthio derivatives (42) has been reported (Japanese Kokai, 1978).

Because of low yields, these syntheses are of limited practical importance; however, they do provide a variation in the synthesis of nocardicin from penicillin.

B.   Acid Chloride–Imine Cycloaddition

One of the most direct routes to β-lactams is based on the well-known cycloaddition of ketene precursors with imines, a procedure originally adapted to the synthesis of epipenicillin by Bose et al. (1968). This method has been utilized in the synthesis of important β-lactam antibiotics and nuclear analogs (Ratcliffe and Christensen, 1973a,b).

The Fujisawa group was the first to demonstrate the total synthesis of nocardicin by this method (Kamiya, 1977, 1978; Kamiya et al., 1979). The starting material in their work was the thioimidate 43 which was derived from D-p-hydroxyphenylglycine. This compound reacted smoothly with phthalimidoacetyl chloride and triethylamine to give a stereoisomeric mixture of azetidinones 44 and 45. The methylthio group in both azetidinones was trans to the phthalimido group, as expected from previous results (Bose et al., 1974). Desulfurization of the mixture with

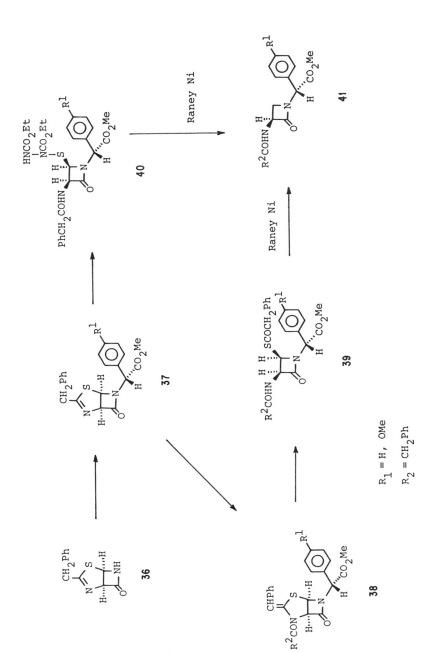

$R_1 = H$, OMe

$R_2 = CH_2Ph$

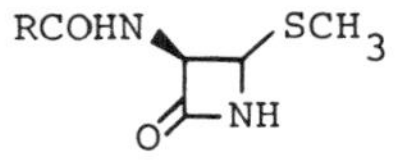

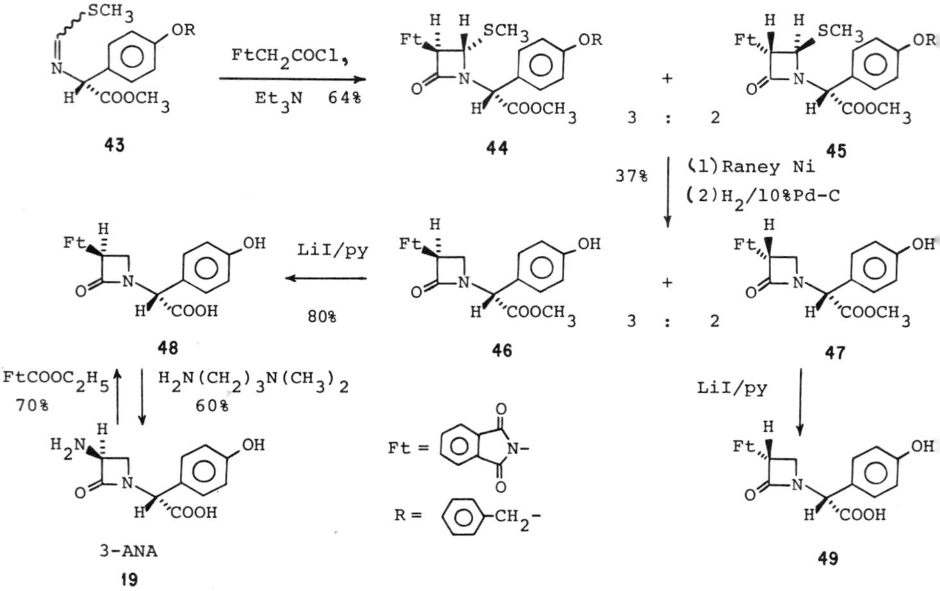

Raney nickel, followed by hydrogenation on Pd–C, gave a mixture of 4-unsubstituted azetidinones **46** and **47** in a ratio of 3:2. After separation, these compounds were hydrolyzed with lithium iodide in refluxing pyridine to give good yields of 3-phthalimidonocardicinic acid (**48**) and its epimer (**49**). The use of azidoacetyl chloride gave the analogous azidoazetidinones of general structure **50** (a 3β/3α epimer ratio of 2:1). The desired β epimer is always obtained as a main product in this reaction. Hydrogenation of **50,** followed by acylation, gave the acylamino derivative (**51**) which was then converted to nocardicin (**52**) by desulfurization. Compound **52** was also obtained by catalytic hydrogenation of oxazoline (**53**) which was derived by treatment of **51** with chlorine followed by cyclization with base (T. Kamiya *et al.,* unpublished data).

Although recent elegant modifications have been achieved, the cycloaddition approach still has some disadvantages in that separation or resolution of isomers and subsequent removal of substituents at C-4 are

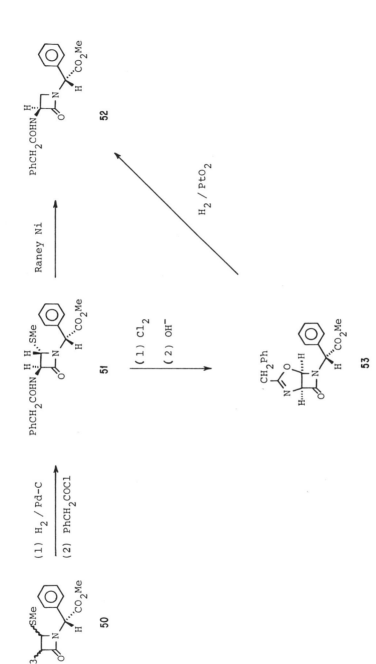

required to obtain nocardicin. In order to prepare 4-unsubstituted azetidinones directly by the cycloaddition procedure, utilization of formaldimines as a starting material may be possible. Formaldimines exist
usually as trimeric compounds, hexahydro-s-triazines. Therefore, if the
formaldimines are recovered from the hexahydro-s-triazines in a reaction,
then azetidinones with no substituent at C-4 will be produced.

A convenient and easy cycloaddition reaction that provides nocardicins
in one step from optically active hexahydro-s-triazines has been devised
by the Fujisawa group (Kamiya, 1978; Kamiya et al., 1978). The starting
material was the condensation product of benzyl D-p-benzyloxophenyl-
glycinate and formaldehyde, namely, hexahydro-s-triazine (54). When
54 was treated with boron trifluoride etherate in methylene chloride at
room temperature, followed by reaction with a phthalimidoacetyl chloride–pyridine complex at −78°C, a stereoisomeric mixture of the azetidinones 55 and 56 in a ratio of 3:1 was obtained in high yield. The
desired isomer (55) was separated by simple recrystallization. Removal
of the benzyl group by hydrogenation and subsequent removal of the
phthaloyl group by dimethylaminopropylamine afforded 3-ANA (19) in
good yield. This new method is superior to the earlier one and is also
generally applicable to the synthesis of nocardicin analogs. The p-hy-
droxyphenyl group in nocardicins was replaced as shown in Table XI.

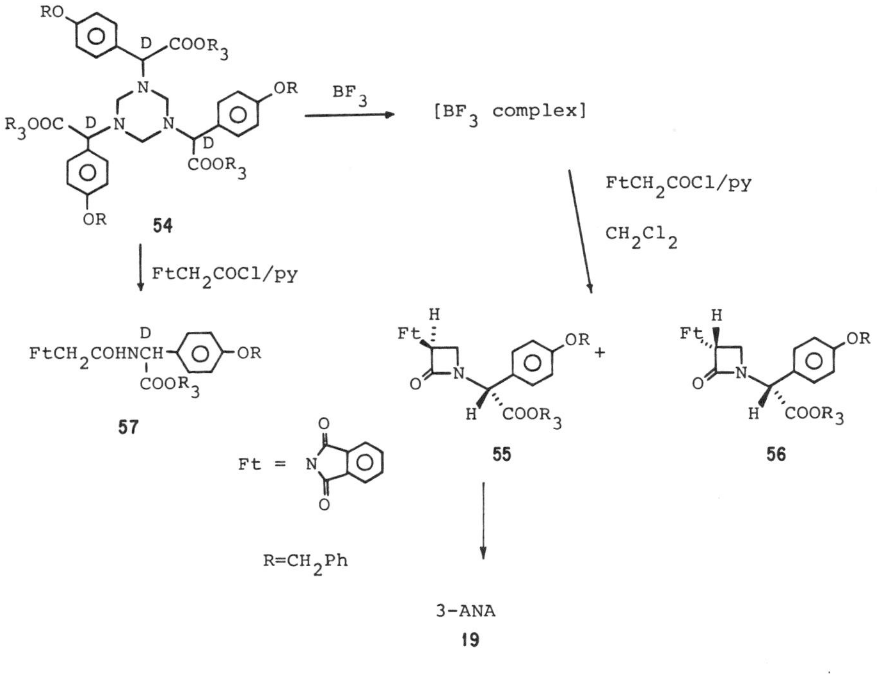

TABLE XI Nocardicin Analogs by Cycloaddition Reaction

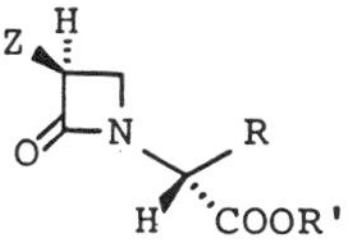

a	b

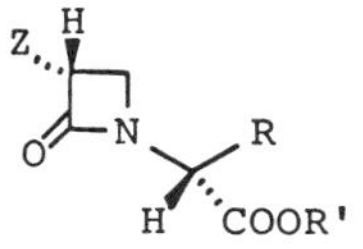

Compound[a]	Reaction temp. (°C)	Condition time (hr)	Yield of mixture (%)	Ratio of a to b	Isolation yield of II (%)
1	0	2	80	7:2	35
2	0	2	72	3:1	47
3	−35 ~ 0	2.5	42	2:1	—
4	−78 ~ 0	2.5	51	10:1	43
5	−78 ~ 0	2.5	65	7:2	32
6	−78 ~ 0	2.5	39	3:1	17
7	−78 ~ 0	2.5	36	3:1	—
8	−78 ~ 0	2.5	—	—	35

[a] Structures:

	R	R'	Z
1	Ph	CH_3	Ft
2	Ph	CH_2Ph	Ft
3	Ph	CH_2Ph	N_3
4	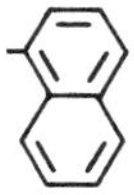 naphthyl	CH_3	Ft
5	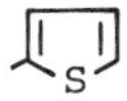 thienyl	CH_3	Ft
6	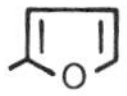 furyl	CH_3	Ft
7	$CH_2S—Ph$	CH_3	Ft
8	H	CH_2Ph	Ft

The mechanism of this cycloaddition reaction is not clear. In the presence of boron trifluoride etherate, however, the formaldimine appears to exist to some extent as a boron trifluoride complex in equilibrium with the hexahydro-s-triazine. The former could react with acid chloride via the cycloaddition process to give the azetidinone. The necessity for boron trifluoride in this reaction was shown by the fact that hexahydro-s-triazine yielded the N-acylglycine derivative 57 as a sole product in the absence of boron trifluoride etherate. The stereochemistry of the products is governed by the substituents of both reactants. Apparently, hexahydro-s-triazine derived from α-naphthylglycine gave the largest stereoselectivity in the reaction with phthaloylacetyl chloride, while azidoacetyl chloride showed a relatively low stereoselectivity as shown in Table XI. The biological properties of these derivatives will be discussed later.

The synthesis of 3-ANA has thus been achieved. The next target was total synthesis of the nocardicin side chains. The first synthesis was accomplished by the Fujisawa group (Kamiya, 1977, 1978; Kamiya *et al.*, 1979). The starting material for synthesis of the side chain was the α-phthalimidobutyrolactone **58**. Condensation with *p*-hydroxyacetophenone sodium salt in diglyme produced phthalimido acid **59** which was then converted to amino acid **60** by acid hydrolysis. Protection of the amino group with the *tert*-butoxycarbonylating reagent, BOC-ON (Itoh *et al.*, 1975), followed by resolution with cinchonidine, produced the optically active + -acid **62**. Esterification with diazomethane followed by oxidation yielded the protected ketoacid **64**. Removal of the protecting groups gave the ketoacid **11** which was identical to the natural sample derived from nocardicin A.

The protected amino acid (**64**) was converted to the mixed anhydride with ethyl chloroformate and then treated with silylated 3-ANA to yield protected nocardicin D (**65**). Removal of the protecting groups by hydrolysis afforded nocardicin D in 43% overall yield from 3-ANA. The final step in the total synthesis of nocardicin A was oximination of the carbonyl group in nocardicin D. Nocardicins are relatively stable under alkaline conditions in comparison with other fused β-lactams; nocardicin D gave a direct 60% yield of nocardicin A by treatment with hydroxylamine.

The general use of this route was exemplified by the preparation of nocardicin A analogs such as the thienyl and phenyl derivatives **66** and **67**. Similarly, nocardicins E and G were also synthesized by acylation of the protected acids **68** and **69**, followed by deprotection.

C.   Cyclization of β-Haloamide

The obvious synthesis of an azetidinone, dehydrohalogenation of 3-halogenopropranoamide, is not readily achieved because of competitive elimination and heretofore has not been regarded as an attractive route to azetidinones. However, two approaches have been reported, both avoiding competitive elimination. This was first accomplished by incorporating C-3 and C-4 into a five-membered ring to control the stereochemistry. Baldwin and co-workers (1975), in the synthesis of penicillin, achieved the ring closure of chlorothiazolidine (**73a**) to the azetidinone **74** with a strong base without β-elimination. The remarkable resistance to β-elimination can be explained by the fact that the C–3—X and C–2—H bonds are not coplanar. This method has been extended to the syn-

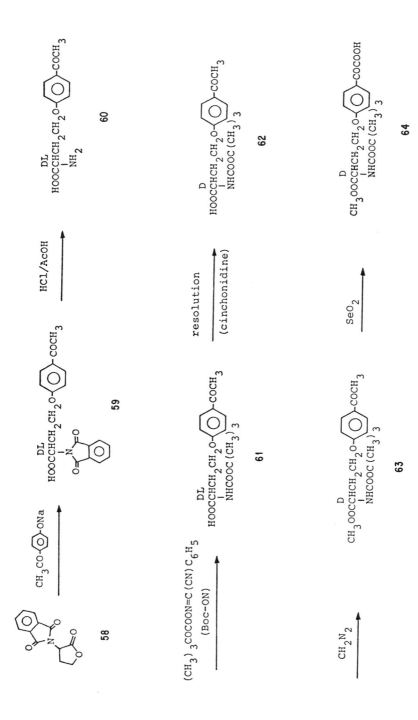

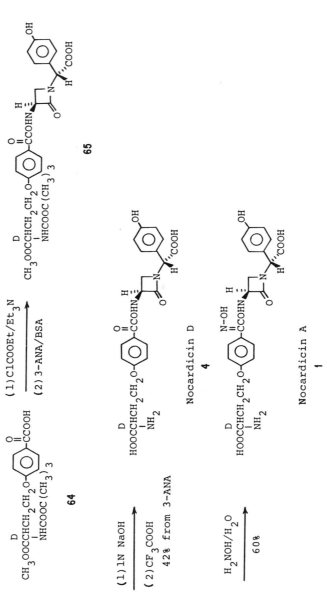

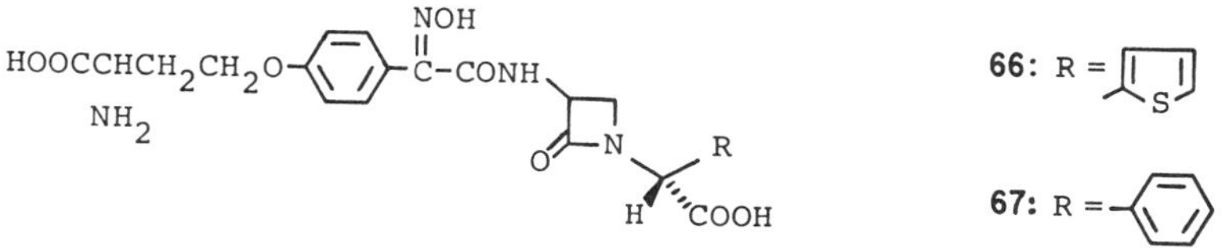

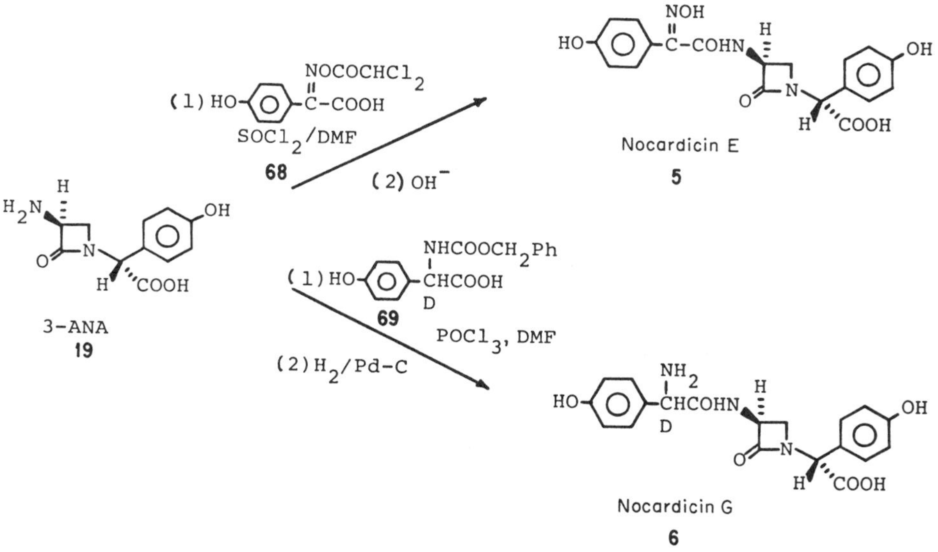

HOOCCHCH$_2$CH$_2$O—⟨benzene⟩—C(=NOH)—CONH (azetidinone ring with R, COOH)
   NH$_2$

66: R = ⟨thiophene⟩

67: R = ⟨benzene⟩

(1) HO—⟨O⟩—C(=NOCOCHCl$_2$)—COOH
SOCl$_2$/DMF
68
(2) OH$^-$

Nocardicin E
5

H$_2$N (azetidinone with OH phenyl, COOH)
3-ANA
19

(1) HO—⟨O⟩—CHCOOH
        NHCOOCH$_2$Ph
69   D
POCl$_3$, DMF
(2) H$_2$/Pd–C

Nocardicin G
6

thesis of nocardicin derivatives (United States Patent, 1979). By using this procedure, the Lilly group synthesized nocardicins A and D (Koppel *et al.*, 1978). The starting material was the condensation product of thiazolidine **70** and protected D-*p*-hydroxyphenylglycine (derivative **71**). Treatment with benzoylperoxide introduced the benzoyloxy group at C-3 of the cysteine moiety stereoselectivity to give the benzoate **72**. This was then converted to the chloro derivative **73** by treatment with dry, gaseous hydrogen chloride. Ring closure was readily achieved by treatment with sodium hydride in methylene chloride–dimethylformamide to give the isomeric mixture of **75** and **76** in a ratio of 3:1. Fortunately, it was found that crystallization of the mixture from aqueous pyridine gave only the desired crystalline isomer. This epimerization seemed to be very rapid even in the presence of weak bases. Thus the desired product (**75**) could be obtained selectively in good yield by this β-lactam ring closure reaction. Oxidation of **75** with mercuric acetate in aqueous tetrahydrofuran at room temperature gave the oxazoline (**77**). However, when the thiazoline (**75**) was treated with mercuric acetate in acetic acid, the

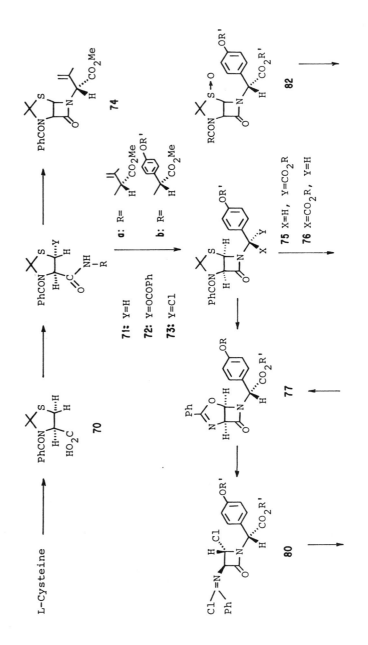

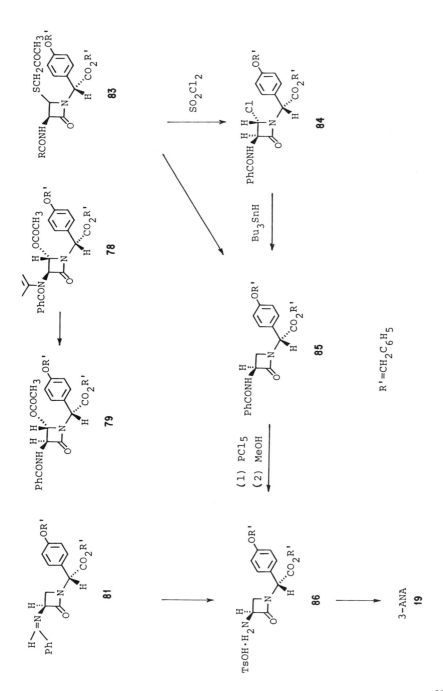

R'=CH$_2$C$_6$H$_5$

203

acetate (**78**) was obtained. Selective removal of the isopropenyl group at the amide with aqueous hydrochloric acid produced the amide (**79**). Treatment of **79** with hydrogen chloride in methylene chloride again gave the oxazoline (**77**) (United States Patent, 1979). Treatment of **77** with phosphorus pentachloride followed by quenching of the reaction with pyridine gave the chloroazetidinone (**80**). Reduction with tributyltin hydride in the presence of azobisisobutyronitrile produced the Schiff base (**81**). Similarly, reduction of chloroazetidinone (**84**) gave the nocardicin derivative **85**. The chloroazetidinone (**84**) was obtained by the reaction of sulfuryl chloride and thioketone (**83**), which was derived from the *S*-oxide (**82**) by rearrangement followed by acid hydrolysis. Selective hydrolysis of the Schiff base (**81**) with *p*-toluenesulfonic acid hydrate in ethyl acetate gave 3-ANA salt **86** in 34% overall yield from **73**. Reductive removal of the benzyl group of the 3-ANA ester gave 3-ANA.

Cooper and co-workers (1978) have also reported synthesis of the side chain of nocardicin A from D-methionine. The starting material was the optically active *tert*-BOC methionine (**87**). This compound was treated with trimethylsilyl chloride followed by methyl iodide to give the quaternary salt **88**. Treatment with potassium *tert*-butoxide produced a good yield of D-homoserine lactone (**89**). Hydrolysis of lactone **89** with aqueous potassium hydroxide gave, after lyophilization, the potassium salt (**90**) which was converted to the benzhydryl ester (**91**) by treatment with benzhydryl bromide in the presence of 18-crown-6. Coupling of the glyoxylic ester (**92**) with homoserine (**91**) was achieved by using triphenylphosphine–diethylazodicarboxylate to give the ether (**93**). Finally, hydrolysis of ether **93** with sodium hydroxide in aqueous dioxane gave the protected side chain (**94**) in high yield. By using the method described earlier (Section VII,B), syntheses of nocardicins A and D were also achieved.

The second approach involves selective cyclization of β-halopropanoamides to azetidinones under controlled conditions. As described above, the yields of the cyclization product were generally low because of the competing elimination. However, Wasserman *et al.* (1979a) have reviewed the experimental conditions that might favor the desired cyclization over the competing elimination. It was noted that the cyclization was markedly dependent on the concentration of the reactants and the rate of addition of amide to base. Synthesis of 3-ANA by this method has been reported (Wasserman and Hlasta, 1978). The starting material, 3-chloropropionamide (**96**), was prepared from methyl *p*-(benzyloxy)phenylmalonate (**95**). When **96** in dimethyl-formamide–dichloromethane (0.1 *M*) was added slowly to a suspension of sodium hydride in the same solvent at 25°C, azetidinone **97** was obtained in good yield. In a more concentrated solution, the reaction gave a

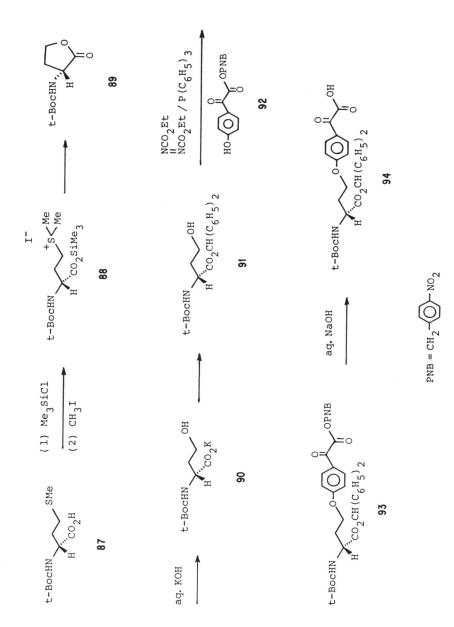

PNB = CH₂—⟨ ⟩—NO₂

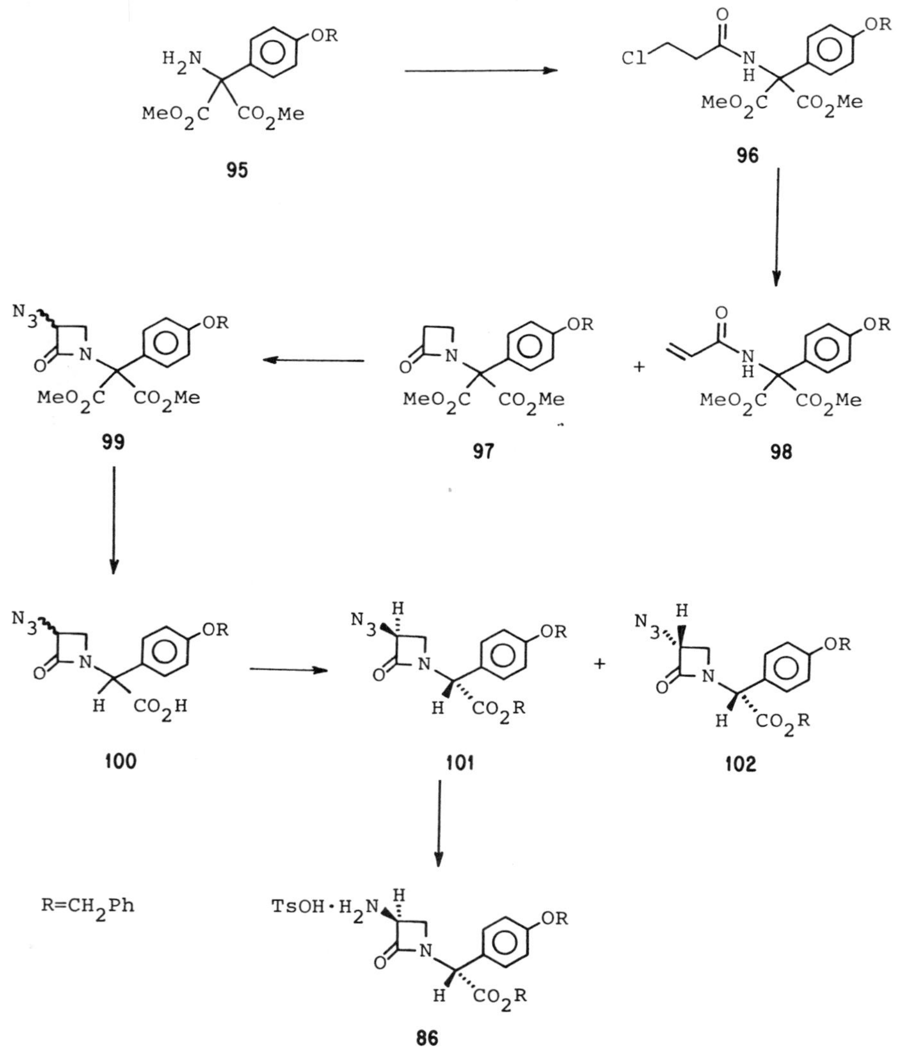

substantial amount of the elimination product **98.** Treatment of **97** with LDH in tetrahydrofuran, followed by treatment with *p*-toluenesulfonyl azide and then trimethylsilyl chloride gave the azide azetidinone **99** in good yield. Hydrolysis with sodium hydroxide in methanol followed by acidification resulted in decarboxylation with the formation of carboxylic acid (**100**) as a 1:1 mixture of diastereomers. Treatment with benzyl bromide and triethylamine gave a mixture of the benzyl esters **101** and **102** which were separated by high-pressure liquid chromatography. Reduction of each isomer with hydrogen sulfide gave 3-ANA ester **86** and its epimer. The final conversion of the 3-ANA ester (**86**) to 3-ANA by reduction had previously been reported by the Lilly group (Koppel *et al.*, 1978).

Recently, Mattingly *et al.* (1979) have reported a mild, easy N—C-4 bond closure that provides 4-unsubstituted *N*-hydroxy-2-azetidinones as precursors in the synthesis of 3-ANA.

Internal displacement of halide by amide nitrogen is not energetically favorable unless the amide is first converted to its conjugate base. The latter conversion requires a strong base. Consequently, additional protective steps must be taken to avoid competitive elimination as described above. Thus, β-halo *N*-alkoxyamide was expected to allow selective N—H ionization and subsequent cyclization to *N*-hydroxyazetidinone in the presence of base because the N—H bond of *O*-acyl- and *O*-alkylhydroxamic acids has a pK of 6–10. The starting materials in this work were the condensation products **105** and **106** of *O*-benzylhydroxylamine

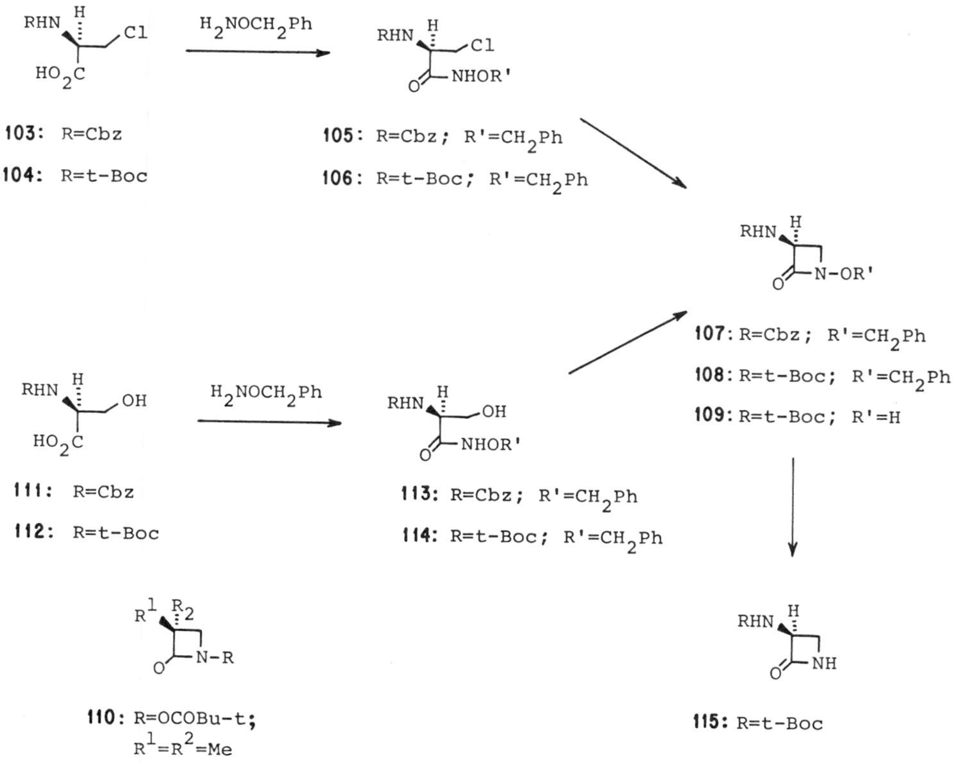

103: R=Cbz

104: R=t-Boc

105: R=Cbz ; R'=CH$_2$Ph

106: R=t-Boc ; R'=CH$_2$Ph

107: R=Cbz ; R'=CH$_2$Ph

108: R=t-Boc ; R'=CH$_2$Ph

109: R=t-Boc ; R'=H

111: R=Cbz

112: R=t-Boc

113: R=Cbz ; R'=CH$_2$Ph

114: R=t-Boc ; R'=CH$_2$Ph

110: R=OCOBu-t;
R^1=R^2=Me

115: R=t-Boc

and *N*-carbobenzoxy (**103**) or *N-tert*-butoxycarbonyl-L-β-chloroalanine (**104**). Cyclization of each of the hydroxamates with sodium hydride in dimethylformamide–dichloromethane at 50°C gave the azetidinones **107** and **108** in high yield. No dehydrohalogenation and racemization products were detected. Thus the hydroxamates might be converted selectively to their conjugate base and subsequently cyclized to azetidinones. Gentle catalytic hydrogenation of **108** gave a quantitative yield of the *N*-hydroxyazetidinone (**109**). With lithium carbonate as an alternate base, cyclization was also achieved. Compound **110** was prepared in this manner. A simpler route to azetidinones **107** and **108** was also demonstrated. Treatment of the hydroxamates **113** and **114** [prepared from *N*-carbobenzyloxy- (**111**) or *N-tert*-butylcarbonyl-L-serine (**112**) and *O*-benzylhydroxylamine] with diethyl azodicarboxylate and triphenylphosphine and followed by chromatography gave the azetidinones **107** and **108** in high yields. These products were identical in all respects to those obtained from **105** and **106**. Reduction of *N*-hydroxyazetidinone (**109**) with titanium trichloride in buffered aqueous methanol afforded azetidinone **115**. By using a procedure similar to that previously described, the synthesis of 3-ANA and nocardicin has been described (Miller *et al.*, 1979).

D. Cyclopropanone Ring Expansion

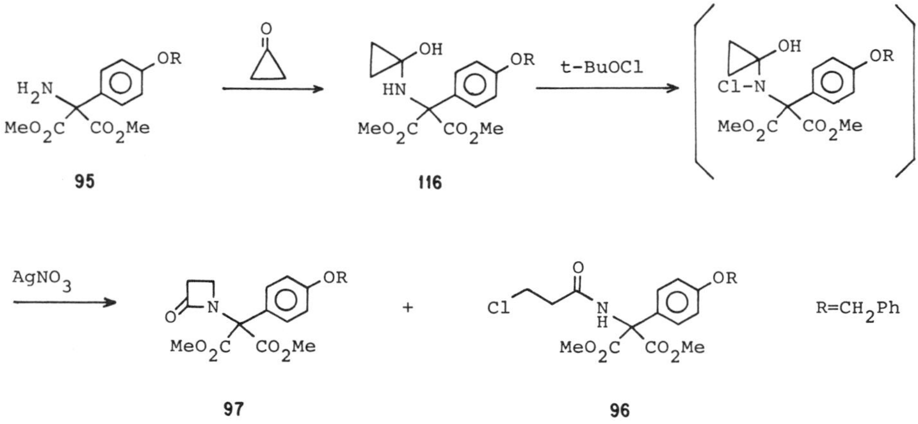

The synthesis of azetidinones by cyclopropanone ring expansion (Wasserman and Glazer, 1975) has been applied to the synthesis of 3-ANA (Wasserman and Hlasta, 1978). The starting material, alkylaminocyclopropanol (**116**), was prepared by the reaction of cyclopropanone with the amine **95**. Chlorination with *tert*-butyl hypochloride, followed by treatment with silver nitrate, gave the azetidinone **97** with the chloroamide **96** as a by-product. Conversion of both **96** and **97** to 3-ANA has already been described (Section VII,C).

E. Oxidative Decarboxylation of Azetidine Carboxylates

Wasserman and co-workers (1977; Wasserman and Lipshutz, 1976) have reported a new method for the formation of azetidinones by the oxidative decarboxylation of azetidine-2-carboxylic acids. Synthesis of 3-ANA by this method has been reported (Wasserman *et al.*, 1979b). The starting material, azetidine diester **119**, was obtained as a mixture of diastereomers from the reaction of dibromoester **117** with aminoester **118**. After selective hydrolytic cleavage of the *tert*-butyl group with anhydrous trifluoroacetic acid, the intermediate azetidine carboxylic acid monoester (**120**) thus formed was converted directly to the iminium salt (**121**) by treatment with oxalyl chloride followed by perchloric acid.

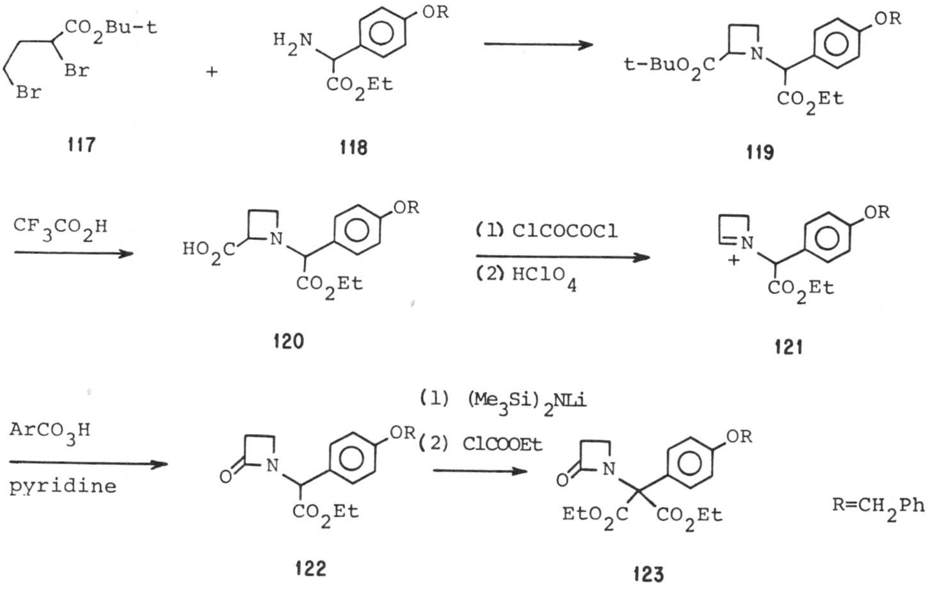

Oxidation with *m*-chloroperbenzoic acid in the presence of pyridine produced azetidinone **122** in 53% overall yield from **119**. Selective carboethoxylation with hexamethyldisilazide and ethyl chloroformate gave the azetidinone malonate (**123**). As previously described, azidomalonate can be converted to 3-ANA (Section VII,C). The procedure outlined here, utilizing an azetidine carboxylate as a precursor of azetidinone, provides an alternate route to 3-ANA and to nocardicins.

F. Cyclization of 3-Amino Propionic Acid Derivatives

Cyclization of 3-aminopropionic acid derivatives to azetidinones was not readily achieved. Few examples of this method have been reported for norcardicin (Kamiya, 1978). Cyclizing agents which have been reported are thionyl chloride, dicyclocarbodiimide, and bromine with triphenylphosphine for the acid (**124**) and the Grignard reagent for the ester (**125**). Catalytic hydrogenation, followed by acylation of the amino azetidinone **126** thus obtained, gave deoxynocardicin.

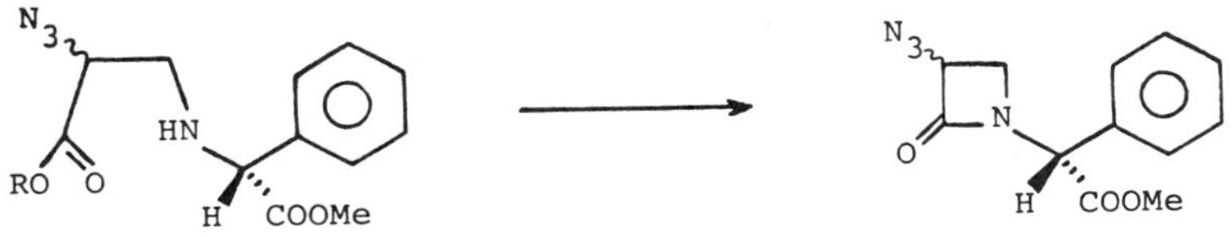

124: R=H

125: R=CH$_3$

126

α:β = 1:1

G. Passerini Reaction

A number of β-lactams have been synthesized by means of an extension of the Passerini reaction. This method has been applied to the synthesis of nocardicin. The starting material, Schiff bases (**127**), was reacted with isocyanide to give a stereoisomeric mixture of nocardicin amides of general structure **128**. Selective hydrolysis of amide to carboxylic acid has not been reported (Japanese Kokai, 1979a).

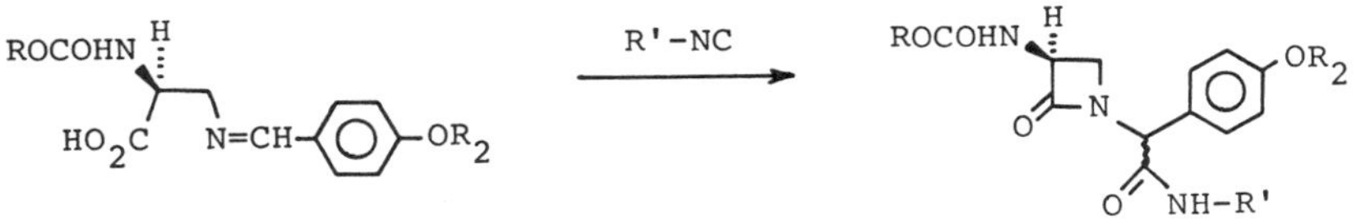

127

128

R=Bu-t, CH$_2$CCl$_3$, CH$_2$Ph

R^1=Bu-n, Ph

R^2=H, CH$_2$Ph

H. Insertion of Carbon Monoxide into Bromoaminopropenes

A novel synthesis of β-lactams has been reported by Mori and co-workers (1979). This method is based on the insertion of carbon monoxide into various 2-bromo-3-aminopropenes in the presence of a catalytic amount of palladium acetate and triphenylphosphine. K. Chiba and co-workers (personal communication) extended this approach to the synthesis of nocardicin. The starting material was the condensation product **130** of *p*-hydroxyphenylglycine derivative **129** and 2,3-dibromopropene. Treatment with carbon monoxide in the presence of a catalytic amount of palladium acetate and triphenylphosphine gave the α-methylene azetidinone **131** in good yield. Oxidation and subsequent treatment with hydroxylamine gave the oxime **135**. Acetylation and catalytic hydrogenation gave the *N*-acetylnocardicinic acid (**136**).

VIII. Structure Activity Relationships

Nocardicin has been demonstrated to possess a relatively high potency against gram negative bacteria, a low order of toxicity in animals, and cell wall biosynthesis inhibitory activity. However, its mode of action differs from that of penicillins and cephalosporins. This prompted massive efforts to develop effective new derivatives. As described above, a number of derivatives have been prepared by direct modification of nocardicins and also by total synthesis of analogous compounds. The differences in *in vitro* antibacterial activity resulting from changes in structure are summarized in this section.

A. Comparison of Nocardicin A and Its Congeners

The antibacterial activity of nocardicin A and its congeners is shown in Table XII. Nocardicin A is most active against gram-negative organisms. The activity of nocardicins C–E is relatively weak, whereas nocardicins F and G are devoid of antibiotic activity. This clearly indicates that the oxime with the syn configuration and the homoserine moiety in nocardicins are important for biological activity. This effect is quite general and will be repeatedly observed in other compound groups discussed below.

B. Nocardicin A, C, and D Derivatives

Table XIII lists some substituted variants of nocardicins A and D, which are usually less active than the unsubstituted compounds.

Table XIV shows the change in activity seen with substituted variants of nocardicin C. Almost all these compounds show reduced activity. Only the acyl derivatives of the α-amino group in nocardicin C produce a somewhat higher activity than that of the parent nocardicin C.

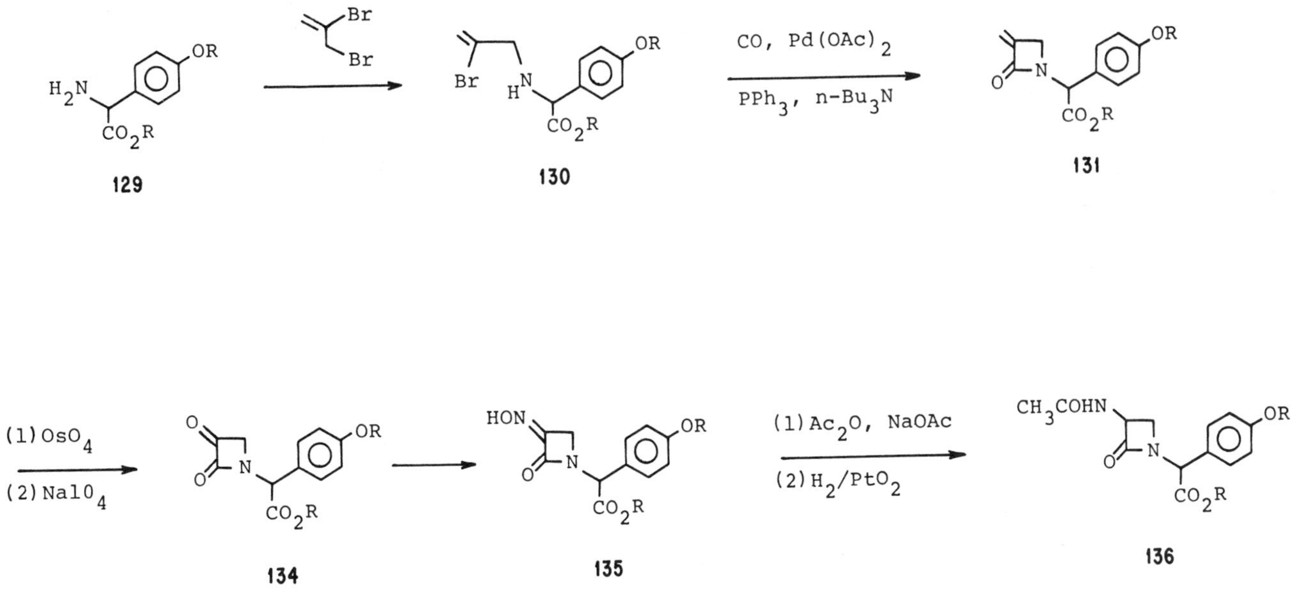

OR

CO₂R

131

OR

CO₂R

CH₃COHN

136

CO, Pd(OAc)₂

PPh₃, n-Bu₃N

(1) Ac₂O, NaOAc

(2) H₂/PtO₂

OR

CO₂R

H
N

Br

130

OR

CO₂R

HON

135

Br
Br

(1) OsO₄

(2) NaIO₄

OR

CO₂R

134

OR

CO₂R

H₂N

129

R=CH₂Ph

TABLE XII Antibacterial Activity of Nocardicins

Test organism[a]	MIC (μg/ml)					
	A	C	D	E	F	G
Pseudomonas aeruginosa NCTC 10490	2.5	50	800	12.5	100	>400
Proteus vulgaris IAM 1025	3.1	400	12.5	>400	>400	>400
Escherichia coli NIHJ JC-2	100	400	50	>400	>400	>400
Bacillus subtilis ATCC 6633	50	200	200	>400	>400	>400
Staphylococcus aureus 209p JC-1	>800	>800	>800	>800	>400	>400

[a] Agar dilution streak method (heart infusion agar, 37°C, 18 hr).

C. Various Nocardicins

In Table XV a series of acetamide derivatives of 3-ANA is shown. All members of this group are relatively weak antibacterial agents. The changes in biological activity again indicate that the oxime and homoserine moieties play an important role in the activity.

D. Various Nocardicin Analogs

Replacement of the *p*-hydroxyphenyl function of nocardicin by other aromatic groups is possible by several methods (Section VII). Table XVI lists examples of this type of compound. In general, these compounds are as active as or more active than the parent *p*-hydroxyphenyl compound against both gram-negative and gram-positive organisms with the exception of the furanyl and naphthyl derivatives.

Tables XVII and XVIII indicate trends toward variation in biological activity with change in the *p*-hydroxyphenyl function of nocardicins A and D. These modifications in structure produce little change in antibacterial activity. When compared to other nocardicin derivatives, nocardicin A analogs retain significant gram-negative activity. This again indicates the ability of the nocardicin A side chain to enhance gram-negative bacterial inhibition.

Several related compounds have been reported, such as **138** (Hakimelahi and Just, 1979) and **137** (T. Kamiya, unpublished data), which are almost inactive.

TABLE XIII Nocardicin A and D Derivatives: Paper Disk Method (mg/ml)

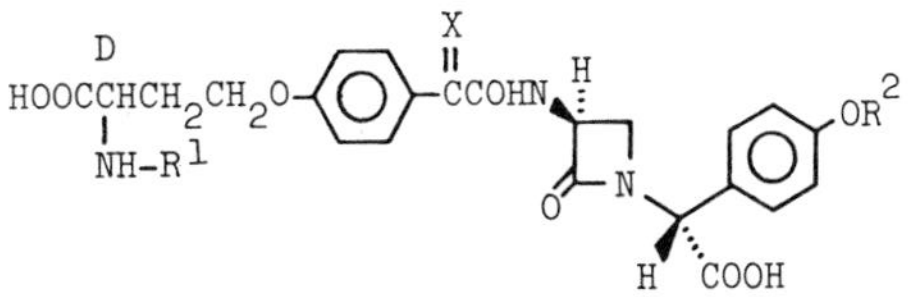

R¹	R²	X	P. aeruginosa 10490	E. coli NIHJ	Es-114	P. vulgaris	S. aureus	B. subtilis
H (Nocardicin A)	H	N—	0.025	0.8	0.0063	0.25	—	0.1
H	H	N—OCH$_3$	0.16	1.25	0.04	0.16	5	5
H	H	N—OCH$_2$C$_6$H$_5$	5	—	0.15	10	—	10
H	CH$_2$C$_6$H$_5$	N—OH	0.6	1.25	0.02	2.5	2.5	10
H	CH$_3$	NηOCH$_3$	10	—	0.3	1.25	—	—
NHCONH$_2$	H	NNHCONH$_2$	10	2.5	0.6	10	—	10
NOCH$_2$CO$_2$H	H	NOCH$_2$COOH	0.6	2.5	0.075	2.5	—	—
COCH$_3$	H	NηOH	0.15	—	0.6	5	—	10
CH(CH$_3$)$_2$	H	HηOH	0.15	10	0.039	0.6	10	10
H	H	O	0.1	0.2	0.025	0.25	10	10
COCH$_3$ (Nocardicin D)	H	O	10	—	1.25	5	—	—

TABLE XIV Nocardicin C Derivatives: Paper Disk Method (mg/ml)

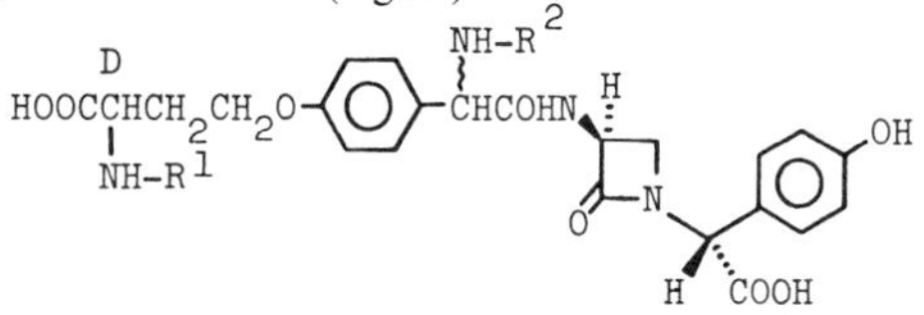

R¹	R²	P. aeruginosa 10490	E. coli NIHJ	Es-114	P. vulgaris	S. aureus	B. subtilis
H	H (Nocardicin C)	0.625	5	0.316	5	—	2.5
COCH₃	H	0.6	—	—	—	—	—
H	CONHC₆H₅	0.6	10	0.02	2.5	10	2.5
H	COCH₂C₆H₅	—	10	2.5	2.5	—	10
H	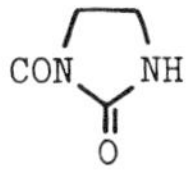 CON⟨ring⟩NH=O	0.15	0.6	0.15	—	—	2.5

TABLE XV Various Nocardicins: Paper Disk Method (mg/ml)

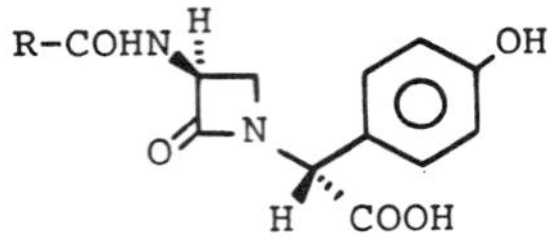

R	P. aeruginosa 10490	E. coli NIHJ	Es-114	P. vulgaris	S. aureus	B. subtilis
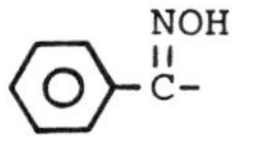 (phenyl)-C(=NOH)-	0.6	10	0.6	2.5	0.6	2.5
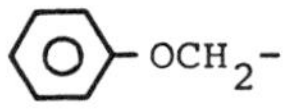 (phenyl)-OCH$_2$-	0.375	>3	3	>3	3	0.75
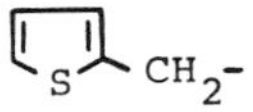 (thienyl)-CH$_2$-	5	10	2.5	2.5	10	0.025
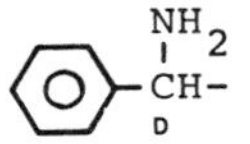 (phenyl)-CH(NH$_2$)- D	1.25	5	5	5	5	5
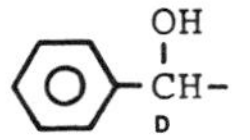 (phenyl)-CH(OH)- D	>5	>10	>10	5	1.25	1.25
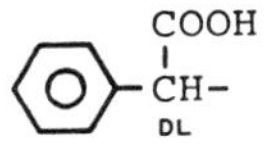 (phenyl)-CH(COOH)- DL	0.6	>10	>10	>10	>10	>10

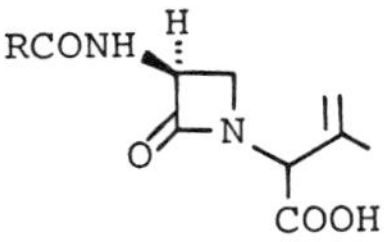

137

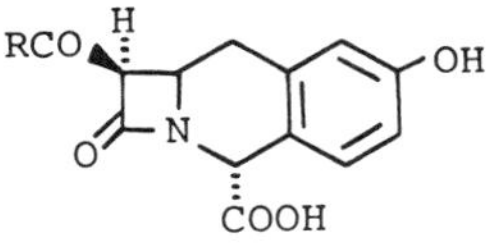

138

$$R = \begin{array}{c} HOOC \\ H_2N \end{array}\!\!> CH-CH_2CH_2O\!-\!(phenyl)\!-\!C(=NOH)-$$

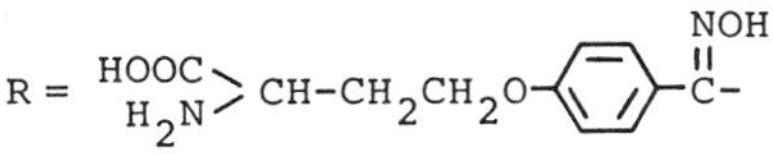

E. Conclusion

Modifications of the naturally occurring nocardicin A have been studied, and several hundred compounds have been prepared. The only useful antibiotic in this series is nocardicin A. In order to maintain an effective level of activity, only limited modification of nocardicin A is possible.

TABEL XVI   Nocardicin Analogs: Paper Disk Method (mg/ml)

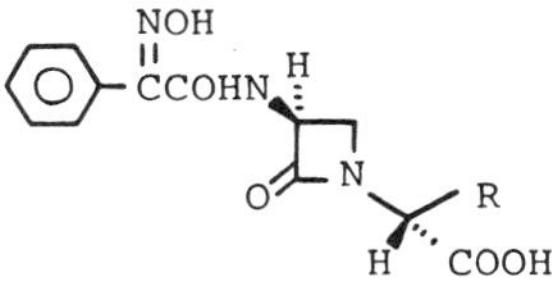

R	P. aeruginosa 10490	E. coli NIHJ	Es-114	P. vulgaris	S. aureus	B. subtilis
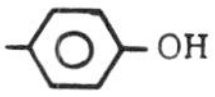 (phenyl)-OH	0.6	10	0.6	2.5	0.6	2.5
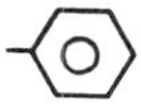 (cyclohexyl)	1.25	2.5	0.3	5	0.075	0.6
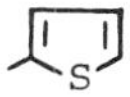 (thiophene-S)	0.15	2.5	0.15	>10	0.0375	0.15
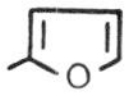 (furan-O) (dl)	2.5	10	1.25	>10	0.6	1.25
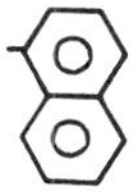 (bicyclic) (dl)	>10	>10	>10		0.6	>10

TABLE XVII   Nocardicin A Analogs: Paper Disk Method (mg/ml)

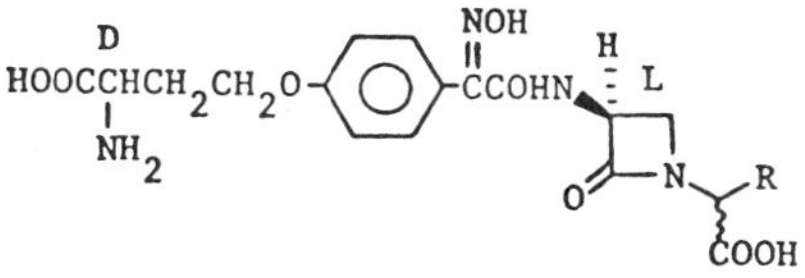

R	Stereo- chemistry at 5- position	P. aeruginosa 10490	E. coli NIHJ	Es-114	P. vulgaris	S. aureus	B. subtilis
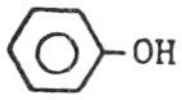 (phenyl)-OH	D	0.025	0.8	0.0063	0.25	—	0.1
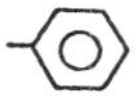 (cyclohexyl)	DL	0.04	5	0.005	0.6	1.25	2.5
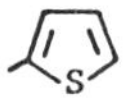 (thiophene-S)	DL	0.04	0.3	0.0025	0.6	0.6	2.5

TABLE XVIII   Nocardicin D Analogs: Paper Disk Method (mg/ml)

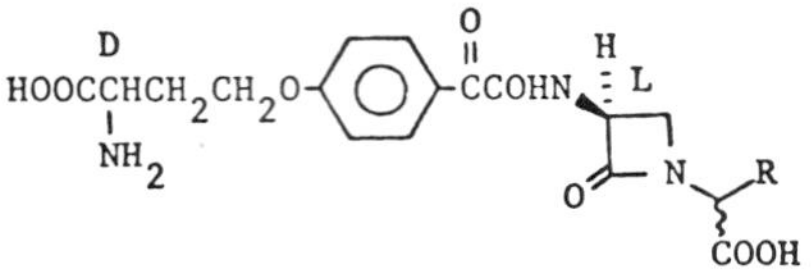

$$HOOCCHCH_2CH_2O-\langle O\rangle-CCOHN-[\text{β-lactam}]-N-CH(R)-COOH$$

R	Stereo-chemistry at 5-position	P. aeruginosa 10490	E. coli NIHJ	Es-114	P. vulgaris	S. aureus	B. subtilis
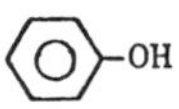 —⟨O⟩—OH (4-hydroxyphenyl)	D	0.25	0.5	0.016	0.25	10	10
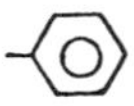 —⟨O⟩ (phenyl)	DL	5	1.25	0.01	2.5	—	—
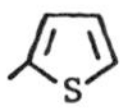 ⟨S⟩ (thienyl)	DL	5	1.25	0.005	2.5	—	10

IX.   Mechanism of *in Vivo* Activity of Nocardicin A

A.   Introduction

The antibacterial activity of an antibiotic against a given microorganism is usually expressed quantitatively as the minimum inhibitory concentration (MIC) or the minimum bactericidal concentration (MBC) in conventional medium. These values, however, are frequently affected by medium, inoculum size, pH, etc. Changes in antibacterial activity in the presence of serum and other components of the living body have been intensely discussed mainly from the viewpoint of protein binding and stability.

Furthermore, the penetration of an antibiotic into the infected organ and its retention in the tissues, as well as the interaction between the protective function of the living body and the antibiotic, must be fully considered in investigating the *in vitro* and *in vivo* activities of an antibiotic. In all cases, the *in vitro* antibacterial activity of an antibiotic must be properly evaluated in correlation with its *in vivo* activity. The *in vitro* activity of conventional β-lactam antibiotics is comparatively well reflected in their therapeutic effect on experimental infections. However, there is a distinct discrepancy between the *in vitro* and *in vivo* antibacterial activities of nocardicin A. The *in vitro* antibacterial activity of nocardicin A is greatly influenced by the kind of medium used (Nishida *et al.*, 1977), as well as factors such as potassium phosphate and sodium chloride in the medium. The former increases its activity, whereas the latter markedly inhibits it. The influence of these factors differs according to the organism (Kojo *et al.*, 1977). The elucidation of the discrepancy between the *in vitro* and *in vivo* activities of nocardicin A might not only explain the mechanism of the *in vivo* activity of the drug but also provides a focus on problems in evaluating β-lactam antibiotics in general.

B. Profile of *in Vitro* and Therapeutic Activities of Nocardicin A on Bacterial Infections in Mice

The *in vitro* activity of nocardicin A was compared with its *in vivo* activity using *Pseudomonas aeruginosa* and *Proteus mirabilis* as the test organisms. Table XIX shows that *P. aeruginosa* 191 and 161 were both resistant to nocardicin A on heart infusion agar (MIC > 800 μg/ml) but were sensitive (MIC = 25 μg/ml) and resistant (MIC = 800 μg/ml), respectively, on antibiotic medium no. 3 agar. When the therapeutic activity of nocardicin A against infections due to the above two strains was compared in mice, the drug was effective against strain 191 [50% effective dose (ED$_{50}$) = 24.5 mg/kg)] but ineffective against strain 161 (ED$_{50}$ > 250 mg/kg). *Proteus mirabilis* 60 and 100 were resistant to nocardicin A (MIC = 100 and 200 μg/ml, respectively) on heart infusion agar but were sensitive (MIC = 6.25 and 12.5 μg/ml, respectively) on antibiotic medium no. 5 agar. In tests in mice, nocardicin A was effective against infections due to both of the above strains of *P. mirabilis* (ED$_{50}$ = 4.5 and 5.2 mg/kg, respectively).

These results clearly indicate that the MIC values of nocardicin A on heart infusion agar did not accurately reflect its therapeutic activity

TABLE XIX Relation Between *in Vitro* and Therapeutic Activities of Nocardicin A in Experimental Bacterial Infections in Mice[a]

Organism	ED$_{50}$ (mg/kg)	MIC (μg/ml)	
		Heart infusion agar	Antibiotic medium no. 3[b] or no. 5[c] agar
Pseudomonas aeruginosa 191	24.5	>800	25[b]
Pseudomonas aeruginosa 161	>250	>800	800[b]
Proteus mirabilis 60	4.5	100	6.25[c]
Proteus mirabilis 100	5.2	200	12.5[c]

[a] Given subcutaneously 1 hr after challenge.

TABLE XX Therapeutic Activity of Nocardicin A and Carbenicillin in Experimental Bacterial Infections in Mice[a]

Organism	ED$_{50}$ (mg/kg)		MIC (μg/ml)	
	Nocardicin A	Carbenicillin	Nocardicin A	Carbenicillin
Pseudomonas aeruginosa 708	2.5	14.1	12.5	12.5
Proteus mirabilis 504	21.6	167.6	12.5	0.78
Proteus vulgaris 629	9.6	117.1	12.5	1.56
Proteus inconstans 21	6.7	54.0	3.13	0.78

[a] Given subcutaneously 1 hr after challenge.

(ED$_{50}$), but the MIC values on antibiotic medium no. 3 or no. 5 agar correlated well with its therapeutic activity.

The *in vitro* antibacterial and therapeutic activities of nocardicin A for *P. aeruginosa* and *Proteus* species were compared with those of carbenicillin (Table XX). The MIC of nocardicin A against *P. aeruginosa* 708 was almost the same as that of carbenicillin, but the ED$_{50}$ of nocardicin A was about five times lower than that of carbenicillin. Likewise, the MIC values of nocardicin A against *Proteus* species were about 4–16 times higher than those of carbenicillin, but the ED$_{50}$ values of nocardicin A were about 8–12 times lower than those of carbenicillin.

The strong therapeutic activity of nocardicin A was confirmed not only by the survival rate in systemic infection in mice but also by the decrease in viable cells of the liver and kidneys of mice after challenge with *P. mirabilis* (Table XXI). Mice in groups of four were injected intraperitoneally with 3.2 × 10^6 cells of *P. mirabilis* 563, and 22 mg/kg of no-

TABLE XXI Bactericidal Effect of Nocardicin A and Carbenicillin on Viable Cells in Liver and Kidneys of Mice Infected with *Proteus mirabilis* 563

Tissue	Antibiotic[a]	Dose (mg/kg)	Mean viable cells per gram of tissue 9 hrs after therapy
Liver	Nocardicin A	22	6.0 × 10^5
	Carbenicillin	22	9.2 × 10^7
	Control	0	1.0 × 10^8
Kidneys	Nocardicin A	22	6.1 × 10^5
	Carbenicillin	22	2.7 × 10^8
	Control	0	3.2 × 10^8

[a] Given subcutaneously 1 hr after challenge.

cardicin A or carbenicillin was administered subcutaneously 1 hr later. Viable bacterial cells in liver and kidney tissues were counted 9 hr after dosing. Nocardicin A markedly decreased the viable bacterial cells in these tissues under these conditions, but the viable cell counts of the carbenicillin-treated group were almost the same as those of the untreated control group.

These findings show that the *in vitro* antibacterial activity of nocardicin A is not outstanding and is less potent than that of carbenicillin. However, the *in vivo* activity of nocardicin A is more potent than that of carbenicillin against experimental infection in mice.

These results suggest that the *in vivo* activity of nocardicin A cannot be accurately expressed by comparison of MICs with those of carbenicillin. Values obtained with antibiotic medium no. 3 or 5 show the most potent antibacterial activity of nocardicin A.

To explain the gap between the *in vitro* and *in vivo* activities of nocardicin A, the pharmacokinetics in mice were compared with that of carbenicillin (Table XXII). The serum, hepatic, and renal concentrations

TABLE XXII Mean Serum, Hepatic, and Renal Concentrations and Urinary Excretion of Nocardicin A and Carbenicillin in Mice[a]

	Mean peak concentration in			Mean urinary excretion, 0–24 hr	
Antibiotic	Serum (μg/ml)	Liver (μg/g)	Kidney (μg/g)	Concentration (μg/ml)	Recovery (%)
Nocardicin A	32.8	297	35	148	47.9
Carbenicillin	28.2	45	36	236	56.7

[a] Given in subcutaneous doses of 40 mg/kg.

and urinary excretion were determined in mice given the test drugs subcutaneously in doses of 40 mg/kg. The concentration of nocardicin A was almost the same as that of carbenicillin in the serum and in renal excretion in mice, whereas the hepatic concentration of nocardicin A was about seven times higher than that of carbenicillin. It is generally known that a serum concentration higher than the MIC of an antibiotic for a susceptible organism is required for the antibiotic to be effective against experimental systemic infection in mice. In view of the above, the finding that MIC and ED_{50} values were, respectively, 12.5 μg/ml and 2.5 mg/kg for infections due to *P. aeruginosa* 708 (Table XX) cannot be explained entirely by the results of pharmacokinetic studies in mice given 40 mg/kg.

C. Effect of Nocardicin A on Bactericidal Action of Fresh Serum and
    Polymorphonuclear Leukocytes

To explain the gap between the *in vitro* and *in vivo* activities of nocardicin A, the optimal medium for determining *in vitro* antibacterial
activity was selected, and the pharmacokinetics in mice given the drugs
were investigated as described above. To determine the host–parasite–drug
relationship, the bactericidal activity of nocardicin A was investigated
in the presence of the protective factors of the living body, e.g., serum
bactericidal factors, and polymorphonuclear leukocytes (PMNs).

1. *Fresh Serum*

The *in vitro* antibacterial activity of antipseudomonal agents such as
polymyxin, gentamicin, and colistin decreases in the presence of the
serum (Davis *et al.*, 1971). The bactericidal activity of carbenicillin, a
β-lactam antibiotic, in fresh serum is almost the same as that of the drug
in serum-free media (Nishida *et al.*, 1977). The bactericidal activity of
nocardicin A in fresh serum has also been investigated (Table XXIII).

TABLE XXIII Bactericidal Activity of Nocardicin A against *Pseudomonas aeruginosa*
7095 in the Presence of 20% Fresh Rabbit Serum

Nocardicin A (μg/ml)	Fresh serum	No. of residual viable cells per milliliter
0	Without	8.0×10^6
	With	5.0×10^7
12.5	Without	2.0×10^5
	With	1.5×10^3
50	Without	9.5×10^3
	With	9.0×10^1

Fresh rabbit serum was added to antibiotic medium no. 3 broth to produce
a final 20% concentration, 12.5 or 50 μg/ml of nocardicin A was added,
and the medium was inoculated with *P. aeruginosa* to obtain an inoculum
size of 10^6 cells/ml. After incubation at 37°C for 5 hr with shaking, the
viable cell count was compared with that in the medium without the
serum. These findings indicated that the bactericidal activity of nocardicin
A was enhanced markedly in the presence of fresh serum. Table XXIV
depicts the investigation for determining if the synergism of the drug and
fresh serum against *P. aeruginosa* was attributable to a heat-labile or
a heat-stable factor in the serum. The procedure employed inactivated
serum heat-treated for 30 min at 56°C. The results show that the bac-

TABLE XXIV   Effect of Fresh Serum and Heat-Inactivated Serum on the Bactericidal Activity of Nocardicin A against *Pseudomonas aeruginosa*

Medium	No. of residual viable cells per milliliter
Broth plus nocardicin A	1.0×10^4
Fresh serum plus nocardicin A	1.0×10^1
Inactivated serum plus nocardicin A	8.5×10^3

tericidal activity of nocardicin A was enhanced by the addition of fresh serum but not by inactivated serum. This finding suggests that the enhanced bactericidal activity of nocardicin A is attributable to heat-labile components, e.g., complement in the serum. Synergism was also obtained when fresh human serum was used.

2.   Polymorphonuclear Leukocytes

Like a serum bactericidal factor, PMNs are known to play an important role in host defense. The bactericidal activity of nocardicin A was investigated in the presence of PMNs (Table XXV).

TABLE XXV   Bactericidal Activity of Nocardicin A in the Presence of Rabbit PMNs

Organism	Nocardicin A (μg/ml)	PMNs	No. of residual viable cells per milliliter
Pseudomonas aeruginosa	25	Without	1.5×10^7
		With	2.0×10^4
Escherichia coli	25	Without	1.5×10^7
		With	2.0×10^3
Proteus vulgaris	25	Without	2.5×10^6
		With	3.0×10^3

PMNs obtained from rabbits given glycogen intraperitoneally were suspended in Hank's balanced salt solution to obtain a 9×10^6 cells/ml suspension which was inoculated with 6×10^6 bacterial cells/ml, and 25 μg/ml of nocardicin A was added. After incubation at 37°C for 4 hr the bactericidal activity was evaluated in comparison with that observed in the absence of PMNs. The surviving viable cell count of *P. aeruginosa* was about 10^7 cells/ml in the absence of PMNs but decreased markedly to about 10^4 cells/ml in the presence of PMNs. Similar effects were obtained in *E. coli* and *Proteus vulgaris*, and also in human leukocytes (Nakano *et al.*, 1978). This finding suggests that nocardicin A acts synergistically with PMNs for bactericidal activity.

D. Discussion

Nocardicin A is a new monocyclic β-lactam antibiotic which has an excellent therapeutic effect on bacterial infections in mice, although its *in vitro* antibacterial activity is weak when tested on conventional media. The correlation between the *in vitro* and *in vivo* activities of nocardicin A has been investigated. There is an appreciable correlation between the ED_{50} of the drug against bacterial infections in mice and its MIC on antibiotic medium no. 3 or 5 agar. However, the *in vivo* activity of nocardicin A cannot be completely explained by its *in vitro* activity on these media or by its pharmacokinetics in mice when compared with carbenicillin. The interaction between nocardicin A and both serum bactericidal components as well as PMNs was investigated. The bactericidal activity of nocardicin A was found to be enhanced in the presence of these factors. At an early stage of the investigation, it was found that nocardicin A, unlike immunopotentiators, did not directly stimulate the immune system of the host. Considering the interaction between nocardicin A and PMNs, it was found that *P. mirabilis* pretreated with nocardicin A was more sensitive to blood than were nontreated bacteria. Invasion of the nocardicin A-pretreated bacterial cells into the blood of mice after intraperitoneal inoculation was more markedly prevented than that of nontreated cells (Nishida *et al.,* 1978). These findings strongly suggest that the cell walls of bacteria are damaged by nocardicin A. As a result of this damage, bacteria are readily affected by the bactericidal activity of serum and by phagocytosis and the intracellular killing activity of PMNs.

It is clear from a series of experiments that the *in vitro* activity of antibiotics in conventional medium, expressed as the MIC or MBC, is not always reflected in the *in vivo* activity. Therefore the correlation between the *in vitro* and *in vivo* activities of antibiotics can only properly be evaluated by determining the *in vitro* antibacterial activity under conditions where host defense mechanisms operate. Nocardicin A is the first antibiotic that requires this evaluation wherein the host–parasite–drug relationship is considered.

References

Aoki, H., Sakai, H., Kohsaka, M., Konomi, T., Hosoda, J., Kubochi, Y., Iguchi, E., and Imanaka, H. (1976). *J. Antibiot.* **29,** 492.
Aoki, H., Kunugita, K., Hosoda, J., and Imanaka, H. (1977). *Jpn. J. Antibiot.* **30,** Suppl., p. s207.

Baldwin, J. E., Au, A., Christie, M., Haber, S. B., and Hesson, D. (1975). *J. Am. Chem. Soc.* **97**, 5957.

Bose, A. K., Spiegelman, G., and Manhas, M. S. (1968). *J. Am. Chem. Soc.* **90**, 4506.

Bose, A. K., Manhas, M. S., Chib, J. S., Chawla, H. P. S., and Dayal, B. (1974). *J. Org. Chem.* **39**, 2877.

Brain, E. G., Eglington, A. J., Nayler, J. H. C., Pearson, M. J., and Southgate, R. (1976). *J.C.S. Perkin I* p. 447.

Cama, L. D., and Christensen, B. G. (1974). *J. Am. Chem. Soc.* **96**, 7582.

Cooper, R. D. G., and Jose, F. L. (1970). *J. Am. Chem. Soc.* **92**, 2575.

Cooper, R. D. G., Jose, F., McShane, L., and Koppel, G. A. (1978). *Tetrahedron Lett.* p. 2243.

Davis, S. D., Iannetta, A., and Wedgwood, R. J. (1971). *J. Infect. Dis.* **123**, 392.

Foglio, M., Franceschi, G., Lombardi, P., Scarafile, C., and Arcamone, F. (1978). *J.C.S. Chem. Commun.* p. 1101.

Hakimelahi, G. H., and Just, G. (1979). *Can. J. Chem.* **57**, 1939.

Hashimoto, M., Komori, T., and Kamiya, T. (1976a). *J. Am. Chem. Soc.* **98**, 3023.

Hashimoto, M., Komori, T., and Kamiya, T. (1976b). *J. Antibiot.* **29**, 890.

Hosoda, J., Konomi, T., Tani, N., Aoki, H., and Imanaka, H. (1977). *Agric. Biol. Chem.* **41**, 2013.

Itoh, M., Hagiwara, D., and Kamiya, T. (1975). *Tetrahedron Lett.* p. 4393.

Itoh, M., Hagiwara, D., and Kamiya, T. (1977). *Bull. Chem. Soc. Jpn.* **50**, 718.

Japanese Kokai Tokkyo Koho (1978). No. 78 71,058; *C.A.* **89**, 163383.

Japanese Kokai Tokkyo Koho (1979a). No. 79 125,651; *C.A.* **92**, 146583.

Japanese Kokai Tokkyo Koho (1979b). No. 79 151,960; *C.A.* **93**, 7995.

Kamiya, T. (1977). *In* "Recent Advances in the Chemistry of β-lactam Antibiotics" (J. Elks, ed.), pp. 281–294. Chem. Soc., London.

Kamiya, T. (1978). *In* "Bioactive Peptides Produced by Microorganisms" (H. Umezawa, T. Takita, and T. Shiba, eds.), pp. 87–104. Kodansha, Tokyo and Wiley, New York.

Kamiya, T., Oku, T., Nakaguchi, O., Takeno, H., and Hashimoto, M. (1978). *Tetrahedron Lett.* p. 5119.

Kamiya, T., Hashimoto, M., Nakaguchi, O., and Oku, T. (1979). *Tetrahedron* **35**, 323.

Kojo, H., Mine, Y., Nishida, M., and Yokota, T. (1977). *J. Antibiot.* **30**, 926.

Komori, T., Kunugita, K., Nakahara, K., Aoki, H., and Imanaka, H. (1978). *Agric. Biol. Chem.* **42**, 1439.

Koppel, G. A., McShane, L., Jose, F., and Cooper, R. D. G. (1978). *J. Am. Chem. Soc.* **100**, 3933.

Kurita, M., Jomon, K., Komori, T., Miyairi, N., Aoki, H., Kuge, S., Kamiya, T., and Imanaka, H. (1976). *J. Antibiot.* **29**, 1243.

Mattingly, P. G., Kerwin, J. F., and Miller, M. J. (1979). *J. Am. Chem. Soc.* **101**, 3983.

Miller, M. J., Mattingly, P. G., and Kerwin, J. F. (1979). *Nat. Meet. Am. Chem. Soc., 178th, Washington, D.C., Org. Chem. Sect.* No. 129. (Abstr.)

Mori, M., Chiba, K., Okita, M., and Ban, Y. (1979). *J.C.S. Chem. Commun.* p. 698.

Nakano, H., Imanaka, H., Nishida, M., and Kamiya, T. (1978). *In* "Principles and Techniques of Human Research and Therapeutics, A Series of Monographs" (F. G. McMahon, ed.), Vol. 15, pp. 209–240. Futura, New York.

Nishida, M., Mine, Y., Nonoyama, S., Kojo, H., Goto, S., and Kuwahara, S. (1977). *J. Antibiot.* **30**, 917.

Nishida, M., Mine, Y., and Nonoyama, S. (1978). *J. Antibiot.* **31**, 719.

Ratcliffe, R. W., and Christensen, B. G. (1973a). *Tetrahedron Lett.* p. 4645.

Ratcliffe, R. W., and Christensen, B. G. (1973b). *Tetrahedron Lett.* p. 4649.
Strominger, J. L., and Tipper, D. J. (1965). *Am. J. Med.* **39**, 708.
United States Patent (1979). No. 4,147,699.
United States Patent (1979). No. 4,180,507.
Wasserman, H. H., and Glazer, E. (1975). *J. Org. Chem.* **40**, 1505.
Wasserman, H. H., and Hlasta, D. J. (1978). *J. Am. Chem. Soc.* **100**, 6780.
Wasserman, H. H., and Lipshutz, B. H. (1976). *Tetrahedron Lett.* p. 4613.
Wasserman, H. H., Lipshutz, B. H., and Wu, J. S. (1977). *Heterocycles* **7**, 321.
Wasserman, H. H., Hlasta, D. J., Tremper, A. W., and Wu, J. S. (1979a). *Tetrahedron Lett.* p. 549.
Wasserman, H. H., Tremper, A. W., and Wu, J. S. (1979b). *Tetrahedron Lett.* p. 1089.

4

The Chemistry of Thienamycin and Other Carbapenem Antibiotics

RONALD W. RATCLIFFE AND GEORG
ALBERS-SCHÖNBERG

I. Structures of Natural Carbapenem Compounds

A. Introduction

In 1976, almost five decades after the discovery of penicillin and two decades after cephalosporin, three biogenetically novel, microbial β-lactam compounds were reported: the weakly antibacterial *nocardicin A* (**1**) (Volume 2, Chapter 3) (Aoki *et al.*, 1976); the β-lactamase inhibitor *clavulanic acid* (**2**) (Volume 2, Chapter 6) (Brown *et al.*, 1976; Howarth

Chemistry and Biology of
β-Lactam Antibiotics, Vol. 2

et al., 1976); and thienamycin (**3**) (Kahan *et al.*, 1976; Albers-Schönberg *et al.*, 1976; Kropp *et al.*, 1976; U.S. Pat. 3,950,357). The later is of particular interest as a potent, broad spectrum antibiotic with natural stability against β-lactamases and acting by inhibition of bacterial cell wall synthesis.

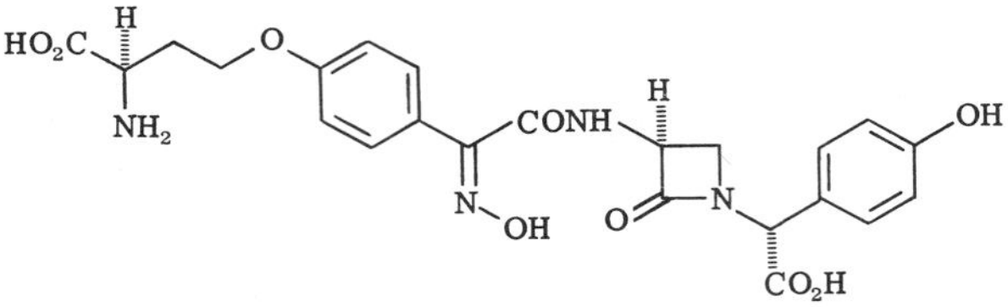

1

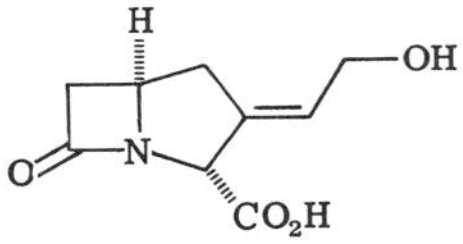

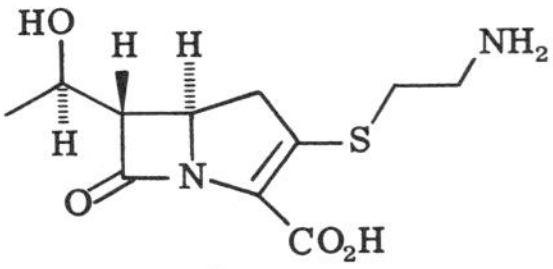

2   **3**

The present chapter is concerned solely with thienamycin and the growing list of its more recently reported analogs, in particular MC-696-SY2-A, the olivanic acids or epithienamycins, the PS group of compounds, and the carpetimycins. Collectively these products are derivatives of *carbapenem carboxylic acid* (**4a**), so-called to indicate the replacement of the sulfur atom of penicillin (a penam) by a carbon atom (Johnston *et al.*, 1978). All biologically active members of the class contain the unsaturated carbapen-2-em carboxylic acid nucleus (**4b**). In the following, we will briefly catalog the presently known carbapenems and discuss their isolation, structure determination, and stereochemical assignment. The bulk of the chapter will then review chemical derivatizations of the natural products and the synthetic approaches to carbapenem compounds as they have been developed in several laboratories.

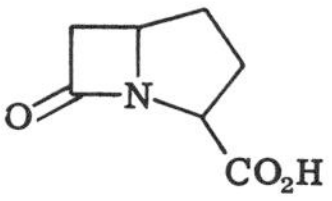

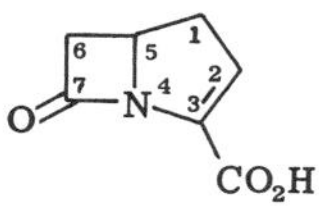

4a   **4b**

B. Summary of Known Natural Carbapenem Compounds

Thienamycin (**3, 5a**) is a metabolite of *Streptomyces cattleya* (U.S. Pat. 3,950,357; Kahan *et al.*, 1976, 1979), but has been named to denote the then novel β-thioenamin chromophore. It is a zwitterionic compound carrying an aminoethylthio substituent in the 2-position and a 1-hydroxyethyl substituent in the 6-position of the carbapenem nucleus (Albers-Schönberg *et al.*, 1976, 1978). The absolute stereochemistry at the three chiral centers is 5*R*, 6*S*, and 8*R*. A minor component of the fermentation broth is *9-northienamycin* (**5b**) with 5*R* and 6*S* configurations (U.S. Pat. 4,247,640; K. E. Wilson and A. J. Kempf, unpublished results, 1978).

5a R = CH$_3$
5b R = H

Merck, in searching for inhibitors of bacterial cell wall synthesis, and Beecham, in searching for β-lactamase inhibitors, independently discovered and named a group of derivatives of stereoisomers of thienamycin. The *olivanic acids*, named by Beecham in the traditional manner after the producing organism *Streptomyces olivaceus,* consisted initially only of the sulfated β-lactamase inhibitors MM 17880 (**6a**) (Corbett *et al.*, 1977), MM 13902 (**6b**), and MM 4550 (**6c**) (Brown *et al.*, 1977), and only more recently included the nonsulfated antibiotics MM 22380 (**6d**), MM 22381 (**6f**), MM 22382 (**6e**), and MM 22383 (**6g**) (Brown *et al.*, 1979; Box *et al.*, 1979). Merck, which focused first on antibacterial properties and stereochemical differences, named the same metabolites of *Streptomyces flavogriseus* variants the *epithienamycins* A (**6d**), B (**6e**), C (**6f**), D (**6g**), E (**6b**), and F (**6a**) (Stapley *et al.*, 1977, 1981; Cassidy *et al.*, 1977, 1981). At the same time, two further minor components elaborated by *S. cattleya* were identified as **7a** (Belg. Pat. 848,346) and **7b** (U.S. Pat. 4,162,323). Compounds **6** and **7** appear in stereochemically identical pairs carrying either the *N*-acetylaminoethylthio (*n* = 4) or *N*-acetylamino-*trans*-ethenylthio (*n* = 2) substituent at C-2. The β-lactamase inhibitors (**6a–c**) are sulfate esters of the C-8 hydroxyl group and have 5*R*, 6*R*, and 8*S* configurations. MM 4550 (**6c**) is furthermore oxidized to the sulfoxide of unknown chirality; this compound is missing from the series of epithienamycins. The nonsulfated olivanic acids/epithienamycins (**6d–g**) are two pairs with 5*R*, 6*R*, and 8*S* and 5*R*, 6*S*, and 8*S* configurations,

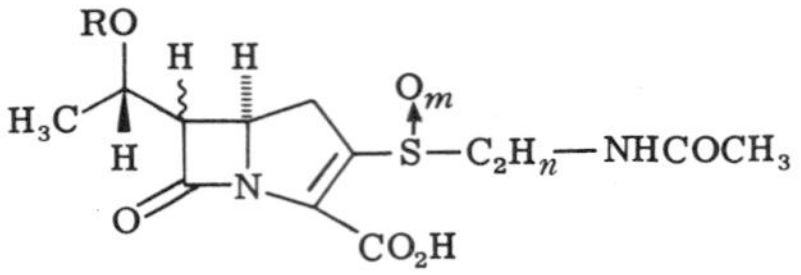

6a   R = SO₃H, m = 0, n = 4, 6α-H
6b   R = SO₃H, m = 0, n = 2, 6α-H
6c   R = SO₃H, m = 1, n = 2, 6α-H
6d   R = H, m = 0, n = 4, 6α-H
6e   R = H, m = 0, n = 2, 6α-H
6f   R = H, m = 0, n = 4, 6β-H
6g   R = H, m = 0, n = 2, 6β-H
6h   2, 3-dihydro-6d

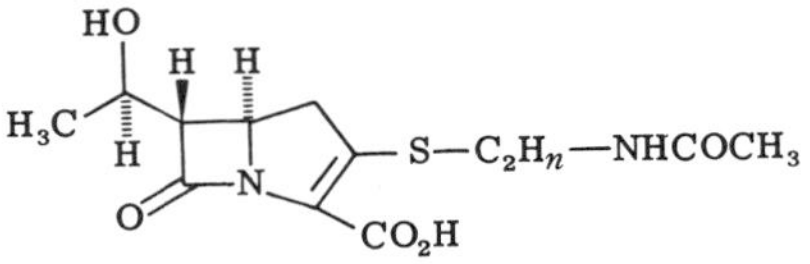

7a n = 4
7b n = 2

respectively. The pair of thienamycin derivatives (7a–b), as the parent compound, have 5R, 6S, and 8R configurations.

MC-696-SY2-A has been reported as a metabolite of S. fulvoviridis by the Institute of Microbial Chemistry, Tokyo, in collaboration with Meiji and the Japan National Institute of Health (Maeda et al., 1977). It is most likely identical with MM 4550 (6c). It was reported as a β-lactamase inhibitor of unknown structure as early as 1973 (Umezawa et al., 1973).

Sanraku-Ocean/Panlab's PS-1 to 4 and Sankyo's 17927 group of compounds (Ger. Offen. 2,809,235) also have structures (6) with R = H but have not been defined stereochemically. Sankyo's 17927 A₁ is most likely identical to epithienamycin A (6d), 17927 A₂ with epithienamycin B (6e), and 17927 D (6h) is a 2,3-dihydro derivative of 17927 A₁.

PS-5 (Okamura et al., 1978, 1979; Yamamoto et al., 1980), PS-6, and PS-7 (Shibamato et al., 1980) have also been reported by Sanraku-Ocean in collaboration with Panlabs as minor components in cultures of S. cremeus, subsp. auratilis A271. PS-5 (8a) and PS-7 (8b) lack the C-8 hydroxyl group, whereas PS-6 (8c) replaces it by a second methyl group. The configurations at C-5 and C-6 of these compounds are R and R, respectively; the compounds, like thienamycin, are trans-substituted about the β-lactam ring. Most recently, the Tokyo Research Laboratories of the Kowa Company reported carpetimycins A (9a) and B (9b) as metabolites of a not further identified Streptomyces species (Mori et al.,

1980; Nakayama *et al.*, 1980). These compounds provide further examples of a C-6 isopropyl substituent, but now include the C-8 hydroxyl group. The configurations at C-5 and C-6 of the carpetimycins are the same as those of the sulfated olivanic acids. Carpetimycin B (**9b**) is 8-methyl-MM 4550 if one assumes the same *R*-sulfoxide chirality for both compounds; carpetimycin A (**9a**) is the corresponding C-8 alcohol.

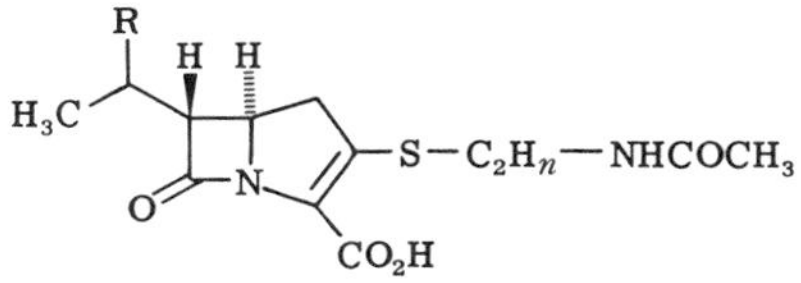

8a R = H, n = 4
8b R = H, n = 2
8c R = CH$_3$, n = 4

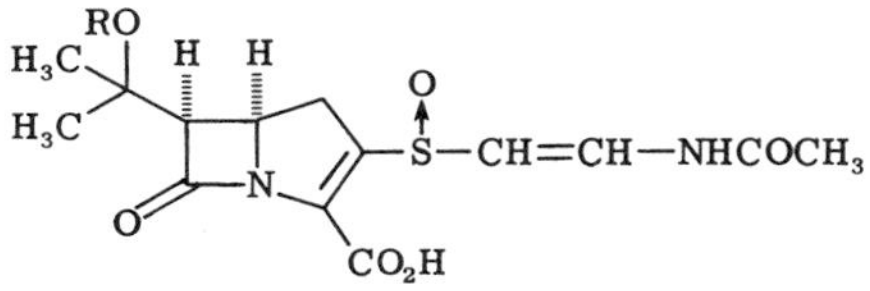

9a R = H
9b R = SO$_3$H

These correlations among the various compounds are summarized in Table I and partial structures **10, 11, 12,** and **13**. So far, there is no evidence for a naturally occurring carbapenem derivative with 5*R*, 6*R*,8*R* configurations.

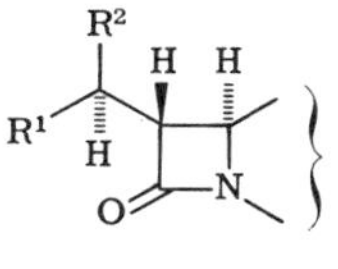

10

Thienamycin
N-Acetylthienamycin   } R^1 = CH$_3$
N-Acetyl-11, 12-dehydrothienamycin } R^2 = OH
9-Northienamycin   R^1 = H; R^2 = OH
PS-5
PS-7   } R^1 = H; R^2 = CH$_3$
PS-6   R^1 = R^2 = CH$_3$

TABLE I Identities and Stereochemical Assignments of Natural Carbapenem Compounds

	Compound			H-5/H-6	C-5	C-6	C-8
(5a)	Thienamycin			trans	R	S	R
(5b)	9-Northienamycin			trans	R	S	S
(6a)	Epithienamycin F ,	Olivanic Acid MM 17880		cis	R	R	S
(6b)	Epithienamycin E ,	Olivanic Acid MM 13902		cis	R	R	S
(6c)		Olivanic Acid MM 4550 ,	MC 696-SY2-A	cis	R	R	S
(6d)	Epithienamycin A ,	Olivanic Acid MM 22380 ,	17927 A$_1$	cis	R	R	S
(6e)	Epithienamycin B ,	Olivanic Acid MM 22382 ,	17927 A$_2$	cis	R	R	S
(6f)	Epithienamycin C ,	Olivanic Acid MM 22381		trans	R	S	S
(6g)	Epithienamycin D ,	Olivanic Acid MM 22383		trans	R	S	S
(6h)		17927 D		cis	R	R	S
(7a)	N-Acetylthienamycin			trans	R	S	R
(7b)	N-Acetyl-11,12-dehydrothienamycin			trans	R	S	R
(8a)		PS-5		trans	R	R	
(8b)		PS-7		trans	R	R	
(8c)		PS-6		trans	R	R	
(9a)	Carpetimycin A			cis	R	R	
(9b)	Carpetimycin B			cis	R	R	

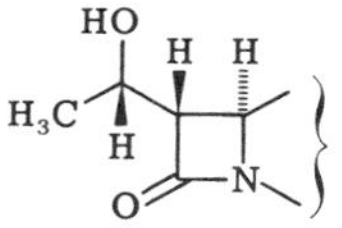

11

Epithienamycin C/MM 22381
Epithienamycin D/MM 22383

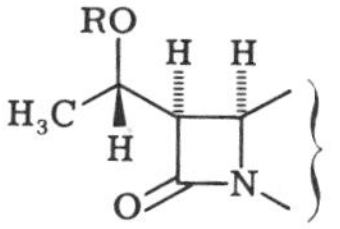

Epithienamycin A/MM 22380/17927A$_1$ }
Epithienamycin B/MM 22382/17927A$_2$ } R = H
17927D }
Epithienamycin E/MM 13902 }
Epithienamycin F/MM 17880 } R = SO$_3$H
MC-696-SY2-A/MM 4550 }

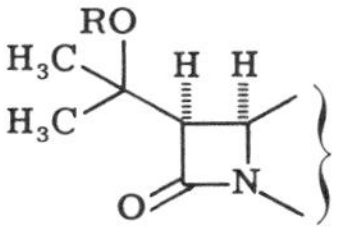

12

13

Carpetimycin A   R = H
Carpetimycin B   R = SO$_3$H

C. Isolation of Carbapenems from Fermentation Broth

The carbapenem ring system is highly strained and the β-lactam is consequently very reactive, particularly outside a narrow pH range near neutrality which has to be maintained throughout an isolation process. Lengthy procedures have been published, often only in schematic outline, describing the use of ion-pair extraction, ion-exchange and gel filtration methods. The reader is referred to the original reports on thienamycin (Kahan *et al.*, 1979) and northienamycin (U.S. Pat. 4,247,640), *N*-acetyl-(U.S. Pat. 4,165,379) and *N*-acetyl-11,12-dehydrothienamycin (U.S. Pat. 4,162,323), sulfated (Hood *et al.*, 1979) and nonsulfated olivanic acids (Box *et al.*, 1979), epithienamycins (U.S. Pat. 4,141,986; 4,162,324; Cassidy *et al.*, 1981), PS-5 (Okamura *et al.*, 1979), PS-6, and PS-7 (Shibamato *et al.*, 1980), carpetimycins (Nakayama *et al.*, 1980), and MC-696-SY2-A (Umezawa *et al.*, 1973).

D. Structure Determinations

1. *Spectroscopic Analyses and Degradations*

The first carbapenem structure to be reported was that of thienamycin (U.S. Pat. 3,950,357), and detailed accounts of this analysis including stereochemical assignments by chemical and crystallographic methods

have been given (Albers-Schönberg *et al.*, 1976, 1978). Low broth titers
and the inherent instability of the antibiotic had created major difficulties
in the isolation of the antibiotic and made it necessary to begin the
structure determination with derivatizations of only partially purified
material. It had been observed that the characteristic ultraviolet absorption of biologically active samples near 300 nm could be abolished together with bioactivity by treatment with typical β-lactam reagents such
as hydroxylamine or cysteine (Kahan *et al.*, 1976). Together with the
known mode of action of the antibiotic by interference with bacterial cell
wall synthesis, this immediately brought the classical β-lactam antibiotics
to mind and directed the attention to two components that appeared with
sulfur isotope peak ratios in field-desorption mass spectra of partially
purified antibiotic (MH^+ 273 and 333). Acetylation and esterification then
led to the isolation of three pure, sulfur-containing products (**15–17**) that
showed intense ultraviolet absorption near 310 nm. On the basis of their
mass spectra the products were hypothetically related to each other by
assuming that, either during the derivatization or during the last chromatographic purification step using an acetate buffer, acetolysis of a very
reactive carboxyl function, probably a lactam, occurred; the initially
formed mixed anhydride would acetylate the newly generated basic nitrogen function (Scheme 1). Field-desorption mass spectra of pure thienamycin, when this eventually became available, showed a molecular ion
peak at *m/e* 273; ^{13}C-NMR spectra showed a total of 11 carbon atoms
and ^1H-NMR spectra 12 nonexchangeable protons (Tables II and III);
quantitative energy-dispersive X-ray fluorescence analysis (EDAX) confirmed one sulfur atom per molecule; and the ultraviolet absorption maximum was found at 297 nm.

The elucidation of the thienamycin structure, naturally, revolved
around the question of whether or not the antibiotic contained a β-lactam
ring. Infrared absorption of **15** at 1779 cm^{-1}, similar to that of cephalosporin esters, and the absorption of thienamycin itself at 1765 cm^{-1},
similar to that of cephalosporin C, were regarded as strong evidence in
favor of a β-lactam despite the much higher ring strain, as compared to
cephalosporins, of the eventually proposed structure. It could be ar-
gued—and was subsequently substantiated by literature data (see Volume
1, Chapter 5)—that replacement of a sulfur substituent in the 4-position
of an azetidin-2-one by carbon, hydrogen, or even oxygen substantially
lowers the β-lactam carbonyl frequency.

A second argument for a β-lactam function in **15** was provided by a
mass spectral fragmentation that could be interpreted by analogy to the
well-known β-lactam cleavages of penicillins and cephalosporins (Richter
and Biemann, 1964, 1965), provided a two-carbon substituent R = C_2H_5O

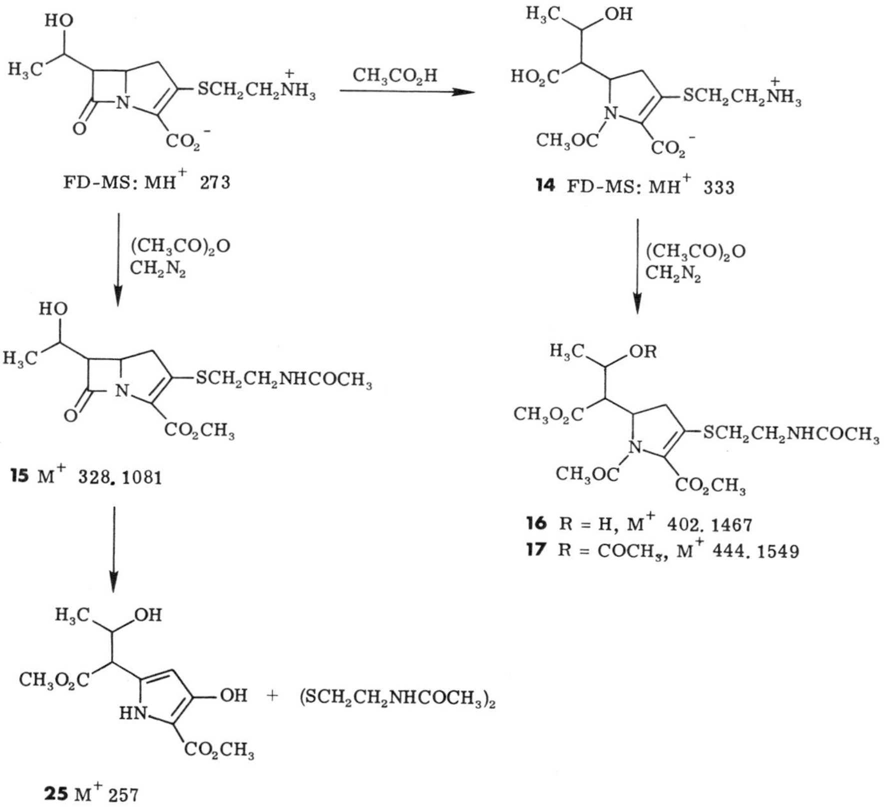

Scheme 1

was assumed instead of the classical *N*-acylamino substituent (Scheme 2). The argument was valid because a detailed comparison of the mass and NMR spectra of **15, 16,** and **17** independently proved the presence of such a substituent adjacent to the reactive carboxyl group, as follows:

Derivative **15** gave mass spectral fragments of *m/e* 86, $C_4H_6O_2$, and *m/e* 243, $C_{10}H_{15}N_2O_3S$([$^2H_3$]acetyl analog: *m/e* 246), whereas **16** and **17**

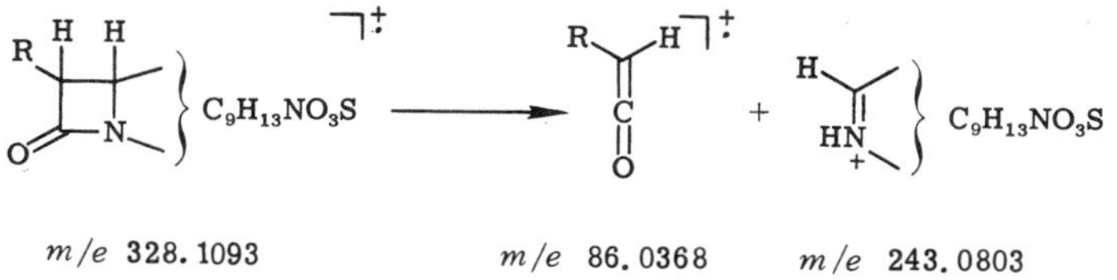

Scheme 2

TABLE II ¹H-NMR Absorptions of the Natural Carbapenem Compounds[1]

Compound	C-1-H$_2$	C-5-H	C-6-H	C-8-H	C-9-H$_3$	CH$_n$–S	CH$_n$–NH	C-14-H$_3$
(5a) Thienamycin[a]	3.15 m	4.20 m	3.39 dd J = 2.7, 6	4.20 m	1.27 d J = 6.5	3.15 m	3.15 m	
(5b) 9-Northienamycin[b]	3.08–3.22 m	4.22 dt J = 2.5–3, 8	3.58 m J(5,6) = 2.5–3	3.91 dd, J = 4.0, 12 3.96 dd, J = 4.5, 12		3.08–3.22 m	3.08– 3.22 m	
(7a) N-Acetylthienamycin[c]	3.17 m	3.96 m	3.37 dd J = 3, 6	3.96 m	1.27 d J = 6.5	2.93 m	3.39 m	1.98 s
(7b) N-Acetyl-11,12-dehydrothienamycin[d]	3.10 dd, J = 8.7, 17.5 3.21 dd, J = 9.5, 17.5	4.22 m	3.39 dd J = 2.5, 6	4.22 m	1.29 d J = 6.5	6.07 d J = 13.5	7.19 d J = 13.5	2.08 s
(6f) Epithienamycin C[e] Olivanic Acid MM 22381[f]	3.13 m	4.13 m	3.42 dd J = 2.5, 6 J(5,6) = 3	4.13 m	1.29 d J = 6.5	2.92 m	3.39 m	1.98 s
(6g) Epithienamycin D[e] Olivanic acid MM 22383[f]	3.04 dd, J = 9, 17 3.12 dd, J = 9, 17	4.16 m	3.41 dd J = 3, 5 J(5,6) = 3	4.16 m	1.29 d J = 6.5	6.00 d J = 13.5	7.11 d J = 13.5	2.05 s
(6d) Epithienamycin A[e] Olivanic acid MM 22380[f] 17927 A$_1$[g]	3.18 m	4.14 m	3.63 dd J = 5.2, 9.8 J(5,6) = 5.5–6	4.14 m	1.35 d J = 6.5	2.97 m	3.41 m	1.98 s

236

(6e) Epithienamycin B[e]	3.08 dd, J = 9.8, 18; 3.15 dd, J = 9.8, 18	4.19 m	3.61 dd J = 5, 9.6	4.19 m	1.33 d J = 6.5	6.03 d J = 13.8	7.13 d J = 13.8	2.06 s
Olivanic acid MM 22382[f] 17927 A$_2$			J(5,6) = 5.5–6 3.6 dd					
(6a) Epithienamycin F[e] Olivanic acid MM 17880[h]	3.27 m	4.34 m	3.89 dd J = 5.4, 9.2 J(5,6) = 6	4.83 m	1.55 d J = 6.5	3.03 m	3.43 m	2.02 s
(6b) Epithienamycin E[e]	3.06 dd, J = 9, 18 3.32 dd, J = 9, 18	4.29 m	3.84 dd J = 5, 10	4.85 m	1.50 d J = 6.5	6.07 d J = 13.8	7.16 d J = 13.8	2.04 s
Olivanic acid MM 13902[i,*]	2.94 dd, J = 9.5, 18 3.29 dd, J = 8.5, 18	4.25 m	3.78 dd J = 5.5, 9	4.75 m	1.47 d J = 6	5.87 d (d$_6$-DMSO) J = 14	6.98 dd (d$_6$-DMSO) J = 10, 14	2.00 s
(6c) Olivanic acid MM 4550[i,*]	2.99 dd, J = 10.5, 18 3.46 dd, J = 9.0, 18	4.37 m	3.88 dd J = 6, 9	4.97 m	1.45 d J = 6.5	6.24 d (d$_6$-DMSO) J = 14	7.18 dd (d$_6$-DMSO) J = 11, 14	2.05 s
MC 696-SY2-A[k]	3.05 dd, J = 10, 18 3.50 dd, J = 9, 18	4.48 m	3.96 dd J = 6, 8	4.90 m	1.50 d J = 6	6.49 d J = 14	7.59 d J = 14	2.12 s
(8a) PS-5[l,**]	2.88–3.58 m	2.88–3.58 m	4.04 dt J = 3, 9.2	1.72–2.00 m	1.06 t J = 7	2.88–3.58 m	2.88–3.58 m	2.05 s
(8b) PS-7[m,**]	2.45–3.30 m	2.45–3.30 m	3.90 dt J = 3, 9	1.54–1.84 m	0.91 t J = 7	5.97 d J = 14	7.14 d J = 14	2.01 s
(8c) PS-6[m,**]	2.80–3.60 m	2.80–3.60 m	4.00 dt J = 3, 9	1.96–2.20 m	0.94 d, 0.98 d J = 7	2.80–3.60 m	2.80–3.60 m	1.95 s

(continued)

TABLE II [1](Continued)

Compound	C-1-H$_2$	C-5-H	C-6-H	C-8-H	C-9-H$_3$	CH$_n$-S	CH$_n$-NH	C-14-H$_3$
(9a) Carpetimycin A"	3.06 dd, $J = 11, 17$ 3.95 dd, $J = 8, 17$	4.50 m	3.84 d $J = 5.5$		1.35 s, 1.43 s	6.44 d $J = 14$	7.62 d $J = 14$	2.16 s
(9b) Carpetimycin B"	3.14 dd, $J = 11, 18$ 3.94 dd, $J = 8, 18$	4.56 m	4.02 d $J = 5.5$		1.67 s, 1.75 s	6.47 d $J = 14$	7.65 d $J = 14$	2.17 s

[1] Spectra were recorded at 100 or 300 MHz in D$_2$O; reference for most compounds is reported or assumed to be internal DSS, in some cases internal TMS–CD$_2$–CD$_2$–COONa (**) or CH$_3$CN at δ2.00 (*); coupling constants are given in Hertz. Chemical shifts for MC 696-SY2-A and the carpetimycins are corrected to internal DSS by subtracting 0.48 δ from values reported relative to external TMS. References: (a) Albers-Schönberg et al. (1976, 1978); (b) K. E. Wilson et al. (unpublished data); U.S. Pat. 4,247,640: (c) F. M. Kahan et al. (unpublished data); U.S. Pat. 4,165,379; Cassidy et al. (1981); (d) U.S. Pat. 4,162,323; U.S. Pat. 4,162,323; (e) Cassidy et al. (1977, 1981); (f) Brown et al. (1979); U.S. Pat. 4,165,379; (g) Ger. Offen. 2,809,235; 2,811,514; (h) Corbett et al. (1979); Hood et al. (1977); (i) Brown et al. (1977); Hood et al. (1979); (k) Maeda et al. (1977); (l) Okamura et al. (1978, 1979); (m) Shibamoto et al. (1980); (n) Mori et al. (1980); Nakayama et al. (1980).

TABLE III ^{13}C-NMR Absorptions of Natural Carbapenem Compounds^a

	Thienamycin	PS-5	MM 13902	MM 4550	MC 696-SY2-A
C-9	21.0 q	11.4 q	19 q	19 q	19.1 q
C-14	—	22.6 q	23 q	23 q	23.0 q
C-1	39.6 t**	39.9 t*	37 t	29 t	29.6
C-5	53.3 d	55.6 d	54 d	55 d	54.6
C-6	65.8 d*	60.2 d	58 d	59 d	59.0
C-8	65.9 d*	22.5 t	74 d	74 d	73.7
C-11	29.4 t	31.5 t	103 d	112 d	112.1
C-12	40.1 t**	40.0 t*	131 d	135 d	135.0
C-2	132.8 s	130.4 s	128 s	139 s*	141.1*
C-3	137.6 s	141.1 s	144 s	140 s*	139.1*
C-10	166.1 s	169.3 s	169 s	166 s	166.1
C-7	180.3 s	184.0 s	178 s	177 s	177.7
C-13	—	175.0 s	172 s	173 s	173.5

^{a} All spectra were recorded on sodium or barium (MC 696-SY2-A) salts, resp. on the zwitterionic thienamycin (pD 6.8) in D$_2$O; chemical shifts are given relative to internal dioxane at 67.4 ppm. Starred assignments are interchangeable.

lost 117 (C$_4$H$_6$O$_2$ + OCH$_3$) and 159 (C$_4$H$_6$O$_2$ + OCH$_3$ + C$_2$H$_2$O) mass units, respectively, to give m/e 285 (243 + CH$_2$CO; ^{2}H$_3$: m/e 291). Therefore, m/e 86 of **15** had to contain the reactive carbonyl group and a hydroxyl group of thienamycin, whereas the protected zwitterionic functionalities remained part of the m/e 243 fragments (amide I and II bands of **15** at 1631 and 1548 cm^{-1} and the mass spectral loss of acetamide from m/e 243 specify a secondary amide). This is summarized in partial structure **18** for derivative **16**. The C$_3$H$_5$ substructure had to be a saturated chain to which the five hydrogens and three other substituents could be attached in four different ways of which only **19** was compatible with NMR spectra of thienamycin and its derivatives. The 100-MHz spectrum

18

19

20

of the antibiotic showed a methyl doublet at δ 1.27, a narrow six-proton multiplet centered at δ 3.15, a methine doublet-of-doublets at δ 3.39, and two overlapping methine multiplets at δ 4.20. Double-irradiation at the frequency of the lower field methine signals reduced the methyl doublet and the methine signal at δ 3.39 to singlets. The lower field methine multiplet of **15** in [²H₆]dimethyl sulfoxide was resolved into a multiplet at δ 3.95 and a doublet-of-triplet at δ 4.12. Thus, a string of five hydrogen-bearing carbon atoms as shown in partial structure **20** was defined. Combining **18, 19,** and **20,** considering likely chemical shifts and incorporating the ¹³C-NMR information on thienamycin (Table III), resulted in partial structure **21** for the derivative **15.**

Partial structure **21** accounted for five of the seven medium and high-field ¹³C-NMR signals of thienamycin, leaving the signals of two de-shielded methylene groups to be assigned. ¹H-NMR spectra of **15** in [²H₆]DMSO showed an amidic, exchangeable NH triplet at δ 8.22. The signal of the adjoining methylene group was not resolved from other absorptions but could be observed by itself at δ 3.16 in the spectrum of **16** in CDCl₃ as a triplet after exchange of the amide proton. This implied a X—CH₂—CH₂—NHCOCH₃ substructure in which X is another de-shielding group. Analogous conclusions were drawn from mass spectra of **15** and **16.** Both compounds showed abundant fragments of m/e 86.0593, C_4H_8NO, and m/e 118.0336, C_4H_8NOS, both containing reagent-derived acetyl groups and interpreted in terms of —CH₂—CH₂NHCOCH₃ and —S—CH₂—CH₂—NHCOCH₃ substructures. The original observation pointing to such a substituent in thienamycin had been the finding of β-aminoethylsulfonic acid (taurine) in amino acid analyses following peracid oxidation. Amino acid analyses of complex microbial metabolites must be interpreted with much caution, but in this case all data appeared to be consistent, and partial structure **21** could thus be elaborated to **22.**

21

22

The structural elements of **22** can be assembled to give two different ring systems, the fused β-lactam **23** and the azabicyclo[2.2.1]heptene **24,** each with two substitutional isomers at the double bond. At the time of the analysis, **24** was not considered as an alternative. It would, through

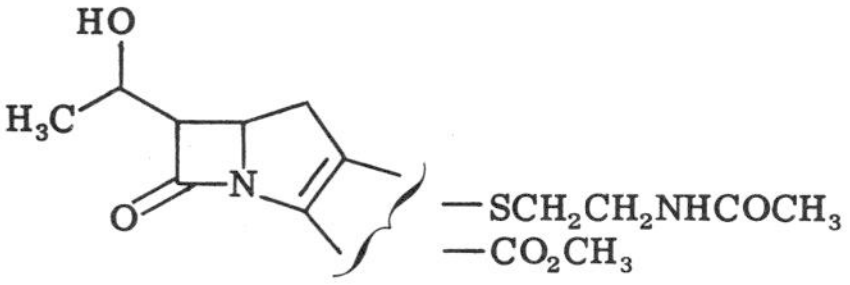

23 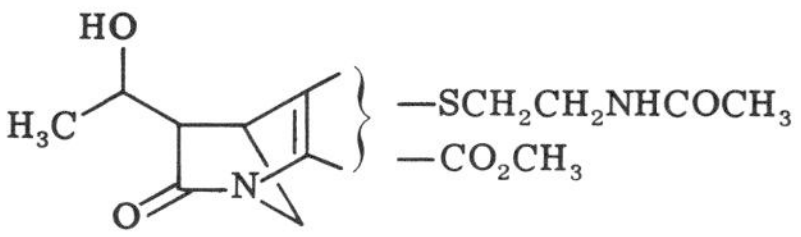   **24**

a highly favored retro-Diels–Alder fragmentation, give the identical or tautomeric fragments m/e 86 and 243 as **15**. However, the fragmentations of **16** seem less likely for the corresponding isomeric structure. Moreover, **24** appears incompatible with the observed infrared and ^{1}H-NMR data and is not likely to undergo the extremely facile acetolysis reaction of thienamycin. The final thienamycin structure was unambigously established by methanolysis of **15** at room temperature under conditions permitting air oxidation, which resulted in the 3-hydroxypyrrol-2-carboxylic ester derivative **25**. The structure of **25** was ascertained by spectroscopic comparison with model compound **26** which was synthesized from glycine ethyl ester and ethyl acetoacetate. Compound **24** would have led to the isomeric pyrrol **27** for which the C-5 hydrogen signal is expected near δ 6.5 as reported for **28**. Compound **25** also unambiguously determines the double bond substitution.

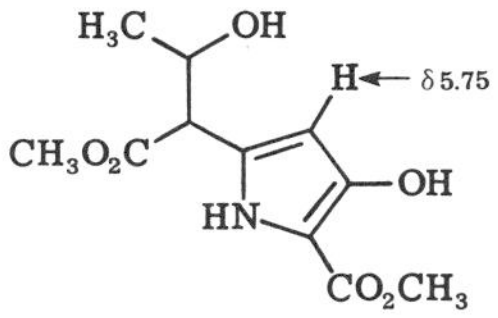

25 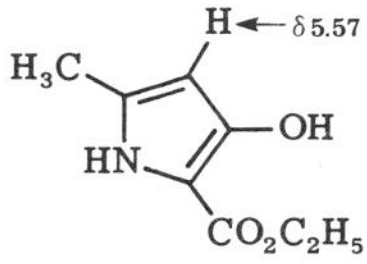   **26**

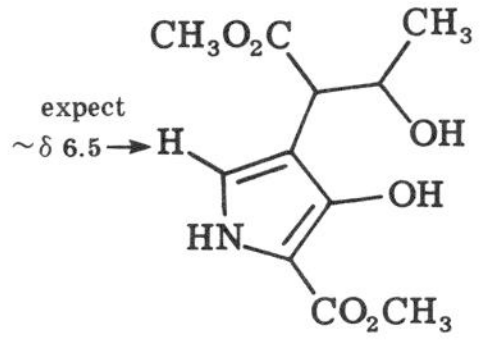

27 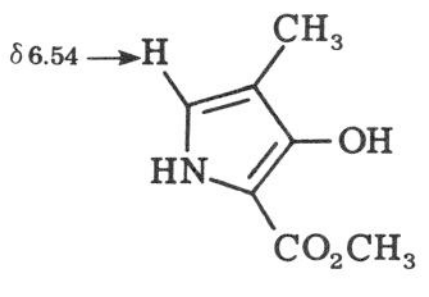   **28**

In the course of the described structure determination, crystals of **15** were obtained from dilute solutions in dry, aprotic solvents. These were suitable for a single-crystal X-ray analysis that fully confirmed all conclusions. This analysis will be discussed in the section on stereochemistry.

It would be redundant to recount in detail the analyses of all natural carbapenems. Hydroxyethyl-substituted β-lactam substructures were in all cases assigned on the basis of infrared absorption in 1750–1770 cm^{-1} region (Table IV) (in some cases supported by higher frequency absorptions of the corresponding esters) and of NMR evidence for the characteristic sequence of hydrogen-bearing carbon atoms. Also, the mass spectral β-lactam cleavage has provided useful information, particularily on the novel C-6 isopropyl analogs. The presence of a sulfate ester group was deduced variously from combustion analyses, electrophoretic mobilities, infrared absorptions in the 1220 cm^{-1} region, and low- and high-resolution mass spectra. Attachment of the sulfate ester group at C-8 was inferred from downfield chemical shift changes, com-

TABLE IV   Optical Characteristics of Natural Carbapenem Compounds

	β-Lactam CO (cm^{-1}, KBr)	Ultraviolet absorption [λ_{max}nm, (ε)]	$[\alpha]_D^{20-27}$ (c, H$_2$O)
(5a) Thienamycin[a]	1765	296.5 (7900)	+82° (0.1)
(5b) 9-Northienamycin[b]	1764	297	
(7a) N-Acetylthienamycin[c]	1750	301 (8480)	
(7b) N-Acetyl-11,12-dehydrothienamycin[d]		307.5	
(6f) Epithienamycin C[e]		300	
Olivanic acid MM 22381[f]	1750	301 (7930)	
(6g) Epithienamycin D[e]		308 (15390), 228 (14660)	
Olivanic acid MM 22383[f]	1750	309 (13933), 229 (13933)	
(6d) Epithienamycin A[e]		299 (7222)	
Olivanic acid MM 22380[f]	1750	298 (8131)	
(6e) Epithienamycin B[e]		308 (15700), 288 (14950)	
Olivanic Acid MM 22382[f]	1750	308 (13627), 288 (13290)	
(6a) Epithienamycin F[e]		300 (8274)	
Olivanic acid MM 17880[g]	1750	298 (8410)	
(6b) Epithienamycin E[e]		308 (14500), 228 (13800)	
Olivanic acid 13902[h]	1750	307 (15520), 227 (14640)	−81° (1.0)
(6c) Olivanic acid MM 4550[h]	1765	287 (12110), 240 (13560)	−137° (0.52)
MC 696-SY2-A[i]	1765–1770	280 (12000), 240 (15300)	−109° (0.56)
(8a) PS-5[k]	1760	301 (7970)	+77.3° (1.59)
(8b) PS-7[l]	1755	308 (13900), 226 (14300)	+62° (0.23)
(8c) PS-6[l]	1750	300 (9003)	+55° (0.22)
(9a) Carpetimycin A[m]	1770	288 (10500), 240 (12915)	−27° (1.7)
(9b) Carpetimycin B[m]	1770	285 (15870), 240 (15350)	−145° (1.0)

References: (a) Kahan *et al.* (1979); U.S. Pat. 3,950,357; (b) Wilson *et al.* (unpublished data); U.S. Pat. 4,247,640; (c) U.S. Pat. 4,165,379; U.S. Pat. 4,165,379; (d) U.S. Pat. 4,162,323; U.S. Pat. 4,162,323; (e) Cassidy *et al.* (1981); (f) Brown *et al.* (1979); Box *et al.* (1979); (g) Corbett *et al.* (1977); Hood *et al.* (1979); Brown *et al.* (1979); (h) Brown *et al.* (1977); (i) Maeda *et al.* (1977); (k) Okamura *et al.* (1979); Yamamoto *et al.* (1980); (l) Shibamoto *et al.* (1980); (m) Mori *et al.* (1980); Nakayama *et al.* (1980).

pared to the nonsulfated analogs, of about 0.6 ppm for C-8 hydrogen and about 0.2 ppm for C-6 hydrogen and the methyl protons (Table II). Epithienamycins E and F (Table I) were isolated as ammonium salts for direct mass spectrometric analysis as trimethylsilyl derivatives. The spectra showed strong signals for bistrimethylsilyl sulfate ions and 8,6- or 8,9-ene-lactam structures with no changes indicated in the pyrroline and thioether substructures (Cassidy *et al.*, 1981).

The acylated β-aminoethylthio and β-aminoethenylthio substituents were mostly inferred from spectroscopic data, but in at least one case also by degradation to dehydrotaurine and taurine (Maeda *et al.*, 1977). NMR evidence for an unsaturated substituent is the striking replacement of two-thirds of the complex methylene absorption of the saturated compounds in the δ 2.8–3.5 range by olefinic signals of a deshielded trans-disubstituted double bond; simultaneously, the AB signal pattern for the ring methylene group becomes interpretable. The absence of mass spectral fragments, which represent the loss of acetamide, from mass spectra of the 11,12-dehydro derivatives has been reported for the trimethylsilyl derivatives of the epithienamycins B, D, and E (Cassidy *et al.*, 1977, 1981) and for PS-7 (Shibamoto *et al.*, 1980). Spectra of PS-7 methyl ester instead show a pronounced loss of ketene typical for vinyl acetates. Unsaturation in the thioether substituent is also reflected in a bathochromic shift of about 8 nm and a 75% increase of the molecular extinction at the long-wavelength ultraviolet absorption maximum and in the appearance of an equally intense absorption near 228 nm (Table IV). Elemental analyses of MM 4550 and MC-696-SY2-A were ambiguous about the exact number of oxygen atoms in the molecule. The sulfoxide group of MC-696-SY2-A was deduced by oxidation to the sulfone with peracid and reduction to the sulfide with stannous chloride, with concomitant ultraviolet absorption changes. In the case of MM 4550, differences in the circular dichroism spectra compared to MM 13902 were interpreted in support of a sulfoxide because of the groups chirality. The most recently reported X-ray analysis of the *p*-bromobenzyl ester of carpetimycin A (Nakayama *et al.*, 1980) undoubtedly provides the strongest evidence for such a group.

In the following paragraphs we summarize three degradation sequences which in each case yielded important additional information on the compounds.

1. Partial hydrolysis of MC-696-SY2-A (Maeda *et al.*, 1977) (**6c**) and tautomerization of the resulting enamine gave (Scheme 3) the diastereomeric imines **29**. Reduction with Raney nickel gave *N*-ethylacetamide and derivative **30** whose "positive ninhydrin test suggested the presence of a proline moiety." Removal of the sulfate ester and esterification of

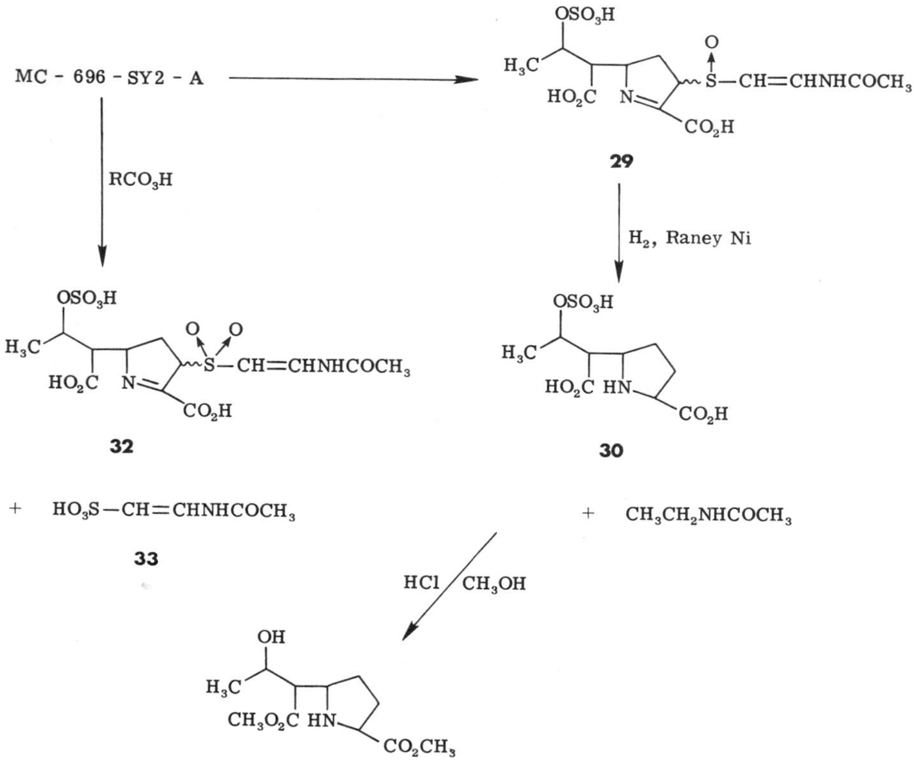

Scheme 3

the carboxylic acid group yielded **31** which was amenable to mass spectral analysis. Oxidation of the antibiotic with peracid gave the already mentioned sulfone (**32**) and *N*-acetyldehydrotaurine (**33**) which was reduced catalytically for identification. Most products are reported with their ^{1}H- and ^{13}C-NMR characteristics. No mass spectral details are provided.

2. An interesting, quantitative degradation of the carbapenem system (Scheme 4) was discovered by the Beecham group (Corbett *et al.*, 1977) and used for the structure determination of MM 17880 by analogy to MM 13902. Warming of the carboxymethyl esters of these compounds for 2 hr to 70°C in dimethyl sulfoxide (DMSO) resulted in the hydrolysis of the lactam and dehydrogenation of the pyrroline without loss of either the sulfate ester or the thioether substituents. Elimination of the sulfate ester by treatment with DBU, followed by esterification with diazomethane then gave **34** which was analyzed mass spectrometrically (reported

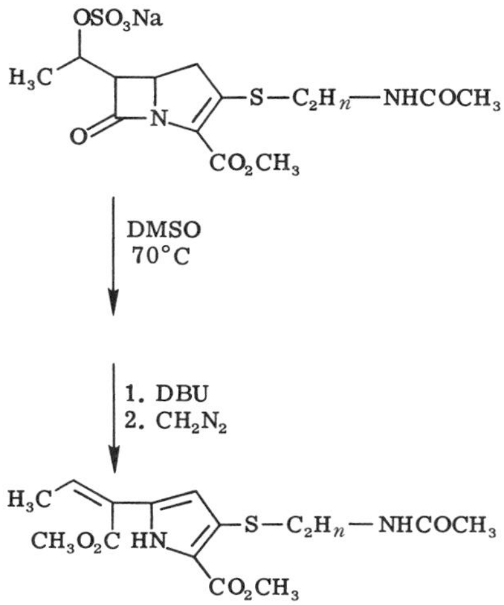

Scheme 4

fragments: m/e 84/86, $C_2H_nNHCOCH_3$; $M-C_4H_{5/7}NO$; $M-CH_3CONH_2$). The degradation in DMSO is reminiscent of the degradation of N-acetylthienamycin methyl esters to the pyrrol (25).

3. ^{1}H-NMR analysis of the methyl ester of PS-5 (Yamamoto *et al.*, 1980) established the usual sequence of five hydrogen-bearing carbon atoms, except for the absence of the C-8 hydroxy group (Scheme 5). The remainder of the proton signals could be assigned to a β-substituted N-ethylacetamide group and a methyl ester. These results, ^{13}C-NMR, and mass and infrared spectral data suggested structure **8a**; and a step-by-step degradation aimed at the determination of the absolute configuration at C-6, constituted an almost complete independent structure proof. The p-nitrobenzyl ester (**35**) was treated with ozone to give the thioester (**36**) which was converted to the acid with mercuric trifluoroacetate and esterified with diazomethane to **37**. Treatment with m-chloroperbenzoic acid converted **37** to the diacyl peroxide (**38**) which under mild conditions underwent a "carboxy inversion" rearrangement to the carbonic anhydride (**39**). Hydrolysis and lactonization then yielded **40**.

2. Stereochemical Assignments

The known natural carbapenem compounds have two or three chiral centers at C-5, C-6, and C-8. The absolute configuration at C-5 has been shown in four independent studies, including that of thienamycin, to be R, providing a molecular geometry of the ring system analogous to that

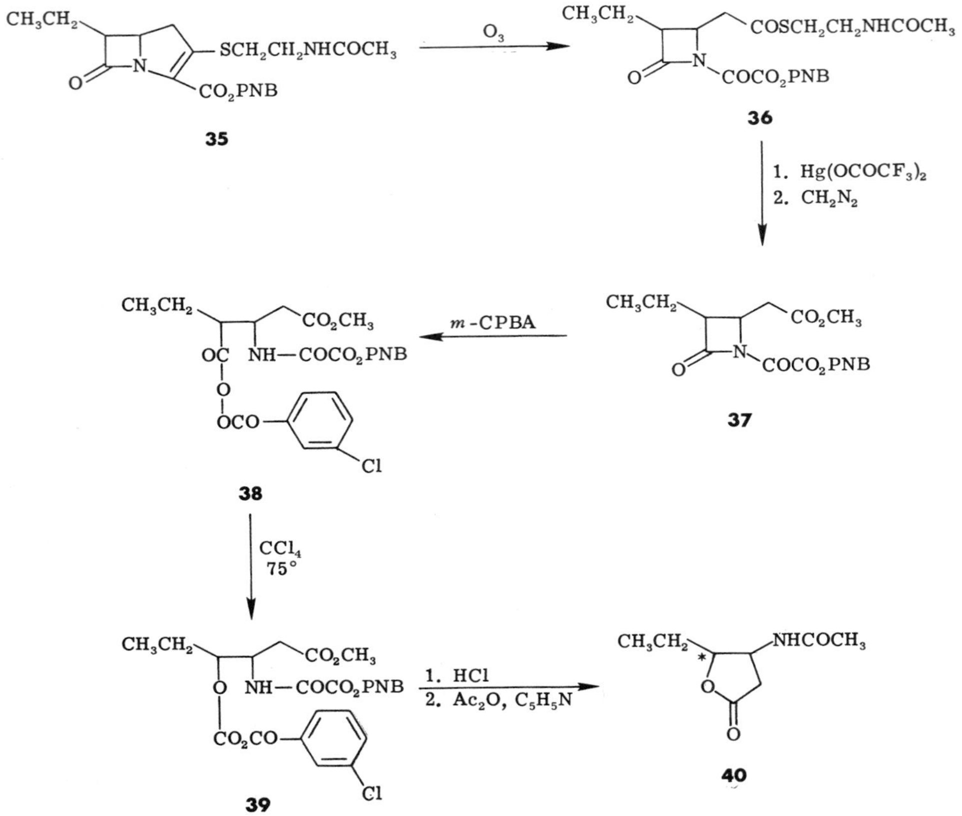

PNB = p-nitrobenzyl

Scheme 5

of both the older β-lactam antibiotics and clavulanic acid. A comparison of the circular dichroism spectra of thienamycin (U.S. Pat. 3,950,357) and several epithienamycins (Cassidy et al., 1981) with that of cephalosporin C (Demarco and Nagarajan, 1972) seemed to confirm the correlation, but insufficient data are available to test its generality and limitations. However, totally synthetic (±)-thienamycin was shown to have half the potency of natural (+)-thienamycin (Johnston et al., 1978), and we therefore assume that all biologically active carbapenems have the 5R configuration. Rules have been established for the determination of relative configurations at C-5 and C-6 by NMR spectroscopy. Determinations of the configurations at C-8, however, were difficult. Close spectroscopic similarities between epimers and the sensitivity of the spectroscopic data to pH and solvent differences made it impossible to compare data from different laboratories. In several cases differences were determined or identities established by NMR analyses of mixed samples. In the following we first summarize those reported assignments based on direct analyses of individual compounds rather than on indirect evidence. We will then show how the remaining correlations of Table I were derived.

Relative configurations at all three chiral centers of (+)-thienamycin were determined by X-ray crystallographic analysis of the acetyl methyl ester (**15**) (Hirshfield and Hoogsteen, cited in Albers-Schönberg *et al.*, 1978). Absolute configurations were determined by several chemical transformations (Hensens and Ratcliffe *et al.*, cited in Albers-Schönberg *et al.*, 1978). Mesylation of *N*-benzyloxycarbonylthienamycin benzyl ester and elimination of methylsulfonic acid gave the enelactam (**41**).

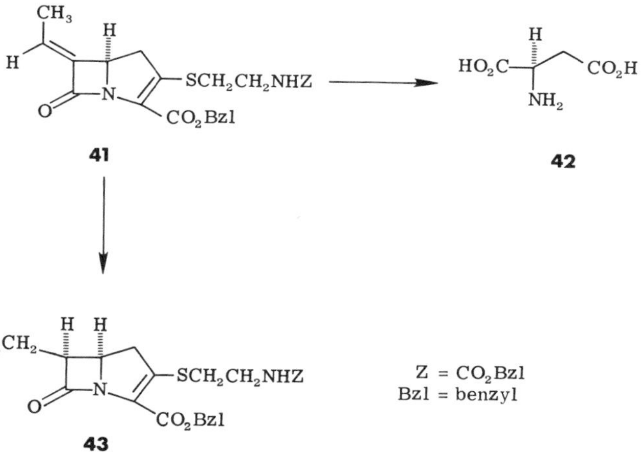

Ozonolysis of **41** followed by peroxide treatment and acid hydrolysis then gave D-(−)-aspartic acid (**42**) in 69% yield. The configuration of D-(−)-aspartic acid corresponds to the *R* configuration at C-5 of the carbapenem nucleus. Thienamycin and the minor metabolites of *S. cattleya* all showed small $J_{5,6}$ coupling constants of ≤3 Hz, intermediate between the values for cis- and trans-situated protons on the β-lactams of isomeric penams and cephems. In order to determine characteristic *J* values for *cis*- and *trans*-carbapenems, the enelactam (**41**) was catalytically reduced to the 6-ethylcarbapenem (**43**). Reduction was expected to occur from the less-hindered exo face and to result in *cis*-β-lactam stereochemistry. For penams and cephems the larger coupling constant had always been associated with cis configuration, and the significant increase of the *J*

value from 2.5 Hz for *N*-benzyloxycarbonylthienamycin benzyl ester to 5.5 Hz for **43** showed that this correlation holds also for carbapenems. NMR spectra of the C-8 ester (**44**) of *N*-benzyloxycarbonylthienamycin benzyl ester prepared with *R*-(+)-α-methoxy-α-trifluoromethylphenyl-acetyl chloride [*R*-(+)-MTPA] showed the C-9 methyl signal upfield and the C-5 hydrogen, C-6 hydrogen, and CF$_3$ signals downfield relative to the same signals in the spectra of the diastereomeric ester (**45**) derived from *S*-(−)-MTPA. According to Mosher's rule (Dale and Mosher, 1973; Sullivan *et al.*, 1973), which was shown to apply to the same derivatives (**46** and **47**) of a 6-hydroxyethylpenam of known absolute stereochemistry

44 from *R*-(+)-MTPA
45 from *S*-(−)-MTPA

46 from *R*-(+)-MTPA
47 from *S*-(−)-MTPA

(DiNinno *et al.*, 1977), these data imply the *R* configuration at C-8 of thienamycin. Acylation of the C-8 hydroxyl group with racemic α-phenylbutyric anhydride and hydrolysis of the excess anhydride gave dextrorotatory α-phenylbutyric acid in 18% optical purity, also indicating the *R* configuration according to Horeau's rule (see Horeau, 1977, and references cited therein). Finally, the same conclusions could be drawn from the NMR spectra of the diastereomeric α-phenylbutyryl esters that resulted from this experiment. Figure 1 shows a stereoscopic view of the X-ray structure of *N*-acetyl-(+)-thienamycin methyl ester in the correct 5*R*, 6*S*, 8*R* absolute configuration. Figure 2 summarizes the numerical bond distance and bond angle values which were determined in this analysis.

In the olivanic acid group of compounds, the absolute configurations of MM 22383 (**6g**) were determined to be 5*R*, 6*S*, and 8*S* by single-crystal X-ray analysis of the *p*-bromobenzyl ester. X-ray analysis of the *p*-bromobenzyl ester of carpetimycin A (**9a**) established 5*R* and 6*R* configurations for the two compounds of this group; the same analysis revealed the *R*-sulfoxide stereochemistry. No details of these analyses have been reported. Finally, the absolute configuration at C-6 of PS-5 was determined to be *R* (the same geometry as in thienamycin; note the change in nomenclature due to the absence of the C-8 oxygen) by applying

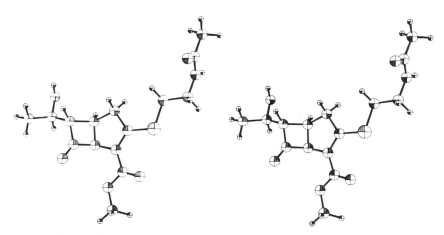

Fig. 1. Stereoscopic view of *N*-acetylthienamycin methyl ester (**15**).

Hudson's rule (Hudson, 1910; Witkop, 1956) to the lactone (**40**) which predicts a positive rotation if the configuration at the starred center is *R*. The experimental value was $[\alpha]_D = 63.3°$. The "carboxy inversion" reaction (Denney and Sherman, 1965) by which the compound was generated had previously been shown to proceed with retention of configuration (Barton *et al.*, 1973). The *trans*-β-lactam configuration of PS-5 was predictable from the NMR coupling constant $J_{5,6} = 3$ Hz.

On the basis of 5,6-coupling constants (Table II) which we now regard as reliable criteria, the four thienamycins from *S. cattleya*, epithienamycins C and D, olivanic acids MM 22381 and MM 22383, and PS-5, PS-6, and PS-7 have trans configurations. The epithienamycins A, B, E, and F, the olivanic acids MM 22380, MM 22382, MM 17880, MM 13902 and MM 4550, MC-696-SY2-A, and carpetimycins A and B have *cis*-β-

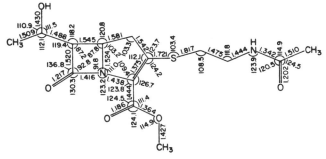

Fig. 2. Bond angles and bond distance in *N*-acetylthienamycin methyl ester (**15**).

lactam stereochemistry. ^{1}H-NMR signals of the C-6 protons of unsulfated 6-hydroxyethylcarbapenems with trans configurations consistently appear near δ 3.4, of those with cis configurations near δ 3.6. This allows one to determine the cis-β-lactam configuration of Sankyo's antibiotic 17927 A$_2$ from a spectrum reproduced in the patent literature (Ger. Offen. 2,809,235); the coupling constant could not be read with certainty.

It remains to discuss the configurations at C-8 of the minor thienamycin analogs 7a and 7b, epithienamycins and olivanic acids, and to clarify the structural relations between epithienamycins and olivanic acids. Three bioconversion experiments are helpful in this task: (1) Addition of N-[^{3}H]acetylthienamycin to S. cattleya cultures resulted in 7% conversion to N-[^{3}H]acetyl-11,12-dehydrothienamycin of the same specific activity as the labeled starting material (P. J. Cassidy et al., unpublished results). (2) Addition of MM 22380 to cultures of a blocked mutant of S. olivaceus resulted in the formation of MM 17880, MM 13902, and MM 4550 (addition of MM 22382 to the mutant culture gave only MM 13902 and MM 4550) (Box et al., 1979). (3) Dehydrogenation of Sankyo's fully saturated (biologically inactive) 17927 D with an appropriate microbial enzyme gave 17927 A$_1$ and A$_2$ (Jpn. Kokai 80 024,129). If one assumes that under these conditions no stereochemical changes at C-8 occur, then these experiments prove stereochemical identity within each of the groups of thienamycins, cis-olivanic acids, and 17927 compounds. We assume that stereochemical identity also applies to the pairs of saturated and unsaturated epithienamycins and trans-olivanic acids for which it has not been explicitly demonstrated. On this basis, the following correlations can be made.

Natural N-acetylthienamycin was found to be identical with semi-synthetic product obtained from thienamycin (J. S. Kahan, unpublished results). Both N-acetylthienamycin and N-acetyl-11,12-dehydrothienamycin must then have 5R,6S,8R configurations. Epithienamycin C has trans-β-lactam configuration but was found to be different from N-acetylthienamycin by NMR analysis of a mixed sample of the two compounds. Epithienamycin C and the unsaturated companion D must therefore have 5R,6S,8S configurations. The same configuration has been determined by X-ray crystallographic analysis for the trans-olivanic acid MM 22383 (Brown et al., 1979). This and the saturated analog MM 22381 must, therefore, be identical to epithienamycins C and D. Enzymatically deacetylated epithienamycin A (U.S. Pat. 4,207,395; Cassidy et al., 1981) having cis-β-lactam configuration ($J_{5,6} = 5$ Hz, $J_{6,8} = 9$ Hz) was found by NMR to be different from a totally synthetic thienamycin (S. M. Schmitt et al., unpublished results, 1978) whose 5R, 6R, and 8R configurations ($J_{5,6} = J_{6,8} = 6$ Hz) were known by X-ray analysis of a synthetic intermediate containing all three chiral centers. The epithiena-mycins A and B must therefore have 5R,6R,8S configurations. Chemical evidence for the reported stereochemical assignments for the olivanic acids (Eur. Pat. Appl. 5,348) consists of stereospecific, base catalyzed eliminations of C-8 sulfate ester or mesylate groups which convert the *trans*-β-lactam compounds to (Z)-enelactams (**48**) and the *cis*-β-lactam

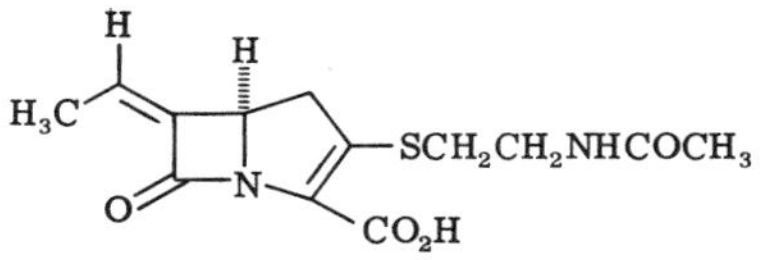

compounds to (E)-enelactams (**49**). Both results require 8S configura-tions. Finally, direct comparison of epithienamycin E with an authentic sample of MM 13902 by NMR analysis of a mixed sample established their identity, and by analogy the identity of epithienamycin F with MM 17880. Thus, the epithienamycins and olivanic acids are identical groups of carbapenems with both *cis*- and *trans*-β-lactam stereochemistry but uniformly 8S configuration. One can then summarize this section on the stereochemistry of the natural carbapenem compounds as follows:

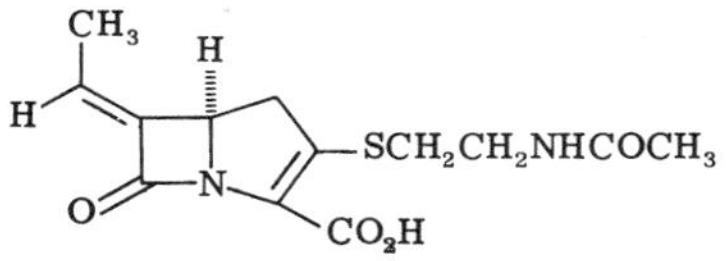

1. Only compounds with 5R configuration have been reported and are likely to have biological activity.

2. *trans*-β-Lactam configuration is compatible with either 8R or 8S configuration.

3. *cis*-β-Lactam configuration has been found exclusively with 8S con-figurations (with the trivial exception of C-8 achiral compounds); in other words, no natural carbapenems with 5R,6R,8R stereochemistry have been reported.

4. Sulfate esters and sulfoxides are known only with *cis*-β-lactam/8S configuration. The sulfoxide chirality has been analyzed in only one case and found to be R.

II. Chemical Modification of the Natural Carbapenem Antibiotics

A. Introduction

The discovery of the naturally occurring carbapenem antibiotics has opened a new and exciting chapter in β-lactam chemistry. By analogy with the classical penicillins and cephalosporins, a major proportion of the initial effort in carbapenem research has been directed toward natural product modification with the goals of defining coherent structure–activity relationships and, ultimately, of developing clinically important products. However, certain fundamental structural differences between the classical antibiotics and the carbapenem compounds has necessitated somewhat different approaches to chemical modification.

The most obvious structural difference between the classical β-lactam antibiotics and the carbapenem natural products is the absence of a ring sulfur atom and the establishment of a more strained pyrroline–azetidinone ring system. The amide bond in this ring system is expected to be highly reactive due to both ring strain and the electron-withdrawing effects associated with the adjacent double bond, thereby limiting potential chemical modification to relatively nonvigorous methods. Another striking difference between the penicillins and cephalosporins and the carbapenem antibiotics is the absence of a cis-substituted 6(7)-amido group. All of the carbapenem antibiotics possess a 6-alkyl or substituted alkyl substituent and this side chain can be either cis or trans oriented with respect to the substituents about the azetidinone ring. The most common 6-substituent is the 1-hydroxyethyl group and its sulfated variant, with the configuration at the hydroxy-bearing carbon being either R or S. Finally, all carbapenem-based natural products are ring substituted at the 2-position by either an aminoethylthio or (E)-aminoethenylthio group, and the amino group is acetylated in most cases. Another variation involves oxidation of the side-chain sulfur to the corresponding sulfoxide. Thus, in contrast to the penicillins and cephalosporins in which the majority of chemical derivatization involved amide side-chain replacements or C-3 modifications, the carbapenems offer several novel functional groups as targets for chemical manipulation. The most obvious of these are the hydroxyethyl and aminoethylthio groups and their variants.

From a biological point of view, the carbapenem antibiotics also differ considerably from the naturally occurring penicillins and cephalosporins. Many of the new natural products already possess potent activity against a broad range of gram-positive and gram-negative organisms. For example, thienamycin is an exceedingly potent antibiotic which is active against most β-lactamase-producing strains including *Pseudomonas* species. Several members of the carbapenem family have also been found to exhibit β-lactamase inhibitory activity and consequently to protect the antibacterial activity of penicillin. For these reasons the chemical effort in the carbapenem area takes on a somewhat different perspective. In addition to defining and modifying the structural parameters leading to potent, broad-spectrum antibacterial activity and β-lactamase stability, derivatization should lead to compounds having increased stability and pharmacological properties suitable for therapeutic use. Other goals include maximizing β-lactamase inhibitory activity and developing derivatives having oral activity. The recent discovery of mammalian peptidases, and particularly renal dehydropeptidases, capable of rapidly destroying carbapenem antibiotics has added the further goal of imparting stability to these enzymes via chemical modification.

Most of the derivatization studies conducted on the carbapenem natural products have been reported by Merck researchers working with thienamycin and by the Beecham group working with the related olivanic acids. An effort by Sanraku-Ocean involving the antibiotics PS-5 and PS-7 has also appeared. The remainder of this section summarizes these chemical derivatization programs.

B. Thienamycin Derivatives

1. *General Considerations*

Thienamycin (**5a**), *N*-acetylthienamycin (**7a**), and *N*-acetyldehydrothienamycin (**7b**) are the only naturally occurring carbapenem antibiotics possessing the trans-oriented (*R*)-1-hydroxyethyl side chain. Biological comparison of thienamycin with other carbapenem natural products has revealed that this configuration of the 6-side chain, trans-*R*, provides maximum β-lactamase stability and antibacterial potency. Also of importance is the fact that thienamycin and northienamycin (**5b**) remain the only reported natural products incorporating a nonacetylated aminoethylthio side chain. As will be seen, a basic side chain of this type plays a significant role in extending antibacterial activity, particularly with respect to antipseudomonal activity. The aminoethylthio group has also been implicated in the high concentration instability of thienamycin presumably caused by intermolecular aminolysis of the β-lactam amide.

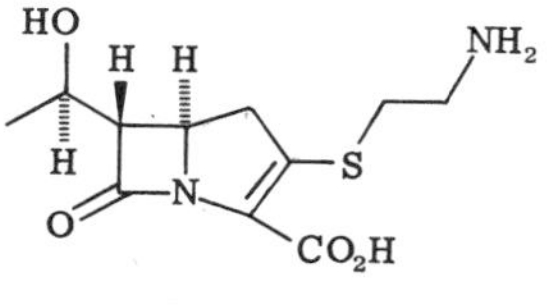

5a

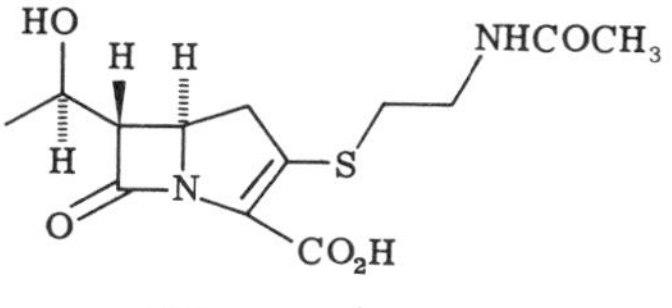

7a

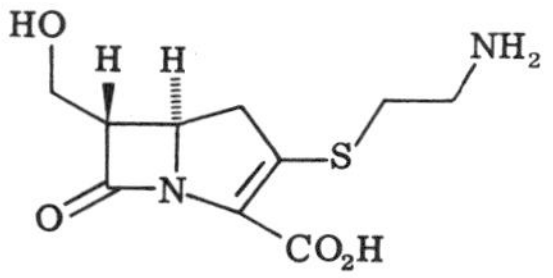

5b

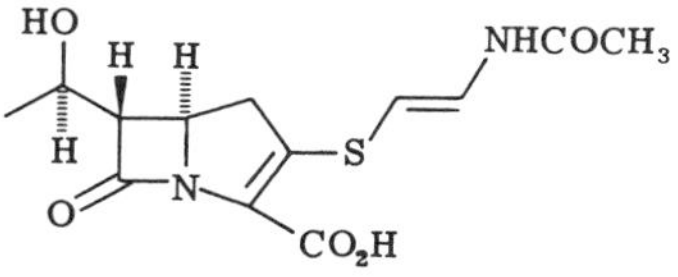

7b

Derivatization of the amino group, with the goal of maintaining or improving antibacterial activity while imparting chemical stability, therefore became an attractive pathway to potential clinical candidates.

Because of the sensitivity of the strained bicyclic carbapenem nucleus to both basic and acidic conditions, reagents and reaction conditions should be as mild as possible. For multistep processes involving more profound molecular changes, amino and carboxyl protecting groups capable of cleavage under mild and neutral conditions are required. Finally, the relative reactivities of the peripheral functional groups are of paramount importance in designing strategy and setting synthetic goals. In the case of thienamycin, the functional groups may be ranked in order of decreasing reactivity by the sequence amino, carboxyl, hydroxyl, and thio, an order also reflected in the number of derivatives in each class.

The carbapenem antibiotics and their derivatives containing an unoxidized 2-thio side chain exhibit a strong UV absorption maximum near 300 nm which is extinguishable by hydroxylamine or cysteine. This chromophore plays a unique role in assaying chemical reactions and monitoring purification of thienamycin and other carbapenem derivatives. Water-soluble products are generally purified by ion-exchange chromatography using Dowex 50 (sodium cycle), by chromatography on a neutral polystyrene resin such a XAD-2, or by gel-permeation chromatography on BioGel P-2. The purified products thus produced are usually isolated as lyophilized powders or solid residues.

Electrophoresis followed by bioautography is another convenient method of assaying product homogeneity and monitoring chemical reactions involving transformation of the amino and carboxyl groups. For those derivatives or intermediates incorporating an esterified carboxyl group, rapid chromatography on silica gel using UV visualization is most often employed in product purification.

2. Derivatives of the Amino Group

The largest class of thienamycin derivatives arose from modification of the amino group. The principle structural variations in this class include N-acylation, N-alkylation, N-imidoylation, and combinations thereof.

Acetylation of thienamycin (**5a**) with acetic anhydride in dimethylformamide (U.S. Pat. 4,165,379) provided *N*-acetylthienamycin (**7a**), a compound identical to the natural product isolated from *S. cattleya*. A more general route leading to a variety of *N*-acyl derivatives (**50**) involves reactions of thienamycin with acid chlorides and acid anhydrides under Schotten–Bauman conditions (Ger. Offen. 2,652,675). This route provided the amide, thioamide, urethane, and sulfonamide derivatives listed in Table V. An alternative to the Schotten–Bauman methods, which is particularly useful when anhydrous conditions are desired, involves si-

TABLE V   *N*-Acyl Derivatives of Thienamycin (**50**)

Method A: R = COCH$_2$OCH$_3$, COCH$_2$OC$_6$H$_5$, COCH$_2$Cl, COCH$_2$Br, COCH(OCHO)C$_6$H$_5$,
COCH$_2$N$_3$, COCH(N$_3$)C$_6$H$_5$, COCH$_2$CH$_2$N$_3$, CO$_2$CH$_2$CH$_3$, CO$_2$CH$_2$CCl$_3$,

CO$_2$CH$_2$—⟨benzene ring⟩—NO$_2$, CO$_2$CH$_2$—⟨benzene ring with O$_2$N⟩ , COSC$_6$H$_5$, CSOC$_6$H$_5$, CSC$_6$H$_5$

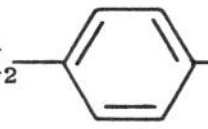

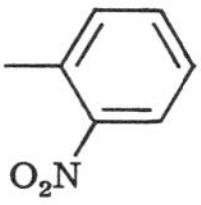

Method B: R = COC(CH$_3$)$_2$CH$_2$Br, COCH$_2$—⟨benzene ring⟩—NHC(=NH)NH$_2$,

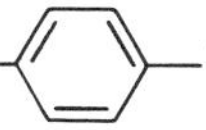

CO—⟨benzene ring⟩—Br, CO$_2$CH$_3$, CO$_2$CH$_2$C$_6$H$_5$, SO$_2$C$_6$H$_5$

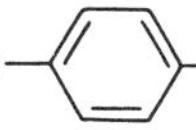

Method C: R = CO$_2$C(CH$_3$)$_2$CH$_2$Br, CO$_2$CH$_2$—⟨benzene ring⟩—NO$_2$, SO$_2$NH$_2$, PO(OCH$_3$)$_2$,

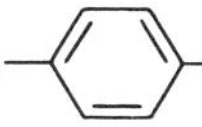

PS(OCH$_3$)$_2$, PS(SCH$_3$)$_2$, CONHCH$_3$

lylation of thienamycin to tris(trimethyl)silyl derivative (**51**) followed by acylation and mild aqueous hydrolysis (Ger. Offen. 2,652,675). As shown in Table V, this method was useful for preparing phosphonoamino, thio-phosphonoamino, and sulfamoylamino derivatives. The tris(trimethyl)silyl intermediate (**51**) also reacts with isocyanates, such as methyl isocyanate,

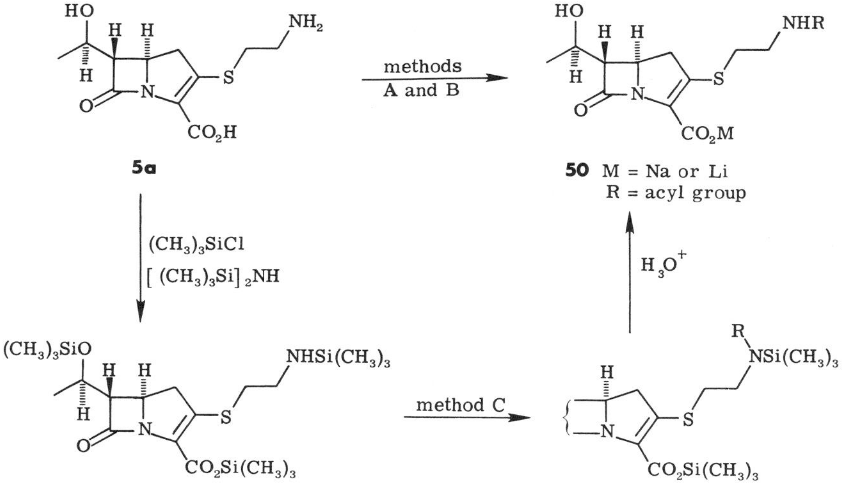

5a

(CH$_3$)$_3$SiCl
[(CH$_3$)$_3$Si]$_2$NH

51

methods
A and B

50 M = Na or Li
R = acyl group

H$_3$O$^+$

method C

Method A: RCl or R$_2$O, NaHCO$_3$, dioxane-H$_2$O or THF-H$_2$O
Method B: RCl, NaOH to pH 8.2-8.5, dioxane-H$_2$O-pH 7 buffer
Method C: RCl, Et$_3$N, THF

to provide ureido derivatives. In most cases the products of Table V were isolated as the sodium salts.

Several of the amide derivatives listed in Table V were further functionalized (Ger. Offen. 2,652,675) leading in many cases to extended side chains bearing a basic group. For example, catalytic reduction of azidoamide **52** gave the β-alanyl derivative **53** which was converted to the highly crystalline amidine **54**. Compound **54** is related to the guanidine analog **55** which was prepared by direct acylation of thienamycin with

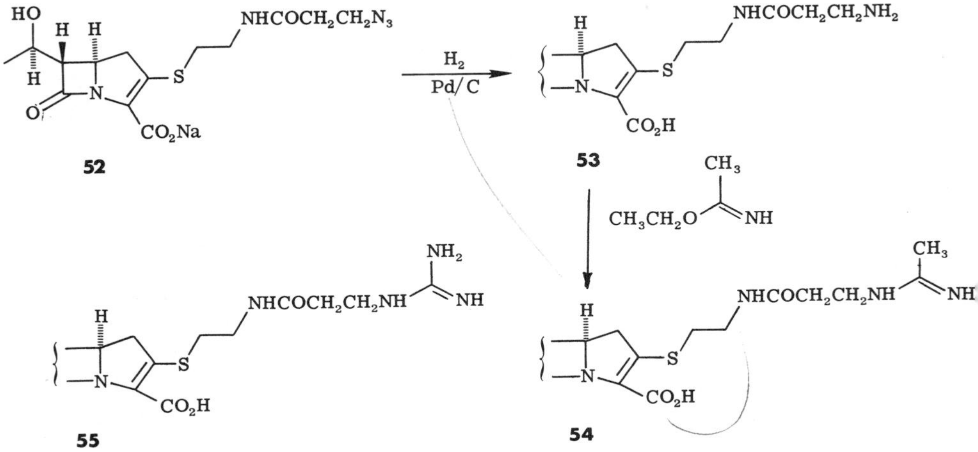

the appropriate acid chloride in DMF containing N,N-diisopropylethylamine. The bromoacetamide derivative **56** reacted with a diverse set of nucleophilic reagents to afford derivatives **57–60**.

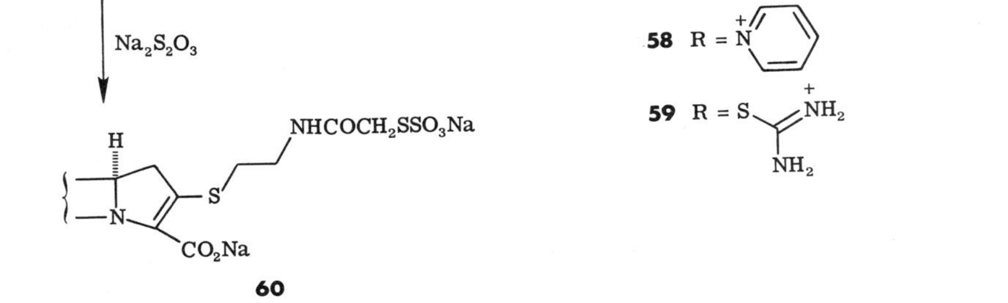

In addition to the chemical acylations discussed above, an enzymatic method employing penicillin amidohydrolase and carboxylic acids is reported (U.S. Pat. 4,135,978) to afford amide derivatives of thienamycin. The same enzymes have also been found to deacylate thienamycin amides under appropriate conditions (U.S. Pat. 4,162,193).

Controlled N-alkylation (Ger. Offen. 2,652,676; Belg. Pat. 866,660) of thienamycin is experimentally difficult since many of the synthetic methods normally employed for mono- or dialkylation are incompatible with the sensitive carbapenem structure or aqueous solvent systems. For example, treatment of thienamycin (5a) with excess dimethyl sulfate in buffered aqueous dioxane produced a mixture of monomethyl (61), dimethyl (62), and trimethyl (63) derivatives which were chromatographically separable. Increasing the amount of dimethyl sulfate afforded additional trimethyl product. The monomethyl derivative was also obtained by desulfurization of thioformamide (64), which was itself prepared by acylation of silylated thienamycin (51). Alkylation of thienamycin with ethyl fluorosulfate in buffered aqueous acetonitrile similarly afforded a mixture of mono- and diethyl derivatives (65 and 66). Attempts to alkylate thienamycin with either p-*tert*-butylbenzyl bromide or p-nitrobenzyl bromide in the polar aprotic solvents HMPA or DMSO afforded mainly N,N-disubstituted esters.

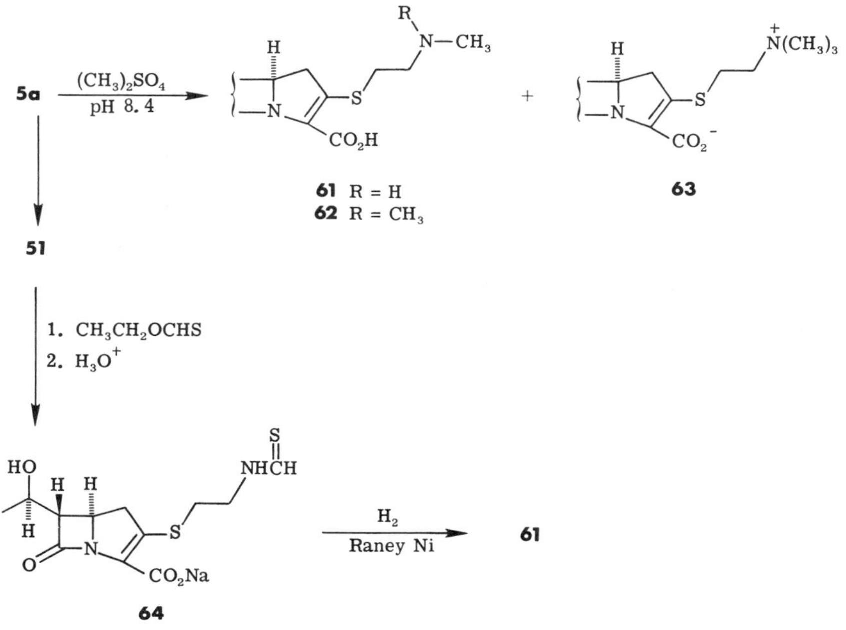

5a $\xrightarrow[\text{pH 9}]{\text{CH}_3\text{CH}_2\text{OSO}_2\text{F}}$

65 R = H
66 R = CH$_2$CH$_3$

The rationale for preparing N-imidoyl (amidino) derivatives (Leanza *et al.*, 1979) of thienamycin was based primarily on two observations. In aqueous solution near pH 7, thienamycin is relatively stable when dilute but unstable at concentrations suitable for therapeutic use. The high concentration instability is presumably due to intermolecular aminolysis of the amide bond by the nucleophilic amino group of the cysteamine side chain. However, a basic side chain also appears necessary for high antipseudomonal activity since the naturally occurring N-acetyl derivative shows greatly reduced antipseudomonal activity when compared to thienamycin. It was therefore considered likely that conversion of the amino group to a more basic functionality, such as an amidino group, would result in derivatives having both antipseudomonal activity and high concentration stability. For zwitterionic structures like thienamycin, a more basic amino derivative would exist to a greater extent in the protonated form and hence be less nucleophilic.

The majority of the N-imidoyl derivatives (**67**) of thienamycin were prepared by treating the parent antibiotic with methyl or ethyl imidates under Schotten–Bauman-like conditions (Belg. Pat. 848,545). The requisite imidates were obtained from the corresponding amines or nitriles using standard methods. In most cases, the amidination reaction was conducted in buffered aqueous dioxane while maintaining the pH near 8.5 by controlled addition of sodium hydroxide. Minor variations included substituting THF or DMF for dioxane or maintaining the basic reaction conditions with excess sodium bicarbonate. When using the more water-sensitive dialkylimmonium chlorides as amidinating reagents, reaction with tris(trimethyl)silyl thienamycin (**51**) proved a useful alternative to derivatives (**68**). Many of the N-imidoyl derivatives of thienamycin, along with the method of preparation, are listed in Table VI.

The amidination reaction has been applied to the preparation of related thienamycin derivatives. For example, the N-methyl- and N-ethylformamidines (**69** and **70**) were prepared by the Schotten–Bauman method (Belg. Pat. 866,661). This process has also been used to convert thienamycin to the N-quanyl derivative (**71**) (U.S. Pat. 4,194,047), albeit in low yield. When the imidate reagent contains additional functionality

TABLE VI N-Imidoyl Derivatives of Thienamycin (**67** and **68**)

Method A: R^1 = H; R^2 = H, CH_3, CH_2CH_3, $CH(CH_3)_2$, $CH_2CH=CH_2$, $CH(CH_3)CH=CH_2$, $CH_2C_6H_5$, CH_2CF_3, CH_2CO_2H, cyclopropyl, $CH_2CH_2SCH_3$, C_6H_5, $N(CH_3)_2$

 R^2 = H; R^1 = CH_3, CH_2CH_3, CF_3, CH_2OCH_3, $CH_2CH_2N_3$

 R^1 = CH_3; R^2 = CH_3

Method B: R^2 = H; R^1 =

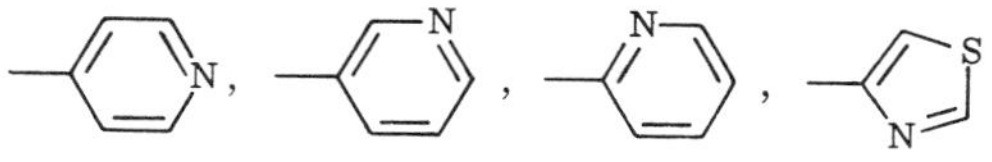

Method C: R^3 = CH_3, $(CH_2)_5$

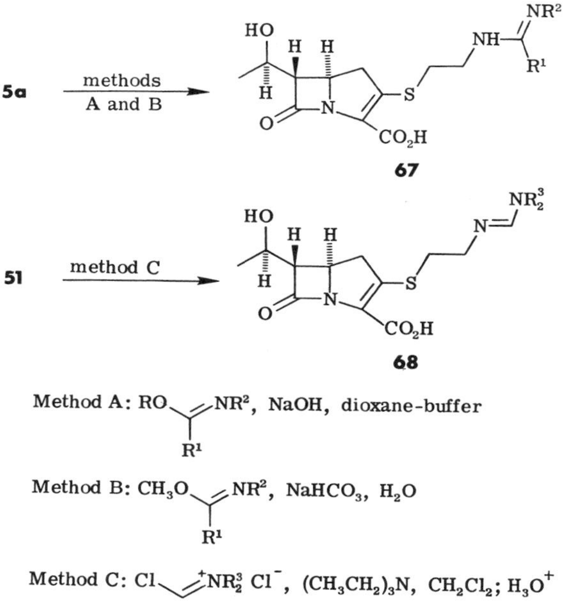

Method A: RO⎯NR², NaOH, dioxane-buffer
         |
         R¹

Method B: CH₃O⎯NR², NaHCO₃, H₂O
          |
          R¹

Method C: Cl⎯⁺NR₃² Cl⁻, (CH₃CH₂)₃N, CH₂Cl₂; H₃O⁺

capable of secondary reactions, heterocyclic derivatives (U.S. Pat. 4,-189,493) such as imadazoline (**72**) and imadazole (**73**) were obtained.

Of the various N-imidoyl derivatives of thienamycin described in this section, the N-formimidoyl derivative (**74**) has been selected for clinical evaluation. Extensive *in vitro* and *in vivo* evaluation (Kropp *et al.*, 1980) has shown that this compound retains the antibacterial spectrum of thienamycin and is two- to fourfold more potent against *P. aeruginosa* spp. The N-formimidoyl derivative has been obtained as a stable, crystalline solid (Eur. Pat. Appl. 6,639) which shows greatly improved high concentration solution stability (Leanza *et al.*, 1979). N-formimidoylthienamycin (**74**) has been given the Merck designation MK-787.

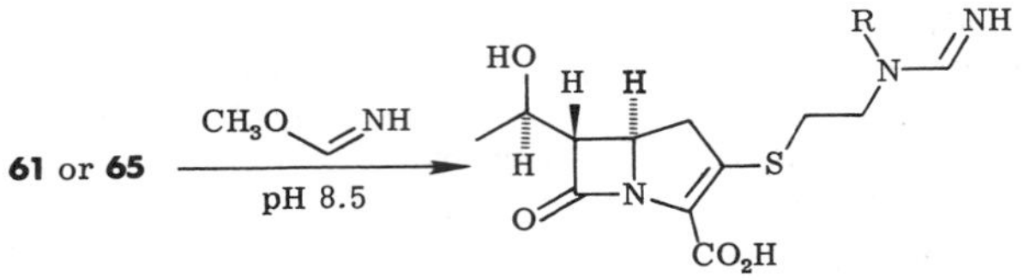

69 R = CH$_3$
70 R = CH$_2$CH$_3$

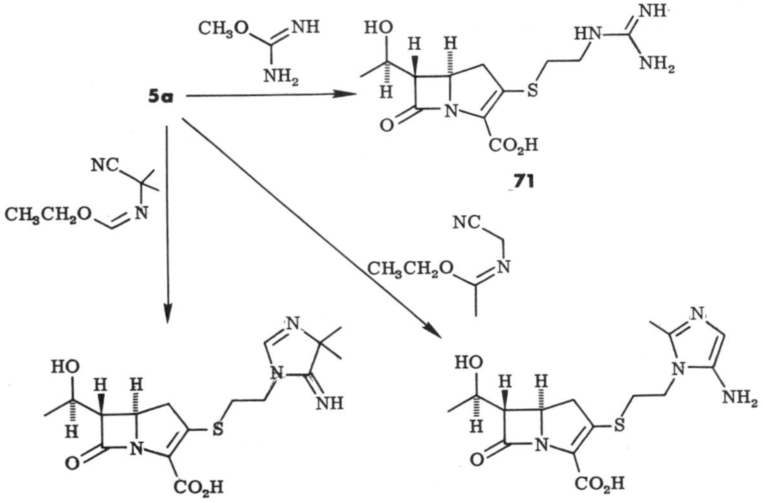

71

72

73

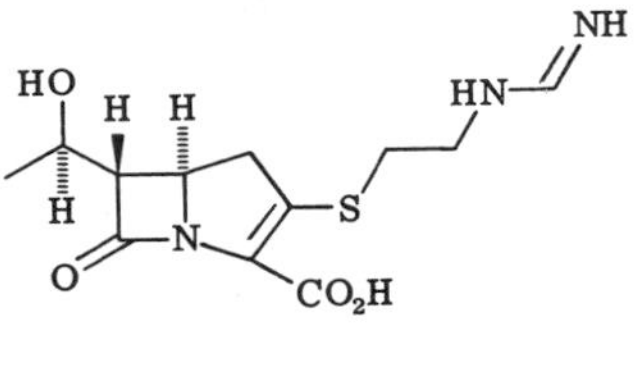

74

3. Derivatives of the Carboxyl Group

The most common and easily accessible carboxyl derivatives of thienamycin are esters, and mainly esters of N-acyl derivatives. The ester derivatives have importance as potential oral antibiotics and as protected forms for further chemical alteration. For the latter purpose, the p-nitrobenzyl group is especially useful since it can be removed under mild and neutral hydrogenolytic conditions.

The N-acylthienamycin esters 76 and 77 were prepared by two widely applicable procedures (Ger. Offen. 2,652,674; U.S. Pat. 4,181,733), namely alkylation of the lithium or sodium carboxylates (75) in an aprotic solvent such as HMPA or by reaction of the free carboxylic acids with a diazoalkane. Representative examples of the products afforded by these methods are given in Table VII. The preparation of N-(benzyl-oxycarbonyl)thienamycin benzyl ester and N-(p-nitrobenzyloxy-carbonyl)thienamycin p-nitrobenzyl ester, diprotected derivatives having special utility for further functional group manipulations, have also been reported (Belg. Pat. 865,786).

Thienamycin esters bearing an unacylated aminoethylthio side chain have been prepared by two methods. Direct esterification of thienamycin in aqueous dioxane at pH 5 with diazoalkanes provided the esters (78) which were isolated as their Schiff base adducts (79) with salicylaldehyde (U.S. Pat. 4,172,144). Reductive removal of the p-nitrobenzyloxycar-

TABLE VII N-Acylthienamycin Esters (76)

Method	R^1	R^2
A	$COCH_2N_3$	$CH_2C_6H_5$, CH_2—⟨benzene⟩—$C(CH_3)_3$, $CH_2OCOC(CH_3)_3$, $CH_2CH=C(CH_3)_2$ 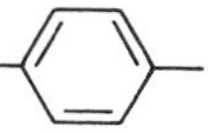
A	$PS(OCH_3)_2$	$CH_2OCOC(CH_3)_3$
A	$CO_2C(CH_3)_2CH_2Br$	CH_2—⟨benzene⟩—NO_2, CH_2CO—⟨benzene⟩—Br 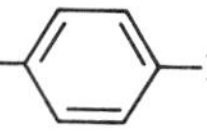 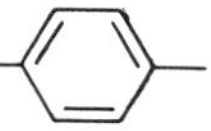
A	CO_2CH_2—⟨benzene⟩—NO_2 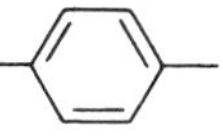	CH_2—⟨benzene⟩—NO_2, CH_2—⟨benzene⟩—$C(CH_3)_3$, CH_2—⟨benzene⟩—OC_6H_5 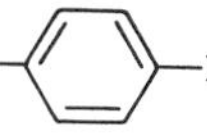 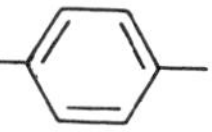 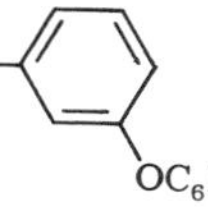
A	CO_2CH_2—⟨benzene⟩—OCH_3 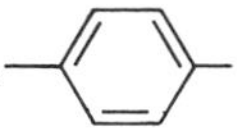	CH_2—⟨benzene⟩—$C(CH_3)_3$ 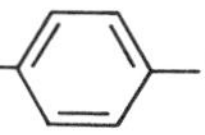
A	CO_2CH_2—⟨benzene, O_2N⟩ 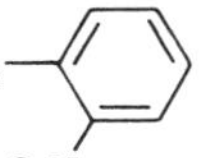	CH_2CO—⟨benzene⟩—Br 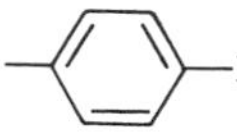
A, B	$CO_2CH_2C_6H_5$	$CH_2C_6H_5$
B	$COCH_2Br$	CH_3, $CH_2C_6H_5$
B	CO_2CH_2—⟨benzene⟩—OCH_3 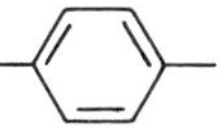	$CH(C_6H_5)_2$

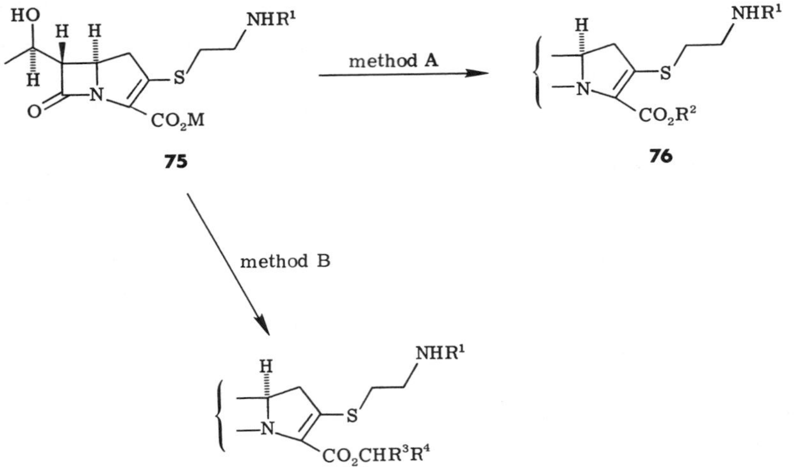

Method A: M = Li or Na, R^2Cl or R^2Br, HMPA
Method B: M = H, $R^3R^4C{=}N_2$, EtOAc

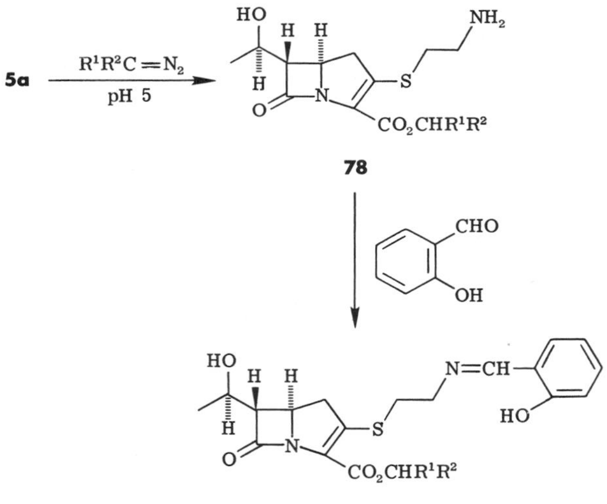

$R^1 = H$, $R^2 = C_6H_5$
$R^1 = R^2 = C_6H_5$

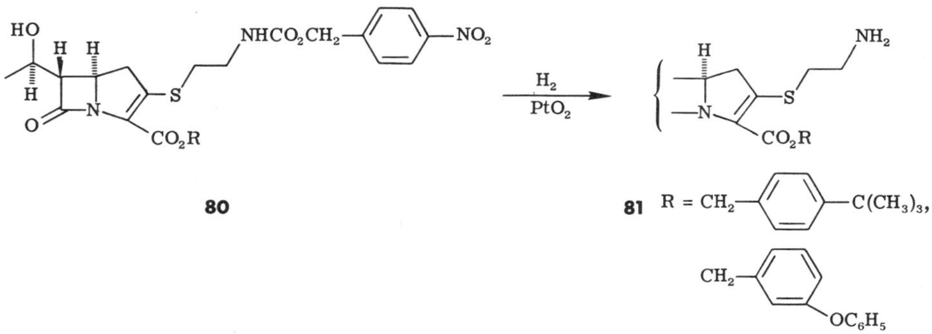

80

81 R = CH_2—⟨⟩—$C(CH_3)_3$,

CH_2—⟨⟩—OC_6H_5

bonyl group of **80** gave the free amino esters (**81**) (U.S. Pat. 4,181,733). These products proved unstable and polymerized on storage.

4. Derivatives of the Hydroxyethyl Group

Modification of the hydroxyethyl group of several N-acylthienamycin esters via O-acylation and O-alkylation has been described (Ger. Offen. 2,652,680; 2,724,560). The general process is exemplified for the diprotected derivatives (**82**). Acetylation with acetic anhydride in pyridine gave the O-acetyl derivative (**83**) and reaction with excess diazomethane

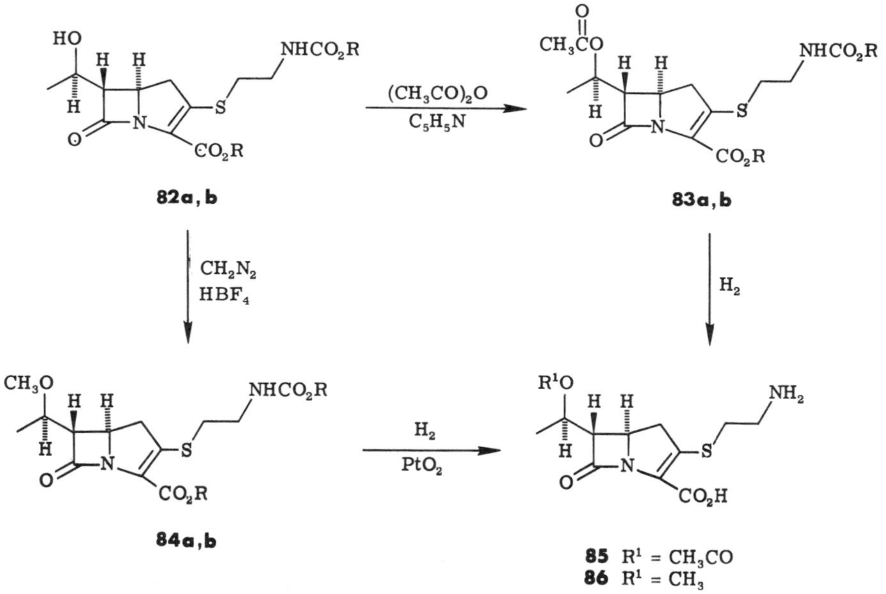

82a,b

$(CH_3CO)_2O$
C_5H_5N

83a,b

CH_2N_2
HBF_4

H_2

84a,b

H_2
PtO_2

85 $R^1 = CH_3CO$
86 $R^1 = CH_3$

a : R = benzyl
b : R = p-nitrobenzyl

in the presence of a catalytic amount of fluoboric acid gave the O-methyl derivative (**84**). Removal of the protecting groups by hydrogenolysis was best effected in the p-nitrobenzyl series, yielding O-acetylthienamycin (**85**) and O-methylthienamycin (**86**).

Complete removal of the hydroxyl group was accomplished by a three-step process (Belg. Pat. 865,786). Treatment of **82** with methanesulfonyl chloride and triethylamine afforded the mesylate (**87**) which underwent stereospecific trans elimination on base treatment to give the anhydro derivative (**88**). In the p-nitrobenzyl ester series, hydrogenation of **88b** provided deshydroxy thienamycin (**89**), presumably as a mixture of isomers. In the benzyl series, selective reduction of the exocyclic double bond to provide a cis-6-ethyl benzyl ester has been reported (Albers-Schönberg et al., 1978).

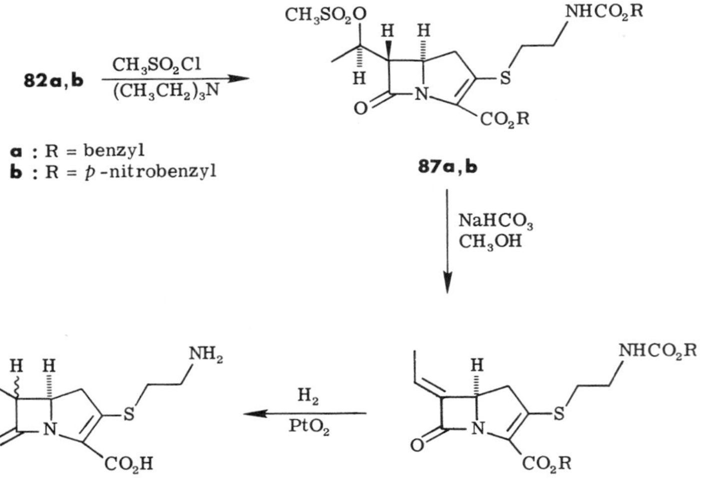

5. *Oxidation and Removal of the Aminoethylthio Side Chain*

The sulfur side chain of thienamycin and several of its derivatives is readily oxidized to the corresponding sulfoxide and sulfone side chains by a variety of reagents (Neth. Pat. 7,702,183; U.S. Pat. 4,123,547; Eur. Pat. Appl. 1,264; 1,265; U.S. Pat. 4,150,145). Two of these oxidative methods are illustrated for the preparation of thienamycin sulfoxide (**91**). Oxidation of bis-p-nitrobenzyl-protected intermediate **82b** with m-chloroperbenzoic acid gave the sulfoxide (**90**) as a single diastereomer which was deblocked to **91** by hydrogenolysis. By contrast, direct oxidation of thienamycin (**5a**) with sodium hypochlorite in water provided **91** as

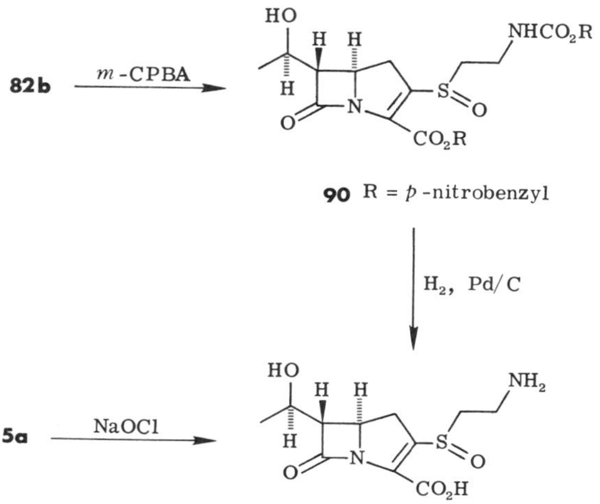

90 R = p-nitrobenzyl

91

a mixture of isomers. The sulfoxide derivative was found to be more labile in aqueous solution than its parent.

An unusual class of thienamycin derivatives, descysteaminylthienamycin (**93**) and its derivatives (**94**), has been prepared (Shih *et al.*, 1978; U.S. Pat. 4,196,211; Ger. Offen. 2,820,055; Belg. Pat. 867,227) in a sequence involving reductive cleavage of the ring carbon to sulfur bond as the key step. The phenoxyacetyl derivative (**92**) was selected for the process because the acyl group reduces the nitrogen nucleophilicity of the by-product and facilitates the separation of the by-product from **93**. Descysteaminylthienamycin was found to possess *in vitro* antibacterial activity comparable to thienamycin against gram-positive bacteria and the *Enterobacteriaceae* and approximately one-third of the thienamycin activity against *Pseudomonas* strains (Shih *et al.*, 1978). It is noteworthy that extended reduction of **92** produces a bioactive substance thought to be the dihydro product (**95**) (Ger. Offen. 2,820,055; Belg. Pat. 867,227).

6. *Isomerization of the Double Bond*

N-Acylthienamycin esters (**76**) were equilibrated (U.S. Pat. 4,146,633) to mixtures of starting material and the double bond isomer (**96**) on exposure to strong bases in aprotic solvents. The exo orientation of the carboxyl group as shown in structure **96** is based on thermodynamic considerations and analogy to related examples in early Merck synthetic work (Schmitt *et al.*, 1980b). Deblocking of derivative **96a** to isothienamycin (**97**) was accomplished in two stages, namely hydrogenolysis of the benzyl ester followed by hydrolysis of the bromo Boc group. Com-

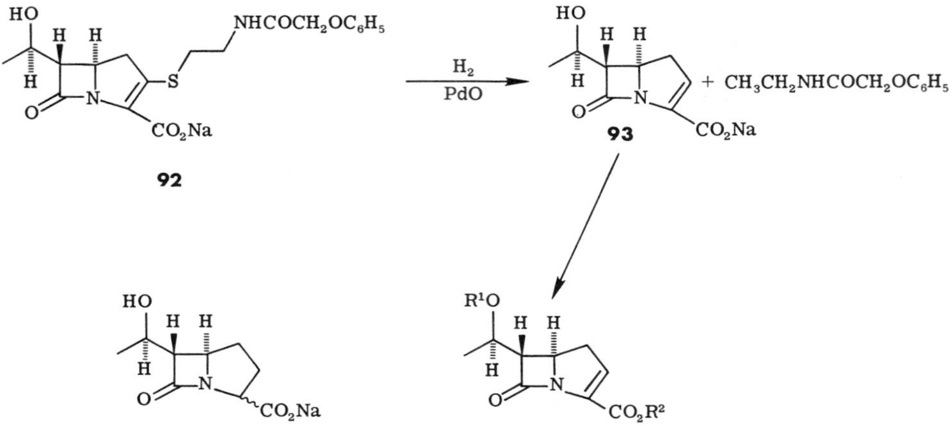

96a $R^1 = C(CH_3)_2CH_2Br$; R^2 $CH_2C_6H_5$
96b $R^1 = R^2 = p$-nitrobenzyl
96c $R^1 = R^2 = CH_2C_6H_5$

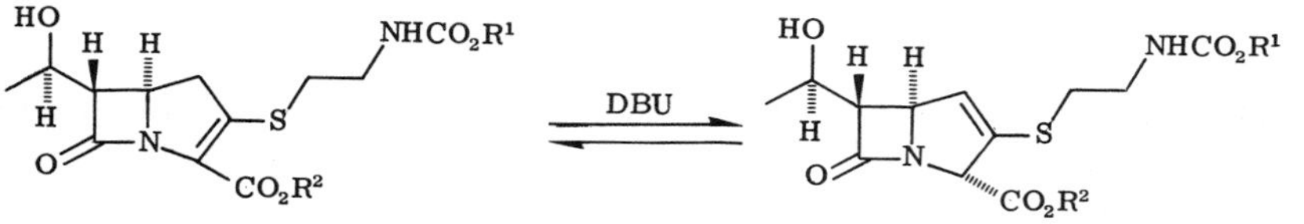

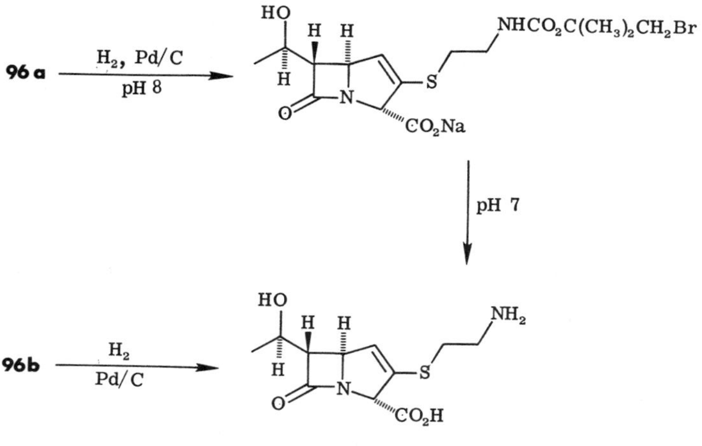

pound **97** was also obtained by hydrogenolysis of bis-*p*-nitrobenzyl derivative **96b**.

C. Derivatives of the Olivanic Acids

1. *General Considerations*

Various strains of *Streptomyces* have been found to produce a complex of structurally related carbapenem compounds that exhibit broad-spectrum antibacterial activity and possess β-lactamase inhibitory properties. The structures of the compounds isolated from *S. olivaceus*, to which the Beecham group has given the name olivanic acids, are shown in Table VIII. Identical or related compounds have been isolated by re-

TABLE VIII Olivanic Acids and Related Compounds

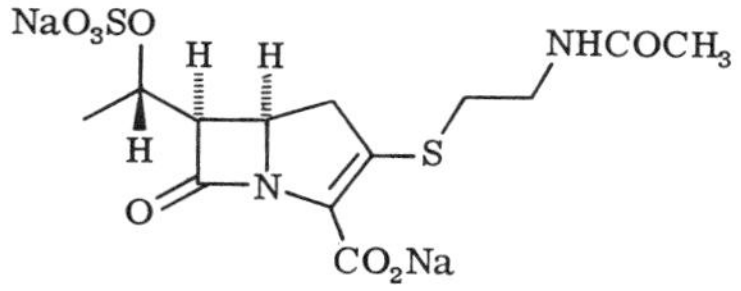

6a Beecham MM 17880
Merck Epithienamycin F

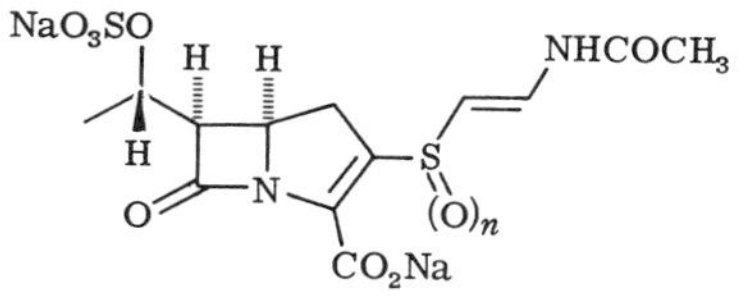

6b *n* = 0, Beecham MM 13902
Merck Epithienamycin E
6c *n* = 1, Beecham MM 4550
Meiji 696-SY2-A

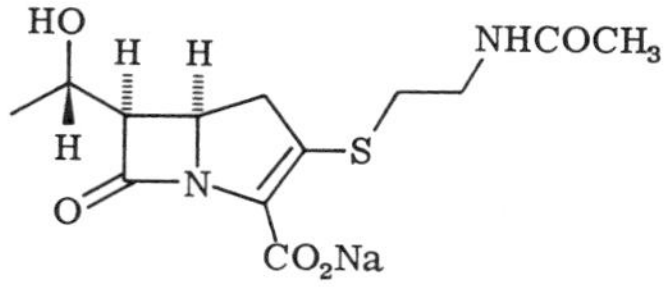

6d Beecham MM 22380
Merck Epithienamycin A
Sankyo 17927 A$_1$

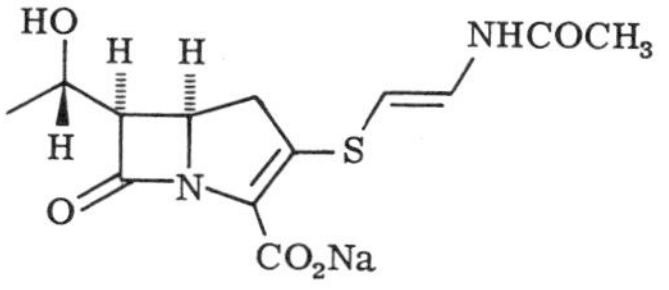

6e Beecham MM 22382
Merck Epithienamycin B
Sankyo 17927 A$_2$

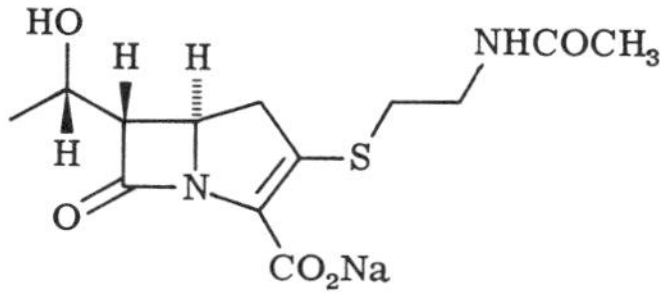

6f Beecham MM 22381
Merck Epithienamycin C

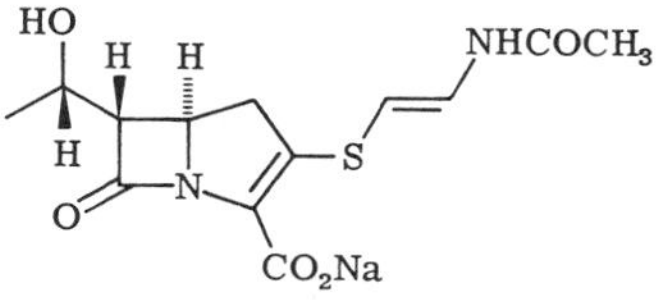

6g Beecham MM 22383
Merck Epithienamycin D

searchers at Merck, Meiji, Sanraku Ocean, and Sankyo; equivalent structures are indicated in Table VIII when known or inferred.

All of the olivanic acids have two common structural features that set them apart from thienamycin. The aminothio side chain, whether saturated or unsaturated, is invariably N-acetylated and the chiral center of the hydroxyethyl side chain always has the S configuration. Whereas thienamycin is trans substituted about the azetidinone ring, olivanic acids MM 17880 (**6a**), MM 13902 (**6b**), MM 4550 (**6c**), MM 22380 (**6d**), and MM 22382 (**6e**) are cis substituted. Olivanic acids MM 22381 (**6f**) and MM 22383 (**6g**) are differentiated from the other members of the complex by their trans stereochemistry. Olivanic acids MM 17880 and MM 13902 are the sulfate esters of MM 22380 and MM 22382, and MM 4550 is the sulfoxide of MM 13902. The structural differences among the olivanic acids and thienamycin, namely the substitution, orientation, and configuration of the hydroxyethyl group and the nature of the N-acetylaminothio side chain, naturally affect the biological properties of the parent antibiotics and their derivatives.

The derivatization of the olivanic acids has been studied almost exclusively by the Beecham group. Their chemical effort was guided by the nature and relative reactivities of the various functionalities and has centered about esterification of the carboxyl group, modification of the hydroxyethyl group by acylation, elimination, reduction, and replacement, and halogenation or isomerization of the *trans*-acetamidoethenylthio side chain. The reported Merck effort in this area has been limited to enzymatic deacetylation of epithienamycins A and C (Belg. Pat. 848,349) and epithienamycin E (Ger. Offen. 2,805,724).

As previously discussed in the thienamycin section, the long-wavelength UV absorption near 300 nm for the olivanic acids and their derivatives greatly facilitates product location and isolation. Most of the final products described in this section were isolated as solid residues after chromatography on Biogel P2 polyacrylamide beads. Intermediate, organic-soluble materials were generally purified by column chromatography on silica gel. Because of the diversity of natural products within the olivanic acid class, general structural representations will be used to describe most of the chemical transformations.

2. *Derivatives of the Carboxyl and Sulfooxy Groups*

Esterification of the carboxylic acid group of the olivanic acids serves two functions. The resulting esters might be expected to have oral activity or to act as prodrugs having improved pharmacodynamic properties. Esterification also provides for organic-soluble, protected intermediates which can be further modified and subsequently deblocked to the derivatized antibiotic. The olivanic acids possessing the sulfooxyethyl side chain are also capable of being esterified or converted to organic-soluble salt forms amenable to further chemical modification.

The most commonly employed method for esterifying the olivanic acids involves treatment of the sodium carboxylates with an alkylating agent in DMF (Eur. Pat. Appl. 4,132; Belg. Pat. 857,781). The process is represented in general form for the preparation of esters **98** and **99** from the natural products **6a–c** and **6d–g**. In the case of the sulfooxyethyl olivanic acids (**6a–c**), the carboxylic acid is selectively esterified; alkylation of the sulfooxy group requires more forcing conditions. Typical esters prepared by this method include the methyl, allyl, benzyl, *p*-bromobenzyl, *p*-iodobenzyl, *p*-nitrobenzyl, *p*-bromophenacyl, pivaloyloxymethyl, and phthalidyl. Preparation of the *p*-carbomethoxybenzyl and *t*-butyldiphenylsilyl esters by related procedures has also been described (Eur. Pat. Appl. 5,348). As will be seen, the *p*-nitrobenzyl ester is the most effective choice for a removable covering group. It is usually cleaved by atmospheric pressure hydrogenation in aqueous dioxane with palladium on charcoal as the catalyst. Subsequent addition of sodium bicarbonate and chromatography on Biogel P2 provides the products as sodium carboxylates.

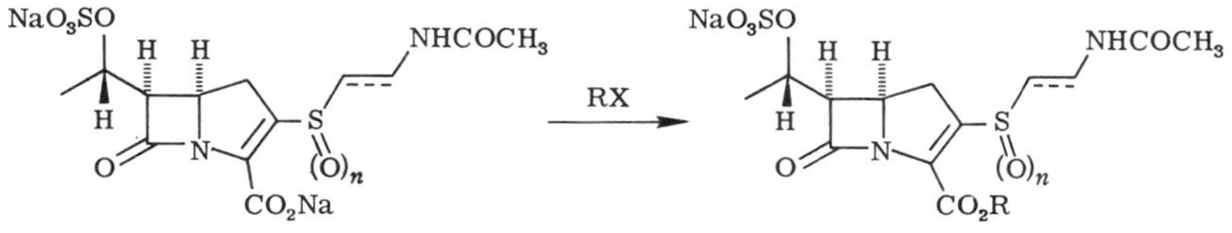

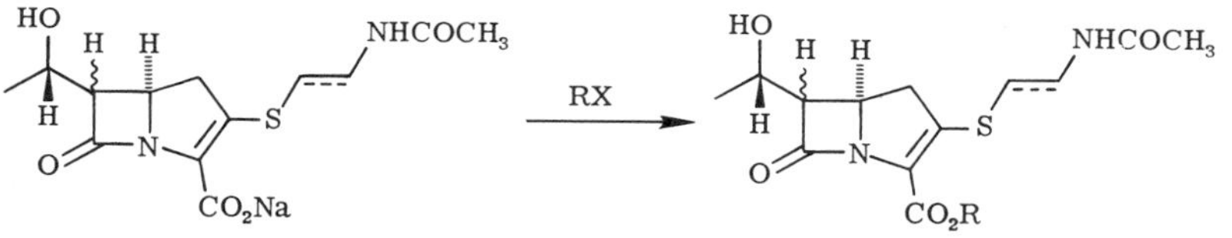

The sulfooxy group of the carboxylate esters (**98**) has been alkylated by two methods. Exchanging the sodium salt of **98** with a highly lipophilic ammonium salt, such as *N*-cetyl-*N*-benzyldimethylammonium chloride, affords the organic-soluble, ammonium sulfooxy derivatives (**100**) (Belg. Pat. 857,781; Eur. Pat. Appl. 5,348; 7,753). These materials can be ethylated with triethyloxonium tetrafluoroborate in methylene chloride to provide the sulfate esters (**101**) (Eur. Pat. Appl. 5,348; 7,753). Alternatively, the sodium salts (**98**) can be suspended in methylene chloride and directly ethylated to yield **101.** Intermediate **100** in which the *N*-cetyl-*N*-benzyldimethylammonium group has been replaced by other lipophilic ammonium or phosphomium salts has been described (Belg. Pat. 857,-781). Similarly, treatment of olivanic acids **6b** and **6c** with *N*-cetyl-*N*-benzyldimethylammonium chloride affords the organic-soluble diammonium salts (**102**) (Belg. Pat. 857,781; Eur. Pat. Appl. 7,753).

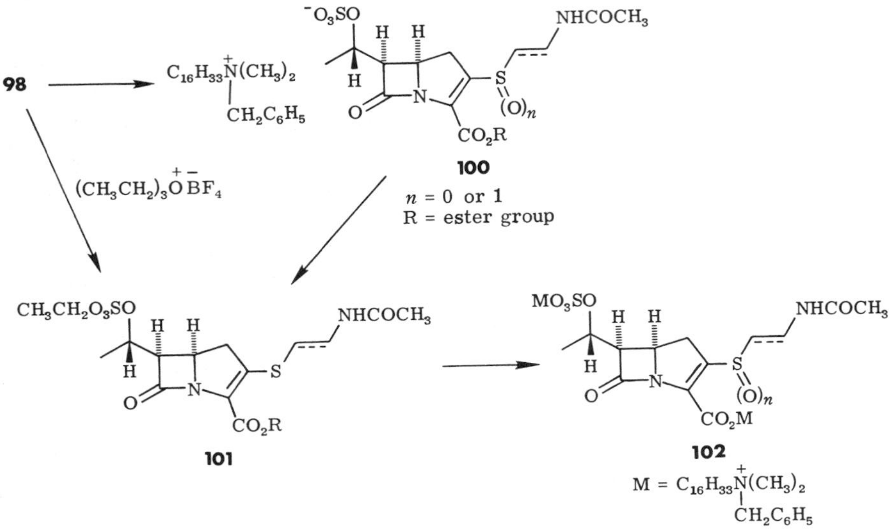
98
$C_{16}H_{33}\overset{+}{N}(CH_3)_2$
$CH_2C_6H_5$
^-O_3SO
NHCOCH$_3$
H H
H
S
(O)n
N
O
CO$_2$R
100
n = 0 or 1
R = ester group
$(CH_3CH_2)_3\overset{+}{O}\,\overset{-}{B}F_4$
$CH_3CH_2O_3SO$
101
MO_3SO
CO$_2$M
102
$M = C_{16}H_{33}\overset{+}{N}(CH_3)_2$
$CH_2C_6H_5$

3. *Modification of the Hydroxy(sulfooxy)ethyl Side Chain*

Modification of the hydroxy(sulfooxy)ethyl side chain of the olivanic acids has taken three main forms: acylation, elimination, and replacement of the oxygen function. The *O*-acyl derivatives are obtained by acylation of the esterified hydroxyethyl olivanic acids. The sulfated olivanic acids, as their salt and ester forms, are particularly suited to elimination and replacement of the side-chain oxygen group. Carboxyl-deblocked final products are usually obtained by hydrogenolysis of the *p*-nitrobenzyl ester, although the *p*-carbomethoxy group has also shown limited utility in this connection.

Acylation (Eur. Pat. Appl. 7,152) of the benzyl and *p*-nitrobenzyl esters of olivanic acids MM 22380, MM 22382, and MM 22383, as represented by the general structure **99**, with acetic anhydride or acetyl and phenylacetyl chlorides in pyridine afforded the *O*-acyl derivatives (**103**) (R^1 = methyl or benzyl). Similar treatment with methyl isocyanate provided the *N*-methyl carbamoyl derivative (**103**) (R^1 = methylamino). The sodium salts of the products (**104**) were obtained by catalytic hydrogenation

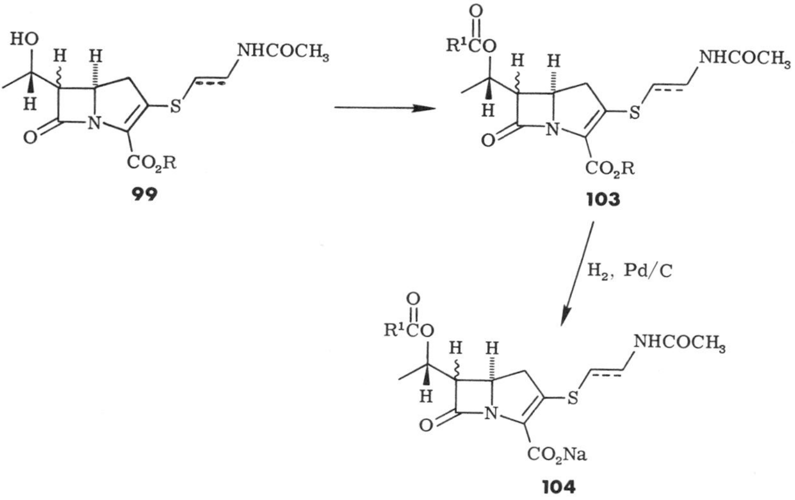

99 → **103**

H₂, Pd/C

104

$R^1 = CH_3, CH_2C_6H_5, CH_3NH$

of the *p*-nitrobenzyl esters in aqueous dioxane followed by neutralization with sodium bicarbonate.

Acylation of the hydroxyethyl derivatives (**99**) with methanesulfonyl chloride and triethylamine afforded the reactive mesylates (**105**) (Eur. Pat. Appl. 5,348). These derivatives underwent stereospecific antielimination on treatment with bases such as potassium carbonate or diazabicycloundecene (DBU), the trans compounds providing the (*Z*)-enelactams (**106**) and the cis compounds providing the (*E*)-enelactams (**107**).

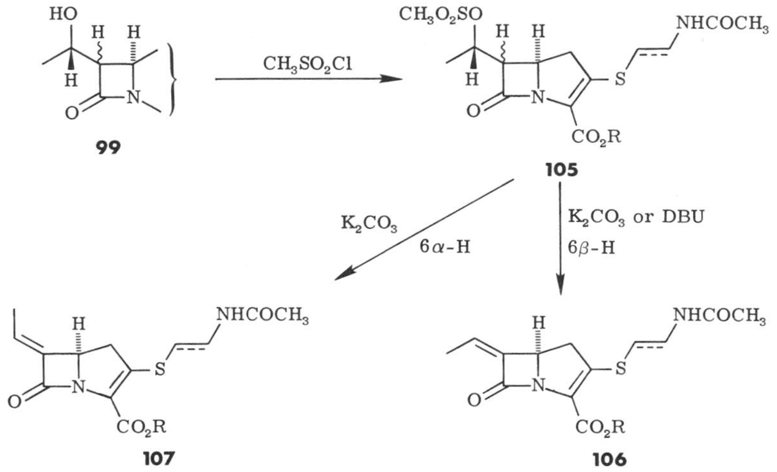

99 → **105**

CH₃SO₂Cl

K₂CO₃   6α-H

K₂CO₃ or DBU   6β-H

107   **106**

The intermediate mesylates wherein R is *p*-nitrobenzyl were deblocked to the corresponding sodium carboxylates.

The enelactams, as represented by structure **110**, have also been obtained from derivatives of the sulfooxyethyl olivanic acids (Eur. Pat. Appl. 5,348). Exposure of sodium sulfooxyethyl derivatives (**108**) to potassium carbonate in DMF, ammonium salts (**109**) to DBU in methylene chloride, or ethyl sulfates (**101**) to either DBU or triethylamine in methylene chloride led to mixtures of enelactams (**110**) in which the *E* isomer (**107**) predominates. These mixtures could be used without separation for further derivatization studies.In contrast to the nonstereospecific eliminations, treatment of **101** with either potassium carbonate or potassium acetate afforded solely the *E* isomer (**107**). The ester groups R employed in these transformations were methyl, benzyl, *p*-bromobenzyl, *p*-nitrobenzyl, and *p*-carbomethoxybenzyl.

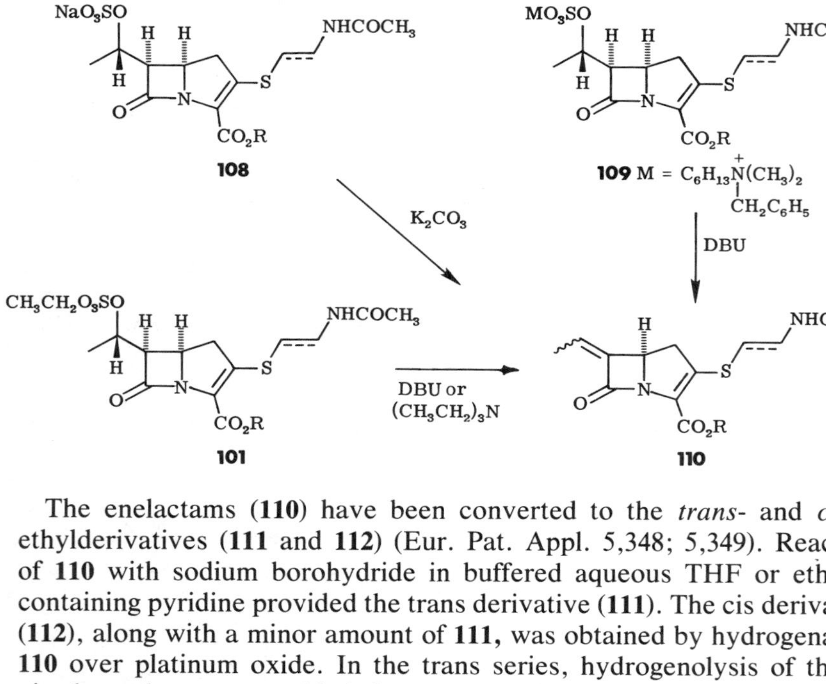

The enelactams (**110**) have been converted to the *trans*- and *cis*-6-ethylderivatives (**111** and **112**) (Eur. Pat. Appl. 5,348; 5,349). Reaction of **110** with sodium borohydride in buffered aqueous THF or ethanol containing pyridine provided the trans derivative (**111**). The cis derivative (**112**), along with a minor amount of **111**, was obtained by hydrogenating **110** over platinum oxide. In the trans series, hydrogenolysis of the *p*-nitrobenzyl esters provided the parent antibiotics (**111**, R = Na); one of which is equivalent to the natural product PS-5 (**8a**). In the cis series, the deblocked products (**112**, R = Na) were obtained by electrolytic cleavage of the corresponding *p*-carbomethoxybenzyl esters.

Replacement of the hydroxyl or sulfooxy group by a thio group has been accomplished by two methods (Eur. Pat. Appl. 5,348). Treatment of enelactams (110) with mercaptans and potassium carbonate in DMF yielded the trans adducts (113) which are diastereomeric at the newly created chiral center. The mercaptans that have been used in this Michael-type process include methyl, ethyl, allyl, acetamidoethyl, carbomethoxymethyl, and phenyl mercaptans. The phenylthio adducts (114) have also been prepared in a stereospecific manner by reacting hydroxyethyl intermediates (99) with N-phenylthiosuccinimide in the presence of tributylphosphine. This reaction presumably involves *in situ* activation of the hydroxyl group followed by displacement with inversion. A series of deblocked 6-hydrocarbylthioethyl derivatives (113 and 114, R = Na) was obtained by hydrogenolysis of the corresponding *p*-nitrobenzyl esters.

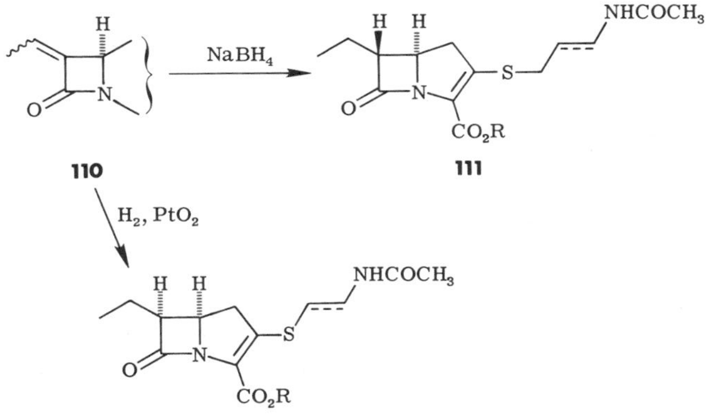

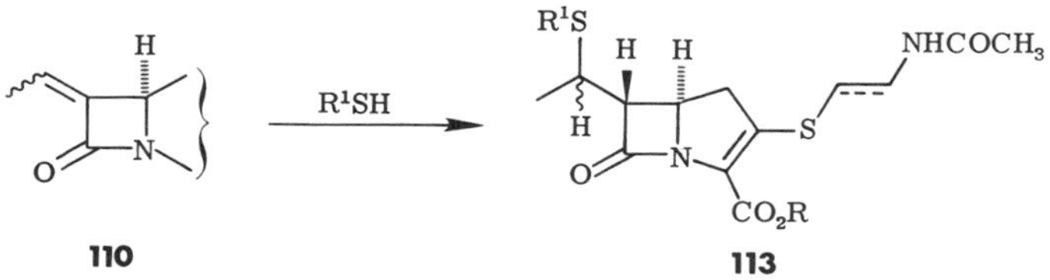

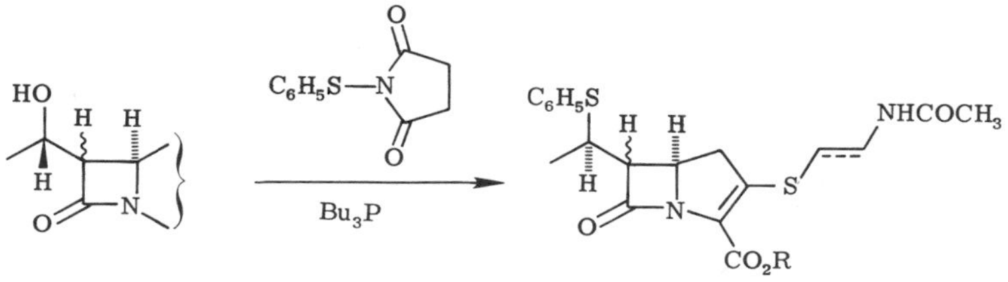

4. Isomerization and Halogenation of the Acetamidoethenylthio Side Chain

Two modifications of the *trans*-acetamidoethenylthio side chain, namely isomerization and halogenation, have been reported. These transformations are illustrated for the general structure **115** which represents a variety of olivanic acid derivatives, both sulfated and nonsulfated, incorporating the unsaturated side chain.

The isomerization of the side-chain double bond from the *E* to the *Z* configuration was accomplished by treating **115** with mercuric chloride in buffered aqueous acetonitrile (Eur. Pat. Appl. 8,885). The reaction was usually performed on the benzyl and *p*-nitrobenzyl carboxylates but has also been carried out on MM 13902 (**6b**) itself. In the *cis*-azetidinone series, both the hydroxyethyl and sulfooxyethyl analogs were isomerized to **116,** and in the trans series the hydroxyethyl derivative **116** was prepared. Hydrogenolysis of the *p*-nitrobenzyl esters provided the deblocked products as the corresponding sodium carboxylates.

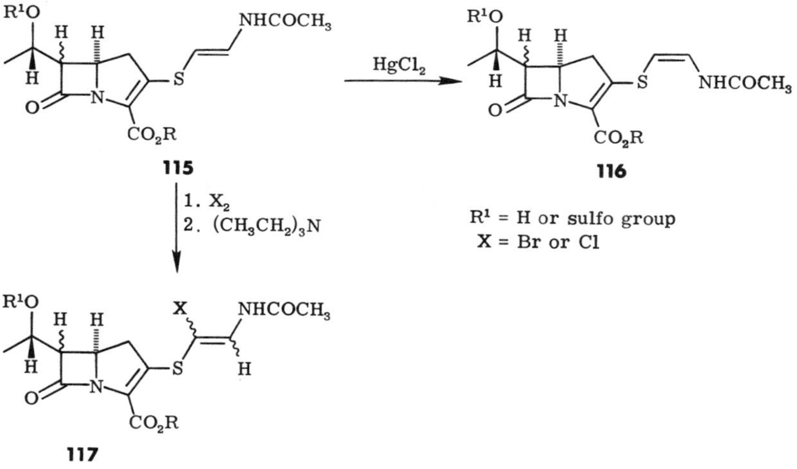

115

116

R¹ = H or sulfo group
X = Br or Cl

117

Halogenation of the unsaturated side chain of a variety of olivanic acid derivatives has been described (Eur. Pat. Appl. 7,753). The derivatives (**115**) were treated with either bromine or chlorine at low temperature followed by warming in the presence of a base to give the products (**117**) as mixtures of the double bond isomers. Since the reactions were conducted in an organic solvent, usually methylene chloride and carbon tetrachloride, R was an ester group or the lipophilic ammonium cation. Variations of the R¹ group included hydrogen and sulfo esters and salts.

5. Oxidiation of the Sulfur Atom

Oxidation of olivanic acids MM 17880 (**6a**) and MM 13902 (**6d**) with *m*-chloroperbenzoic acid in water gave diastereomeric mixtures of the corresponding sulfoxides (Ger. Offen. 2,728,097). In the latter case, one of the isomers was identical to the naturally occurring olivanic acid MM 4550 (**6c**) (Brown *et al.*, 1977).

D. Derivatives of PS-5

PS-5 (**8a**), a carbapenem antibiotic isolated from fermentations of *S. cremeus* subsp. *auratilis,* is active against a variety of gram-positive and gram-negative bacteria and shows inhibitory activity against β-lactamases produced by various bacteria. The structure of PS-5 differs most noticibly from that of thienamycin and the olivanic acids by the lack of an oxygen functionality in the 6-ethyl side chain. Derivatization of PS-5 is therefore limited to modification of the carboxyl group and the acetamidoethylthio side chain, both of which have been reported.

Esters of PS-5 (**118**) were prepared by reacting the parent antibiotic, as its sodium salt, with an alkyl halide in DMF (Jpn. Kokai 79 084,589; Eur. Pat. Appl. 2,058). The trityl and triethylmethyl derivatives so obtained were deacetylated (Eur. Pat. Appl. 2,058) via the imino halide–imino ether route to provide desacetyl PS-5 (**119**). This compound was also obtained by enzymatic deacetylation of PS-5 using *Protaminobacter ruber* extracts (Eur. Pat. Appl. 2,058) or L- and D-aminoacylases (Jpn. Kokai 80 042,536). Oxidation of PS-5 with *m*-chloroperbenzoic acid in water afforded the sulfoxide (**120**) (Jpn. Kokai 79 135,790).

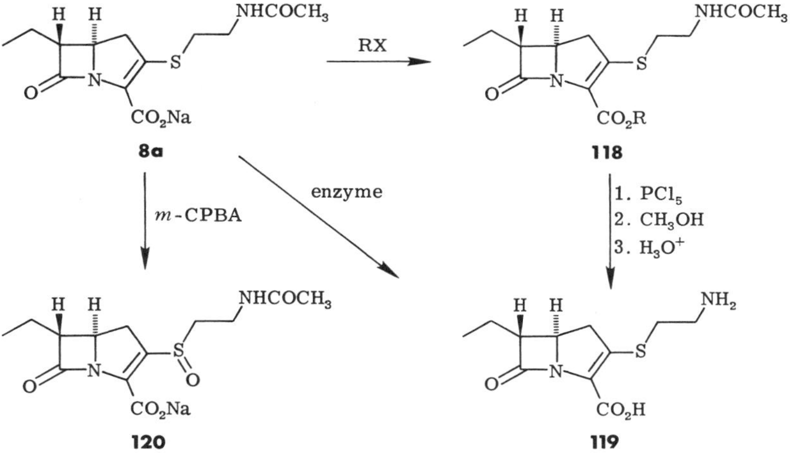

III.   Total Synthesis of Carbapenem Antibiotics

A.   Introduction

The decade of the 1970s has witnessed a dramatic expansion of research activity directed toward the total synthesis of both classical and
nonclassical β-lactam antibiotics. Impetus for this effort has come from
many directions of which several deserve special comment. The classical
work of Sheehan, Woodward, and Bose and their co-workers, as well
as the Roussel effort, showed that the total synthesis of penicillins and
cephalosporins was not only conceptionally possible but tactically feasible. Familiarization with the early synthetic techniques, coupled with
the desire to explore and expand classical structure–activity relationships, led chemists to develop new synthetic strategies and methods
capable of producing diverse structural types not obviously available via
natural product modification. Examples of synthetic achievements that
have added to our understanding of the structural features necessary for
antibacterial activity include the carba-, oxa-, and isocephems, the oxa-
penams, and the penems. More recently, the discovery of several novel,
naturally occurring, β-lactam compounds (nocardicins, clavulanic acid,
and the carbapenem family as represented by thienamycin and the olivanic acids) has generated significant interest in synthesizing these compounds and structurally related analogs.

The genesis of much of the synthetic activity in the carbapenem area
is rooted in the unparalleled biological properties as well as the highly
functionalized and unusual ring system associated with the natural products. The carbapenem antibiotics, as represented by structure **121**, exhibit
potent antibacterial activity and substantial β-lactamase inhibitory activity. The major structural differences between the carbapenem antibiotics
and the classical penicillins and cephalosporins mentioned earlier (see
p. 252) lead to unique synthetic challenges.

The objectives of carbapenem total synthesis are multipurpose. Syntheses
directed toward the natural products are primarily demonstrations of

121

R^1 = H, CH$_3$, OH, OSO$_3$H
R^2 = CH$_2$CH$_2$NH$_2$,
    CH$_2$CH$_2$NHCOCH$_3$,
    CH=CHNHCOCH$_3$

methodology for constructing the bicyclic nucleus and for appending the peripheral side chains. More importantly, the synthetic strategies evolving from these studies should allow for rapid analog synthesis, particularly those analogs involving replacement of the hydroxyethyl and cysteamine groups. Total synthesis provides a unique opportunity for studying the effects of profound side-chain modification or replacement on biological activity, and general routes to substituted carbapenems become particularly attractive goals in this respect and offer the hope of providing novel product candidates.

Although fermentation is almost invariably used for the manufacture of complex natural products whenever applicable, the low fermentation yields thus far reported for the naturally occuring carbapenem antibiotics make total synthesis an attractive alternative for the development of clinically important compounds. This factor adds the additional objective of developing operationally simple, inexpensive, and high-yielding routes.

The evolution of the synthetic strategies directed toward the carbapenem antibiotics is guided by two primary problems: the construction of the bicyclic nucleus and the introduction of substituents at the 2- and 6-positions, the most challenging of these clearly being the synthesis of the strained ring system. Its construction is best effected under mild, neutral conditions, as late as possible in the synthetic scheme. This notion has lead to routes in which the azetidinone ring is elaborated first, thereby allowing flexibility in its method of construction. The general process is outlined schematically for structures 122 and 123 in which R^2 and R^3 are groups that separately or together represent latent functionality capable of subsequent elaboration into the fused pyrroline ring.

122 **123**

A notable distinction between carbapenem synthesis and the synthesis of β-lactam antibiotics possessing an additional heteroatom in the second ring can be made. The latter class often uses the heteroatom as a pivotal point around which the bicyclic nucleus is formed. The lack of the second heteroatom in the carbapenem nucleus forces further constraints on potential methods for synthesizing the nucleus and encourages development of new methodology. Thus far three general approaches which utilize formation of the C-2—C-3 bond or the C-3—N-4 bond as the ultimate step in the ring-forming process have been described.

A second strategy element guiding most carbapenem syntheses involves the introduction of the peripheral substituents at positions C-2 and C-6. Since the carboxyl group at C-3 is generally assumed to be required for antibacterial activity, its incorporation will be treated as invariant. Those syntheses directed toward preparing hydroxyethylated products must address the question of the relative and, ultimately, the absolute stereochemistry at the three contiguous chiral centers—ring carbons C-5 and C-6 and the hydroxyethyl center. Stereocontrolled routes that avoid troublesome isomer separations or carrying along diastereomeric mixtures are favored. Since a paramount goal in developing synthetic routes to carbapenems is analog synthesis, flexible routes that allow for facile replacement of the hydroxyethyl and aminoethylthio side chains are most desirable. This objective is readily achieved by attachment of the requisite side chains onto an azetidinone precursor before construction of the bicyclic system, thereby minimizing the manipulations of the labile products. One notable exception to this strategy, addition of thio side chains to C-2 of the carbapenems, has been explored with great success.

The remainder of this section will describe the efforts of several industrial and academic groups to solve the considerable synthetic challenges presented by the carbapenem antibiotics. Several elegant and general solutions offering great potential for both analog synthesis and development into commercially important processes have appeared in a relatively short time. Future developments should greatly facilitate the defining of structure–activity relationships in this area of intense research activity.

B.   Total Synthesis of Natural Products

1.   *Synthesis of (±)-Thienamycin and (±)-8-Epithienamycin by C-2—C-3 Bond Formation*

The first total synthesis of a carbapenem natural product [(±)-thienamycin (**5a**)] was communicated by Johnston and co-workers (1978). Subsequent publications by this group (Bouffard *et al.,* 1980; Schmitt *et al.,* 1980a) have detailed their work and its extension to the synthesis of (±)-8-epithienamycin (**144**). The basic scheme followed from three major strategic elements: elaboration of a monocyclic β-lactam into an intermediate containing the peripheral functionality of thienamycin, cyclization to a carbapenam ring system by forming the C-2—C-3 bond, and final transformation into the fully functionalized carbapenem system. A minor strategy element was the desire to introduce the hydroxethyl side chain in a stereochemically indiscriminant manner so that thienamycin stereoisomers could also be obtained.

The requisite monocyclic β-lactam (124) was obtained by condensing 1-acetoxybutadiene with chlorosulfonyl isocyanate. Reduction of the double bond, cleavage of the acetate, and cyclization to the bicyclic acetonide (125) provided an intermediate ideally suited for introduction of the hydroxyethyl side chain via an aldol process. Treating the lactam enolate of 125 with excess acetaldehyde smoothly provided a mixture of all four diastereomers of 126 in near quantitative yield. Chromatography readily separated the trans isomers, which constituted 89% of the mixture, from the cis isomers. The trans isomers were expected to predominate since electrophilic attack on the lactam enolate should occur preferentially from the more accessible exo face of the bicyclic acetonide.

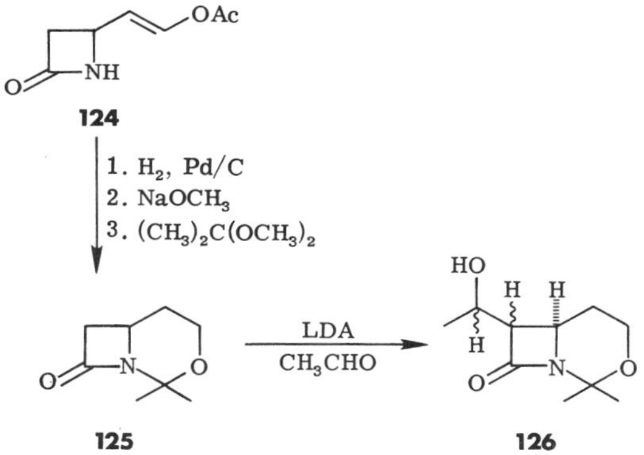

The trans and cis isomers of 126 were readily distinguished by NMR spectroscopy; the vicinal coupling constants of the azetidinone protons being 1.5 and 5 Hz for the trans and cis isomers, respectively. In the cis series, the relative configuration at the hydroxyl-bearing carbon atom of the major isomer was shown to be R^* by single crystal X-ray analysis of the derived O-p-nitrobenzyloxycarbonyl derivative. Only a trace of the cis-S^* isomer was produced in the aldol reaction. In the trans series, the relative configuration at the hydroxyl center was established by converting 127 to a separable mixture of mesylates 128 and 129 which then underwent stereospecific elimination to the enelactams 130 and 131. By assuming a trans coplanar elimination mechanism, enelactam 130 was related to the minor trans-R^* isomer (127a) and enelactam 131 to the major trans-S^* isomer (127b).

Previous model work (Schmitt et al., 1980b) had shown that azetidinone (132) could be cyclized to the carbapenam (133) by successive bromination and base-induced malonic ester-type alkylation. Subsequent dehydrobromination, decarboalkoxylation, and double bond isomerization yielded the carbapen-2-em (134). Since this method of ring closure

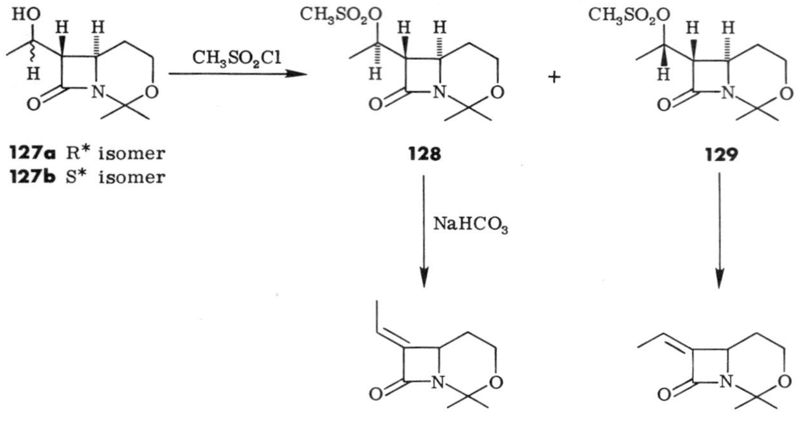

127a R* isomer
127b S* isomer

128

129

130

131

CH₃SO₂Cl

NaHCO₃

was destined to become the key feature of the present synthesis, methods for converting **127** to a monocyclic intermediate containing protected hydroxy, amino, and carboxyl groups were required. The *p*-nitrobenzyl group was chosen as a common protecting group since all three functionalities could then be simultaneously deblocked under mild hydrogenolytic conditions at the final stage of the synthesis.

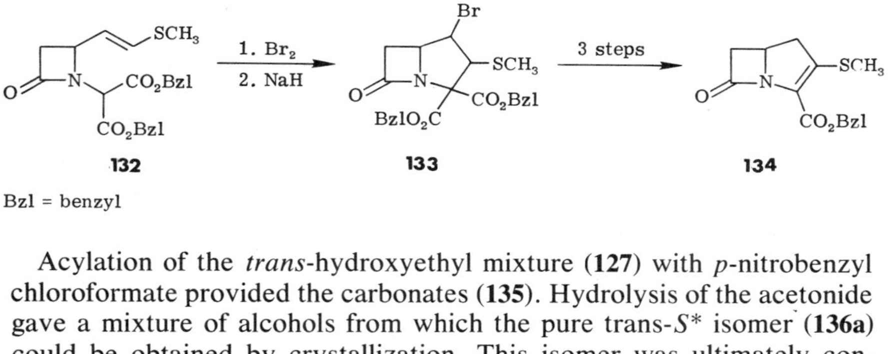

132

1. Br₂
2. NaH

133

3 steps

134

Bzl = benzyl

Acylation of the *trans*-hydroxyethyl mixture (**127**) with *p*-nitrobenzyl chloroformate provided the carbonates (**135**). Hydrolysis of the acetonide gave a mixture of alcohols from which the pure trans-*S** isomer (**136a**) could be obtained by crystallization. This isomer was ultimately converted to (±)-8-epithienamycin. The mother liquors from the crystallization, which constituted a 3:2 mixture of the trans-*R** (**136**) and trans-*S** isomers, were employed in the synthesis of (±)-thienamycin. For the sake of simplicity, the isomerically pure route leading to 8-epithienamycin will be discussed first.

Oxidation of **136a** afforded an aldehyde intermediate which was converted to the dithioacetal (**137**) with *N*-(*p*-nitrobenzyloxy-carbonyl)cysteamine. One of the thio residues was eliminated by suc-

127 $\xrightarrow{\text{RCl}}$ **135** $\xrightarrow{\text{H}_3\text{O}^+}$ **136a** S* isomer
136b R* isomer

RO, H H

RO, H H, OH

$R = CO_2CH_2\!\!-\!\!\langle\!\!\bigcirc\!\!\rangle\!\!-\!\!NO_2$

cessive treatment of **137** with bromine and base; the product thioenol ether (**138**) was obtained primarily as the *E* isomer. The remainder of the carbon framework was introduced by condensing **138** with bis-*p*-nitrobenzyl ketomalonate followed by chlorination and reduction. With compound **139** all of the peripheral functionality had been introduced in a protected form and the stage was set for the critical ring-forming reaction.

Successive treatment of **139** with bromine and triethylamine produced a diastereomeric mixture of carbapenams (**140**). Dehydrobromination of **140** gave **141** which was monodecarboalkoxylated to carbapen-1-em (**142**) with lithium iodide in collidine at 120°C. None of the carbapen-2-em isomer (**143**) was obtained in the latter reaction, presumably because it was unstable to the reaction conditions. Exposure of **142** to *N,N*-diiso-propylethylamine in DMSO afforded an 85:15 mixture of **142** and **143** which could be separated chromatographically. Recycling of the re-covered **142** led to workable yields of **143**. Final deblocking of the three *p*-nitrobenzyl protecting groups by catalytic hydrogenation gave (±)-8-epithienamycin (**144**).

For the synthesis of (±)-thienamycin, the 3:2 trans-*R**–trans-*S** mix-ture (**136**) was converted by the methods just described in the trans-*S** series to a mixture of bicyclic products (**141** and **145**). The trans-*R** isomer (**145**) was separated by preparative TLC and transformed into (±)-thienamycin (**5a**) by the same sequence of reactions used in the preparation of (±)-8-epithienamycin from **141**. Racemic thienamycin was found to possess approximately half the antibacterial potency of the natural product against a variety of microorganisms (Schmitt *et al.*, 1980a) and (±)-8-epithienamycin showed reduced antibacterial potency by comparison to (±)-thienamycin.

A more practical route to the azetidinone (**149**), a key intermediate in the (±)-thienamycin synthesis, has been reported (Ger. Offen. 2,751,-597). Silylation of the readily available 4-vinylazetidinone gave the N-protected derivative (**146**). Hydroxyethylation of **146** via the aldol procedure provided a mixture of diastereomers (**147**) which could be sep-arated into the trans and cis forms. Acylation of the trans mixture gave

136a
1. $CrO_3 \cdot 2\,C_5H_5N$
2. $HSCH_2CH_2NHR$
137
1. Br_2
2. Et_3N
138
1. R_2CO
2. $SOCl_2$
3. Bu_3P
139
1. Br_2
2. Et_3N
140
AgF
141
LiI
142
i-Pr_2NH
143
H_2
Pd/C
144
R = CO_2CH_2—C₆H₄—NO_2

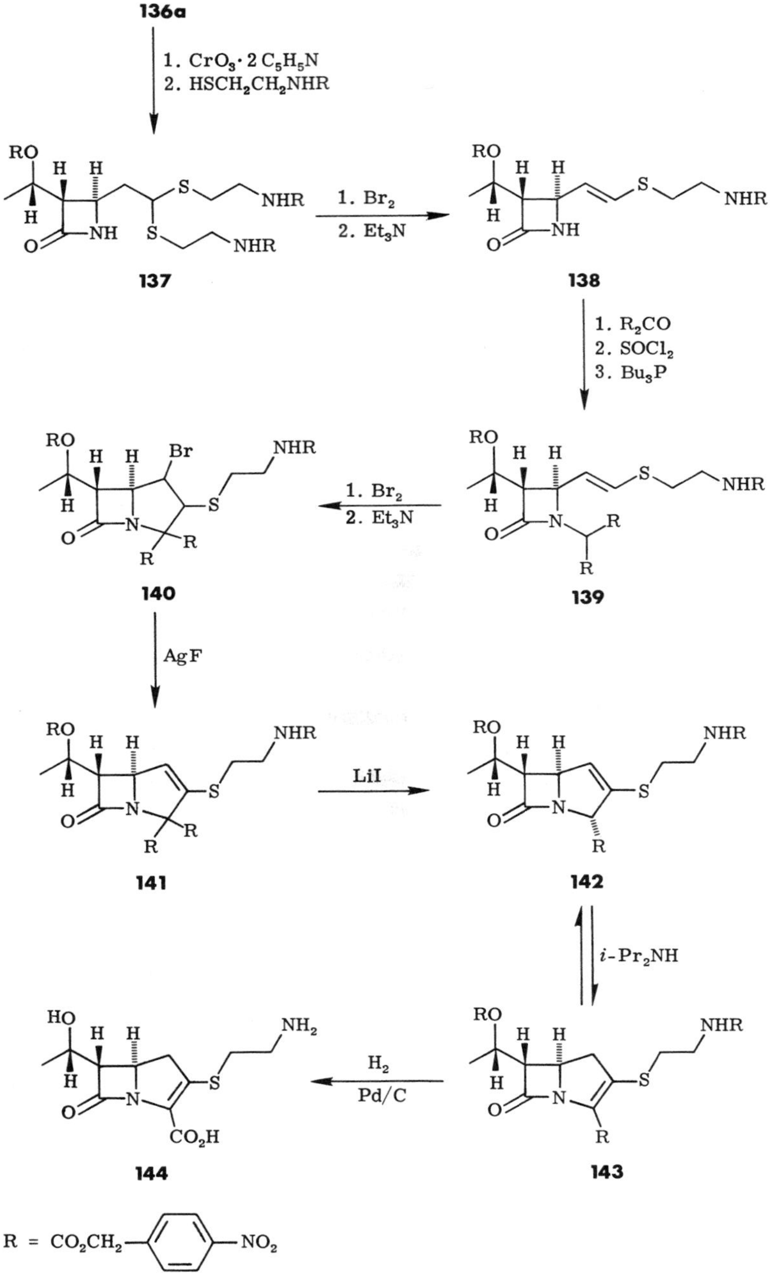

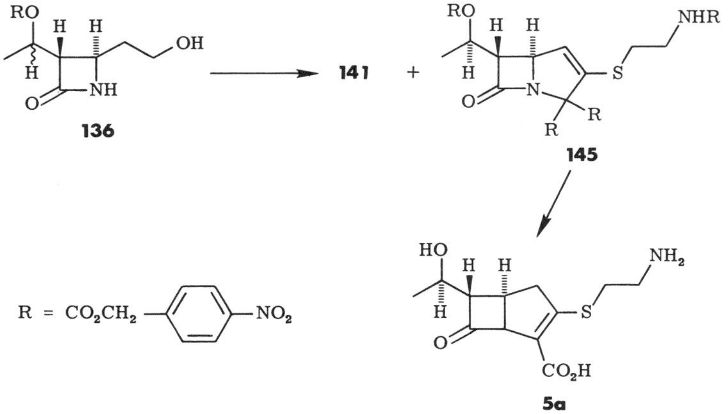

the corresponding carbonates from which the desired R^* isomer (**148**) was separated. Compound **148** was converted to intermediate **149** by hydrolytic removal of the silyl group followed by reaction of the double bond with N-(p-nitrobenzyloxycarbonyl)ethanesulfenyl bromide and base. This sequence has the further advantage of providing intermediate **149** uncontaminated with the S^* isomer (**138**).

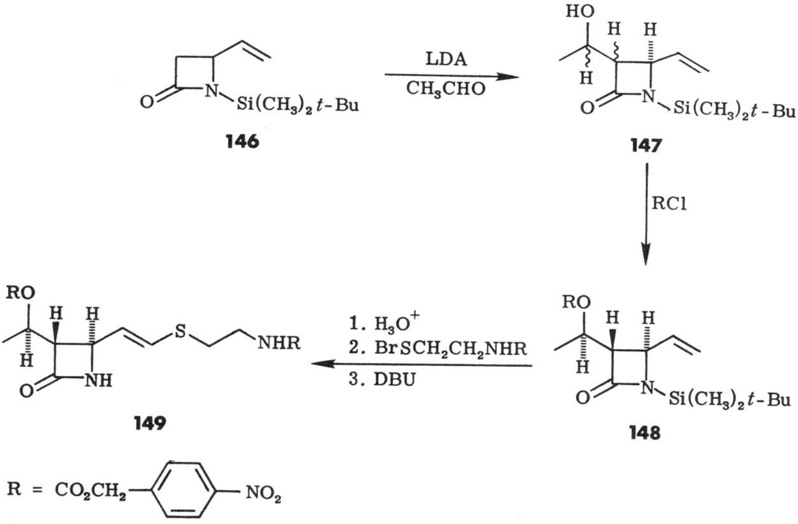

Kametani and associates (1980a,b) have devised a short synthesis of key intermediates that contain all the chiral centers of ($\pm$)-thienamycin and ($\pm$)-8-epithienamycin. The relative stereochemistry was established at an early stage by use of a dipolar cycloaddition reaction between a nitrile oxide and a crotonate ester. In the best case, *t*-butyl crotonate was observed to react both regio- and stereoselectively with the nitrile oxide (150) to give mainly the isoxazoline (151a). Catalytic reduction of 151a gave a 1:1 mixture of amino esters (152a) which, without separation, was selectively cyclized to azetidinone (153) by successive treatment with trimethylsilyl chloride, ethyl magnesium bromide, and aqueous ammonium chloride. Acylation of 153 followed by acetal exchange with *N*-(*p*-nitrobenzyloxycarbonyl)cysteamine provided 154, an intermediate for (±)-thienamycin.

When methyl crotonate was substituted for *t*-butyl crotonate, the initial cycloaddition was less regioselective, reduction of the resulting isoxazoline was less stereoselective, and cyclization of the amino ester mixture via the Grignard method produced lower yields of 153 along with a cis azetidinone product. Saponification of the intermediate amino ester mixture (152b) followed by dicyclohexylcarbodiimide-mediated ring closure afforded mixtures of azetidinones 153 and 155. The major product (155) resulted from epimerization at C-3 in both the hydrolysis and ring-forming reactions. This material was converted to dithióacetal 137, an intermediate in the (±)-8-epithienamycin synthesis.

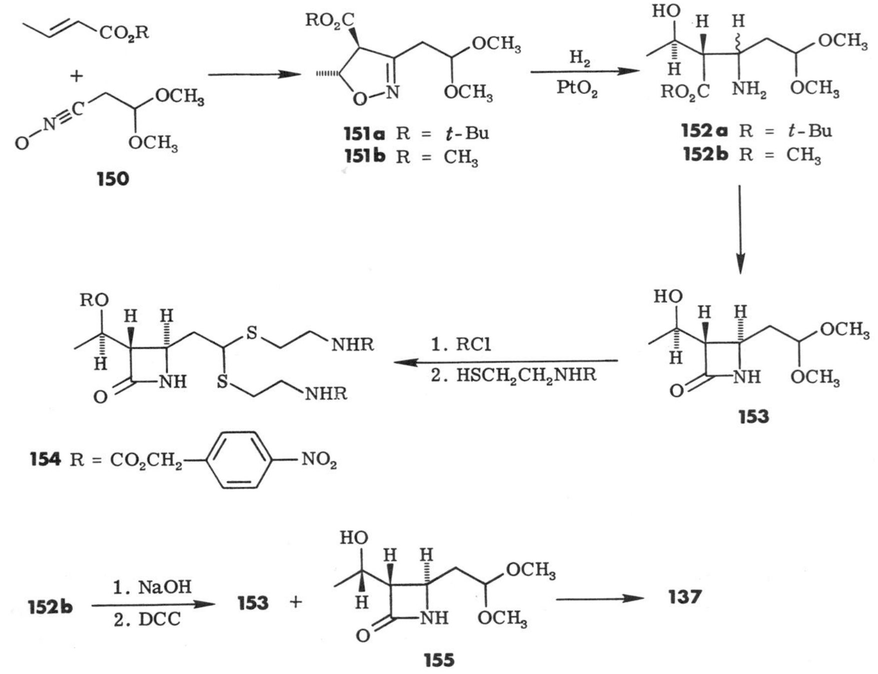

151a R = *t*-Bu
151b R = CH₃

150

152a R = *t*-Bu
152b R = CH₃

1. RCl
2. HSCH₂CH₂NHR

153

154 R = CO₂CH₂⟨benzene ring⟩NO₂

152b → (1. NaOH 2. DCC) → 153 + 155 → 137

2. Synthesis of (+)-Thienamycin by C-3—N Bond Formation

An alternative synthetic approach to thienamycin that differs from the racemic route primarily in the method of ring construction has been devised and developed by Merck chemists. The pivotal reaction in the new scheme involves a novel and highly efficient carbene insertion reaction which produces the bicyclic nucleus by forming the C-3—N bond. In a model study delineating this approach, Ratcliffe and co-workers (1980) prepared the racemic α-diazo-β-keto ester (156) and studied its decomposition under a variety of photolytic and catalytic conditions. On heating in benzene solution with a catalytic amount of rhodium(II) acetate, 156 was converted to the bicyclic ketoester (157) in near quantitative yield. The utility of 157 for the preparation of 2-thio-substituted carbapen-2-ems (159) was demonstrated by its conversion to vinyl tosylate (158) followed by addition of N-protected cysteamine.

156	157	158 R = OTs
		159 R = SCH$_2$CH$_2$NHCO$_2$PNB

The efficiency of the diazo ring closure in the model series prompted consideration of the carbene approach for the synthesis of thienamycin and analogs and as a potential commercial route to carbapenem antibiotics. From a strategic viewpoint, the carbene insertion reaction allows for construction of most of the structure and all of the stereochemistry prior to formation of the strained and reactive bicyclic ring system. Syntheses directed toward thienamycin and its derivatives must, therefore, primarily address the problem of introduction of the hydroxyethyl side chain with the appropriate stereochemistry at the three chiral centers. For analog syntheses involving replacement of the hydroxyethyl group, a common branching point suitable for introduction of various side chains via alkylation or acylation procedures would be appropriate. Since the cysteamine side chain would be introduced near the end of the synthesis, its replacement by other thio side chains should be a trivial exercise. Two synthetic pathways incorporating these elements—one designed primarily for analog synthesis and the other as a practical approach to thienamycin—that share several common features including the ring forming reaction have emerged.

A stereocontrolled, enantiomerically specific synthesis of (+)-thienamycin has been described by Salzmann and co-workers (1980a,b). Since this synthesis was designed to eventually prepare analogs, a key element in the plan was the elaboration of a monocyclic β-lactam intermediate capable of substitution at the pro-C-6 position via enolate chemistry. An additional requirement of producing thienamycin and analogs having the correct absolute configuration lead to the choice of L-aspartic acid as the starting material. The chiral center of aspartic acid, which was destined to become the C-5 bridgehead position of the carbapenem nucleus, would be used to control the introduction of the remaining chiral centers.

Dibenzyl aspartate was cyclized to the azetidinone (160) in 65–70% yield by treating its N-trimethylsilyl derivative with one equivalent of *tert*-butyl magnesium chloride. The dibenzyl ester was chosen for this transformation because the product crystallized directly from the reaction mixture. Reduction of the ester function of 160 with sodium borohydride, followed by conversion of the resulting alcohol to the mesylate and iodide, and finally N-silylation provided the chiral azetidinone alkylating agent (161).

The objectives at this junction in the synthetic pathway were to introduce a masked carboxyl group suitable for future elaboration into the diazo ketoester side chain and to provide a product having only the pro-C-6 position enolizable. In the first report (Salzmann *et al.*, 1980a) this was accomplished by alkylating lithium tri(methylthio)methide with 161. However, because of the difficulties encountered in transforming the tri(methylthio)methyl group into a carboxyl group by direct means, an alternative solution was sought and found. Reaction of 161 with 2-lithio-2-trimethylsilyl-1,3-dithiane gave the substituted dithiane (162) in good yield (Salzmann *et al.*, 1980b).

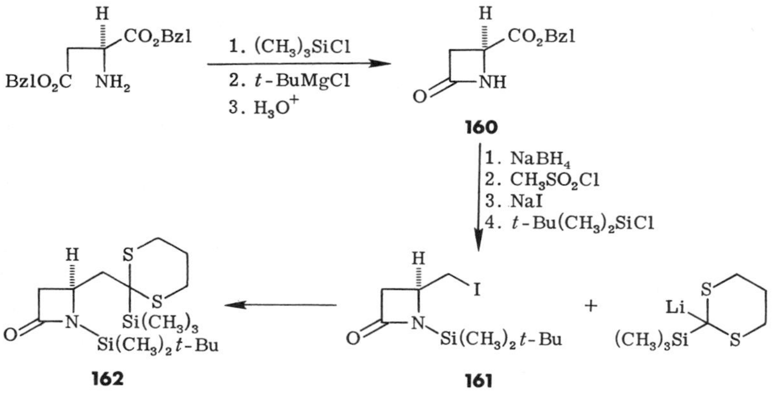

Condensation of the enolate derived from 162 with acetaldehyde gave approximately a 1:1 mixture of trans-R and trans-S isomers (163 and 164) along with a small amount of the cis-R isomer. Stereocontrol could be achieved by oxidizing the aldol mixture to the thermodynamically preferred *trans*-acetyl derivative (165). Alternatively, 165 could be produced directly by acylating the enolate of 162 with acetylimidazole. Reduction of 165 with potassium selectride in ether gave a 9:1 mixture of 163 and 164. Stereoselection in favor of the desired trans-*R* isomer is presumably related to selective hydride delivery from the sterically less-hindered β-face of a chelated structure such as 166.

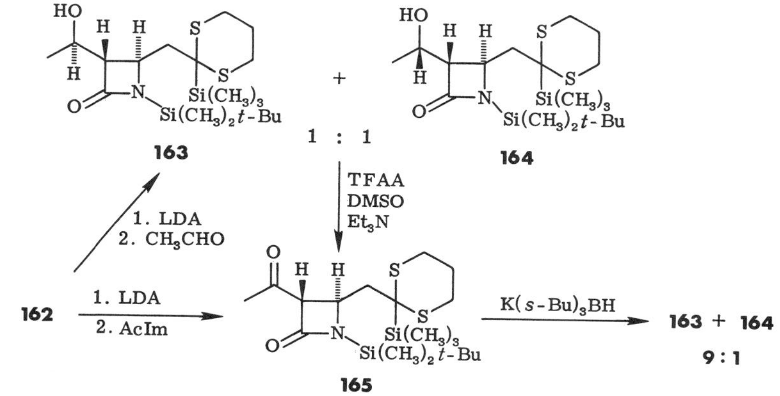

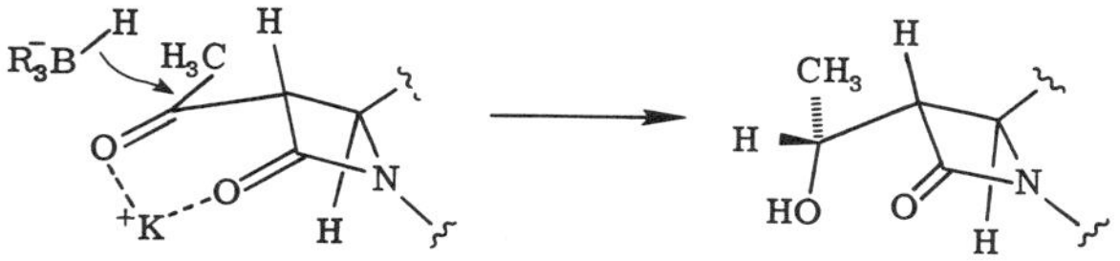

Compound 163 was converted to the carboxylic acid (167) via a two-step procedure. Standard dithiane hydrolysis provided a trimethylsilyl ketone intermediate which underwent a facile Baeyer–Villiger oxidation on treatment with hydrogen peroxide. The requisite ketoester intermediate 168 was obtained by condensing the imidazolide derivative of 167 with the magnesium salt of mono-*p*-nitrobenzyl malonate. Removal of the *N*-silyl protecting group followed by diazo exchange from *p*-carboxybenzenesulfonyl azide provided the cyclization precursor (169).

From this point onward, the synthetic route is common with the Merck Process Research approach to be discussed shortly, and development of the remaining reactions was carried out principally by chemists in Process Research. As in the model case, thermolysis of 169 in the presence of rhodium acetate smoothly produced the bicyclic ketoester (170). Introduction of the cysteamine residue was accomplished by converting

170 to the vinyl tosylate (**171**) prior to base-mediated addition of *N*-(*p*-nitrobenzyloxycarbonyl)cysteamine. This procedure was eventually developed into a rapid, high-yielding sequence involving *in situ* formation and reaction of the enol phosphate (**172**). Final hydrogenolytic deblocking of the *p*-nitrobenzyl protecting groups of **173** gave (+)-thienamycin (**5a**).

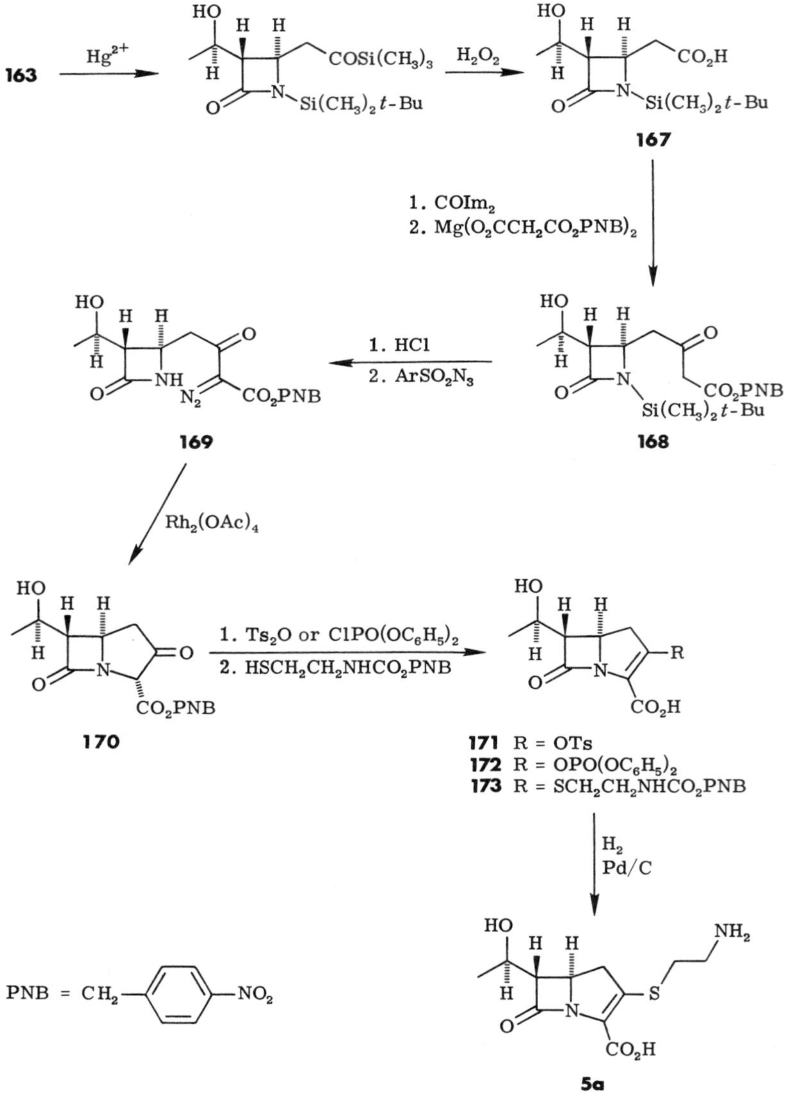

The carbene insertion reaction also formed the cornerstone of a synthesis of thienamycin having potential commercial application. The primary objectives of this effort included high-yielding steps, simple procedures suitable for large scale-up, inexpensive and nontoxic starting materials and reagents, and safety. The basis of the Merck Process Research route that addresses these objectives has been reported by Melillo and co-workers (1980). Further improvements and refinements of the original scheme have been presented by Pines (1981) and are included in the discussion below. This route is characterized by (1) early introduction of the hydroxyethyl group through formation of a highly functionalized, triply asymmetric acyclic derivative; (2) an expedient resolution procedure at an early stage; (3) efficient formation of a monocyclic β-lactam ring using classical diimide chemistry; (4) a clean inversion reaction to correct the relative stereochemistry prior to construction of the bicyclic ring system; and (5) minimal use of protecting groups.

The starting material for this route, acetone dicarboxylate (174), was converted to an enamine with benzylamine and cleanly acetylated with acetic anhydride. The resulting product (175) displayed a rigid structure by virtue of an internal hydrogen bond, thus setting the stage for a stereoselective reduction. Hydride addition to 175 gave a triply asymmetric acyclic product which was conveniently isolated as the crystalline hydrochloride salt of lactone 176 following hydrolysis of the reduction mixture. The lactonization step also introduces a needed chemoselectivity between the two carboxyl groups. The relative stereochemistry of 176 was established by its conversion to model azetidinones and by X-ray analysis of the hydrobromide salt of the (+)-isomer. Unfortunately, the relative stereochemistry at the methyl-substituted carbon was incorrect, thereby necessitating an inversion step at a later stage.

The lactonization reaction also provided an intermediate eminently suitable for an early resolution by a unique procedure. Whereas resolution of 176 with the relatively inexpensive and available (+)-isomer of 10-camphor sulfonic acid gave a highly crystalline salt of the unwanted enantiomer, catalytic reduction of the reserved mother liquors provided a crystalline salt of the desired enantiomer of debenzylated product 177 in greater than 70% yield. By including the hydrogenation step, both enantiomers were effectively obtained with the same resolving agent.

Methanolysis of 177 provided the amino acid (178) which was cyclized in high yield to azetidinone 179 using dicyclohexylcarbodiimide. Saponification of 179 gave the sodium salt (180) which was converted to the ketoester (181) using Masamune's procedure. The one remaining problem, inversion of the side-chain configuration from S to R, was solved at this point by treating 181 with formic acid in the presence of triphenylphosphine and azodicarboxylate. Hydrolysis of the cleanly inverted formate ester provided **182**. Diazo transfer from *p*-dodecylbenzenesulfonyl azide, a less hazardous alternative to the customary reagents, yielded the diazo ketoester (**169**) whose conversion to (+)-thienamycin has already been described.

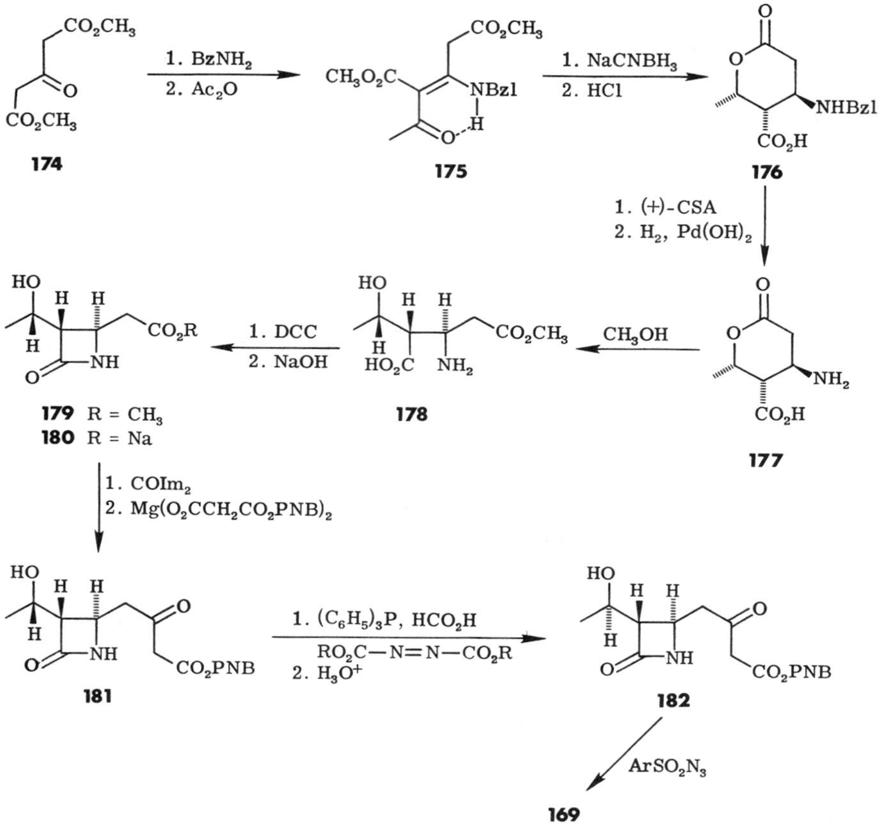

3. Synthesis of (±)-Northienamycin by C-5—C-6 Bond Formation

Northienamycin (**5b**) has been identified as a minor component of the antibiotic complex produced by *Streptomyces cattleya* (K. E. Wilson and A. J. Kempf, unpublished results, 1978), and its total synthesis has been disclosed in the patent literature (Eur. Pat. Appl. 10,312). The key step in the synthetic route to **5b** was the formation of the carbapenam nucleus by photolytic ring contraction of a bicyclic diazopyrrolidine-dione, a method developed by Lowe and co-workers for the construction of several β-lactam systems.

The requisite diazopyrrolidinedione (183) was prepared in a straight-forward, multistep process. Photolysis of 183 in methylene chloride containing water and imidazole as ketene scavengers afforded the carboxylic acid (184) which was reduced to the hydroxymethyl derivative (185) on treatment with diborane. One of the thio groups was oxidatively cleaved using sulfuryl chloride–wet silica gel, and the carbapen-1-em product (186) was base equilibrated to a 1 : 1 mixture of 186 and 187. Separation of the desired carbapen-2-em isomer followed by hydrogenolysis gave (±)-northienamycin (5b).

4. Synthesis of (±)-Olivanic Acid MM 22383 by C-2—C-3 Bond Formation

The Beecham group synthesized olivanic acid MM 22383 (6g) and its 8-epi isomer (7b) (Eur. Pat. Appl. 8,497) as part of an extensive program directed toward preparing 2-thio-substituted carbapenem antibiotics. The general strategy leading to 6g and 7b parallels that previously enumerated; namely, elaboration of a monocyclic β-lactam bearing the structural features of the target molecule followed by ring closure to the bicyclic product. In this case, the carbapenem ring system was constructed using an intramolecular Wittig reaction.

The internal Wittig reaction as applied to β-lactam antibiotic synthesis was introduced by Woodward and associates for cephem synthesis and was subsequently extended by them and others to the synthesis of ox-acephems, carbacephems, and penems. The attractiveness of this route stems from the fact that the bicyclic nucleus is formed under neutral, mild conditions with concomitant introduction of the double bond at the correct location. As will be seen in the next section, the internal Wittig method is by far the most general method for constructing carbapenem molecules having a variety of substituents at the C-2 position.

An azetidinone intermediate containing most of the carbon framework of the olivanic acids was rapidly synthesized from the tetrahydrooxazine (188) (Ponsford and Southgate, 1979; Br. Pat. 2,013,667). Reaction of 188 with diketene gave the ketoamide (189) which underwent diazo exchange with tosylazide to give 190. Irradiation of 190 or exposure to rhodium acetate resulted in cyclization to the *trans*-acetyl compound (191). Reduction of the ketone with sodium borohydride afforded a 1 : 1 mixture of isomers (192). Similar procedures were used to convert 2,2-di-methyltetrahydro-1,3-oxazine (193) to 127, an intermediate prepared by an alternative route in the (±)-thienamycin synthesis (Bouffard *et al.*, 1980).

Compound 192 was converted to aldehyde 194 by successive O-acy-lation, hydrolysis of the spiro aminal, and oxidation of the primary al-

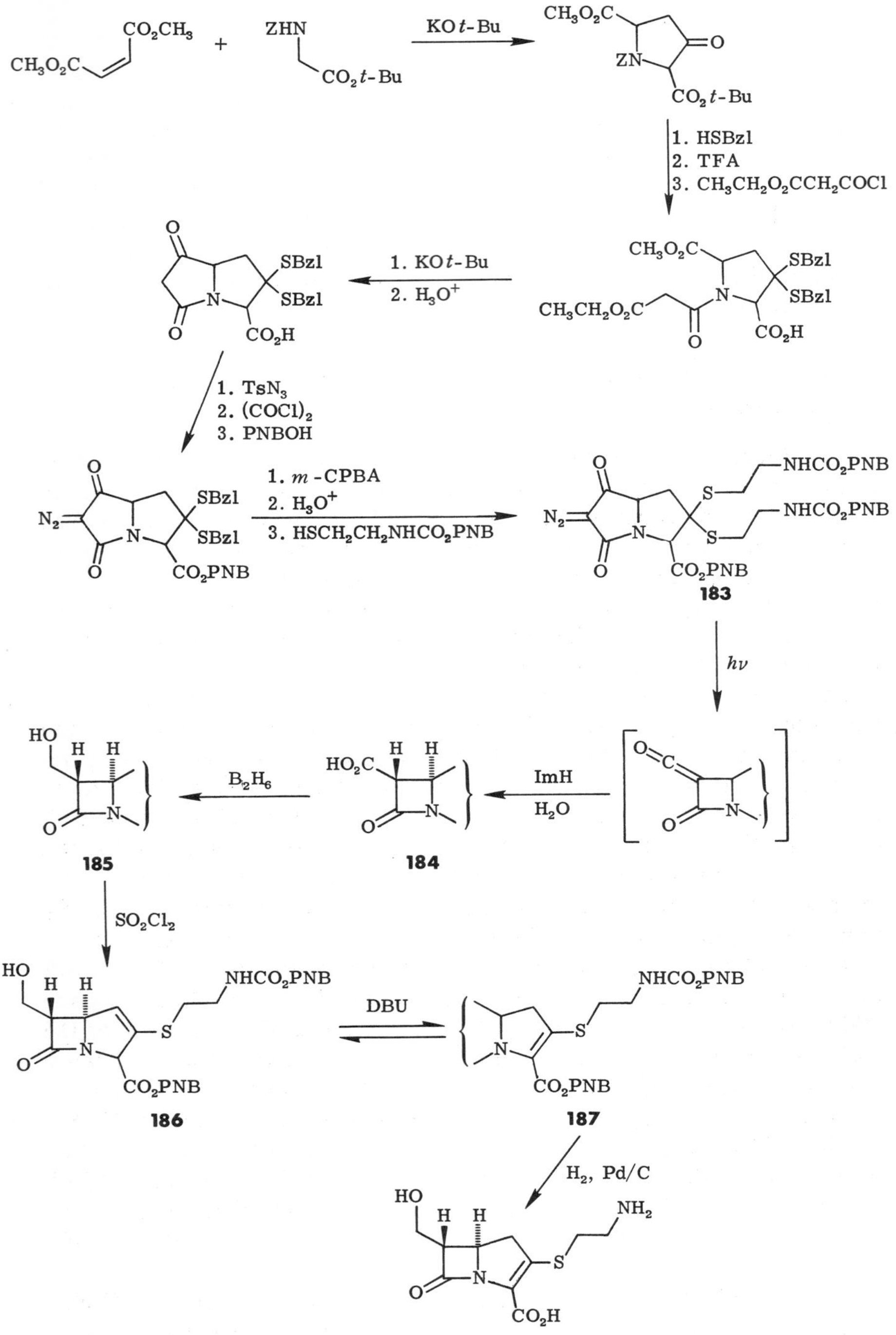

CO2CH3
CH3O2C
+
ZHN
CO2t-Bu
KOt-Bu
CH3O2C
ZN
O
CO2t-Bu
1. HSBzl
2. TFA
3. CH3CH2O2CCH2COCl
CH3O2C
SBzl
SBzl
N
CH3CH2O2C
O
CO2H
1. KOt-Bu
2. H3O+
O
SBzl
SBzl
N
O
CO2H
1. TsN3
2. (COCl)2
3. PNBOH
O
N2
SBzl
SBzl
N
O
CO2PNB
1. m-CPBA
2. H3O+
3. HSCH2CH2NHCO2PNB
O
S
NHCO2PNB
NHCO2PNB
N2
N
S
O
CO2PNB
183
hν
O=C
N
O
ImH
H2O
HO2C
H
H
O
N
184
B2H6
HO
H
H
O
N
185
SO2Cl2
HO
H
H
NHCO2PNB
S
O
N
CO2PNB
186
DBU
NHCO2PNB
S
N
CO2PNB
187
H2, Pd/C
HO
H
H
NH2
S
O
N
CO2H

5b

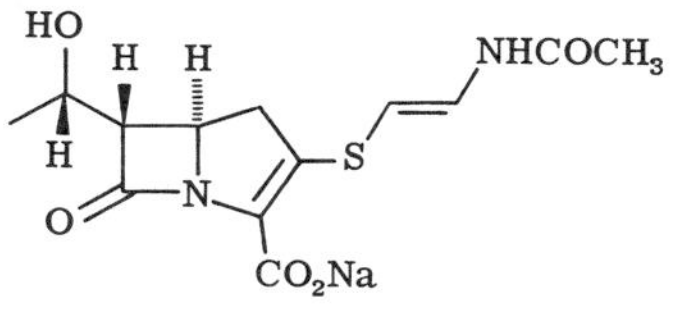

6g 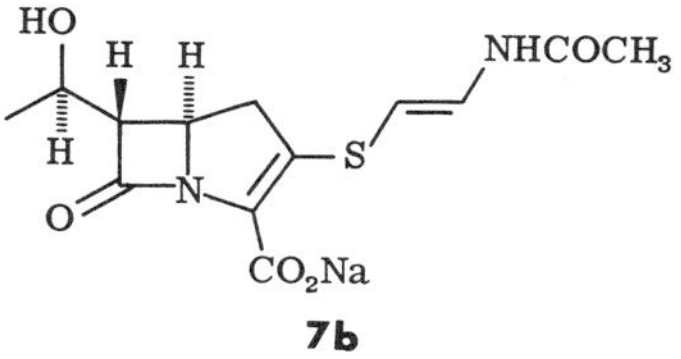   7b

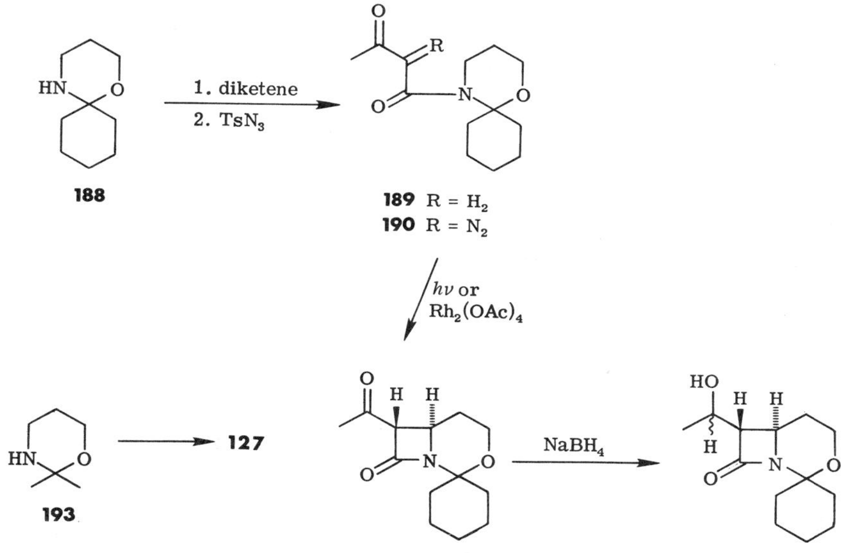

188   189 R = H$_2$
               190 R = N$_2$

$h\nu$ or
Rh$_2$(OAc)$_4$

193   127   191   192

cohol with pyridinium chlorochromate. Reaction of **194** with methoxy-carbonylmethylene triphenylphosphorane provided **195** wherein the olefin group served as a masked carboxyl group. After transformation of **195** in the phosphorane (**196**) by successive treatment with *p*-nitrobenzyl glyoxylate, thionyl chloride, and triphenylphosphine, the carboxyl group was unmasked by ozonolysis using an oxidative work-up. The ozonolysis reaction was conducted in the presence of trifluoroacetic acid in order to protect the phosphorane unit by protonation. Base treatment after the oxidative work-up regenerated the phosphorane. Although the isomers of **197** could be separated, it was found more convenient to accomplish this task following cyclization to the bicyclic products.

Carboxylic acid (**197**), activated as the acid chloride derivative, was condensed with silver (*E*)-acetamidoethenyl mercaptide to provide the thioester (**198**). Heating of **198** in refluxing toluene resulted in cyclization to the carbapenems (**199**). At this stage the isomers could be separated and each deblocked by catalytic hydrogenation to afford **6g** and **7b**.

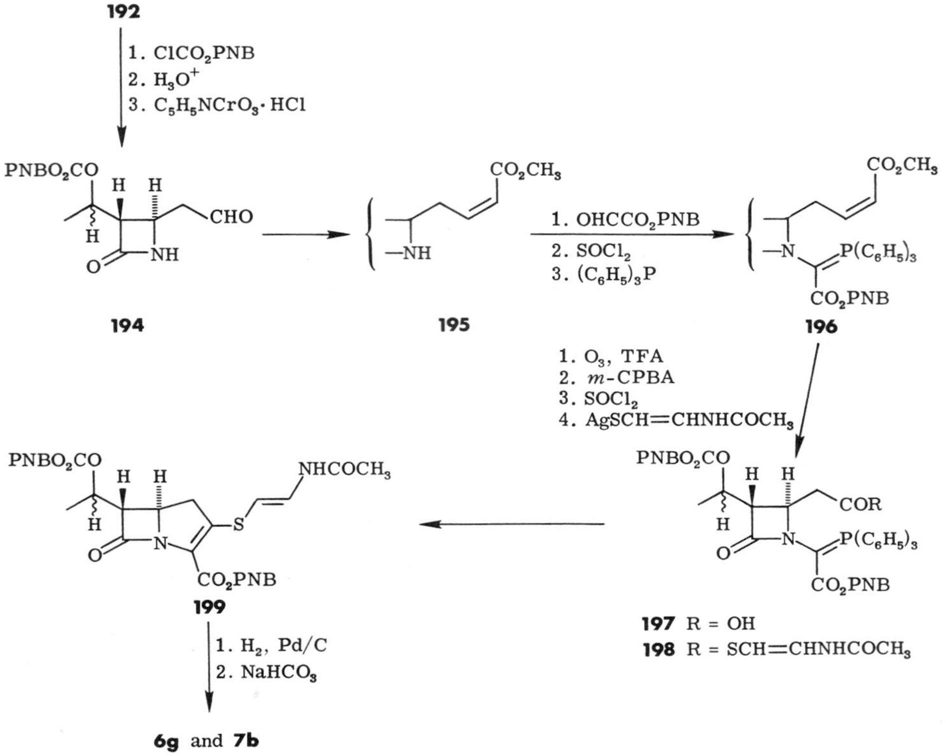

192

1. ClCO₂PNB
2. H₃O⁺
3. C₅H₅NCrO₃·HCl

$$\text{1. ClCO}_2\text{PNB}$$
$$\text{2. H}_3\text{O}^+$$
$$\text{3. C}_5\text{H}_5\text{NCrO}_3\cdot\text{HCl}$$

PNBO₂CO

194

195

1. OHCCO₂PNB
2. SOCl₂
3. (C₆H₅)₃P

CO₂CH₃

P(C₆H₅)₃

CO₂PNB

196

1. O₃, TFA
2. *m*-CPBA
3. SOCl₂
4. AgSCH=CHNHCOCH₃

PNBO₂CO

NHCOCH₃

S

CO₂PNB

199

PNBO₂CO

COR

P(C₆H₅)₃

CO₂PNB

197 R = OH
198 R = SCH=CHNHCOCH₃

1. H₂, Pd/C
2. NaHCO₃

6g and **7b**

C. Total Synthesis of Carbapenem Analogs

In connection with the total synthesis of carbapenem natural products we have seen the development of several distinct approaches for the construction of the bicyclic nucleus and for introduction of the C-2 and C-6 side chains. Most of these approaches are adaptable for preparing analogs not available by natural product modification and were developed primarily with that purpose in mind. However, at this point, very few reports using many of these methods for analog synthesis have appeared. By far the most useful and prevalent approach to analog synthesis has been the internal Wittig method. The utility of the Wittig approach for the construction of diversely substituted carbapenem analogs is the subject of this section.

The basic process, as represented by the conversion of **200** to **201**, is capable of providing a variety of carbapenem analogs. The closure reaction has been accomplished wherein R^2 is hydrogen, alkyl, aryl, and

200   **201**

thio groups and R^1 is hydrogen, alkyl, and substituted alkyl groups. Other variations include C-1 and C-5 methyl substituents, and several of the bicyclic products have been further manipulated to yield additional derivatives.

1. Synthesis of 2-Unsubstituted Analogs

The synthesis of the simplest of all carbapenem antibiotics, sodium carbapen-2-em-3-carboxylate (**207**), was first reported by Cama and Christensen (1978). The synthesis began with the acetoxyethylazetidinone (**202**), an intermediate that had been developed in connection with the Merck ($\pm$)-thienamycin synthesis (Johnston *et al.*, 1978; Bouffard *et al.*, 1980). Compound **202** was converted to the stabilized ylide (**203**) by what now can be considered as routine methodology; that is, by successive treatment with a glyoxylic acid ester, thionyl chloride, and triphenylphosphine. The *o*-nitrobenzyl ester was chosen in this case since a photolytic rather than a hydrogenolytic deblocking procedure was planned as the last step in the sequence. Hydrogenolysis was precluded because of the suspected susceptibility of the ring double bond to reduction.

The stage was set for the crucial ring closure by cleavage of acetate **203** to alcohol **204**. Oxidation of **204** with acetic anhydride in dimethyl sulfoxide at room temperature afforded the aldehyde intermediate (**205**) which spontaneously cyclized to the carbapenem (**206**). The ester was removed by photolysis in the presence of sodium bicarbonate to give the final product (**207**). This material was found to possess significant antibacterial activity, although it was susceptible to hydrolysis by β-lactamases.

Baxter and co-workers (1979) have described an alternative but similar approach to esters of carbapenem **211**. Exposure of 1,4-pentadiene to chlorosulfonyl isocyanate followed by a reductive work-up provided 4-allylazetidinone (**208**). This simple azetidinone is uniquely suited for the Wittig approach as many transformations, including side-chain introduction and ylide formation, can be accomplished prior to generation of the carbonyl group by ozonolysis. In the simplest case, **208** was converted to the phosphorane (**209**) by treatment with a glyoxylate, thionyl chloride, and triphenylphosphine. Selective oxidation of the terminal double bond

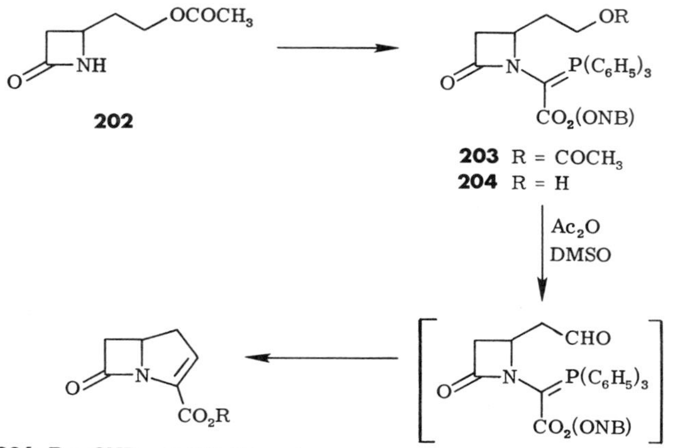
OCOCH$_3$
NH
O
202
OR
N
P(C$_6$H$_5$)$_3$
CO$_2$(ONB)
Ac$_2$O
DMSO
CHO
CO$_2$R

203 R = $COCH_3$
204 R = H

206 R = ONB = *o*-nitrobenzyl
207 R = Na

205

was achieved by ozonolysis in the presence of trifluoroacetic acid; the phosphorane group was protected by protonation. Reduction of the ozonide with triphenylphosphine followed by regeneration of the phosphorane with sodium bicarbonate gave the aldehyde intermediate **210** which spontaneously cyclized to **211.** The benzyl (Baxter *et al.*, 1979), methyl, *t*-butyl, and *p*-nitrobenzyl esters (Ger. Offen. 2,811,514) of **211** were obtained from the corresponding glyoxylate esters. A related approach using glyoxylic acid in the initial phosphorane-forming reaction followed by alkylation eventually afforded the pivaloyloxymethyl and phthalidyl esters of **211** (Ger. Offen. 2,811,514).

Researchers at Shionogi have also employed a side-chain double bond

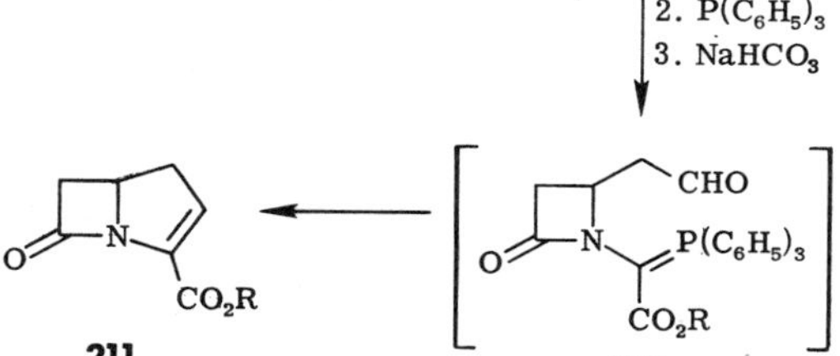
NH
O
208
N
P(C$_6$H$_5$)$_3$
CO$_2$R
209
1. O$_3$, TFA
2. P(C$_6$H$_5$)$_3$
3. NaHCO$_3$
CHO

211

210

as a masked carbonyl unit (Onoue *et al.*, 1979). In this case the requisite azetidinone (**214**) was obtained from a novel coupling reaction of allyl copper (**212**) with the chloroazetidinone (**213**) derived from penicillin. Subsequent modification of both carbon–carbon double bonds afforded the phosphorane (**215**). Acidic hydrolysis of **215** gave a diol that was oxidatively cleaved to an aldehyde intermediate that cyclized to the carbapenem ester (**211**, R = benzhydryl).

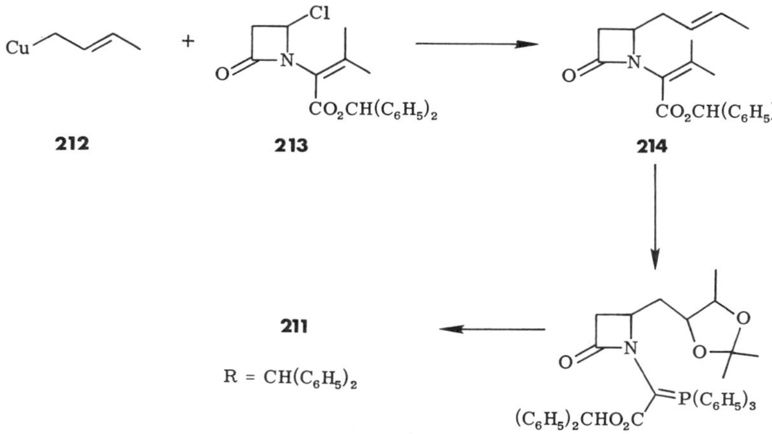

The synthetic approach to carbapen-2-em-3-carboxylic acid (**207**) and its esters (**211**) via the internal Wittig reaction has been extended to a variety of C-6 substituted analogs. In most cases the 6-substituents were introduced by alkylation of a stable azetidinone intermediate prior to establishment of the carbapenem ring system. The processes are illustrated below for the bicyclic azetidinone (**125**) and for the azetidinone phosphorane (**209**).

Alkylation of the lithium enolate of **125** with benzyl bromide or iso-propyl iodide afforded mainly the trans-substituted products (**216a,b**) (Belg. Pat. 860,962). Hydrolysis of the acetonide followed by O-acylation gave the monocylic intermediates (**217a,b**) which were converted to the carbapenem esters (**218a,b**) by essentially the same procedures as previously described for the **202** to **206** conversion. Similarly, condensation of the enolate of **125** with acetone gave mainly compound **219** which was transformed into **220a**. Photolytic removal of the *o*-nitrobenzyl group in the presence of sodium bicarbonate provided the corresponding sodium carboxylate (**220b**).

The conversion of bicyclic intermediate **125** to the hydroxyethylated products **127** via an aldol reaction with acetaldehyde has already been

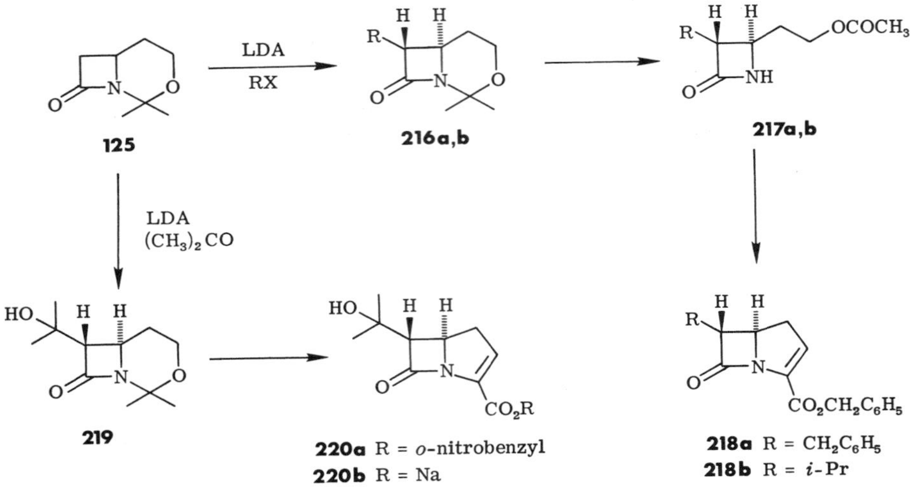

125 →(LDA, RX)→ **216a,b** → **217a,b**

125 →(LDA, (CH₃)₂CO)→ **219** → **220a** R = o-nitrobenzyl / **220b** R = Na

217a,b → **218a** R = CH₂C₆H₅ / **218b** R = i-Pr

discussed. Acylation of **127** with o-nitrobenzyl chloroformate gave a mixture of carbonate derivatives from which the trans-R^* isomer (**221**) was obtained by HPLC (Cama and Christensen, 1978). Compound **221** was converted to the hydroxyphosphorane (**222**) which, upon oxidation with acetic anhydride in dimethyl sulfoxide, gave an aldehyde intermediate that cyclized to the carbapenem (**223**). Photolytic removal of the protecting groups in the presence of sodium bicarbonate provided the sodium salt of (±)-descysteaminyl thienamycin (**224**).

Kametani and co-workers (1980a) have described a related synthesis of diprotected (±)-8-epidescysteaminyl thienamycin (**225**) starting from the azetidinone (**155**). In this case the aldehyde component of the internal Wittig reaction was generated by hydrolysis of the dimethyl acetal. Photolytic deblocking of **225** has not yet been reported.

A sequence of reactions similar to that described for converting **127** to **224**, but staring with derivative **226**, was used to synthesize the ring-methylated analog **227** (Eur. Pat. Appl. 10,317). A synthesis of the aminoethyl analog (**230**) of descysteaminylthienamycin has also been reported (Belg. Pat. 860,962). The side-chain nitrogen functionality was introduced by converting the trans-S^* isomer (**127b**) to a mesylate derivative followed by displacement with azide ion. The resulting azidoethyl product (**228**) was transformed into the diprotected carbapenem (**229**) and photolytically deblocked to provide **230**.

In a manner analogous to that just described for the bicyclic acetonide (**125**), workers at Beecham have converted the phosphorane **209** (R = benzyl) into a series of 6-substituted carbapen-2-em-3-carboxylates (Ger. Offen. 2,811,514). Reaction of **209** with excess lithium N-isopropylcy-

ONB = o-nitrobenzyl

clohexylamide followed by addition of methyl iodide or benzyl bromide gave the trans-alkylated products (231). Similarly, addition of carbonyl compounds such as acetaldehyde, benzaldehyde, acetone, and cyclohexanone to the lithium enolate of 209 provided mixtures of cis- and trans-azetidinones (232). These compounds were converted to the carbapenem derivatives 233, 234, and 235 by employing the procedures previously noted in connection with the synthesis of 211 from 209. In the case of the acetaldehyde addition products, the bicyclic products 234a and 235a were shown to have the $8R^*$ and $8S^*$ configurations, respectively, by X-ray crystallography (Baxter et al., 1979).

The Beecham group has demonstrated an alternative, but somewhat restricted, method for synthesizing C-6 cis-substituted carbapenem de-

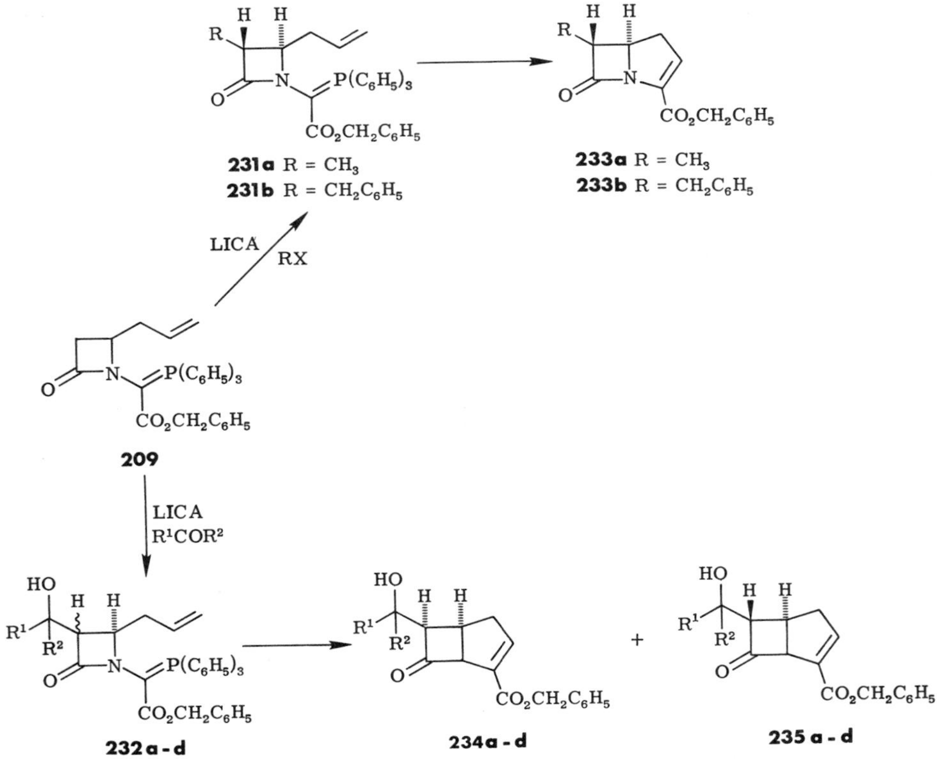

231a R = CH₃
231b R = CH₂C₆H₅

233a R = CH₃
233b R = CH₂C₆H₅

209

232a-d   234a-d   235a-d

Series	R¹	R²
a	H	CH₃
b	H	C₆H₅
c	CH₃	CH₃
d	—(CH₂)₅—	

rivatives (Baxter *et al.*, 1979; Ger. Offen. 2,811,514). The bicyclic β-lactam (**236**), which was derived from 1,4-cyclohexadiene and chlorosulfonyl isocyanate, gave the phosphorane (**237**) which on ozonolysis and cyclization produced the bicyclic product (**238**) having exclusively the cis configuration about the β-lactam. The aldehyde function of **238** was trapped with a variety of stabilized ylide reagents to provide adducts **239.**

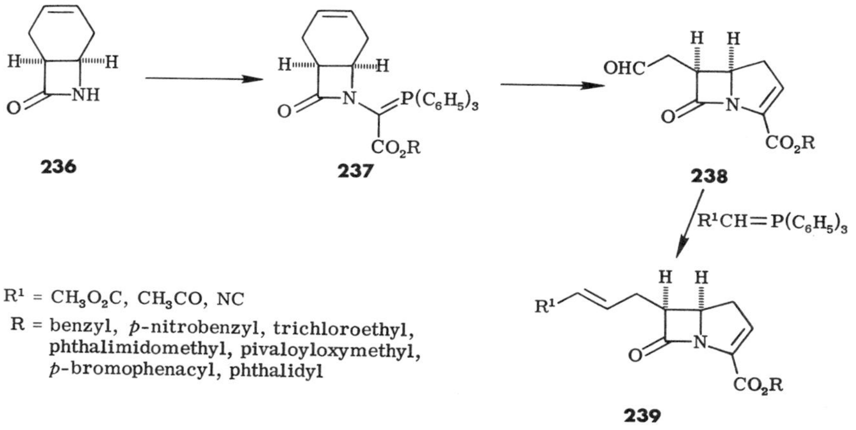

236
237
238
$R^1CH{=}P(C_6H_5)_3$
239
R^1 = CH_3O_2C, CH_3CO, NC
R = benzyl, *p*-nitrobenzyl, trichloroethyl, phthalimidomethyl, pivaloyloxymethyl, *p*-bromophenacyl, phthalidyl

2. *Synthesis of 2-Alkyl and 2-Arylcarbapenem Analogs*

Extension of the Wittig cyclization process to the synthesis of a 2-alkyl carbapenem was first demonstrated by Baxter and co-workers (1979) for the preparation of **242.** Oxypalladation of 4-allylazetidinone (**208**) provided the methyl ketone (**240**) which was converted to the phosphorane (**241**). Whereas the Wittig cyclization occurred spontaneously at room temperature when the carbonyl compound was an aldehyde, the cyclization of ketone **241** to the carbapenem (**242**) required heating for

208
1. $Hg(OAc)_2$
2. $CuCl_2 \cdot H_2O$, $PdCl_2$
240
241
100 °C
242

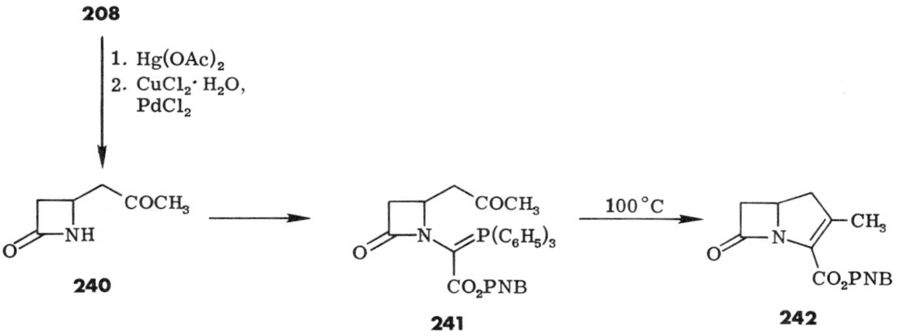

6 hr in toluene at 100°C. An identical approach was employed for the synthesis of the *t*-butyl ester of **242** (Ger. Offen. 2,811,514), but ester deblocking has not been reported in either case.

Cama and Christensen (1980) have developed a general approach for the synthesis of 2-alkyl- and 2-arylcarbapenem analogs via the Wittig method. A pivotal step in the sequence involved the preparation of a ketone intermediate by the reaction of a lithium or magnesium alkyl- or arylcuprate with a thioester. The process is illustrated for the preparation of 2-methyl and 2-phenyl analogs **246a** and **246b.**

The requisite thioester (**243**) was obtained from the primary alcohol (**204**) by Jones oxidation to a carboxylic acid followed by conversion to the acid chloride and treatment with thiophenol. Addition of lithium dimethylcuprate or magnesium diphenylcuprate to **243** gave the ketone intermediates (**244**) which cyclized to the carbapenems (**245**) on heating in xylene solution at 140°C. The 2-methyl analog (**245a**) was photolytically deblocked to **246a,** but this material proved to be too unstable for meaningful antibacterial assay. By contrast, hydrogenolysis of **245b** gave the stable 2-phenyl analog (**246b**), which was found to exhibit antibacterial activity superior to that of the unsubstituted nucleus (**207**).

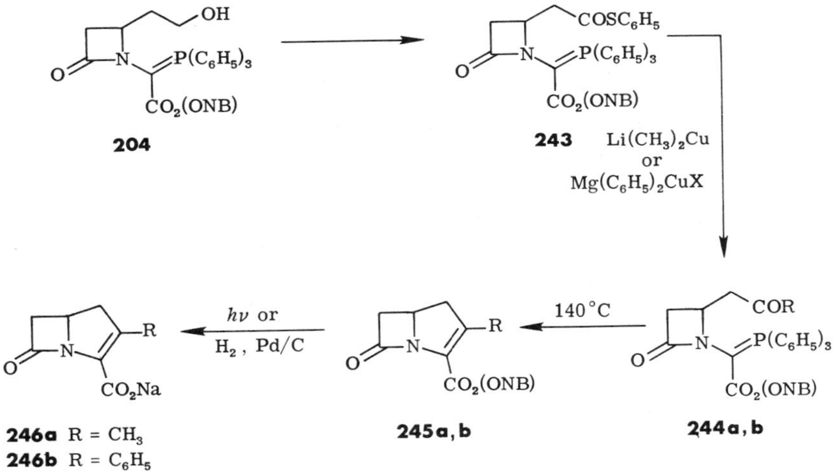

The synthesis of 2-alkyl- and 2-arylcarbapenems via the thioester–Wittig route has been adapted to the preparation of 6-substituted analogs (Belg. Pat. 860,962). For example, the hydroxyethylated intermediate **247** was converted to **248** and the aminoethylated intermediate **249** provided the 2-aryl derivatives **250a,b.**

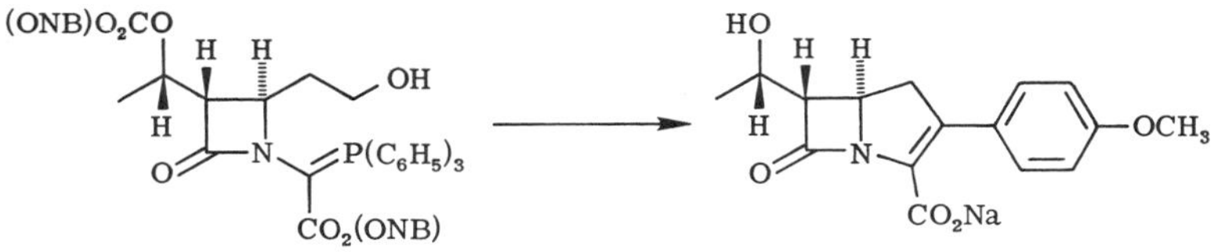

247

248

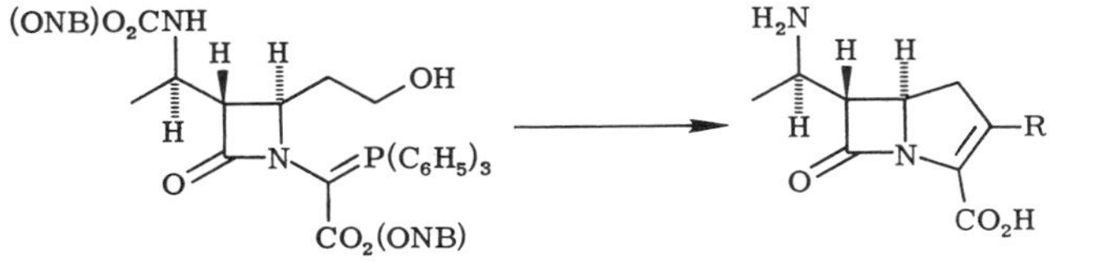

249

250a R = phenyl
250b R = p-methoxyphenyl

3. Synthesis of 2-Thio-Substituted Carbapenem Analogs

The Beecham group has prepared a wide variety of 2-thio-substituted carbapenem analogs by two general routes. The first route, which uses an internal Wittig cyclization on a thioester, has been mentioned previously in regard to the synthesis of olivanic acid MM 22385. This method is generally applicable to the synthesis of alkenylthio and arylthio derivatives, but somewhat limited for the preparation of alkylthio derivatives. The second route employs the Michael addition of thiols to 2-unsubstituted carbapenems followed by oxidation and reintroduction of the C-2—C-3 double bond. The latter route has been used in the synthesis of alkylthio and arylthio derivatives as well as sulfinyl derivatives. The chemistry and types of analogs prepared by the two routes will be described in the remainder of this section.

The intramolecular Wittig reaction using a thioester as the carbonyl component was initially studied with the methylated azetidinone (**251**) (Ponsford *et al.*, 1979; U.S. Pat. 4,153,714). This substance was readily prepared from benzyl 3-methyl-3-butenoate and chlorosulfonyl isocyanate followed by hydrogenolysis of the benzyl ester. Compound **251** was converted to the thioester (**252**) by formation of a mixed phosphonic anhydride or acid chloride followed by treatment with a thallous mercaptide or a mercaptan in the presence of base. The phosphorane (**253**) was established by the usual procedure and heated in toluene under reflux to effect cyclization to carbapenem **254**. The efficacy of the cyclization reaction was found to be influenced by both the thioester group

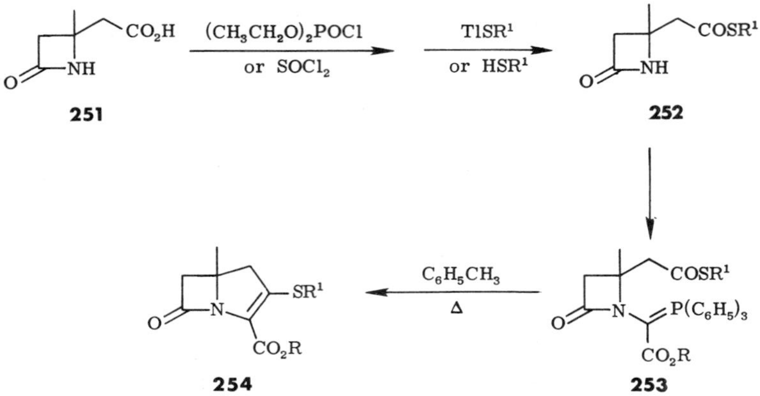

R = C(CH₃)₃; R¹ = CH₂CH₃, CH₂CH₂NHCOCH₃,
            CH₂CO₂CH₃, p-NO₂C₆H₄
R = CH₂C₆H₅; R¹ = p-NO₂C₆H₄
R = p-nitrobenzyl; R¹ = C₆H₅

and the phosphorane ester with the lowest yields being obtained with alkyl thioesters.

Similar procedures were subsequently used to prepare 2-thio-substituted carbapenems (257) lacking the bridgehead methyl group. The phosphorane (209) was subjected to ozonolysis and oxidative work-up with m-chloroperbenzoic acid to give the acid (255). Carboxyl activation followed by addition of mercaptide provided the thioester (256) which was cyclized to the carbapenem (257) on refluxing in toluene solution. The process has been described for the preparation of arylthio analogs (Ponsford et al., 1979; Eur. Pat. Appl. 828), pyrimidinylthio analogs (Eur. Pat. Appl. 8,514), and alkenylthio analogs (Eur. Pat. Appl. 3,740). As in the 5-methyl series, the ease of cyclization was influenced by both the thioester and phosphorane ester, and the yields were generally low (2–39%).

Several of the 2-thio-substituted products having a p-nitrobenzyl ester were deblocked by hydrogenation over palladium on carbon and the products were isolated as either the sodium salts or free acids (258 and 259). Compound 258a was found to be more labile than the 5-methyl analog (258b) and considerably more active against a variety of gram-positive and gram-negative bacteria (Ponsford et al., 1979).

The techniques for converting intermediates 251 and 209 to thio-substituted carbapenems 254 and 257 have been adapted to the synthesis of several 6-substituted-2-thiocarbapenems. For example, azetidinone 197 has been converted to the bis-protected derivative 260a which was deblocked to free acid 260b (Eur. Pat. Appl. 8,514), and intermediates 231a and 232c have provided the bicyclic esters 261 and 262 (Eur. Pat.

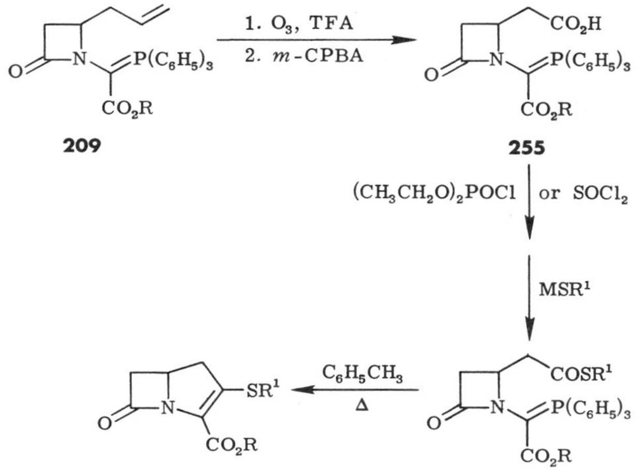

1. O_3, TFA
2. m-CPBA
$(CH_3CH_2O)_2POCl$ or $SOCl_2$
MSR^1
$C_6H_5CH_3$
Δ

209 **255** **257** **256**

M = Li, Na, Tl, or Ag
R = $C(CH_3)_3$; R^1 = C_6H_5, p-$NO_2C_6H_4$
R = $CH_2C_6H_5$; R^1 = C_6H_5, p-$NO_2C_6H_4$, p-$(NHCOCH_3)C_6H_4$, p-$NH_2C_6H_4$, 2-pyrimidinyl, 4-pyrimidinyl, 4,6-dimethyl-2-pyrimidinyl
R = p-nitrobenzyl; R^1 = C_6H_5, 2-pyrimidinyl, 4-pyrimidinyl, 4-methyl-2-pyrimidinyl, 4,6-dimethyl-2-pyrimidinyl, (E)-CH=CHNHCOCH$_3$, (Z)-CH=CHNHCOCH$_3$, (Z)-CH=C(CH$_3$)NHCOCH$_3$
R = pivaloyloxymethyl; R^1 = C_6H_5
R = phthalidyl; R^1 = 2-pyrimidinyl, 4,6-dimethyl-2-pyrimidinyl, (Z)-CH=CHNHCOCH$_3$

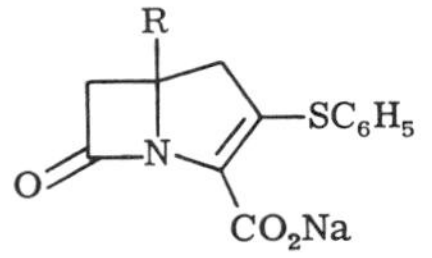

258a R = H
258b R = CH_3

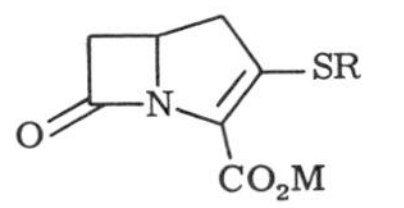

M = H or Na

259 R = 2-pyrimidinyl, 4-methyl-2-pyrimidinyl, (Z)-CH=CHNHCOCH$_3$, (E)-CH=CHNHCOCH$_3$

197

260a R = PNB; R^1 = CO_2PNB
260b R = R^1 = H

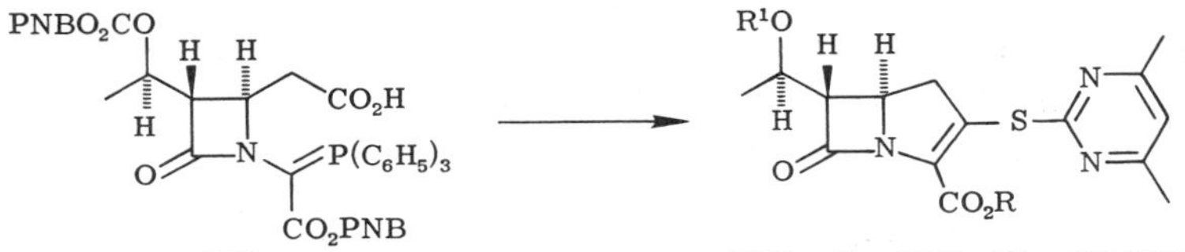

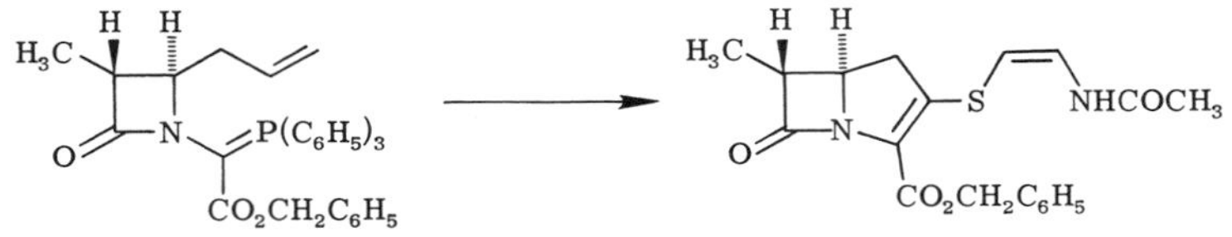

231a → **261**

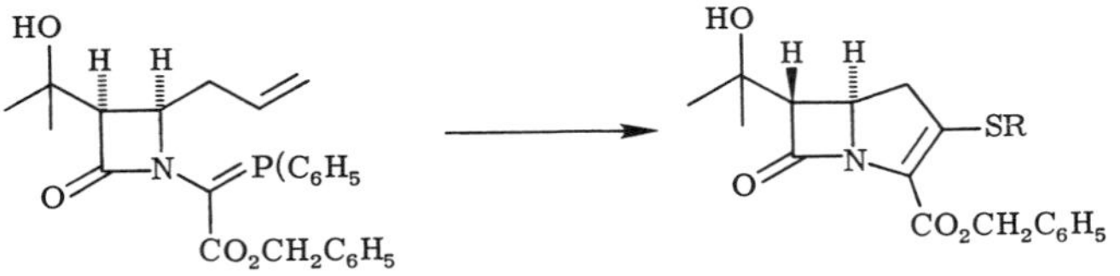

232c → **262a** R = C₆H₅
            262b R = (Z)-CH=CHNHCOCH₃

Appl. 8,497). The utility of the internal Wittig cyclization of a thioester for the synthesis of olivanic acid MM 22385 has been described in the section dealing with natural product syntheses.

The principle drawback of the internal Wittig cyclization as applied to the synthesis of 2-thio-substituted carbapenems is its limitation to arylthio and vinylthio analogs. The paucity of examples wherein alkyl-thio-substituted products are formed is presumably related to the inefficiency of the cyclization process and to the sensitivity of the resulting products to the thermal reaction conditions. Because of these difficulties, an alternative process capable of producing a wide range of 2-thio and 2-sulfinyl analogs was developed. The new process utilizes a base-catalyzed addition of thiols to the readily available 2-unsubstituted carbapenems to afford adducts of the saturated carbapenam ring system. Subsequent oxidation and reintroduction of the ring double bond affords the carbapenem products.

The thiol addition process was first described for the conversion of 2-unsubstituted carbapenems (**263**) to the 2-sulfinyl analogs (**269** and **270**) (Bateson *et al.*, 1980; Eur. Pat. Appl. 2,564). The bicyclic starting materials (**263**), which include compounds **211**, **233**, **234**, **235**, **238** and **239**, were readily accessible via the intramolecular Wittig route previously discussed. A variety of alkyl and aryl mercaptans underwent potassium carbonate-catalyzed Michael addition to **263** giving the saturated adducts **264–266**. Oxidation of adducts **264** and **265** with 2 equiv of iodobenzene dichloride in the presence of pyridine and water gave predominantly the α-chlorosulfoxide (**267**). Brief treatment with diazabicycloundecene effected dehydrochlorination to the unsaturated product **269**. Similar treatment of adduct **266** provided the isomeric product **270**. The 2-sulfinyl-carbapenem analogs, of which representative examples are shown in Table IX, are relatively unstable and decompose on attempted silica gel or florisil chromatography.

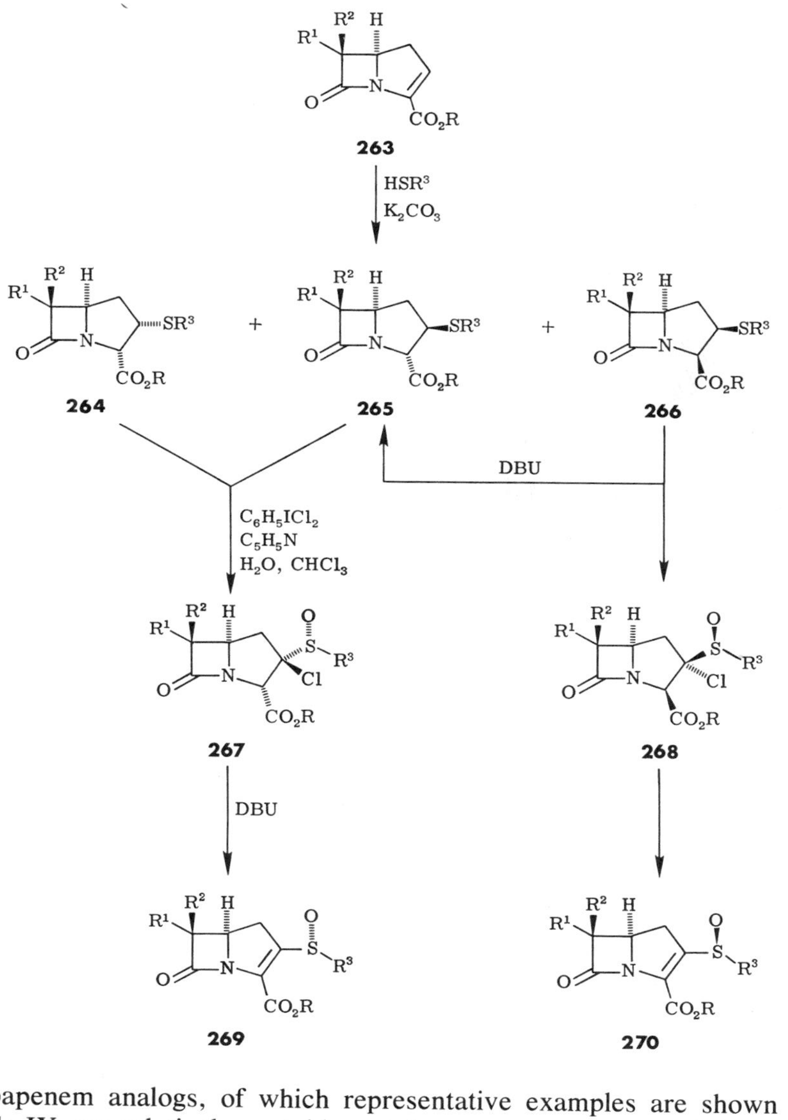

The relative stereochemistry of the saturated intermediates **264–268** was established by X-ray analysis of selected intermediates, by base-catalyzed conversion of **266** to **265,** and by the relative positions of the H-3 proton NMR signals (Bateson *et al.,* 1980). In the patent literature

TABLE IX   2-Sulfinyl Analogs (**269** and **270**)

R^1	R^2	R^3	R
H	H	CH_2CH_3	$CH_2C_6H_5$
H	H	$CH_2CH_2NHCOCH_3$	$CH_2C_6H_5$
H	H	C_6H_5	$CH_2C_6H_5$
H	H	p-$(NHCOCH_3)C_6H_4$	$CH_2C_6H_5$
H	H	CH_2CH_3	p-nitrobenzyl
$CH_2C_6H_5$	H	CH_2CH_3	$CH_2C_6H_5$
(S)-$CH_3CH(OH)$	H	C_6H_5	$CH_2C_6H_5$
CH_3	CH_3	CH_2CH_3	$CH_2C_6H_5$
H	CH_3O_2C—CH=CH—CH_2	C_6H_5	$CH_2C_6H_5$
H	CH_3O_2C—CH=CH—CH_2	CH_2CH_3	p-bromophenacyl

(Eur. Pat. Appl. 2,564; 8,888) the structures of compounds **264** and **265** are interchanged and compound **266** is assigned the α-SR^3 configuration. For this chapter we have adopted the stereochemical assignments as reported by Bateson and co-workers (1980).

An alternative and more useful application of the thiol addition process which ultimately yields 2-thio-substituted analogs (**272**) has been reported in the patent literature (Eur. Pat. Appl. 8,888). By conducting the io-dobenzene dichloride oxidation of the saturated adducts **264** and **265** (R = p-nitrobenzyl) in cold benzene and in the absence of water, carbapen-1-ems (**271**) along with a minor amount of carbapen-2-ems (**272**) were formed directly. Although the mechanism for this transformation is not

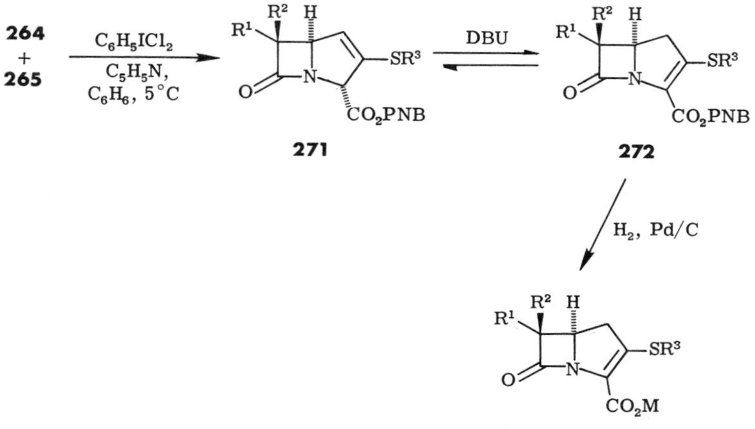

271   **272**

273 M = H, Na, K

clear, the low yield of the products, generally less than 50%, suggests that the carbapen-2-em isomer may be a major product but is destroyed under the reaction conditions. Exposure of the carbapen-1-ems (271) to diazabicycloundecene resulted in partial isomerization of the double bond affording mixtures from which the carbapen-2-ems (272) were chromatographically separable. As noted previously, the equilibration procedure produces mixtures rich in the unwanted isomer.

Several of the 2-thio-substituted carbapenems (272) produced by this method are listed in Table X. Many of these products were hydrogenated over palladium on carbon in aqueous dioxane to afford the deblocked products (273). Alternatively, bioactive esters such as phthalidyl and pivaloyloxymethyl were prepared by deblocking 271 to the corresponding sodium carboxylate followed by realkylation and double bond isomerization. The cis-substituted compounds (272) were obtained from the adducts 264–266 wherein R^1 is hydrogen and R^2 is formylmethyl by appropriate manipulation of the aldehyde group.

The general route outlined for the preparation of analogs 272 has also been applied to the synthesis of the benzyl ester (276) of olivanic acid MM 22381 (Eur. Pat. Appl. 8,888). The only addition to the synthetic sequence was the silylation of the hydroxyethyl side chain of intermediate (274) prior to the oxidative dehydrogenation. In this case the equilibration procedure produced a mixture from which 65% of 275 was recovered and only 8% of 276 was isolated.

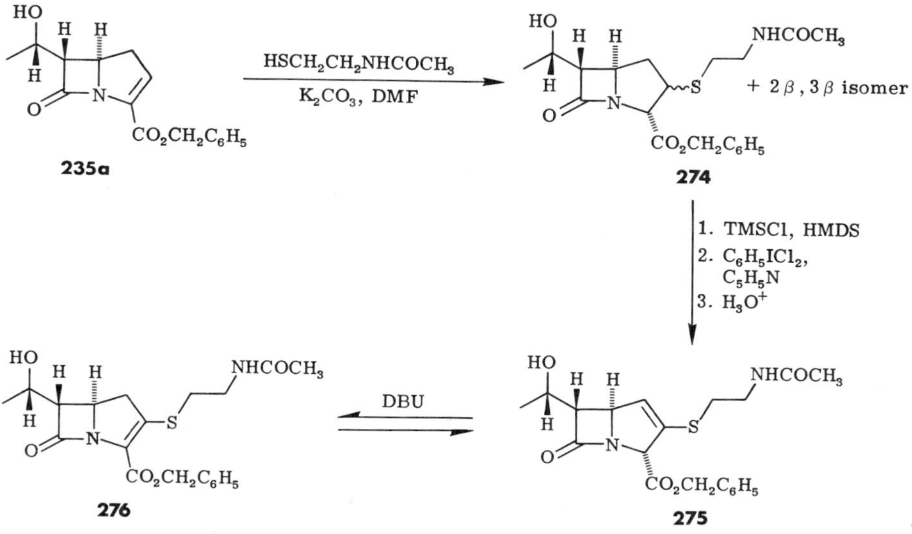

TABLE X 2-Thio Analogs (**272**)

Compound	R^1	R^2	R^3
a	H	H	CH_3
b	H	H	CH_2CH_3
c	H	H	$CH_2C_6H_5$
d	H	H	$CH_2CH_2OCH_3$
e	H	H	$CH_2CH_2CO_2CH_3$
f	H	H	$CH_2CH_2OCONHCH_3$
g	H	H	$CH_2CH_2NHCOCH_3$
h	H	H	$CH_2CH_2NHCO_2$ (p-nitrobenzyl)
i	H	CH_3	CH_2CH_3
j	H	CH_3CH_2	CH_2CH_3
k	H	$CH_3CO_2CH_2CH_2$	CH_2CH_3
l	H	$N_3CH_2CH_2$	CH_2CH_3

References

Albers-Schönberg, G., Arison, B. H., Kaczka, E. A., Kahan, F. M., Kahan, J. S., Lago, B., Maiese, W. M., Rhodes, R. E., and Smith, J. L. (1976). *Intersci. Conf. Antimicrob. Agents Chemother. 16th, Chicago, Ill.* Pap. No. 229. (Abstr.)

Albers-Schönberg, G., Arison, B. H., Hensens, O. D., Hirshfield, J., Hoogsteen, K., Kaczka, E. A., Rhodes, R. E., Kahan, J. S., Kahan, F. M., Ratcliffe, R. W., Walton, E., Ruswinkle, L. J., Morin, R. B., and Christensen, B. G. (1978). *J. Am. Chem. Soc.* **100**, 6491.

Aoki, H., Sakai, H., Kohsaka, M., Konomi, T., Hosoda, J., Kubochi, Y., and Iguchi, E. (1976). *J. Antibiot.* **29**, 492.

Barton, D. H. R., Coates, I. H., and Sammes, P. G. (1973). *J.C.S. Perkin I* p. 599.

Bateson, J. H., Roberts, P. M., Smale, T. C., and Southgate, R. (1980). *J.C.S. Chem. Commun.* p. 185.

Baxter, A. J. G., Dickinson, K. H., Roberts, P. M., Smale, T. C., and Southgate, R. (1979). *J.C.S. Chem. Commun.* p. 236.

Belgian Patent 848,346. Merck and Co., Inc.

Belgian Patent 848,349. Merck and Co., Inc.

Belgian Patent 848,545. Merck and Co., Inc.

Belgian Patent 857,781. Beecham Group Ltd.

Belgian Patent 860,962. Merck and Co., Inc.

Belgian Patent 865,578. Sanraku-Ocean Co., Ltd. and Panlabs, Inc.

Belgian Patent 865,786. Merck and Co., Inc.

Belgian Patent 866,660. Merck and Co., Inc.

Belgian Patent 866,661. Merck and Co., Inc.

Belgian Patent 867,227. Merck and Co., Inc.

Bouffard, F. A., Johnston, D. B. R., and Christensen, B. G. (1980). *J. Org. Chem.* **45**, 1130.

Box, S. G., Hood, J. D., and Spear, S. R. (1979). *J. Antibiot.* **32**, 1239.

British Patent 2,013,667. Beecham Group Ltd.

Brown, A. G., Butterworth, D., Cole, M., Hanscomb, G., Hood, J. D., and Reading, C. (1976). *J. Antibiot.* **29**, 668.
Brown, A. G., Corbett, D. F., Eglington, A. J., and Howarth, T. T. (1977). *J.C.S. Chem. Commun.* p. 523.
Brown, A. G., Corbett, D. F., Eglington, A. J., and Howarth, T. T. (1979). *J. Antibiot.* **32**, 961.
Cama, L. D., and Christensen, B. G. (1978). *J. Am. Chem. Soc.* **100**, 8006.
Cama, L. D., and Christensen, B. G. (1980). *Tetrahedron Lett.* p. 2013.
Cassidy, P. J. (1981). *Dev. Ind. Microbiol.* **22**, 181.
Cassidy, P. J., Stapley, E. O., Goegelman, R., Miller, T. W., Arison, B. H., Albers-Schönberg, G., Zimmerman, S. B., and Birnbaum, J. (1977). *Intersci. Conf. Antimicrob. Agents Chemother., 17th, New York* Pap. No. 81. (Abstr.)
Cassidy, P. J., Albers-Schönberg, G., Goegelman, R., Miller, T. W., Arison, B. H., Stapley, E. O., and Birnbaum, J. (1981). *J. Antibiot.* **34**, 637.
Corbett, D. F., Eglington, A. J., and Howarth, T. T. (1977). *J.C.S. Chem. Commun.* p. 953.
Dale, J. A., and Mosher, H. S. (1973). *J. Am. Chem. Soc.* **95**, 512.
Demarco, P. V., and Nagarajan, R. (1972). In "Cephalosporins and Penicillins: Chemistry and Biology" (E. H. Flynn, ed.), p. 312. Academic Press, New York.
Denney, D. B., and Sherman, N. (1965). *J. Org. Chem.* **30**, 3760.
DiNinno, F., Beattie, T. R., and Christensen, B. G. (1977). *J. Org. Chem.* **42**, 1960.
European Patent Application 828. Beecham Group Ltd.
European Patent Application 1,264. Merck and Co., Inc.
European Patent Application 1,265. Merck and Co., Inc.
European Patent Application 2,058. Sanraku-Ocean Co., Ltd.
European Patent Application 2,564. Beecham Group Ltd.
European Patent Application 3,740. Beechan Group Ltd.
European Patent Application 4,132. Beecham Group Ltd.
European Patent Application 5,348. Beecham Group Ltd.
European Patent Application 5,349. Beecham Group Ltd.
European Patent Application 6,639. Merck and Co., Inc.
European Patent Application 7,152. Beecham Group Ltd.
European Patent Application 7,753. Beecham Group Ltd.
European Patent Application 8,497. Beecham Group Ltd.
European Patent Application 8,514. Beecham Group Ltd.
European Patent Application 8,885. Beecham Group Ltd.
European Patent Application 8,888. Beecham Group Ltd.
European Patent Application 10,312. Merck and Co., Inc.
European Patent Application 10,317. Merck and Co., Inc.
German Offenlegungsschrift 2,652,674. Merck and Co., Inc.
German Offenlegungsschrift 2,652,675. Merck and Co., Inc.
German Offenlegungsschrift 2,652,676. Merck and Co., Inc.
German Offenlegungsschrift 2,652,680. Merck and Co., Inc.
German Offenlegungsschrift 2,724,560. Merck and Co., Inc.
German Offenlegungsschrift 2,728,097. Beecham Group Ltd.
German Offenlegungsschrift 2,751,597. Merck and Co., Inc.
German Offenlegungsschrift 2,805,724. Merck and Co., Inc.
German Offenlegungsschrift 2,809,235. Sankyo Co., Ltd.
German Offenlegungsschrift 2,811,514. Beecham Group Ltd.

German Offenlegungsschrift 2,820,055. Merck and Co., Inc.

Hood, J. D., Box, S. J., and Verrall, M. S. (1979). *J. Antibiot.* **32**, 295.

Horeau, H. (1977). In "Stereochemistry, Fundamentals and Methods" (H. B. Kagan, ed.), p. 51. Thieme, Stuttgart.

Howarth, T. T., and Brown, A. G. (1976). *J. C. S. Chem. Commun.* p. 266.

Hudson, C. S. (1910). *J. Amer. Chem. Soc.* **32**, 338.

Japanese Kokai Tokkyo Koho 79 084,589. Sanraku-Ocean Co., Ltd.

Japanese Kokai Tokkyo Koho 79 135,790. Sanraku-Ocean Co., Ltd.

Japanese Kokai Tokkyo Koho 80 042,536. Sanraku-Ocean Co., Ltd.

Japanese Kokai Tokkyo Koho 80 024,129. Sankyo Co., Ltd.

Johnston, D. B. R., Schmitt, S. M., Bouffard, F. A., and Christensen, B. G. (1978). *J. Am. Chem. Soc.* **100**, 313.

Kahan, J. S., Kahan, F. M., Goegelman, R., Currie, S. A., Jackson, M., Stapley, E. O., Miller, T. W., Miller, A. K., Hendlin, D., Mochales, S., Hernandez, S., and Woodruff, H. B. (1976). *Intersci. Conf. Antimicrob. Agents Chemother., 16th, Chicago, Ill.* Pap. No. 227. (Abstr.)

Kahan, J. S., Kahan, F. M., Goegelman, R., Currie, S. A., Jackson, M., Stapley, E. O., Miller, T. W., Miller, A. K., Hendlin, D., Mochales, S., Hernandez, S., Woodruff, H. B., and Birnbaum, J. (1979). *J. Antibiot.* **32**, 1.

Kametani, T., Huang, S. P., Yokohama, S., Suzuki, Y., and Ihara, M. (1980a). *J. Am. Chem. Soc.* **102**, 2060.

Kametani, T., Nagahara, T., Suzuki, Y., Yokohama, S., Huang, S. P., and Ihara, M. (1980b). *Heterocycles* **14**, 403.

Kropp, H., Kahan, J. S., Kahan, F. M., Sundelof, J., Darland, G., and Birnbaum, J. (1976). *Intersci. Conf. Antimicrob. Agents Chemother., 16th, Chicago, Ill.* Pap. No. 228. (Abstr.)

Kropp, H., Sundelof, J. G., Kahan, J. S., Kahan, F. M., and Birnbaum, J. (1980). *Antimicrob. Agents Chemother.* **17**, 993.

Leanza, W. J., Wildonger, K. J., Miller, T. W., and Christensen, B. G. (1979). *J. Med. Chem.* **22**, 1435.

Maeda, K., Takahashi, S., Sezaki, M., Iinuma, K., Naganawa, H., Kondo, S., Ohno, M., and Umezawa, H. (1977). *J. Antibiot.* **30**, 770.

Melillo, D. G., Shinkai, I., Liu, T., Ryan, K., and Sletzinger, M. (1980). *Tetrahedron Lett.* p. 2783.

Mori, T., Nakayama, M., Iwasaki, A., Kimura, S., Mizoguchi, T., Tanabe, S., Murakami, A., Watanabe, I., Okuchi, M., Itoh, H., Saino, Y., and Kobayashi, F. (1980). *Intersci. Conf. Antimicrob. Agents Chemother., 20th, New Orleans, La.* Pap. No. 165. (Abstr.)

Nakayama, M., Iwasaki, A., Kimura, S., Mizoguchi, T., Tanabe, S., Murakami, A., Watanabe, I., Okuchi, M., Itoh, H., Saino, Y., Kobayashi, F., and Mori, T. (1980). *J. Antibiot.* **33**, 1388.

Netherlands Patent 7,702,183. Merck and Co., Inc.

Okamura, K., Hirata, S., Okumura, Y., Fukagawa, Y., Shimauchi, Y., Kuono, K., Ishikura, T., and Lein, J. (1978). *J. Antibiot.* **31**, 480.

Okamura, K., Hirata, S., Koki, A., Hori, K., Shibamoto, N., Okumura, Y., Okabe, M., Okamoto, R., Kouno, K., Fukagawa, Y., Shimauchi, Y., and Ishikura, T. (1979). *J. Antibiot.* **32**, 262.

Onoue, H., Narisada, M., Uyeo, S., Matsumura, H., Okada, K., Yano, T., and Nagata, W. (1979). *Tetrahedron Lett.* p. 3867.

Pines, S. H. (1981). *IUPAC Symp. Ser., 3rd, Symp. Org. Synth., Madison, Wis.* p. 327.

Ponsford, R. J., and Southgate, R. (1979). *J.C.S. Chem. Commun.* p. 846.

Ponsford, R. J., Roberts, P. M., and Southgate, R. (1979). *J.C.S. Chem. Commun.* p. 847.

Ratcliffe, R. W., Salzmann, T. N., and Christensen, B. G. (1980). *Tetrahedron Lett.* p. 31.

Richter, W., and Biemann, K. (1964). *Monatsh. Chem.* **95**, 766.

Richter, W., and Biemann, K. (1965). *Monatsh. Chem.* **96**, 484.

Salzmann, T. N., Ratcliffe, R. W., Bouffard, F. A., and Christensen, B.G. (1980a). *Philos. Trans. R. Soc. London, Ser. B* **298**, 191.

Salzmann, T. N., Ratcliffe, R. W., Christensen,B. G., and Bouffard, F. A. (1980b). *J. Am. Chem. Soc.* **102**, 6161.

Schmitt, S. M., Johnston, D. B. R., and Christensen, B. G. (1980a). *J. Org. Chem.* **45**, 1142.

Schmitt, S. M., Johnston, D. B. R., and Christensen, B. G. (1980b). *J. Org. Chem.* **45**, 1135.

Shibamoto, N., Koki, A., Nishino, M., Nakamura, K., Kiyoshima, K., Okamura, K., Okabe, M., Okamoto, R., Fukagawa, Y., Shimauchi, Y., Ishikura, T., and Lein, J. (1980). *J. Antibiot.* **33**, 1128.

Shih, D. H., Hannah, J., and Christensen, B. G. (1978). *J. Am. Chem. Soc.* **100**, 8004.

Stapley, E. O., Cassidy, P. J., Currie, S. A., Daoust, D., Goegelman, R., Hernandez, S., Jackson, M., Mata, J. M., Miller, A. K., Monaghan, R. L., Tunac, J. B., Zimmerman, S. B., and Hendlin, D. (1977). *Intersci. Conf. Antimicrob. Agents Chemother., 17th, New York* Pap. No. 80. (Abstr.)

Stapley, E. O., Cassidy, P. J., Currie, S. A., Tunac, J. B., Monaghan, R. L., Jackson, M., Hernandez, S., Mata. J. M., Daoust, D., and Hendlin, D. (1981). *J. Antibiot.* **34**, 628.

Sullivan, G. R., Dale, J. A., and Mosher, H. S. (1973). *J. Org. Chem.* **38**, 2143.

Umezawa, H., Mitsuhashi, S., Hamada, M., Iyobe, S., Takahashi, S., Utahara, R., Osato, Y., Yamasaki, S., Ogawara, H., and Maeda, K. (1973). *J. Antibiot.* **26**, 51.

United States Patent 3,950,357. Merck and Co., Inc.

United States Patent 4,123,547. Merck and Co., Inc.

United States Patent 4,135,978. Merck and Co., Inc.

United States Patent 4,141,986. Merck and Co., Inc.

United States Patent 4,146,633. Merck and Co., Inc.

United States Patent 4,150,145. Merck and Co., Inc.

United States Patent 4,153,714. Beecham Group Ltd.

United States Patent 4,162,193. Merck and Co., Inc.

United States Patent 4,162,323. Merck and Co., Inc.

United States Patent 4,162,324. Merck and Co., Inc.

United States Patent 4,165,379. Merck and Co., Inc.

United States Patent 4,172,144. Merck and Co., Inc.

United States Patent 4,181,733. Merck and Co., Inc.

United States Patent 4,189,493. Merck and Co., Inc.

United States Patent 4,194,047. Merck and Co., Inc.

United States Patent 4,196,211. Merck and Co., Inc.

United States Patent 4,207,395. Merck and Co., Inc.

United States Patent 4,247,640. Merck and Co., Inc.

Witkop, B. (1956). *Experientia* **12**, 372.

Yamamoto, K., Yoshioka, T., Kato, Y., Shibamoto, N., Shimauchi, Y., and Ishikura, T. (1980). *J. Antibiot.* **33**, 796.

5

The Penems

IVAN ERNEST

I. The Penems as Hybrids of Penicillins and Cephalosporins

It is a commonly held belief that the four-membered β-lactam ring is, in general, very labile and easily opened by various nucleophilic agents. As those involved in the β-lactam field know well, this is not always true. Simple monocyclic β-lactams are often stable compounds quite resistant, for example, to alkaline hydrolysis.

Chemistry and Biology of
β-Lactam Antibiotics, Vol. 2

This belief in the lability of β-lactam originates in the chemistry of β-lactam antibiotics. It is true that in these compounds the β-lactam ring is easily attacked by nucleophiles, much in contrast to the behavior of simple monocyclic azetidinones. Thus, rather than speaking of the unstable β-lactam ring in general, it is more appropriate to state that all known naturally occurring bicyclic β-lactam antibiotics and their biologically active synthetic analogs are characterized by an unusual reactivity of their β-lactam system toward nucleophilic agents.

It has been suggested by Tipper and Strominger (1965) and is widely accepted nowadays that the outstanding antibacterial activity of natural β-lactam antibiotics is based on their ability to acylate, by virtue of their reactive β-lactam grouping, the enzymes involved in bacterial cell wall biosynthesis. The above-mentioned general correlation between the biological activity of these compounds on the one hand and the chemical reactivity of their β-lactam system on the other is, in light of this theory, not surprising.

No simple quantitative activity–reactivity relationship is, however, obvious today. Nevertheless, the search for structures with reactive β-lactam rings proved to be useful in designing new biologically active synthetic and semisynthetic derivatives of this class.

What are the reasons for the increased β-lactam reactivity in natural β-lactam antibiotics? In *penicillins,* a rationalization has been given based on their rigid, nonplanar bicyclic structure (Woodward, 1949). Fusion of the four-membered azetidinone with the five-membered thiazolidine ring in these compounds results in a pyramidal geometry of the β-lactam nitrogen (Crowfoot *et al.,* 1949; Sweet and Dahl, 1970) and thus in a distortion of the parallelism of its free-electron pair orbital with the π orbital of the azetidinone carbonyl group. As a consequence, the delocalization of the unshared electron pair into the adjacent carbonyl, by which an amide C(O)—N bond is usually stabilized, is diminished and the stability of the β-lactam lessened in penicillins.

The above-mentioned rationalization does not apply for *cephalosporins,* where the β-lactam nitrogen has an almost planar geometry. Here the increased reactivity of the β-lactam seems to be associated with the presence and the particular (Δ^3) location of the double bond in the six-membered ring. A conjugative interaction of the unshared electron pair of the β-lactam nitrogen with the adjacent double bond competes with its delocalization into the azetidinone carbonyl and, as a consequence, the C(O)—N bond of the β-lactam is cleaved more readily.

To combine both structural elements that appear to be associated with the biological activity of penicillins and cephalosporins, i.e., the five-membered ring and the double bond, in one single structure such as **1** was for a long time an open challenge for synthetic chemists working in the field. With the accelerated developments of recent years in the synthesis of β-lactam antibiotics, the idea of synthesizing such compounds became more realistic and, in 1975, a team at the Woodward Research Institute in Basel announced the first successful synthesis of the novel penem system.

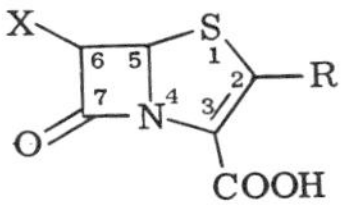

1

II. 6β-Acylamino-(5R)-penem-3-carboxylic Acids

A. Synthesis

As a cross between penicillins and cephalosporins as closely related to both natural classes as possible, the optically active 6β-acylamino-(5R)-penem-3-carboxylic acids (**2**) were synthesized first (Woodward, 1975, 1977b; Ernest *et al.*, 1977b, 1978).

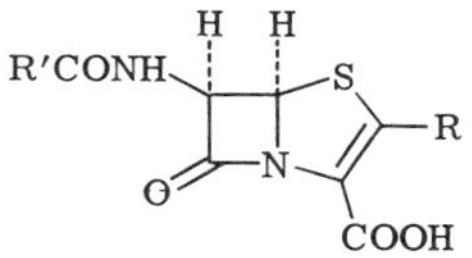

2

For the synthesis of compounds **2**, penicillins proved to be useful, inexpensive, chiral starting materials containing a β-lactam ring with an acylamino side chain and the correct stereochemistry of the chiral centers C-5 and C-6. Their thiazolidine ring had only to be partially degraded to allow construction of the unsaturated ring of the new system.

The key intermediates in the synthesis were the 3-acylamino-4-acyl-thio-2-azetidinones (**7**). One of the ways to prepare these compounds from penicillins is shown in the following scheme:

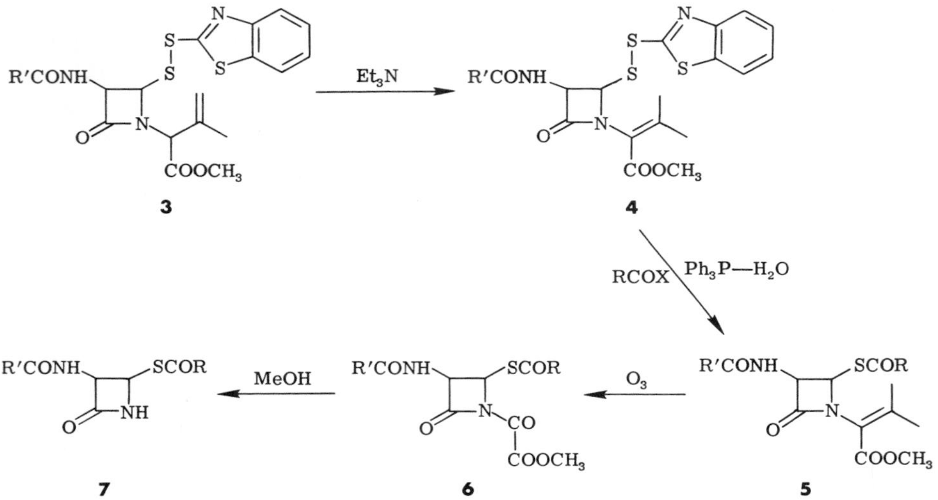

R'CONH S—S [benzothiazole]   —Et₃N→   R'CONH S—S [benzothiazole]
O= N
COOCH₃
3

R'CONH   O= N
COOCH₃
4

RCOX Ph₃P—H₂O

R'CONH SCOR   ←MeOH—   R'CONH SCOR   ←O₃—   R'CONH SCOR
O= NH   O= N   O= N
                            CO
                            COOCH₃   COOCH₃
7   **6**   **5**

The disulfides (**3**), prepared from the esters of penicillin *S*-oxides by heating with 2-mercaptobenzthiazole (Kamiya *et al.*, 1973), were transformed by base-catalyzed isomerization into isomers with the conjugated unsaturated ester grouping (**4**), and these in turn, by reductive acylation (Zn, RCOOH, (RCO)₂O; or Ph₃P, H₂O, RCOX; or NaBH₄, RCOX), into 4-acylthioazetidinones (**5**). Low-temperature ozonolysis of the latter compounds afforded the sensitive *N*-alkoxalyl derivatives (**6**) which, on mild methanolysis, lost the substituent on the nitrogen atom to give N-unsubstituted azetidinones (**7**).

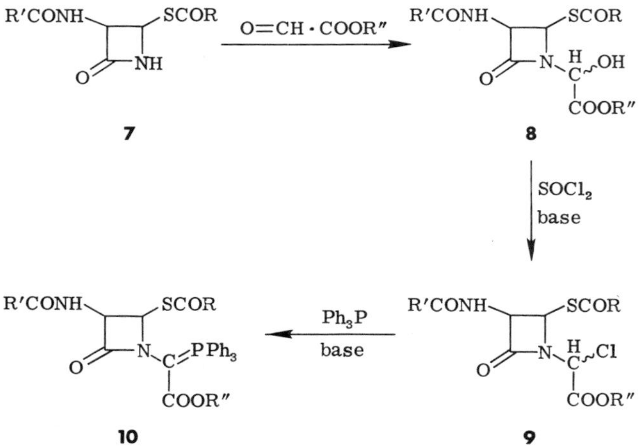

R'CONH SCOR   —O=CH·COOR″→   R'CONH SCOR
O= NH   O= N—C(H)—OH
                                    COOR″
7   **8**

SOCl₂ base

R'CONH SCOR   ←Ph₃P base—   R'CONH SCOR
O= N—C=PPh₃   O= N—C(H)—Cl
      COOR″   COOR″
10   **9**

In a three-step procedure developed some time ago in another connection (Heusler and Woodward, 1969; Woodward *et al.*, 1977), which has since become very popular in the construction of various bicyclic compounds from monocyclic β-lactam intermediates, a stabilized phosphorane grouping was next built up on the azetidinone nitrogen atom of **7**. When the compounds **(10)** thus obtained were heated in toluene at 70–100°C, an intramolecular Wittig condensation occurred between the phosphorane grouping and the thioester carbonyl group, and the esters **(11)** of the novel 6β-acylamino-(5*R*)-penem-3-carboxylic acids were formed with varying ease depending on the substituents R and R″.

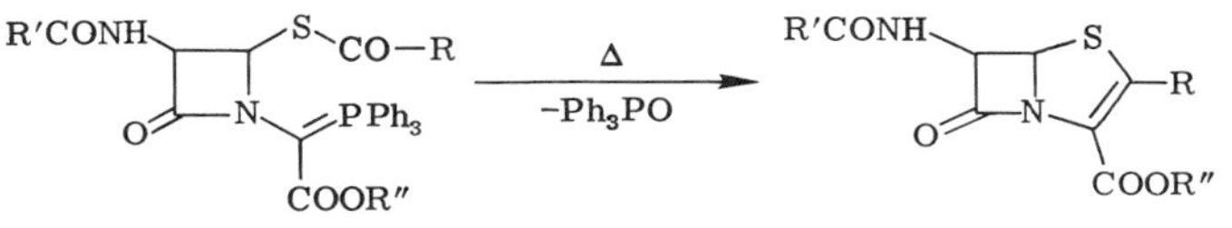

This choice of the Wittig reaction, which formed the penem system under mild and neutral conditions, was very fortunate with respect to the properties of the novel compounds: As discussed in more detail later (Section II,B), the penems proved very sensitive to both acids and bases. This behavior also put serious restrictions on the choice of suitable, readily cleaved ester groupings for ultimate transformation of the esters **(11)** to the free acids **(2)**. Unsatisfactory Wittig reactions with some phosphoranes **(10)** set further limits, making, for example, the trichloroethyl esters of type **11** difficult to obtain. Finally, the problem of preparation of the acids **(2)** was solved by catalytic hydrogenolysis [on a palladium–carbon (Pd–C) catalyst] of the *p*-nitrobenzyl esters **(11a)**.

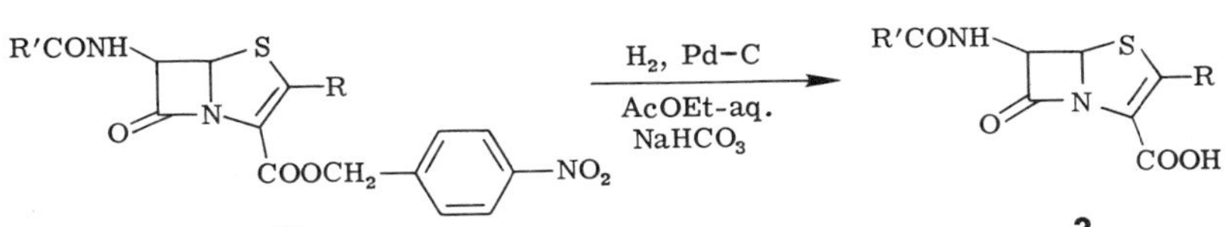

In the above-described way, various 2-alkyl-, 2-aralkyl-, and 2-aryl-substituted penem esters (**11**, R = Me, iPr, CH$_2$Ph, Ph, *p*-C$_6$H$_4$NO$_2$), with 6β-phenoxyacetamido and with 6β-phthalimido side chains, and two free penem acids **(2a,b)** were prepared (Ernest *et al.*, 1976, 1978).

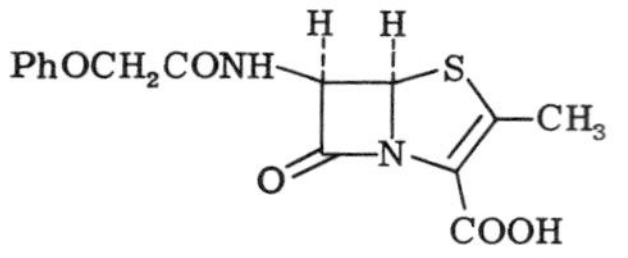

2a 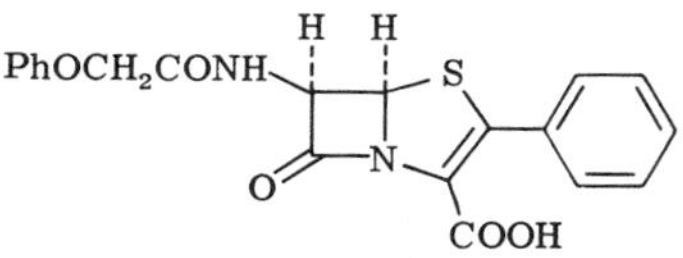   **2b**

For synthesis of the 2-unsubstituted penem-3-carboxylic acid (**2c**), a similar scheme based on an intramolecular Wittig reaction was used. However, for preparation of the phosphorane precursor (**10c**), the general route had to be modified.

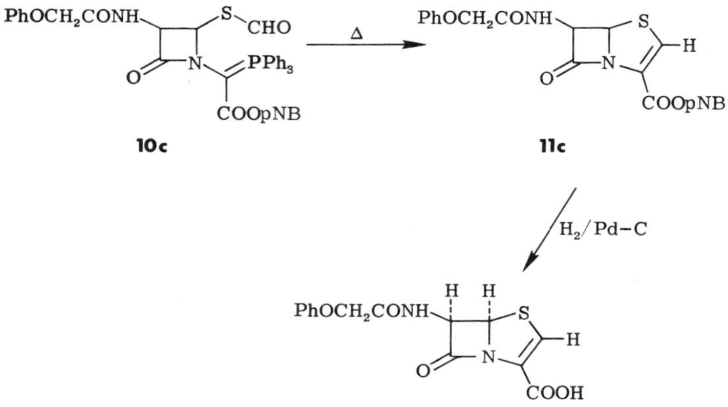

10c   **11c**

2c

The reason for modification of the scheme was the need to replace, in the early stages of the synthesis, the 4-formylthio grouping (as shown in **10c**) by a more stable synthetic equivalent from which the thioformate substituent could be later generated for the ring-closure reaction. In other words, rather than synthesizing the formylthioazetidinone (**12**), the thioacrylate derivative (**15**) was prepared as its more convenient substitute (**4a → 15**).

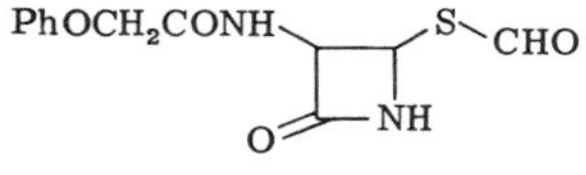

12

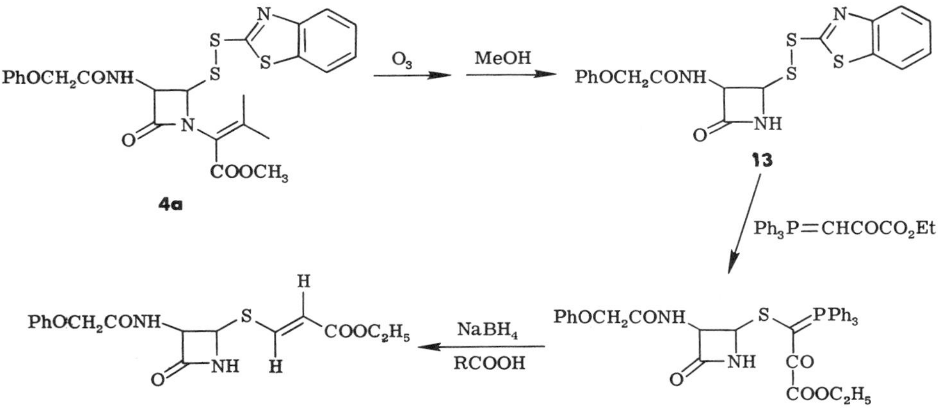

The two last steps (13 → 15) in the preparation of the intermediate (15) are rather unconventional and require some comment. The S—S bond in disulfides of type 13 is readily susceptible to attack by nucleophiles, with resultant cleavage of the linkage and liberation of mercaptobenzthiazole (or its anion). In this manner, the disulfide (13), prepared in two steps from the earlier mentioned intermediate (4a), reacted with ethyl triphenylphosphoranylidene pyruvate to give, along with mercaptobenzthiazole, the azetidinonylthiophosphorane (14). Originally, the latter compound was intended as an intermediate in another synthetic scheme for penems, in which its ketonic carbonyl group would be attacked by the NH group of the azetidinone ring to produce a cyclic intermediate (16) of a Wittig reaction. Subsequent elimination of triphenylphosphine oxide would then have produced a penem ester (Woodward, 1977b; Ernest et al., 1978).

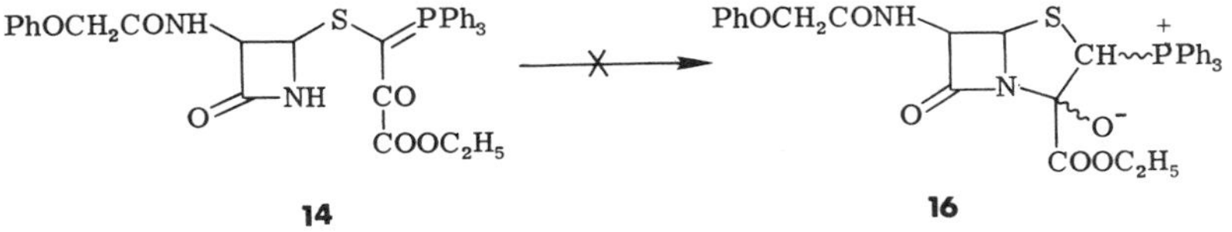

Unfortunately, no such reaction could be realized, probably because of the betaine character of 14 (cf. 14a), making the "carbonyl" carbon atom unreactive toward nucleophilic agents. On the other hand, the compound could be reduced, by sodium borohydride in acidic medium, to the thioacrylate (15) and thus proved to be a useful intermediate in synthesis of the acid (2c).

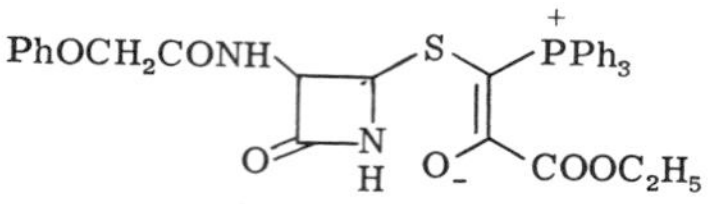

PhOCH$_2$CONH

S

$\overset{+}{P}Ph_3$

O

N
H

O$_-$

COOC$_2$H$_5$

14a

With the previously mentioned three-step procedure, the intermediate (15) was converted to the phosphorane (17). For subsequent ozonolysis of the thioacrylate side chain, which should convert it to the desired formylthio grouping (cf. 10c), the ozone-sensitive phosphorane grouping first had to be protected. Efficient, simple protection was achieved by performing the ozonization in an acidic medium in which 17 was present in its protonated phosphonium form (18). Neutralization of the ozonization mixture with aqueous bicarbonate restored the phosphorane grouping, and the desired precursor (10c) was formed.

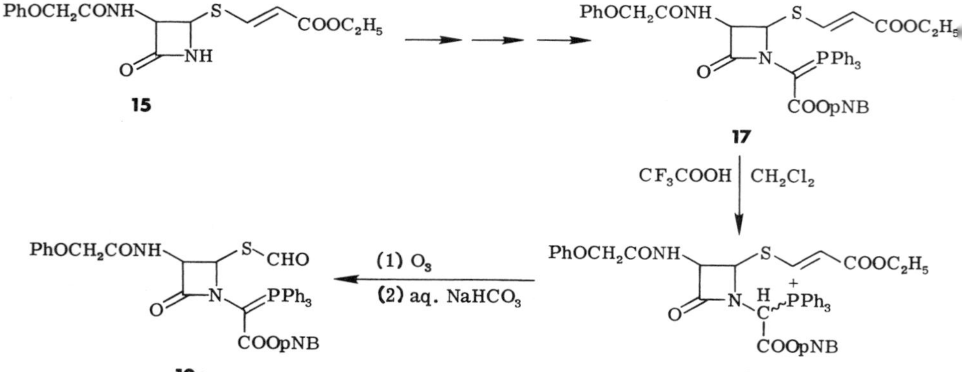

PhOCH$_2$CONH

S

COOC$_2$H$_5$

O

NH

15

$\longrightarrow$ $\longrightarrow$ $\longrightarrow$

PhOCH$_2$CONH

S

COOC$_2$H$_5$

O

N

PPh$_3$

COOpNB

17

CF$_3$COOH | CH$_2$Cl$_2$

PhOCH$_2$CONH

S

CHO

O

N

PPh$_3$

COOpNB

10c

(1) O$_3$

(2) aq. NaHCO$_3$

PhOCH$_2$CONH

S

COOC$_2$H$_5$

O

N

H
$\overset{+}{C}$

PPh$_3$

COOpNB

18

Only a brief heating of the crude phosphorane (10c) in refluxing methylene chloride was needed to accomplish the Wittig ring closure to the penem ester (11c). Its hydrogenolysis afforded then the free, 2-unsubstituted penem acid (2c).

B. Physical Data and Chemical Behavior

For the penem system of the esters (11) and acids (2), the following spectral properties proved characteristic (Ernest *et al.*, 1978).

In the ultraviolet (UV) spectra of the penem-3-carboxylates (11, R = alkyl, R = H) a long-wavelength maximum at about 305 and 308–310 nm, respectively, reflects the conjugation of the sulfur atom through the carbon–carbon double bond to the carbonyl group of the ester function. With the free acids (2a,c), a slight hypsochromic shift of these maxima to 300 and 304 nm, respectively, was observed.

The infrared (IR) spectra of compounds 11 and 2 display a short-wavelength stretching absorption band of the β-lactam carbonyl at 5.54–5.57 μm, suggesting a more strained, more reactive β-lactam system than in cephalosporins and most penicillins.

In the 100-MHz proton magnetic resonance spectra in deuterated chloroform, the cis-disubstituted β-lactam system of the esters (11) is characterized by a closely spaced multiplet, between δ 5.9 and 6.0 ppm, of H-5 and H-6. In a 360-MHz spectrum of p-nitrobenzyl 2-methylpenem-3-carboxylate (11a, R = Me, R' = PhOCH$_2$) this multiplet was resolved to a doublet for H-5 (δ 5.88 ppm, $J_{5,6}$ = 4 Hz) and a doublet of doublets for H-6 (δ 5.96 ppm, $J_{5,6}$ = 4 Hz, $J_{6,NH}$ = 8 Hz). The signal of the methyl group at C-2 of this compound was located at δ 2.21 ppm. In the p-nitrobenzyl ester of the 2-unsubstituted acid (11c), H-2 was represented by a singlet at δ 7.39 ppm.

Not surprisingly, the novel penems proved very labile. In an aqueous phosphate buffer of pH 7.4 at 37°C, the half-life of the 2-methyl-substituted acid (2a) was less than 1 hr (UV evidence), and only a few minutes with the still more labile 2-unsubstituted acid (2c). Also, the 2-phenyl-substituted acid was very labile: In its preparation by two-phase hydrogenolysis of the corresponding p-nitrobenzyl ester, it could be recovered from the aqueous bicarbonate phase only in admixture with β-lactam-free decomposition products and was further decomposed on attempted purification (Ernest et al., 1978).

A characteristic unwelcome feature of the novel penem compounds proved to be their instability to acids. Formic acid, trifluoroacetic acid, or traces of hydrochloric acid induce decomposition of the esters (11) to thiazole-4-carboxylates (19).

This characteristic "vertical" splitting of the penem molecule, the driving force of which is undoubtedly formation of the aromatic thiazole system, also occurred on certain batches of chromatographic silica gel (it could be prevented by using silica gel carefully washed in a neutral solution) and was, to a small extent, observed in some cyclizations of the phosphoranes (10). In the mass spectrum of the methyl ester of the acid (2a), the peaks of both vertical splits belonged, along with the parent peak, to its most characteristic features (Ernest *et al.*, 1976).

C. Biological Activity of the Acids

In an *in vitro* plate diffusion test, 2-methyl-6β-phenoxyacetamido-(5*R*)-penem-3-carboxylic acid (2a) was found active against gram-positive strains (e.g., *Staphylococcus aureus*), thus showing that biological activity was inherent in the new β-lactam system. The level of the biological activity was, however, rather disappointing. A suspicion that this might be a consequence of the low stability of the tested compound was supported by the finding that the still more labile 2-unsubstituted acid 2c was even less active than 2a.

III.   6-Unsubstituted Penem-3-carboxylic Acids

A. Syntheses

1. *Syntheses by the Woodward Research Institute*

a. Racemic 6-Unsubstituted Penem Acids. The first synthesized representatives of the penems (Section II), although very labile, proved sufficiently stable to permit isolation and, although not very active, suggested antibiotic activity to be inherent in the new β-lactam system. This experience raised interest in a more systematic study of the penem class.

The next type of penem to be explored was the 6-unsubstituted penem-3-carboxylic acids (20). It was felt that the fundamental chemistry of the penem system could be best studied with these simple representatives and that they might be relatively easily accessible by total synthesis. It was further of great importance to learn, by preparing the most simple compounds of the class, the degree of intrinsic instability inherent in the penem system. Finally, the appearance upon the scene of clavulanic acid (21) (Howarth *et al.*, 1976) and of thienamycin (22) (Kahan *et al.*, 1976; Albers-Schönberg *et al.*, 1976)—the former compound a potent inhibitor of β-lactamases and the latter a powerful, broad-spectrum antibiotic—raised hopes that interesting biological activity might be found in com-

20   21

pounds **20**, although they lack the acylamino side chain so important for the activity of penicillins and cephalosporins.

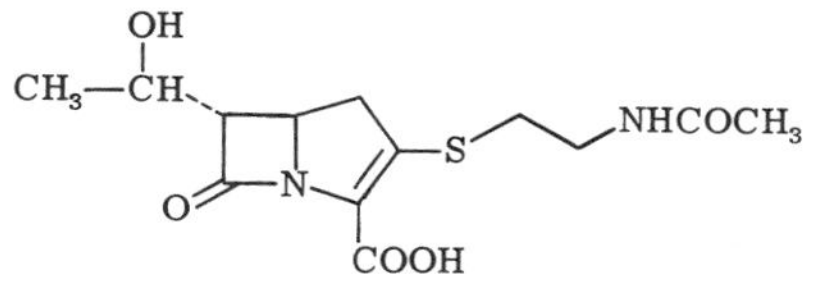

22

The first total synthesis of racemic penem acids of type **20** (Woodward, 1977a; Lang *et al.*, 1979, Gosteli *et al.*, 1978b) was based upon the readily accessible 4-acetoxyazetidinone (**23**) (Clauss *et al.*, 1974) and its ability to undergo facile exchange reactions with nucleophiles. With anions of thiocarboxylic acids, a wide variety of azetidinonyl thioesters (**24**) could be prepared.

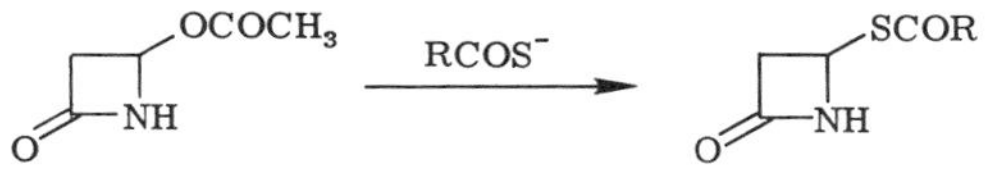

Synthesis of the penem acids (**20**) from these intermediates (**24**) was analogous to that of the 6-acylaminopenems (cf. Section II). In three steps, the versatile phosphorane grouping was attached to the β-lactam nitrogen atom, and the azetidinonylphosphoranes (**25**) thus formed were heated in inert solvents to give, in an intramolecular Wittig reaction, the penem esters (**26**). Finally, hydrogenolysis of the *p*-nitrobenzyl ester grouping on Pd–C afforded racemic 2-substituted penem-3-carboxylic acids (**20**).

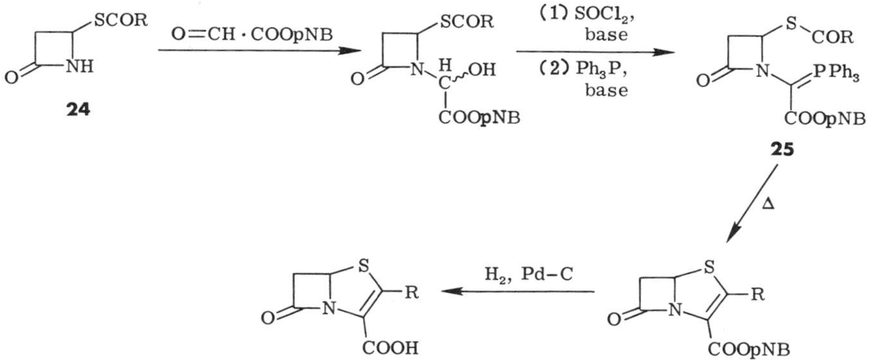

Synthesis of the racemic parent penem acid (**20**, R = H) (Woodward, 1977b; Pfaendler *et al.*, 1979) is in principle also based on that of the corresponding 6-acylamino acid (**2c**) (Section II), however, in contrast to the rather complicated route to the latter, the means of preparing the necessary N-unsubstituted azetidinone intermediate (**27**) was very simple: It was obtained in a single step by treating 4-acetoxyazetidinone (**23**) with the anion of methyl *cis*-β-mercaptoacrylate. The latter reagent was prepared *in situ* by addition, in the presence of hydrochloric acid, of thiourea to methyl propiolate and by alkaline hydrolysis of the isothiuronium salt thus formed.

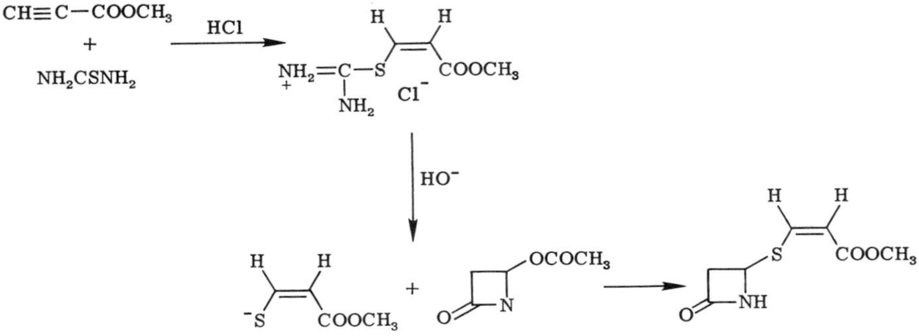

In the following steps of the synthesis, an alternative to the *p*-nitrobenzyl ester, namely, the acetonyl ester, was used for protection of the carboxyl grouping. For the final liberation of the acid (**20**, R = H) the acetonylpenem ester (**28**) could be hydrolyzed under conditions mild enough to preserve the sensitive penem system.

Table I presents various examples of racemic 6-unsubstituted penem-3-carboxylic acids prepared at the Woodward Research Institute. For

TABLE I Examples of Racemic 6-Unsubstituted Penem-3-carboxylic Acids

Structure	R
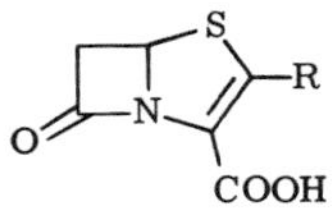 **20**	H, CH$_3$, C$_5$H$_{11}$, CH$_2$Ph, Ph, CH$_2$OCOCH$_3$, CH$_2$SCH$_3$, CH$_2$SC(CH$_3$)$_3$, CH$_2$NHCOCH$_2$OPh, CH$_2$CH$_2$NH$_2$, CH$_2$CH$_2$CH$_2$NH$_2$, SCH$_2$CH$_3$, SCH$_2$CH$_2$NHCOCH$_3$

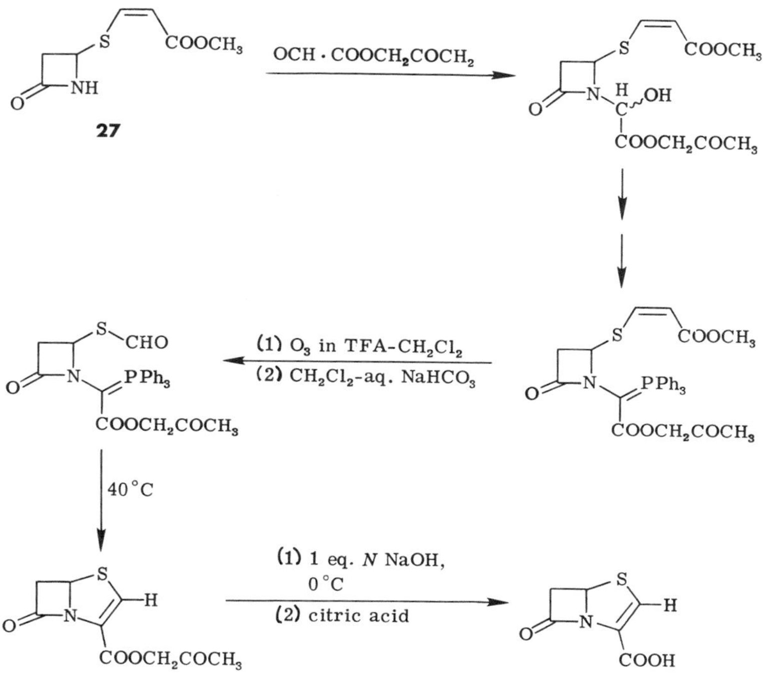

synthesis of the 2-alkylthio-substituted acids (**20**, R = SR′), the general scheme was modified in that the Wittig-type ring closure to the penem system involved the thiocarbonyl group of a trithiocarbonate ester grouping. In preparation of the azetidinone precursor (**29**), a trithiocarbonate ester salt was used as the displacing nucleophile in the reaction with 4-acetoxyazetidinone (Lang *et al.*, 1980; Gosteli *et al.*, 1978b).[*,†]

---

*According to a publication from the Sankyo Central Research Laboratories (Oida *et al.*, 1980), Japanese chemists, obviously unaware of the above-described earlier work by the Woodward Research Institute, used the same route to prepare several 2-alkylthiopenem-3-carboxylic acids. Another claim for this route to 2-alkylthiopenems was recently made by the Schering Corporation. In the corresponding patent (McCombie, 1980), an interesting modification was introduced in the last step: Alkaline salts of the penem acids were obtained by deprotection of the allyl esters with sodium (potassium) 2-ethylhexanoate in nonaqueous media in the presence of triphenylphosphine and tetrakis(triphenylphosphine) palladium.

†In a close analogy to the latter procedure, 2-alkoxypenems were later prepared in the laboratories of the Beecham group by an intramolecular Wittig reaction between a phosphorane and a xanthate grouping (Brain, 1980) (cf. Table V).

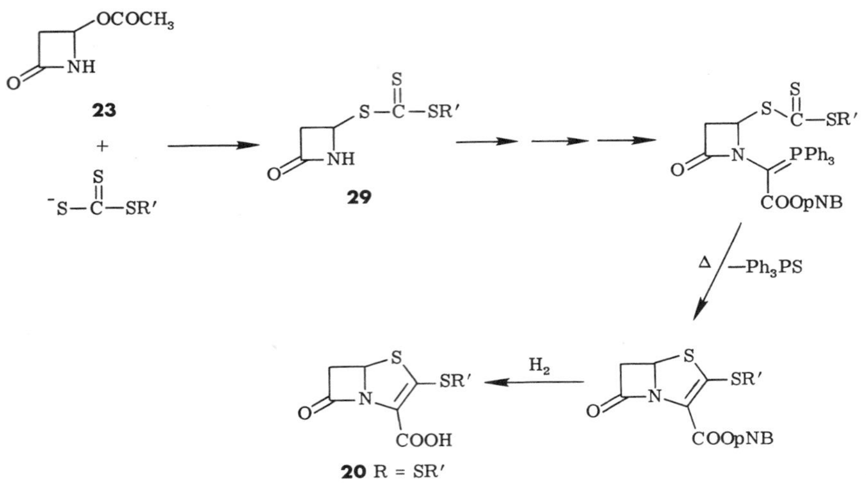

20 R = SR′

b. Optically Active Acids (20). As discussed in more detail below (Section III,B,3), the racemic acids (**20**) displayed activity against a remarkably broad spectrum of bacteria. It was assumed that, in parallel to penicillins and cephalosporins, only the 5*R* component of each racemate was responsible for the biological activity. The correctness of this hypothesis of course had to be proved by preparation of the individual enantiomers. To that purpose, two different approaches were chosen in Basel.

Using in principle the scheme for synthesis of the chiral 6β-acylamino-substituted penem acids from penicillins (Section II,A), the optically active 2-methyl-(5*R*)-penem-3-carboxylic acid (**20a**) was prepared from the natural 6β-amino-(5*R*)-penicillanic acid via methyl (5*R*)-penicillanate S-oxide (**30**) (Ernest *et al.*, 1979).

Another approach to chiral 6-unsubstituted penem acids, based on separation of diastereomeric intermediates, was demonstrated in the synthesis of both enantiomeric parent penem acids (5*R*)-**20b** and (5*S*)-**20b** (Pfaendler *et al.*, 1979). Exchange reaction of 4-acetoxyazetidinone (**23**) with the sodium salt (**31**) of the β-mercaptoacrylic ester of the optically active (−)-menthol led to a 1:1 mixture of the diastereomers (4*R*)-**32** and (4*S*)-**32** which could be separated by fractional crystallization. The independent use of the individual diastereomers in the above-mentioned synthetic scheme for the racemic acid (**20**, R = H) allowed the preparation of both chiral acids.

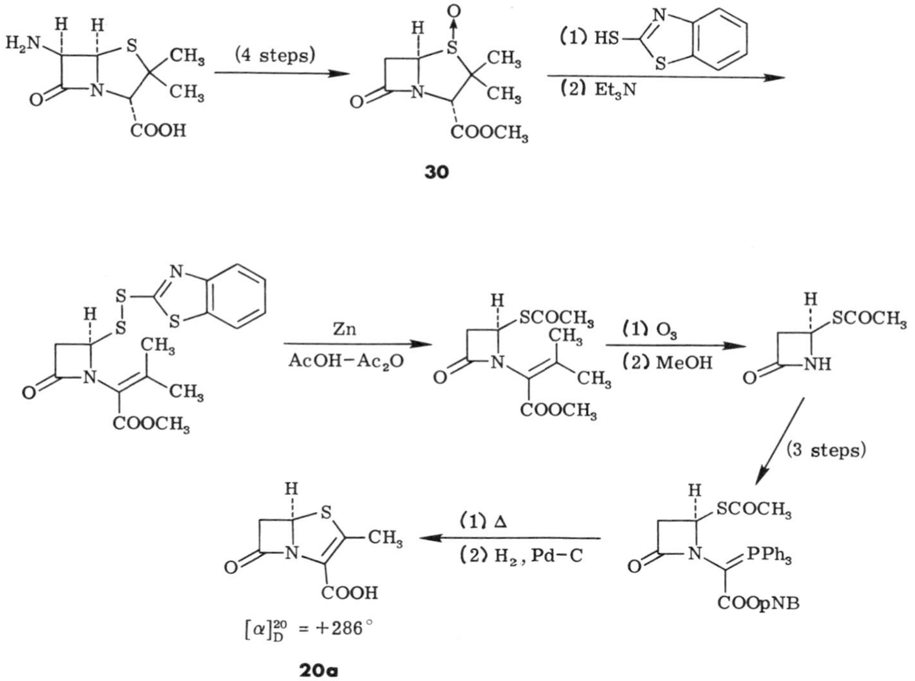

H
H
H_2N
S
CH_3
CH_3
O
N
COOH
(4 steps)
O
H
S
CH_3
CH_3
O
N
$COOCH_3$
30
(1) HS
N
S
(2) Et_3N
N
S
S
H
S
S
CH_3
O
N
CH_3
$COOCH_3$
Zn
$AcOH-Ac_2O$
H
$SCOCH_3$
CH_3
O
N
CH_3
$COOCH_3$
(1) O_3
(2) MeOH
H
$SCOCH_3$
O
NH
(3 steps)
H
$SCOCH_3$
O
N
PPh_3
COOpNB
(1) Δ
(2) H_2, Pd–C
H
S
CH_3
O
N
COOH
$[\alpha]_D^{20}$ = +286°
20a

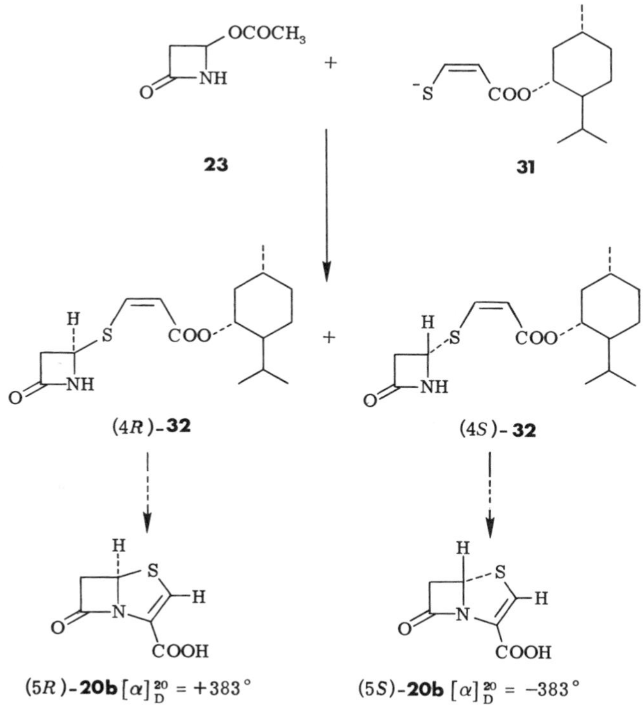

$OCOCH_3$
O
NH
+
^-S
COO
23
31
H
S
COO
O
NH
+
H
S
COO
O
NH
(4R)-32
(4S)-32
H
S
H
O
N
COOH
H
S
H
O
N
COOH
(5R)-20b $[\alpha]_D^{20}$ = +383°
(5S)-20b $[\alpha]_D^{20}$ = −383°

2. The Glaxo Syntheses

a. From Clavulanic Acid. Shortly after the first penem syntheses had been announced, chemists of the Glaxo research group in Greenford introduced the newly described system into their research program directed toward the synthesis of nuclear analogs of clavulanic acid. Two original syntheses of 6-unsubstituted penem acids resulted.

One of the syntheses is based on clavulanic acid as starting material (Cherry *et al.*, 1979; Beels *et al.*, 1979a). Clavulanic acid-derived esters (**33**) were converted, via the betaines (**34**), to the isomeric 1-oxapenems (**35**). The five-membered ring of the latter compounds was easily opened, by heating with butylmercaptan, to give the largely enolized ketoesters (**36**). Subsequent mesylation and chlorinolysis afforded the key intermediates (**38**) which, on treatment with hydrogen sulfide and triethylamine in tetrahydrofuran at 0°C, were converted in good yields to the correspondingly 2-substituted *p*-nitrobenzyl penem-3-carboxylates (**39**).

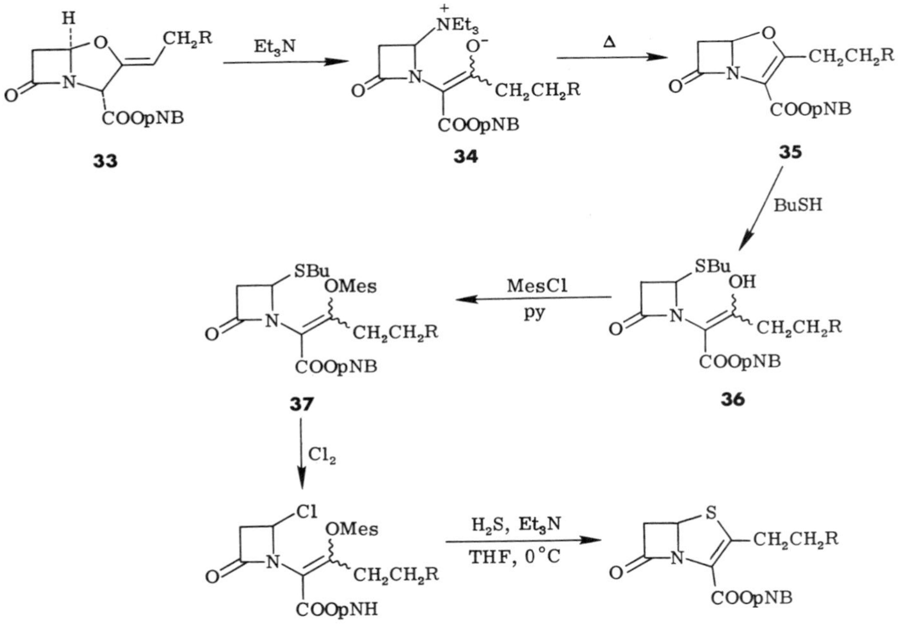

An alternative to the above-mentioned route is based on mesylation of the betaines (**34**) and reaction of the mesylates thus formed with hydrogen sulfide and triethylamine to the thienol betaines (**41**). The latter, on short heating in dichloromethane, eliminate Et₃N and cyclize to the penem esters (39).

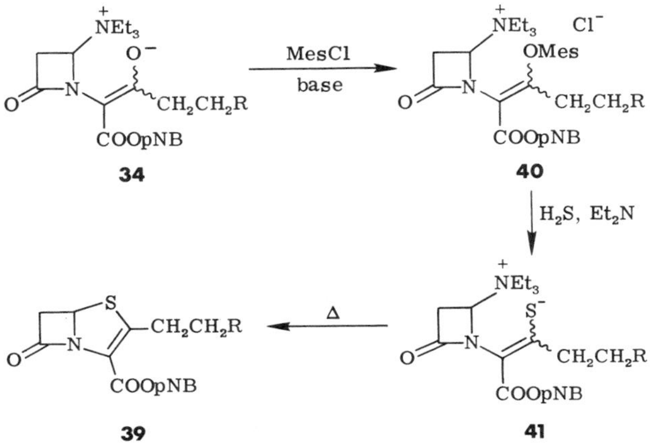

Hydrogenolysis of the *p*-nitrobenzyl ester (39, R = H) produced the free 2-ethylpenem-3-carboxylic acid (42, R = H). With the penem ester [39, R = OCH(CH₃)OC₂H₅], the acetal grouping, by which the hydroxyl group of the starting clavulanic acid had been protected through the whole synthesis, was first hydrolyzed and, if desired, the hydroxyl was alkylated or acylated. In this way, after the final hydrogenolysis of the ester, 2-(β-hydroxyethyl)-, 2-(β-methoxyethyl)-, and various 2-(β-acyl-oxyethyl)-penem-3-carboxylic acids were prepared.*

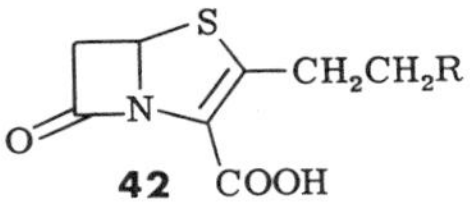

A major drawback of these two routes to penems is the fact that the optical activity of the natural starting material is completely lost in the course of the synthesis and only racemic penem acids result.

  b.   From 6-Aminopenicillanic Acid. Hoping for a route to an optically active penem acid, the Greenford research group modified the above-mentioned synthetic scheme and adapted it for another chiral starting material, namely, 6β-aminopenicillanic acid (6-APA). Accessibility of the

  *A recently published paper by the Glaxo group (Cherry *et al.*, 1980) describes preparation of the potassium salts of 2-(β-acetylthioethyl)- and 2-(β-phenylthioethyl)-penem-3-carboxylic acids starting from the 2-(β-hydroxyethyl) ester (39, R = OH).

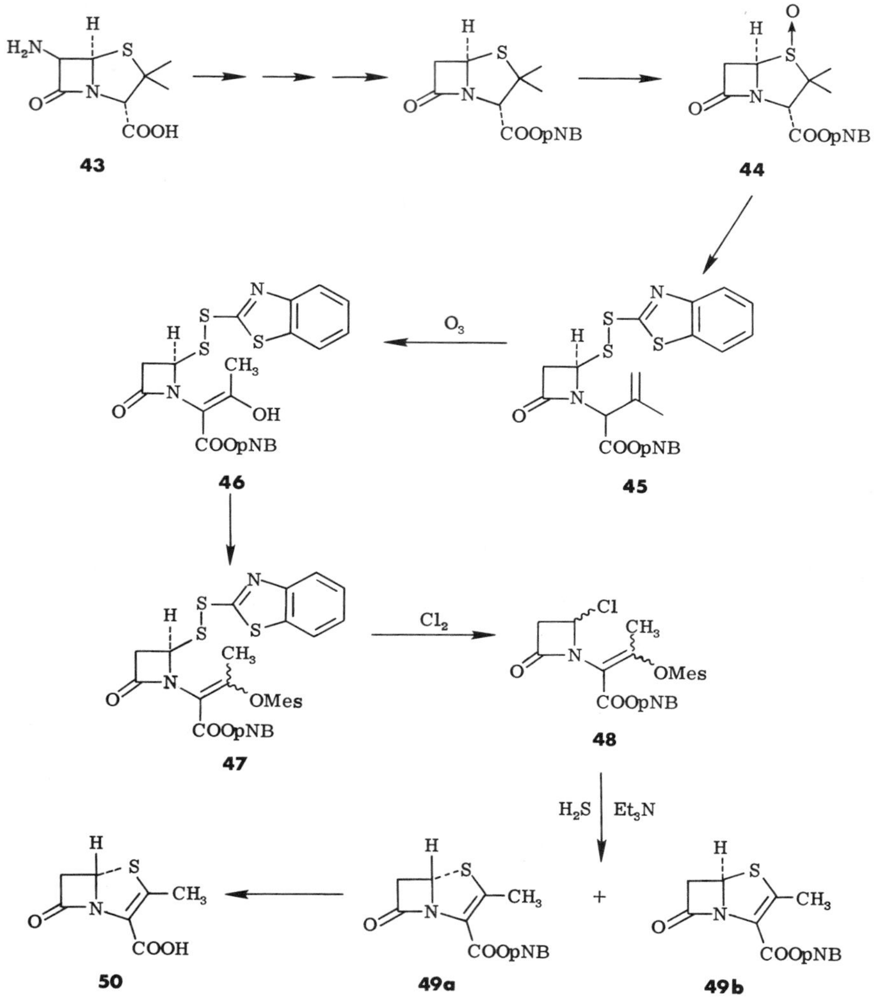

natural 6-APA better than that of clavulanic acid was considered another advantage for the synthesis (Beels *et al.,* 1979a,b).

With a procedure described in Section III,A,1,b, 6-APA (**43**) was converted, via the *p*-nitrobenzyl ester of (5*R*)-penicillanic acid *S*-oxide (**44**), to the disulfide (**45**). Ozonization of the carbon–carbon double bond of the latter intermediate produced the enol ester (**46**) which in turn was treated with methanesulfonyl chloride and triethylamine to give a mixture of both stereomers of the mesylate (**47**). Chlorinolysis of the disulfide grouping of **47** resulted in an isomeric mixture of the chloro compounds

(**48**). When the latter mixture was treated in tetrahydrofuran with hydrogen sulfide and triethylamine, a mixture of enantiomeric penem esters (**49a** and **49b**) was formed from which the prevailing isomer, $[\alpha]_D^{20}$ = − 128° ($CHCl_3$),* could be partially separated by crystallization; as shown by X-ray diffraction analysis, it was the 5*S* isomer (**49a**). Catalytic hydrogenolysis of the ester grouping converted it to the free 2-methyi-(5*S*)-penem-3-carboxylic acid (**50**). The desired 5*R* acid (cf. **20a** in Section III,A,1,b) was obtained only in a "near-racemic" mixture with the 5*S* enantiomer.

3. *The Farmitalia–Carlo Erba Syntheses*

In a paper entitled, "Total Synthesis of Thia Analogs of Clavulanic Acid," Lombardi *et al.* (1979) described the preparation of the methyl and acetoxymethyl esters of the racemic 2-(β-acetoxyethyl)penem-3-carboxylic acid (**52**) (see also Lombardi *et al.*, 1980).†

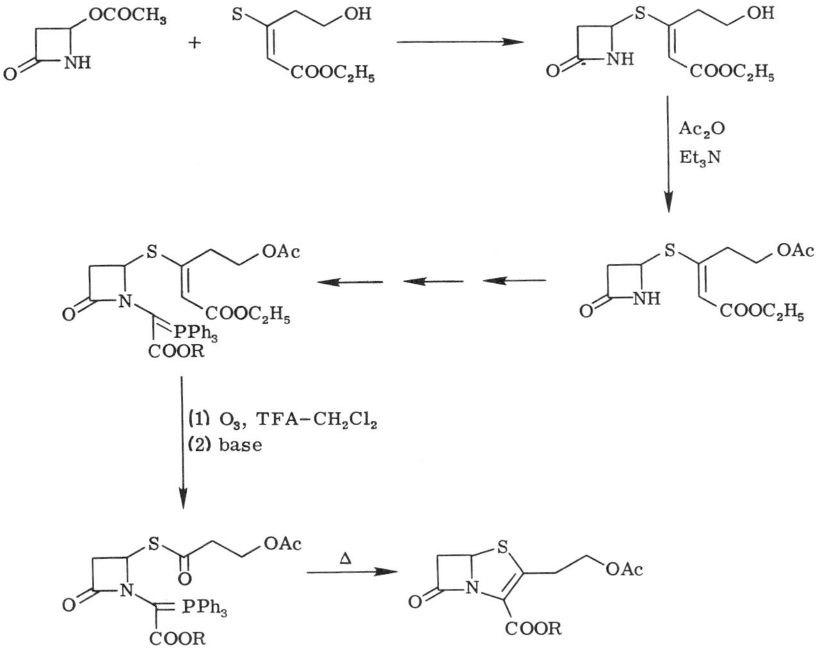

51 **52**

*The (5*R*) enantiomer (**49b**), prepared—as the sole product—from 6-APA in another way by Ernest *et al.* (1979) (Section III,A,1,b), displayed an $[\alpha]_D^{20}$ of + 136° ($CHCl_3$).

†The *p*-nitrobenzyl ester and the potassium salt of 2-(β-acetoxyethyl)-penem-3-carboxylic acid were prepared from clavulanic acid at the Glaxo research laboratories (Section III,A,2,a).

The method used to build up the bicyclic penem system is in principle that of the Woodward Research Institute (cf. Section III,A,1,a).

With the phosphorane (53), similar to the intermediate (51) of the foregoing scheme except for the thiomalonate side chain, the intramolecular Wittig reaction led to the "thiaclavulanoid" (54) with the carbon–carbon double bond in the exocyclic position. When, however, the latter compound was oxidized with m-chloroperbenzoic acid, the double bond moved into the ring and the penem S-oxide (55) was formed.

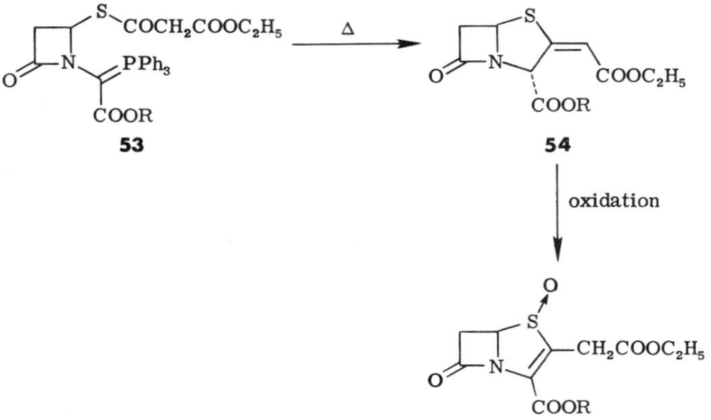

Another synthesis of penems by the Farmitalia research group, this time starting from penicillin, was also published (Foglio et al., 1980a,b; Franceschi et al., 1980). The penem system is again constructed in the way of Woodward, but a different approach is used for formation of the thioester side chain necessary for the ultimate Wittig reaction (see p. 335).

The acetoxymethyl ester (56) as such proved biologically active (Table IV, Section III,C) and thus made unnecessary the last, usually somewhat delicate, step in the synthesis of the penem acids, namely, their liberation from esters.

4. The Contribution of the Bristol-Myers Company

In a patent of the Bristol-Myers Company, Menard and Caron (1979) describe preparation of the racemic and of the (+)- and (−)-forms of 2-methylpenem-3-carboxylic acid (20, R = Me). Their synthesis of the racemic acid, starting from 4-acetoxyazetidinone, is in all details identical with that of the Woodward Research Institute (Section III,A,1,a). New, however, is resolution of the racemate into both enantiomers by means of (+)- and (−)-α-methylbenzylamines.

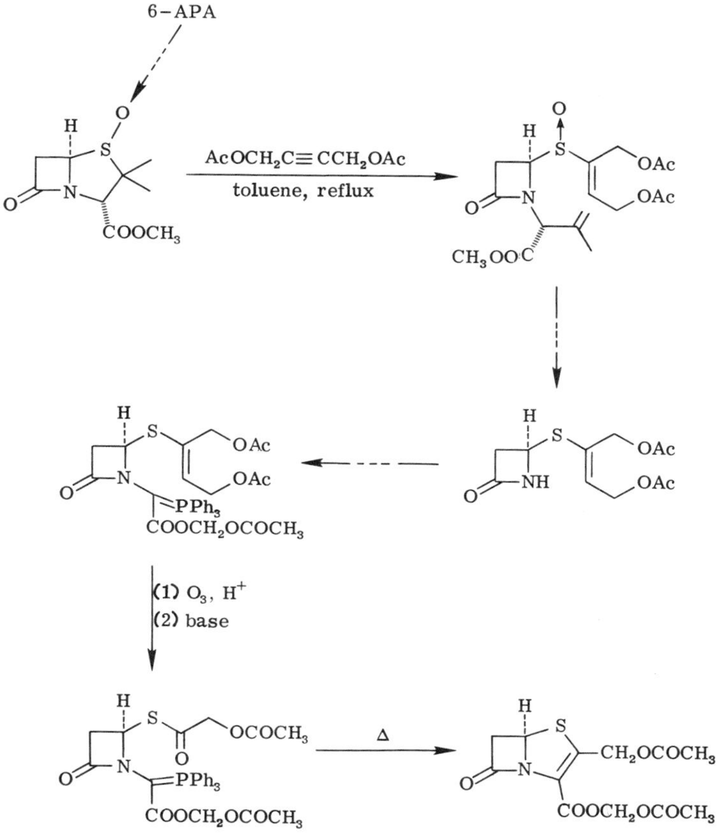

6–APA

AcOCH₂C≡CCH₂OAc

toluene, reflux

(1) O₃, H⁺
(2) base

Δ

56

Two other patents by the Bristol-Myers Company (1980a,b), dealing with 2-substituted and 2,6-disubstituted penem-3-carboxylic acids, are discussed in Section IV,D.

5. The Isopenem Synthesis by Merck

In the recent chemical literature on β-lactams, the interested reader will find still another paper with the word "penems" in its title. It originates from the research laboratories of Merck Sharp & Dohme in Rahway, New Jersey (DiNinno et al., 1979), and describes the realization of an interesting idea of constructing the penem system by closing the five-membered ring between the azetidinone nitrogen and C-3.

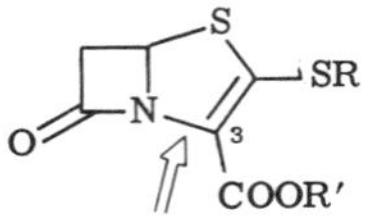

The suggested synthetic route, starting from 4-acetoxyazetidinone (23), consists of only three steps. The exchange reaction between 23 and the sodium thioenolate of alkyl p-nitrobenzyl 1,1-dithiomalonates (57) (a procedure for the preparation of these reagents had to be developed) afforded mixtures of stereoisomeric azetidinone derivatives (58) which in turn, on treatment with N-bromosuccinimide, were transformed into the bromoketene dithioacetals (59).

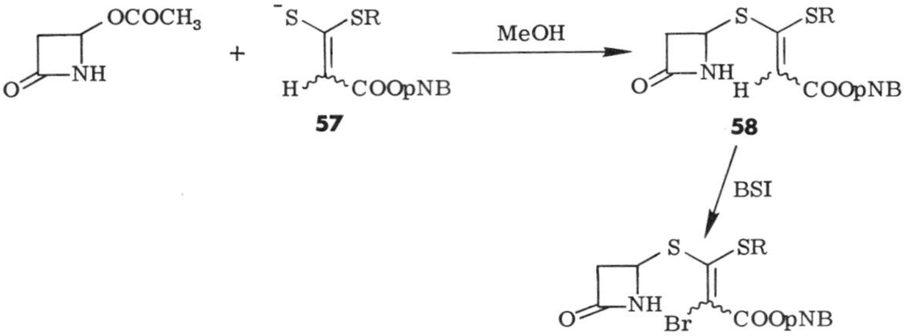

Attempts to cyclize the bromo compounds (59) with lithium diisopropylamide (in tetrahydrofuran at low temperatures) were unsuccessful. When, however, complexed cuprous salts such as $CuI \cdot PBu_3$ or $CuBr \cdot SMe_2$ were used along with the above-mentioned base, β-lactam-containing compounds were isolated in yields of about 40–50%, which were believed to be the desired 2-alkylthiopenem-3-carboxylates. Recently, however, Oida et al. (1980) at the Sankyo Central Research Laboratories in Tokyo found marked discrepancies in the data reported by DiNinno et al. for one of the described compounds (R = Me) with those for p-nitrobenzyl 2-methylthiopenem-3-carboxylate as prepared in Tokyo by the Wittig route (cf. Section III,A,1,a). To clear up the situation, they repeated the Merck synthesis (for R = Me) and submitted the compound thus obtained to an X-ray diffraction analysis. This showed it to be the "isopenem" derivative 60 (R = Me) with a fused isothiazoline ring.

The mechanism of formation of the isopenem system from the bromo compounds (59) is at present a matter of speculation.

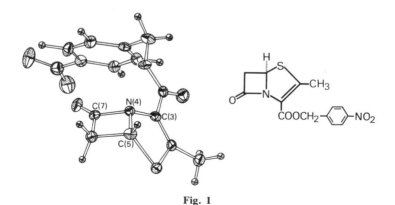

B. Physical Data and Chemical Behavior

1. X-Ray Crystal Structure Analysis

The structure and, with optically active compounds, the absolute configuration of the novel 6-unsubstituted penem acids were corroborated by X-ray diffraction analyses of their esters (Rihs, 1977; Beels *et al.*, 1979b; Pfaendler *et al.*, 1981).

The steric presentation of the molecule of *p*-nitrobenzyl 2-methyl-(5*R*)-penem-3-carboxylate (Fig. 1) as resulting from such a structure determination (Rihs, 1977) reveals, among other interesting features, the pyramidal geometry of the β-lactam nitrogen; the height (0.43 Å) of the

Fig. 1

pyramid formed by the apical N-4 and C-3, C-5, and C-7 lies between the values found for penicillins (0.38–0.40 Å) (Sweet, 1972) and those observed for carbapenems (0.49–0.50 Å) (Albers-Schönberg et al., 1978; Pfaendler et al., 1981). The length of the N-4—C-7 amide bond, with its value of 1.42 Å, substantially exceeds the normal values for amides (1.32–1.34 Å) and also those for cephems (~1.38 Å) but is about the same as that in penicillins.

2. Spectroscopic Data and Stability

The characteristic spectral properties of the penem system as described for 6β-acylamino-substituted compounds (Section II,B) proved typical also for 6-unsubstituted penem-3-carboxylic acids and esters.

In the UV spectra (in EtOH) of 2-alkyl-substituted acids (20, R = alkyl), the long-wavelength maximum lies at about 305–307 nm ($\varepsilon \sim$ 6500) and is shifted to 310 nm in the parent penem acid (20, R = H). Of course, more pronounced shifts result if the substituent in position 2 is conjugated with the penem system, as in 2-phenyl (20, R = Ph; λ_{max} = 323 nm) and 2-ethylmercapto (20, R = SEt; λ_{max} = 325 nm) acids. The long-wavelength maximum is always accompanied by a secondary maximum at 253–260 nm ($\varepsilon \sim$ 3000–3700).

In the IR spectra, the stretching absorption band of the β-lactam carbonyl is at about 5.55–5.60 μm (somewhat higher values and, occasionally, splitting into two distinct bands are found when KBr pellets are used).

The 100-MHz proton magnetic resonance spectra of the acids (20) (in [D_6]DMSO or $CDCl_3$) display a doublet of doublets of H-5 at δ 5.65–5.78 ppm and an ABX system of signals for the two H-6 hydrogens located between δ 3.3 and 3.9 ppm. The coupling constants between H-5 and H-6 are J_{cis} = 4 Hz and J_{trans} = 2 Hz; for the two H-6 hydrogens, the geminal coupling constant of 16 Hz is characteristic.

A remarkable difference between the previously discussed 6β-acyl-aminopenem acids (2) and the 6-unsubstituted compounds (20) was found in the stabilities of the two groups: The 6-unsubstituted acids proved substantially more stable. Whereas the half-lives of the acids (2) in a

	2	20
$t_{1/2}$ (pH 7.4, 37°C)	R = H: <15 min R = CH₃: <60 min	20 hr 100 hr

phosphate buffer of pH 7.4 at 37°C were on the order of minutes, 20–100 hr were typical values for 6-unsubstituted penem-3-carboxylic acids (**20**) (Ernest *et al.*, 1977a).

C. Biological Activity

In sharp contrast to the similarly 6-unsubstituted, biologically inactive penicillanic (**61**) and cephalosporanic (**62**) acids and showing a surprising difference from the only weakly active 6β-acylaminopenem acids (**2**), penem-3-carboxylic acids (**20**) exhibit *in vitro* powerful antibiotic activity against a wide range of microorganisms. In Table II, the minimum inhibitory concentration (MIC) values of five racemic representatives are given in comparison with the corresponding values for cephalexin and penicillin (Lang *et al.*, 1979, 1980).

Also, all other compounds of structure **20**, prepared at the Woodward Research Institute, with different substituents R in position 2 (R = CH_2Ph, CH_2OCOCH_3, CH_2SCH_3, $CH_2CH_2CH_2NH_2$, SCH_2CH_3, $SCH_2CH_2NHCOCH_2$, etc.) were, with some variations in the individual antibiotic spectra, biologically active compounds. In agreement with this are the reports of the Glaxo research group (Cherry *et al.*, 1979) to the effect that the potassium salts of their penem acids (Section III,A,3) exhibit good broad-spectrum antibacterial activity and are stable to the action of certain β-lactamases. Also, the *in vitro* MIC values of various 6-unsubstituted penem acids as described in the patents of Glaxo (Table III), Farmitalia Carlo Erba (Table IV), and the Beecham group (Table V) manifest a high degree of antibacterial activity.

It has been shown in two cases that, as in all known natural β-lactam antibiotics, the above-mentioned biological activity of the acids (**20**) is restricted to the 5*R* enantiomers:

1. The optically active 2-methyl-(5*R*)-penem-3-carboxylic acid, prepared from natural 6-aminopenicillanic acid by a sequence of reactions that preserved the natural *R* configuration on C-5, was tested, along with the (totally synthetic) racemic compound **20** (R = Me), against 24 gram-positive and gram-negative strains. It was found to be twice as active

TABLE II MIC Values (μg/ml) of Racemic 6-Unsubstituted Penem-3-carboxylic Acids[a]

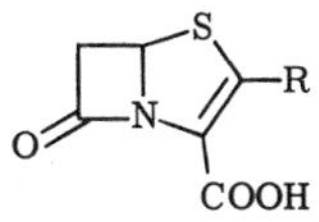

	CH_3	C_6H_5	C_5H_{11}	SC_2H_5	SCH_2CH_2NHAc	Peni-cillin V	Cepha-lexin
	R						
Staphylococcus aureus Smith 14	1	1	0.2	1	4	0.05	1
Staphylococcus aureus 2999	1	4	2	2	32	64	8
Streptococcus pyogenes Aronson K1129	0.5	0.05	0.05	0.5	2	0.05	1
Streptococcus pneumoniae III/84	0.5	0.1	0.05	8	0.5	0.05	0.5
Neisseria meningitidis K1316	0.1	0.1	0.05	8	1	0.5	32
Haemophilus influenzae NCTC 4560	4	4	2	32	16	4	8
Escherichia coli 205	8	8	32	0.5	2	128	8
Salmonella typhimurium 277	4	8	16	0.5	2	64	4
Proteus rettgeri K856	8	4	32	2	>128	>128	128
Pseudomonas aeruginosa K1118	8	—	64	—	—	>128	>128

[a] From Lang *et al.* (1979, 1980).

TABLE III Antimicrobial *in Vitro* Activities of Racemic 2-Substituted Penem-3-carboxylic Acids (**20**)[a]

20

	MIC of the acids (μg/ml)[b]							
Microorganism	a	b	c	d	e	f	g	h
Staphylococcus aureus 853E	0.5	0.5	<0.1	0.5	0.5	<0.1	0.5	1
Micrococcus sp. 1810E	<0.1	0.2	<0.1	0.2	<0.1	<0.1	—	0.2
Escherichia coli 851E	4	4	2	4	2	0.5	31	8
Enterobacter cloacae 1051E	8	16	8	8	8	4	125	16
Enterobacter cloacae 1321E	4	2	2	2	2	0.5	31	8
Klebsiella aerogenes 1522E	8	8	4	4	4	0.5	31	16
Serratia marcescens 1324E	8	62	4	4	8	1	31	8
Hemophylus influenzae 1184E	8	—	2	4	4	1	4	4

[a] From Beels *et al.* (1979a) [Glaxo Group Ltd].
[b] Structures: **a**, R = CH_2CH_2OH; **b**, R = $CH_2CH_2OCOCH_3$; **c**, R = $CH_2CH_2OCONH_2$; **d**, R = CH_2OCH_3; **e**, R = $CH_2CH_2OCH_3$; **f**, R = $CH_2CH_2CH_3$; **g**, R = $CH_2CH_2CH_2CH_3$; **h**, R = CH_3.

as the racemate in 20 cases, whereas equal activity was realized in the remaining 4 instances (Ernest *et al.*, 1979).*

2. In a similar, parallel test with both individual enantiomers and with the racemic form of the simplest penem acid (**20**, R = H) (Section III,A,1,b), the 5*R* enantiomer was found to be highly active, whereas its 5*S* antipode was devoid of any activity against several representative microorganisms (Table VI). The activity of the racemate was accordingly lower than that of the 5*R* acid (Pfaendler *et al.*, 1979).†

An interesting insight into the biological action of the new β-lactam derivatives was obtained from experiments in which their affinity for the penicillin-binding proteins was determined using the method developed by Spratt (1977). It was found that the racemic 2-methyl (**20**, R = Me) and 2-phenylpenem (**20**, R = Ph) acids, as well as the biologically active parent acid (**20**, R = H) of the natural 5*R* series were bound to some of these proteins, whereas the 5*S* enantiomer of the latter showed no

*Similar biological results for the racemic and the 5*R* forms of 2-methylpenem-3-carboxylic acid are given by the Bristol-Myers Company (Menard and Caron, 1979).

†Also, the 5*S* enantiomer of 2-methylpenem-3-carboxylic acid, as described in the Bristol-Myers patent (Menard and Caron, 1979), was found inactive against most strains and displayed only marginal activity against a few sensitive microorganisms.

TABLE IV MIC Values (μg/ml) of Acetoxymethyl Esters of 2-Substituted (5R)-Penem-3-carboxylic Acids Compared to Those of Ampicillin and Cefoxitin[a]

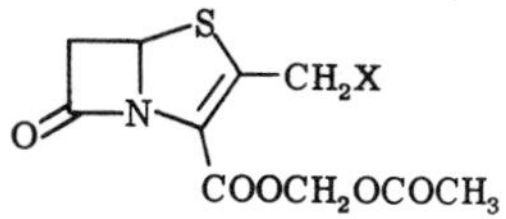

Microorganism	X = OCOCH$_3$	X 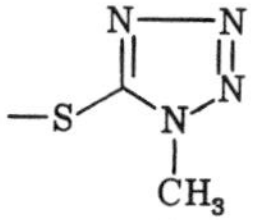 = —S— (triazole, CH$_3$)	Ampicillin	Cefoxitin
Staphylococcus aureus 209P	0.39	0.39	≤0.19	0.78
Staphylococcus aureus 153	1.56	0.78	1.56	0.78
Staphylococcus aureus PV2	0.39	0.78	≤0.19	0.78
Staphylococcus aureux Smith ATCC 13709	≤0.19	0.39	≤0.19	0.78
Streptococcus pyogenes ATCC 12384	3.12	0.78	3.12	1.56
Escherichia coli B	1.56	0.78	0.39	1.56
Escherichia coli V14	1.56	0.78	1.56	3.12
Escherichia coli V23	3.12	0.78	3.12	12.5
Enterobacter sp. V19	12.5	>100	>100	12.5
Klebsiella pneumoniae ATCC 10031	—	3.12	50	0.78
Klebsiella sp. R2	25	—	50	12.5
Proteus vulgaris V15	3.12	6.25	1.56	0.78
Proteus mirabilis V15	0.39	0.78	≤0.19	0.78
Proteus mirabilis 525	3.12	0.78	0.39	1.56
Shigella flexneri	0.39	0.39	≤0.19	0.78
Pseudomonas aeruginosa	3.12	0.39	25	6.25
Salmonella typhimurium	1.56	0.78	0.78	3.12
Salmonella panamae F15	1.56	0.78	0.78	1.56
Salmonella Saint Paul F20	1.56	0.78	0.78	3.12
Salmonella derby F14	3.12	0.78	0.78	3.12
Salmonella montevideo F16	3.12	0.78	0.78	3.12

[a] From Foglio *et al* (1980a) and Franceschi *et al.* (1980) [Farmitalia Carlo Erba Ltd].

TABLE V   Antimicrobial Activities of Racemic 2-Substituted Penem-3-carboxylic Acids[a]

$$\underset{\mathbf{20}}{\text{(penem-3-carboxylic acid, }R\text{, S, N, O, COOH)}}$$

Microorganism	MIC of the acids (μg/ml)[b,c]						
	a	b	c	d	e	f	g
Citrobacter freundii E8	12.5	10	10	25	12.5	5.0	12.5 (0.5)
Enterobacter cloacae N1	12.5	50	100 (62)	–	>50	>50	50 (16)
Escherichia coli 0111	12.5 (16)	10 (31)	25 (8)	25 (31)	5.0 (16)	5.0 (16)	25 (8)
Escherichia coli JT 39	12.5 (31)	10 (62)	50 (31)	100 (250)	>50 (125)	>50 (125)	50 (16)
Klebsiella aerogenes A	6.2 (16)	10 (31)	10 (8)	>100 (62)	25 (16)	50 (62)	50 (8)
Proteus mirabilis C977	25 (31)	25 (62)	10 (8)	25 (31)	12.5 (16)	12.5 (31)	25 (8)
Proteus morganii 1580	50	25	10	>100	>50	>50	>50 (16)
Proteus rettgeri WM16	50	50	50	>100	25	50	>50
Proteus vulgaris WO91	25	50	50	>100	>50	>50	>50
Pseudomonas aeruginosa A	50 (125)	50 (62)	>100 (500)	>100 (>500)	>50 (500)	>50 (>500)	125 (1)
Salmonella typhimurium CT10	12.5	10	25	25	5.0	5.0	12.5
Serratia marcescens US20	25	10	25	100	25	25	25 (16)
Shigella sonnei MB 11967	25	10	50	–	5.0	5.0	12.5 (4)
Bacillus subtilis A	3.1	2.5	2.5	2.5	1.2	1.2	2.5
Staphylococcus aureus Oxford	1.6 (4.0)	2.5 (4.0)	10	2.5 (4.0)	2.5 (2.0)	2.5 (8)	5 (2)
Staphylococcus aureus Russell	3.1 (16)	2.5 (8)	10 (8)	25 (16)	5.0 (8)	12.5 (16)	5 (4)
Staphylococcus aureus 1517	50	25	50 (8)	50	>50	50	>50
Streptococcus faecalis I	>50	100	100	>100	50	50	>50 (62)
Streptococcus pneumoniae CN33	≤0.1	1.0	0.5	0.5	0.2	0.2	0.5
Streptococcus pyogenes CN10	0.4	1.0	2.5	1.0	0.5	0.5	1.25 (1)
Escherichia coli ESS	1.6	10	10	10	2.5	2.5	5 (4)

[a] From Brain (1980) and Perryman (1980) [Beecham Group Ltd].

[b] Structures: **a**, $R = OC_2H_5$; **b**, $R = CH_2OH$; **c**, $R = CH_2OCOCH_3$; **d**, $R = CH_2OCH_2CH_2NHCOCH_3$; **e**, $R = CH_2OCH_2OCH_3$; **f**, $R = CH_2OCH_2NHCOCH_3$; **g**, $R = CH_2NH_2$.

[c] DST agar plus 10% horse blood; values for microtiter using nutrient broth are shown in parentheses. In both cases inoculum consisted of 0.001 ml of a 10^{-2} dilution for gram-positive or a 10^{-4} dilution for gram-negative organisms.

343

TABLE VI Antibacterial *in Vitro* Activities of the Optically Active 5*R*,5*S* and Racemic Forms of Penem-3-carboxylic Acid (**20b**)[a]

	MIC (μg/ml)[b]		
Microorganism	5*R*	Racemic	5*S*
Staphylococcus aureus Smith	4	8	Inactive
Staphylococcus aureus 2999 (resistant)	2	8	Inactive
Escherichia coli 205	2	4	Inactive
Pseudomonas aeruginosa ATCC 12055	4	16	Inactive

[a] From Pfaendler *et al.* (1979).
[b] MIC in VST agar; inoculum ~10^4 cells; pH 7.4.

affinity for any of the penicillin-binding proteins of *Escherichia coli* (Zimmermann, 1978).

IV. Structural Modifications of Penem-3-carboxylic Acids

A. 6-Alkyl and 6,6-Dialkylpenem-3-carboxylic Acids

The occurrence in nature of highly potent antibiotics with an alkyl or α-hydroxyalkyl substituent in position 6 of the 1-carbapenem nucleus (thienamycin, olivanic acid, and compound PS-5; cf. Volume 2, Chapter 4) gave an impetus to attempts to modify the closely related penem system structurally at the same position by synthesizing various 6-alkyl- and 6,6-dialkyl-substituted penem acids.

Some of the procedures developed for the synthesis of 6-unsubstituted penem acids (**20**) (Section III,A,1 and 2) could be successfully adopted for preparation of the (racemic) 6-alkyl- and 6,6-dialkylpenems (Woodward, 1980; Gosteli *et al.*, 1978a).

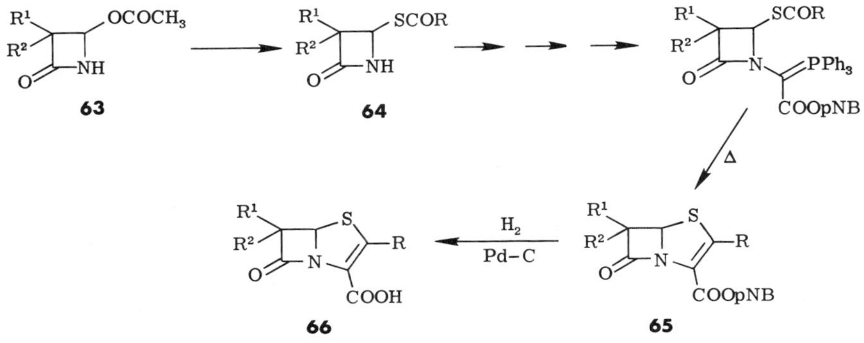

The 3-substituted (or disubstituted) 4-acetoxyazetidinones (63) that are the starting materials of our scheme can be easily obtained by [2 + 2]cycloaddition of 1-alkenyl acetates with chlorosulfonyl isocyanate and by mild hydrolysis of the sensitive N-chlorosulfonylazetidinones (67) thus formed (Clauss *et al.*, 1974).

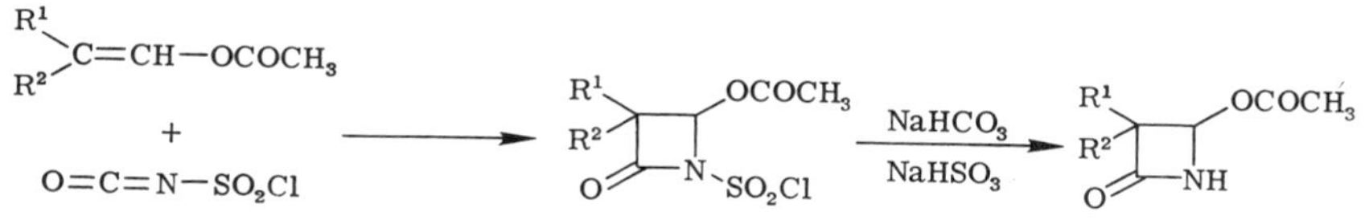

The cycloaddition is highly stereospecific, giving for example, with *cis*-propenyl acetate only the cis-disubstituted azetidinone (63a).

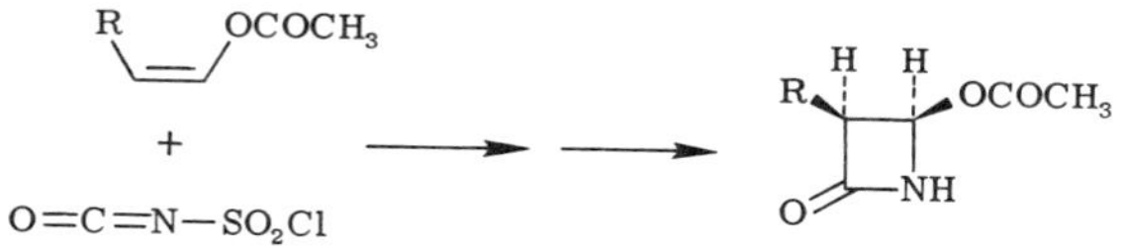

In most cases, the unbranched 1-alkenyl acetates are mixtures of cis and trans isomers and, correspondingly, mixtures of stereomeric 3-alkyl-4-acetoxyazetidinones result. However, for the subsequent exchange reaction with the sulfur nucleophiles, e.g., with anions of the thiocarboxylic acids RCOS⁻, the stereochemistry of the acetoxy precursors (63a,b) is irrelevant, since regardless of the original geometry of the starting material, mainly trans isomers of the 3-alkyl-4-acylthioazetidinones (64b) are formed, suggesting the planar carbonium–immonium ion (68) as a reaction intermediate.

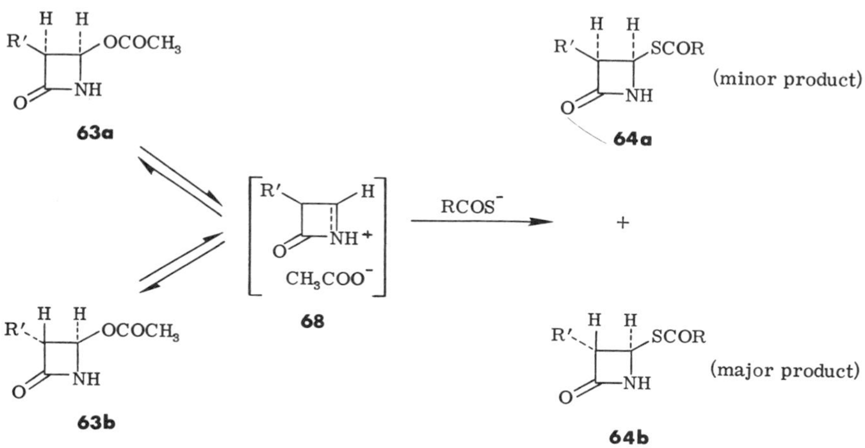

TABLE VII Racemic Penem-3-carboxylic Acids Substituted in Positions 2 and 6[a]

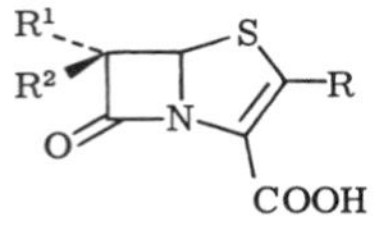

R^1	R^2	R
CH_3	H	CH_3
CH_2CH_3	H	$SCH_2CH_2NHCOCH_3$
H	CH_2CH_3	$SCH_2CH_2NHCOCH_3$
CH_2CH_3	H	$CH_2CH_2CH_2NH_2$
$CH_2C_6H_5$	H	CH_3
$CH(CH_3)_2$	H	CH_3
$CH(CH_3)_2$	H	SCH_2CH_3
OCH_3	H	CH_3
CH_3	CH_3	CH_3
CH_3	CH_3	$n\text{-}C_5H_{11}$

[a] All compounds shown were prepared at the Woodward Research Institute.

For this reason, the trans isomers of the 6-alkylpenem acids (**69**) are more readily accessible than their cis counterparts. In this connection, it is to be remembered that also in thienamycin and in compound PS-5 the carbon side chain at position 6 is disposed in a trans sense.

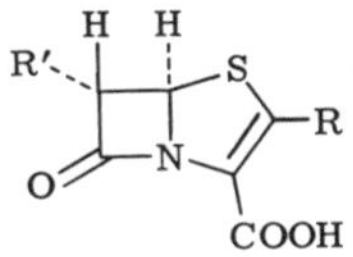

69

Some examples of the racemic penem-3-carboxylic acids substituted in positions 2 and 6 as prepared at the Woodward Research Institute are shown in Table VII.

B. 6α-(α-Hydroxyalkyl)penem-3-carboxylic Acids

In the search for penems with increased biological activity, the α-hydroxyethyl group—the natural side chain of the highly active thienamycin—was thought to be an interesting substituent to examine. The racemic *threo*-6α-(α-hydroxyethyl)penem-3-carboxylic acid (**80a**) having the same stereochemical orientation of the side chain and the same configuration of the chiral center of the hydroxyethyl group as thiena-mycin was synthesized along with its erythro isomer (**80b**) (Woodward, 1980; Pfaendler *et al.*, 1980).

The synthesis involves a novel, versatile bicyclic β-lactam intermediate (**71**) readily prepared from 4-acetoxyazetidinone (**23**) by subsequent base-catalyzed displacement of the acetoxy grouping with 2-mercaptoethanol and ring closure of **70** to the bicycle with acetone dimethylketal using boron trifluoride etherate as catalyst.

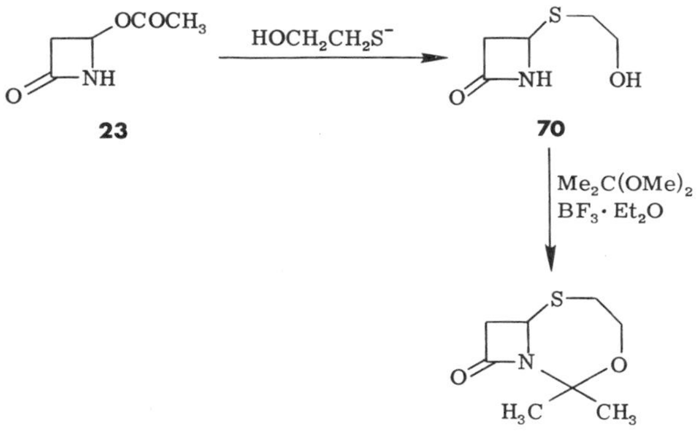

The enolate of the bicyclic intermediate (**71**), prepared *in situ* with lithium diisopropylamide, can be used for introducing various substi-tuents next to the β-lactam carbonyl grouping, Thus, in an aldol-type reaction with acetaldehyde, two trans-oriented (with respect to the seven-membered ring) α-hydroxyethyl derivatives (**72**), epimeric on the carbinol carbon atom, were obtained in a yield of 86%. Without separating the isomers, the hydroxyl group was protected with *p*-nitrobenzyl chloro-formate, and the epimeric carbonates (**73**) thus formed were oxidized on the sulfur atom to give the sulfones (**74**). Subsequent hydrolytic opening of the seven-membered ring gave the β-hydroxyethylsulfonylazetidinones (**75a,b**). At this stage, separation of the epimeric material, by a combi-nation of crystallization and chromatography, was possible, and both pure isomers could be isolated.

By analogy to the mobility of the acetoxy substituent of the azetidinone (**23**), the hydroxyethylsulfonyl grouping of the intermediate (**75a**) was easily displaced by the anion of methyl *cis*-β-mercaptoacrylate, affording compound **76**. With the procedure described for the 6-unsubstituted par-ent penem-3-carboxylic acid (**20**, R = H) (Section III,A,1), the latter intermediate was converted, via **77** → **79**, to the racemic *threo*-6α-(α-

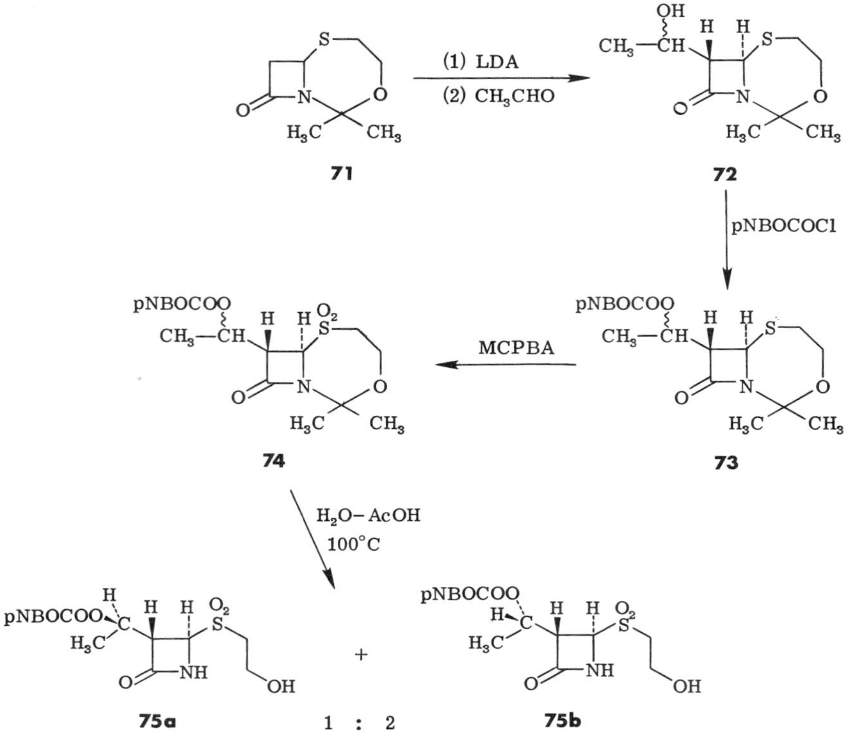

(α-hydroxyethyl)penem-3-carboxylic acid (**80a**). In a similar way, but using the erythro isomer (**75b**), the racemic erythro acid (**80b**) was prepared.

Antimicrobial *in vitro* tests on both acids revealed interesting differences in their biological activity (Section IV,E).

C.   6α-Methoxy-2-methyl-(5*R*)-penem-3-carboxylic Acid

The following synthesis of the optically active 6α-methoxypenem acid (**81**) exemplifies another, rather general, approach to functionalization of position 6 in penems (Gosteli *et al.*, 1980).

With a known procedure, penicillin V was converted to methyl 6-diazopenicillanate (**82**) which, by acid-catalyzed methanolysis, gave methyl 6α-methoxypenicillanate (**83**). In six subsequent steps analogous to the early stages of the synthesis of 6β-acylaminopenem acids (Section II,A), the thiazolidine ring of **83** was degraded and the acetylthioazetidinone (**84**) was formed. Also, the rest of the synthesis of the acid (**81**)

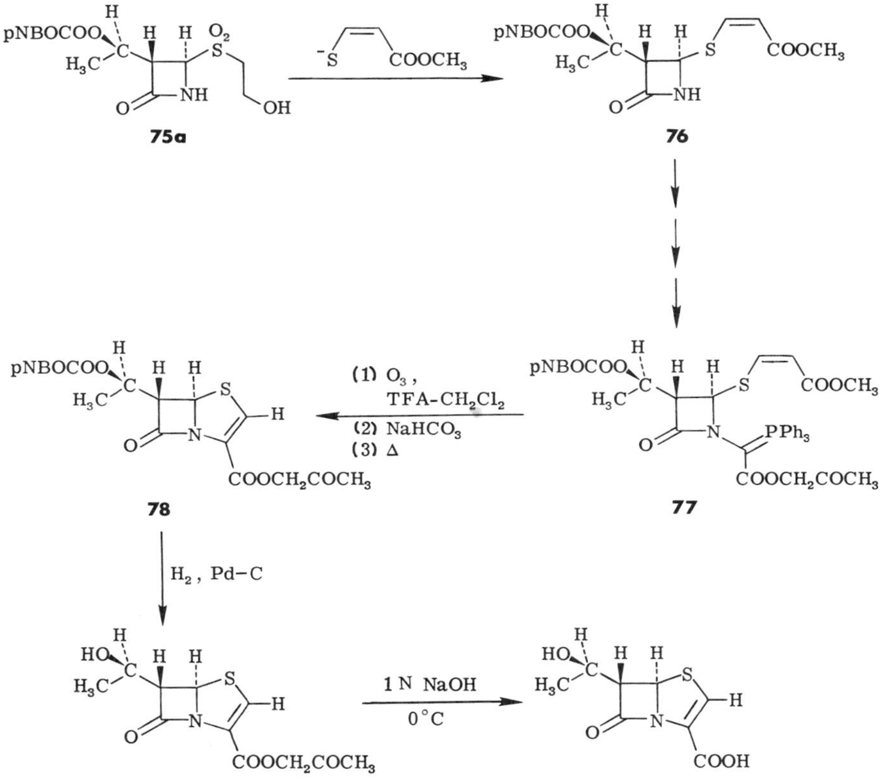

75a → **76**

76 → **77**

78 ← (1) O₃, TFA-CH₂Cl₂ (2) NaHCO₃ (3) Δ ← **77**

78 → H₂, Pd-C → **79**

79 → 1 N NaOH, 0°C → **80a**

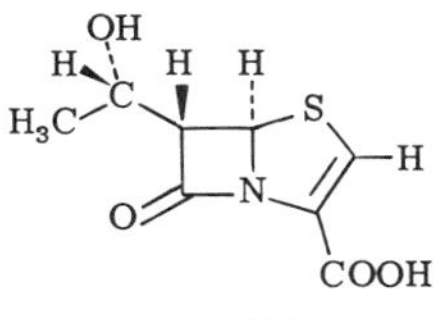

80b

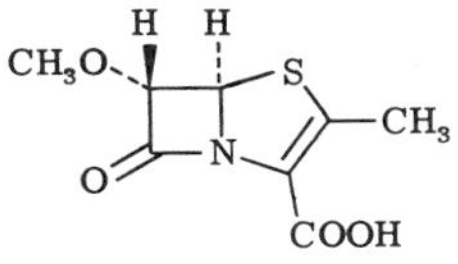

81

followed the general scheme of the penem synthesis as developed at the Woodward Research Institute.

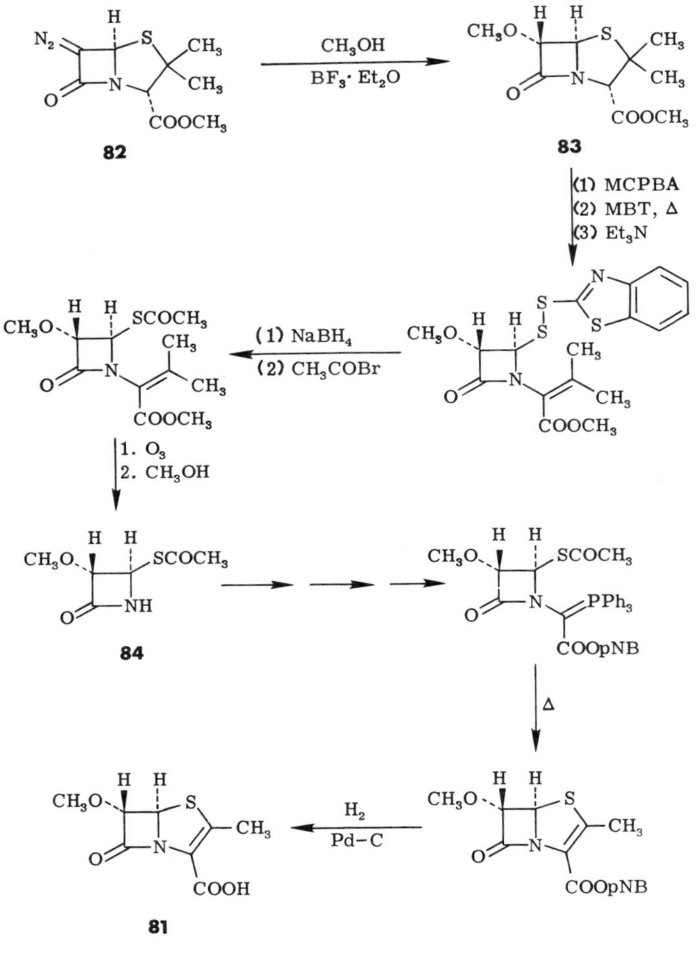

D. Various 2,6-Disubstituted Penem-3-carboxylic Acids

The promising reports—in various lectures of the late R. B. Woodward—on the biological activity of the first synthesized penem acids awoke worldwide interest in this new type of bicyclic β-lactam. Within a short time, great effort was expended at several pharmaceutical companies and at universities in the search for a practical useable penem antibiotic. Some of the work has been published in the form of papers and was discussed in the foregoing sections; another part is now available from the patent literature.

A significant practical contribution was made by the Bristol-Myers Company (1980a,b) whose patents describe the preparation and biological profile of a large number of 2-substituted and 2,6-disubstituted penem-3-carboxylic acids. The synthesis of the bicyclic penem system is based on that of the Woodward Research Institute (Sections III,A, and IV,A). However, several modifications were introduced to make the preparation of various penems possible from common advanced intermediates.

One such modification of the original scheme of Woodward by the Bristol-Myers chemists consists of conversion, by reaction with silver nitrate and pyridine in methanol, of 4-acetylthioazetidinonylphosphorane (**85**) to the silver mercaptide (**86**). The latter common intermediate can be transformed, by acylation with suitable acyl halides, into a multitude of other 4-acylthioazetidinonylphosphoranes (**87**) and, ultimately, into various 2-substituted penems. Instead of the acetylthio compound (**85**), the 4-tritylthioazetidinonylphosphorane (**88**) can be used as well for preparation of the silver mercaptide (**86**); and instead of the silver derivative, a similar mercuric mercaptide may serve as common intermediate in the acylation step.

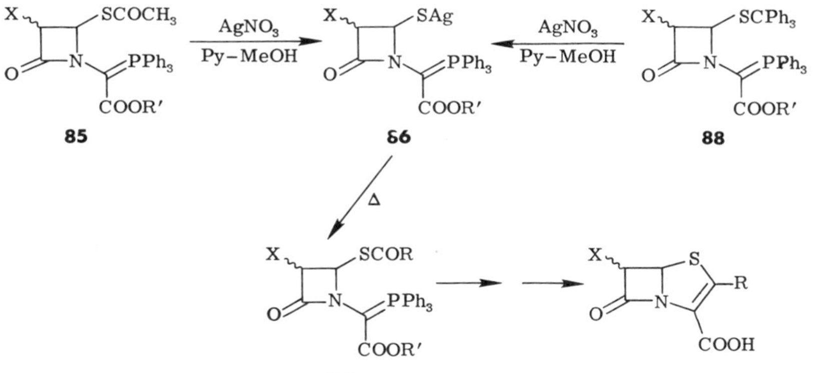

Another enrichment—by the Bristol-Myers chemists—of the methodology for the synthesis of substituted penems is direct introduction of a substituent, e.g., of the α-hydroxyisopropyl grouping, into the C-6 position of a 6-unsubstituted penem acid.

TABLE VIII Antimicrobial *in Vitro* Activities of Racemic 2-Substituted and 2,6-Disubstituted Penem-3-carboxylic Acids[a]

Microorganism	MIC of the acids (µg/ml)							
	a	b	c	d	e	f	g	h
Streptococcus pneumoniae A9585	0.06	0.5	2	1	0.5	0.25	0.004	0.03
Streptococcus pyogenes A9604	0.13	0.5	16	2	4	1	0.004	0.5
Staphylococcus aureus A9537	1	0.5	32	8	4	2	0.008	0.03
Staphylococcus aureus A9537 plus 50% serum	16	16	>32	>63	>63	8	0.06	0.25
Staphylococcus aureus A9606	125	32	2	4	9	4	0.06	0.25
Staphylococcus aureus A15097	>125	>63	8	8	63	8	0.06	0.5
Streptococcus faecalis A20688	125	>63	63	63	125	63	0.5	32
Escherichia coli A15119	16	63	2	32	63	16	0.13	8
Escherichia coli A20 341-1	>125	>63	32	32	125	16	0.13	8
Klebsiella pneumoniae A15130	125	>63	8	63	63	16	0.25	16
Klebsiella species A20468	>125	>63	>63	>125	>125	16	0.5	32
Proteus mirabilis A9900	8	63	4	63	63	32	0.25	2
Proteus vulgaris A21559	63	63	16	63	32	16	0.25	2
Proteus morganii A15153	32	63	8	63	125	32	1	2
Proteus rettgeri A21203	16	63	8	32	32	16	0.25	2
Serratia marcescens A20019	63	63	8	125	63	16	0.5	16
Enterobacter cloacae A9659	125	>63	8	>125	125	32	4	32
Enterobacter cloacae A9656	63	63	8	>125	125	16	0.5	1
Pseudomonas aeruginosa A9843A	125	63	63	>125	>125	>125	16	2
Pseudomonas aeruginosa A21213	125	63	>63	>125	>125	>125	125	—

[a] From Bristol-Myers Company (1980a,b).

[b] Structure: **a**, X = H, R = $CH_2CH_2PO(OCH_3)_2$; **b**, X = H, R = $CH_2CH_2PO(OCH_3)_2$; **c**, X = H, R = $CH_2OCOCH_2NH_2$; **d**, X = CH_3COOCH_2, R = CH_3; **e**, X = CH_3S, R = CH_3; **f**, X = $CH_3CH(OH)$ (R, trans), R = CH_3; **g**, X = $CH_3CH(OH)$ (R, trans), R = CH_3; **h**, X = $CH_3CH(OH)$ (R, trans), R = CH_2NH_2.

⬦···NH_2; **h**, X = $CH_3CH(OH)$ (R, trans), R = CH_2NH_2.

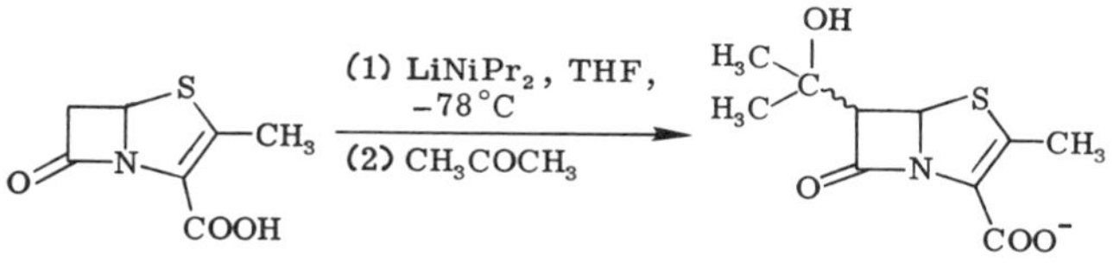

In most cases, however, the biologically interesting α-hydroxyalkyl substituents (Section IV,E) are introduced at an earlier stage of the synthesis (e.g., **90** → **91**).

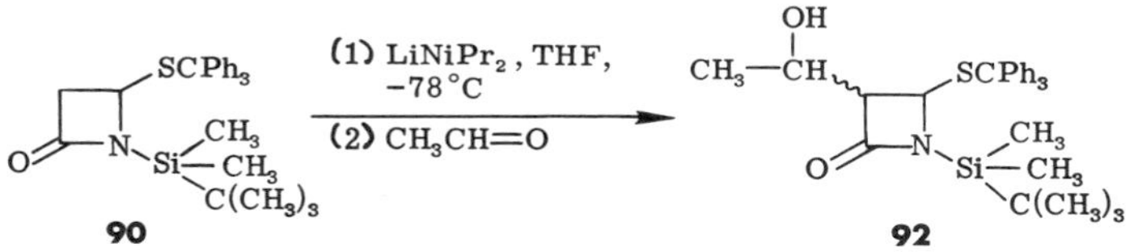

With the use of these and similar methods, a number of penem acids, some of them with promising biological properties, were prepared at the Bristol-Myers laboratories (Table VIII).

The contributions of several other pharmaceutical companies are characterized by extension of the family of penem acids to include new members rather than by innovations in the preparative methodology. Tables IX–XI represent a selection of such compounds and their biological properties as described in various patent applications.

On the other hand, two more original syntheses of 2-substituted 6-acylaminopenem-3-carboxylic esters were developed in addition to that of Woodward (cf. Section II,A). In one of them, the chemists of the Glaxo research laboratories converted penicillin G to the *p*-nitrobenzyl esters of 2-methyl-6β-phenacetamidopenem-3-carboxylic acid (**92**) and of its 5*S* epimer (**93**) (Betty *et al.*, 1980). Their multistep scheme is in principle based on the Glaxo synthesis of 6-unsubstituted penems (cf. Section III,A).

An interesting approach to 2-alkoxy-substituted 6β-acylaminopenems was chosen by the group of L. Ghosez in Louvain. The essential part of their synthesis is formation of the bicyclic β-lactam thiolactone (**95**) from the corresponding penicillin-derived mercapto acid (**94**) and the conversion of **95**, with diazomethane, to the 6β-phenacetamido-2-methoxypenem ester (**96**) (Marchand-Brynaert *et al.*, 1980).

TABLE IX MIC Values (µg/ml) of Racemic 6-Substituted 2-Ethylpenem-3-carboxylic Acids[a]

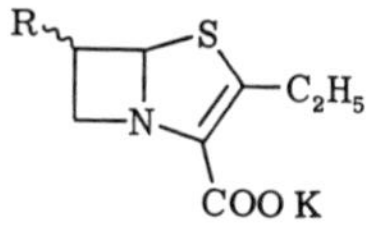

Microorganism	R			α-CH$_2$—CH— (epoxide O)		β-CH$_2$—CH— (epoxide O)	
	H	α-OCH$_3$	β-OCH$_3$	Isomer I	Isomer II	Isomer I	Isomer II
Staphylococcus aureus 853E	<0.1	0.5	16	0.2	4	0.5	2
Escherichia coli TEM 1193E	62	31	250	2	62	62	16
Escherichia coli 1507E	4	31	62	2	62	8	8
Enterobacter cloacae P99 1051E	4	31	125	8	125	62	62
Enterobacter cloacae 1321E	2	31	62	2	62	16	16
Klebsiella aerogenes K1 1082E	>250	31	>250	2	62	>250	>125
Klebsiella aerogenes 1522E	4	31	125	2	62	16	8

[a] From Foxton *et al.* (1980) [Glaxo group].

TABLE X MIC Values of (5R,6S)-2-(2-Aminoethylthio)-6-[(R)-1-hydroxyethyl]penem-3-carboxylic Acid[a]

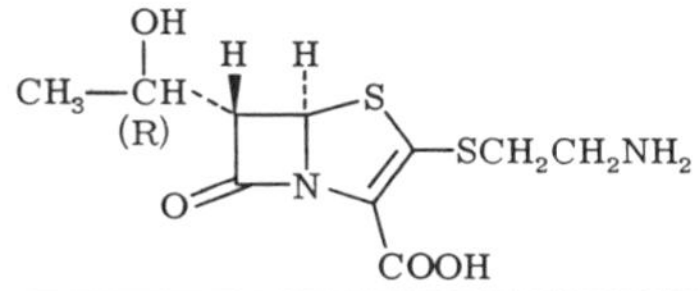

Microorganism	MIC (μg/ml)
Staphylococcus aureus 209P	0.012
Staphylococcus aureus 56	0.012
Escherichia coli NIHJ	0.4
Escherichia coli 609	0.8
Shigella flexneri 2A	0.8
Pseudomonas aeruginosa	6.2
Klebsiella pneumoniae 806	0.8
Klebsiella pneumoniae 846	0.8
Proteus vulgaris	6.2
Salmonella enteritidis	1.5

[a] From Ohki *et al.* (1980) [Sankyo Company, Ltd.].

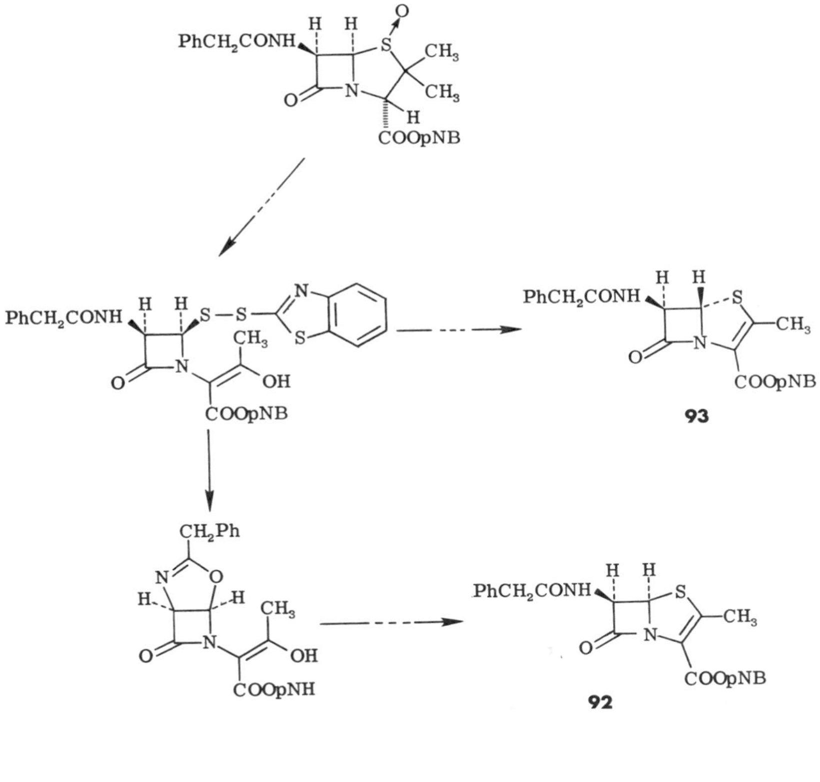

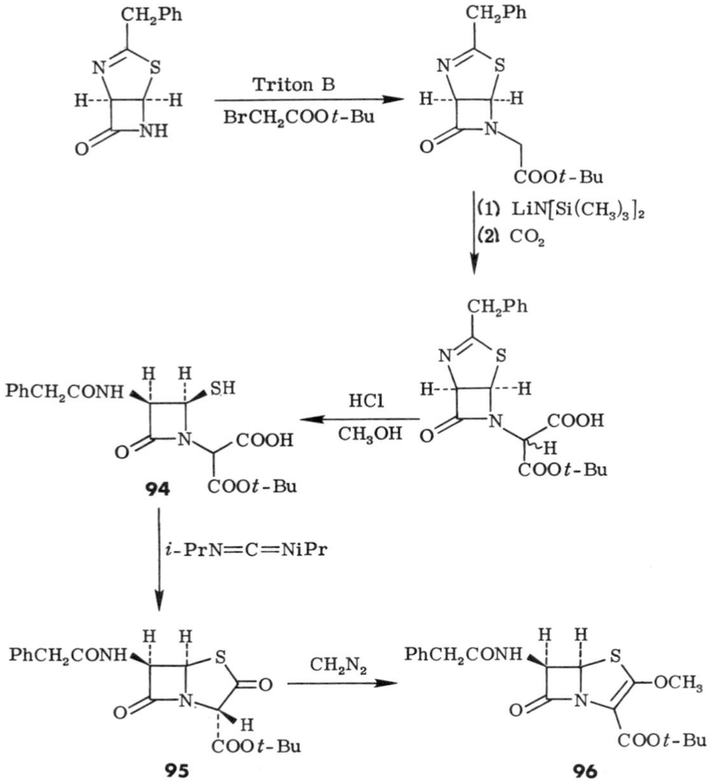

Scheme (reactions):

CH₂Ph thiazoline azetidinone (H---, ---H, O, NH) → Triton B, BrCH₂COO*t*-Bu → CH₂Ph thiazoline azetidinone N-CH₂ COO*t*-Bu

(1) LiN[Si(CH₃)₃]₂
(2) CO₂

↓

CH₂Ph structure with COOH and COO*t*-Bu

HCl, CH₃OH ←

PhCH₂CONH ... SH / N, COOH, COO*t*-Bu **94**

i-PrN=C=NiPr ↓

PhCH₂CONH ... S=O, N, COO*t*-Bu **95**

CH₂N₂ →

PhCH₂CONH ... S—OCH₃, N, COO*t*-Bu **96**

TABLE XI   MIC Values (µg/ml) of 2-(2-Ethoxyethylthio)-penem-3-carboxylic Acids[a,b]

Microorganism	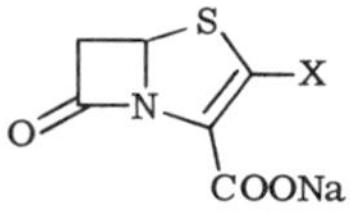 Racemic	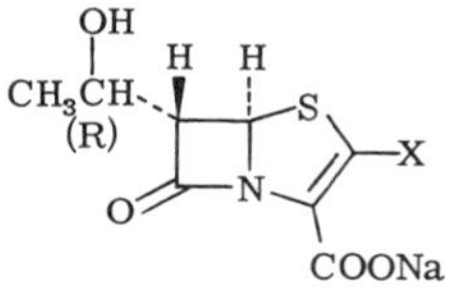 (R) CH₃CH(OH)– COONa	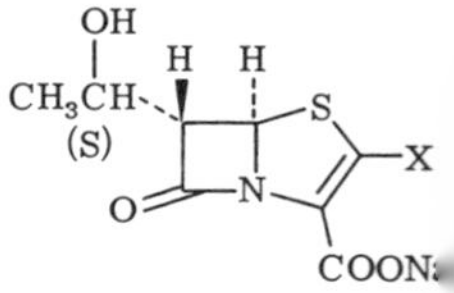 (S) CH₃CH(OH)– COONa
Staphylococcus aureus 209P	0.2	0.05	0.8
Staphylococcus aureus 56	0.8	0.1	1.5
Escherichia coli NIHJ	0.4	1.5	12.5
Escherichia coli 609	200	1.5	12.5
Shigella flexneri	0.4	0.4	3.1
Pseudomonas aeruginosa	>200	>100	>200
Klebsiella pneumoniae	1.5	0.8	6.2
Klebsiella 846	6.2	6.2	100
Proteus vulgaris	6.2	0.4	12.5
Salmonella enteritidis	0.4	0.8	6.2

[a] From Oida (1980) [Sankyo Company, Ltd.].
[b] X = SCH₂CH₂NH₂.

E. Biology and Structure–Activity Relationships in 6-Substituted Penem Acids

The penem family is still too young and the evaluation of its biological potential at this moment too incomplete to allow any far-reaching conclusions about structure–activity relations. Only a few generalizations are now possible.

The 6-monoalkyl-substituted penem acids—most of them the trans-oriented 6α isomers—display in general interesting *in vitro* activity, however, aralkyl and bulky alkyl substituents at this position exert a rather unfavorable effect on the activity spectrum.

The 6,6-dialkylpenem acids ($\mathbf{66}$, $R^1 = R^2 = Me$, $R = Me$ or C_5H_{11}) were found inactive against both gram-positive and gram-negative microorganisms. Since the 2,6,6-trimethylpenem-3-carboxylic acid proved "indefinitely" stable in a phosphate buffer of pH 7.4 at 37°C, the lack of antimicrobial activity of this and similar compounds may be connected with too low a reactivity of their β-lactam system because of a high steric hindrance of its carbonyl grouping (Woodward, 1980). On the other hand, the latter compound exhibited inhibition of β-lactamases (from *Pseudomonas aeruginosa* 18SA and *Enterobacter* P99) (Regos, 1977).

In contrast, too high a β-lactam reactivity may also be detrimental to the measured biological activity if it makes the compound unstable under the conditions of its application. This seems to be the case with the previously discussed 6β-acylaminopenem acids (**2**) and, to some extent, with 6α-methoxy-2-methyl-(5R)-penem-3-carboxylic acid (**81**). Low half-life values of penem acids are usually paralleled by low activity values.

TABLE XI (Continued)

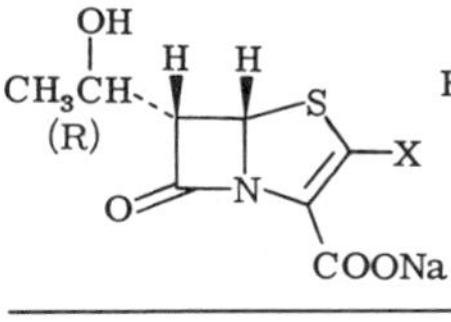 (R) COONa	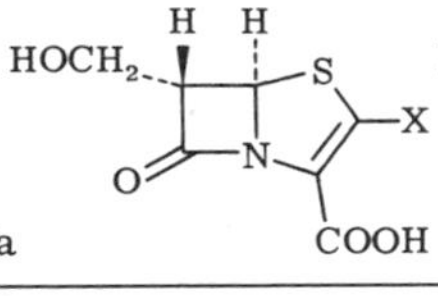 COOH	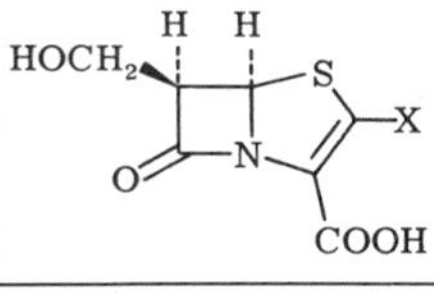 COOH	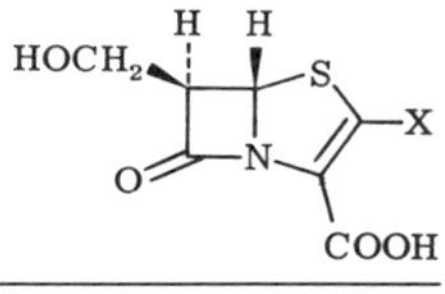 COOH
6.2	0.02	0.4	12.5
12.5	0.1	1.5	50
>200	1.5	3.1	>100
>200	3.1	25	>100
100	3.1	3.1	>100
>200	25	>100	>100
200	3.1	3.1	>100
>200	1.5	3.1	>100
100	6.2	25	>100
100	3.1	3.1	>100

TABLE XII Antibacterial *in Vitro* Activities of the Racemic 6α-(α-Hydroxyethyl)penem-3-carboxylic Acids **80a** and **80b** and of the Racemic Parent Acid **20** (R = H)[a]

Microorganism	MIC (μg/ml)[b]		
	(20, R = H)	(80a)	(80b)
Staphylococcus aureus 10B	8	1	64
Staphylococcus aureus 2999 (penicillin-resistant)	8	1	64
Neisseria gonorrhoeae	8	0.5	32
Escherichia coli 205	4	8	128
Escherichia coli 205 Richmond plus TEM (β-lactamase-producing)	32	8	128
Salmonella typhimurium 277	4	4	64
Enterobacter cloacae P 99	>128	8	>128
Pseudomonas aeruginosa ATCC 12055	16	64	>128

[a] From Pfaendler *et al.* (1980).
[b] MIC in VST agar; inoculum ~10^4 cells; pH 7.4.

Thus a delicate balance between reactivity of the β-lactam system on the one hand and reasonable stability on the other seems to be of importance for high biological activity in this class of compounds. To find such a fortunate balance in a penem, the possibility of modifying both positions C-2 and C-6 offers chemists an inexhaustible number of combinations to test. No clear preferences seem to be obvious at present, and the choice is left to the individual. However, judging from the available data, some workers believe that combination of a polar substituent at position 2 with an α-hydroxyalkyl (or similar) substitution at position 6 might be a good starting point (Tables VIII–XII).

The chances of finding a useful antibiotic among the penems are good, but in the search for it the perseverance and intuition of chemists supported by better knowledge of the penems by biologists will probably be more important than any current oversimplifying structure–activity rules. The case of the two *trans*-(α-hydroxyethyl)penem acids **80a** and **80b**, differing structurally only in the configuration of the chiral center of their hydroxyethyl side chains but very different in their biological activity (Table XII), clearly demonstrates how difficult it is to formulate any structure–activity rules based solely on simple chemical reasoning.

References

Albers-Schönberg, G., Arison, B. H., Kaczka, E., Kahan, F. M., Kahan, J. S., Lago, B., Malese, W. M., Rhodes, R. E., and Smith, J. L. (1976). *Intersci. Conf. Antimicrob. Agents Chemother., 16th, Chicago, Ill.* Pap. No. 229. (Abstr.)

Albers-Schönberg, G., Arison, B. H., Hensens, O. D., Hirshfield, J., Hoogsteen, K., Kaczka, E. A., Rhodes, R. E., Kahan, J. S., Kahan, F. M., Ratcliffe, R. W., Walton, E., Ruswinkle, L. J., Morin, R. B., and Christensen, B. G. (1978). *J. Am. Chem. Soc.* **100**, 6491.

Beels, C. M. D., Cocker, J. D., Ramsay, M. V. J., and Watson, N. S. (1979a). Glaxo Group Ltd., European Patent 0 000 636.

Beels, C. M. D., Abu-Rabie, M. S., Murray-Rust, P., and Murray-Rust, J. (1979b). *J.C.S. Chem. Commun.* p. 665.

Betty, S., Davies, H. G., and Kitchin, J. (1980). *Recent Adv. Chem. β-Lactam Antibiot.*, Spec. Publ. No. 38, p. 349. R. Soc. Chem., London.

Brain, E. G. (1980). Beecham Group Ltd., British Patent 2 042 508A.

Bristol-Myers Company (1980a). German Offenlegungsschrift 2950913.

Bristol-Myers Company (1980b). German Offenlegungsschrift 2950898.

Cheney, L. C., Godfrey, J. C., Crast, L. B., Jr., and Luttinger, J. R. (1966). Bristol-Myers Company, U.S. Patent 3,284,451.

Cherry, P. C., Newall, C. E., and Watson, N. S. (1979). *J.C.S. Chem. Commun.* p. 663.

Cherry, P. C., Evans, D. N., Newall, C. E., and Watson, N. S. (1980). *Tetrahedron Lett.* p. 561.

Christensen, B. G., and DiNinno, F. P. (1978). Merck and Company, Inc., European Patent 0 002 210.

Clauss, K., Grimm, D., and Prossel, G. (1974). *Justus Liebigs Ann. Chem.* p. 539.

Crowfoot, D., Bunn, C. W., Rogers-Low, D. W., and Turner-Jones, A. (1949). *In* "The Chemistry of Penicillin" (H. T. Clarke, J. R. Johnson, and R. Robinson, eds.), p. 310. Princeton Univ. Press, Princeton, New Jersey.

DiNinno, F., Linek, E. V., and Christensen, B. G. (1979). *J. Am. Chem. Soc.* **101**, 2210.

Ernest, I., Gosteli, J., and Woodward, R. B. (1976). Unpublished results.

Ernest, I., Lang, M., Prasad, K., Pfaendler, H. R., Gosteli, J., and Woodward, R. B. (1977a). Unpublished results.

Ernest, I., Gosteli, J., and Woodward, R. B. (1977b). German Offenlegungsschrift 2,655,298.

Ernest, I., Gosteli, J., Greengrass, C. W., Holick, W., Jackman, D. E., Pfaendler, H. R., and Woodward, R. B. (1978). *J. Am. Chem. Soc.* **100**, 8214.

Ernest, I., Gosteli, J., and Woodward, R. B. (1979). *J. Am. Chem. Soc.* **101**, 6310.

Foglio, M., Franceschi, G., Scarafile, C., Arcamone, F., and Sanfilippo, A. (1980a). Farmitalia Carlo Erba Ltd., Belgian Patent 881,862.

Foglio, M., Franceschi, G., Scarafile, C., and Arcamone, F. (1980b). *J.C.S. Chem. Commun.* p. 70.

Foxton, M. W., Newall, C. E., and Ward, P. (1980). *Recent Adv. Chem. β-Lactam Antibiot.*, Spec. Publ. No. 38, p. 281. R. Soc. Chem., London.

Franceschi, G., Foglio, M., Arcamone, F., Sanfilippo, A., and Schioppacassi, G. (1980). *J. Antibiot.* **33**, 453.

Gosteli, J., Ernest, I., Lang, M., and Woodward, R. B. (1978a). European Patent 0 000 258.

Gosteli, J., Ernest, I., and Woodward, R. B. (1978b). German Offenlegungsschrift 2,819,655.

Gosteli, J., Holick, W., Lang, M., and Woodward, R. B. (1980). *Recent Adv. Chem.* β-*Lactam Antibiot.*, Spec. Publ. No. 38, p. 359. R. Soc. Chem., London.
Heusler, K., and Woodward, R. B. (1969). German Offenlegungsschrift 1,935,970.
Howarth, T., Brown, A. G., and King, T. J. (1976). *J.C.S. Chem. Commun.* p. 266.
Kahan, J. S., Kahan, F. M., Goegelman, R., Currie, S. A., Jackson, M., Stapley, E. O., Miller, T. W., Miller, A. K., Hendlin, D., Mochales, S., Hernandez, S., and Woodruff, H. B. (1976). *Intersci. Conf. Antimicrob. Agents Chemother., 16th, Chicago, Ill.* Pap. No. 277. (Abstr.)
Kamiya, T., Teraji, T., Hashimoto, M., Nakaguchi, O., and Oku, T. (1973). *Tetrahedron Lett.* p. 3001.
Lang, M., Prasad, K., Holick, W., Gosteli, J., Ernest, I., and Woodward, R. B. (1979). *J. Am. Chem. Soc.* **101,** 6296.
Lang, M., Prasad, K., Gosteli, J., and Woodward, R. B. (1980). *Helv. Chim. Acta* **63,** 1093.
Lombardi, P., Franceschi, G., and Arcamone, F. (1979). *Tetrahedron Lett.* p. 3777.
Lombardi, P., Franceschi, G., and Arcamone, F. (1980). Farmitalia Carlo Erba Ltd., German Offenlegungsschrift 3,012,975.
McCombie, S. W. (1980). Schering Corporation, European Patent 0 013 662.
Marchand-Brynaert, J., Ghosez, L., and Cossement, E. (1980). *Tetrahedron Lett.* p. 3085.
Menard, M., and Caron, G. (1979). Bristol-Myers Company, U.S. Patent 4,155,912.
Ohki, E., Oida, S., Yoshida, A., Hayashi, T., and Sugawara, S. (1980). Sankyo Company, German Offenlegungsschrift 3,013,997.
Oida, S. (1980). *Recent Adv. Chm.* β-*Lactam Antibiot.*, Spec. Publ. No. 38, p. 330. R. Soc. Chem., London.
Oida, S., Yoshida, A., Hayashi, T., Takeda, N., Nishimura, T., and Ohki, E. (1980). *J. Antibiot.* **33,** 107.
Perryman, B. N. J. (1980). Beecham Group Ltd., European Patent 0 013 067.
Pfaendler, H. R., Gosteli, J., and Woodward, R. B. (1979). *J. Am. Chem. Soc.* **101,** 6306.
Pfaendler, H. R., Gosteli, J., and Woodward, R. B. (1980). *J. Am. Chem. Soc.* **102,** 2039.
Pfaendler, H. R., Gosteli, J., Woodward, R. B., and Rihs, G. (1981). *J. Am. Chem. Soc.* **103,** 4526.
Regos, J. (1977). Res. Dep., Pharm. Div., CIBA-Geigy Ltd. Unpublished results.
Rihs, G. (1977). Phys. Dep., CIBA-Geigy Ltd. Unpublished results.
Spratt, B. G. (1977). *Eur. J. Biochem.* **72,** 341.
Sweet, R. M. (1972). *In* "Cephalosporins and Penicillins: Chemistry and Biology" (E. H. Flynn, ed.), p. 280. Academic Press, New York.
Sweet, R. M., and Dahl, L. F. (1970). *J. Am. Chem. Soc.* **92,** 5489.
Tipper, D. J., and Strominger, J. L. (1965). *Proc. Natl. Acad. Sci. U.S.A.* **54,** 1133.
Woodward, R. B. (1949). *In* "The Chemistry of Penicillin" (H. T. Clarke, J. R. Johnson, and R. Robinson, eds.), p. 440. Princeton Univ. Press, Princeton, New Jersey.
Woodward, R. B. (1975). *Swed. Chem. Soc., Stockholm.* Unpublished lecture.
Woodward, R. B. (1977a). *Acta Pharm. Suec.* **14,** 23.
Woodward, R. B. (1977b). *In* "Recent Advances in the Chemistry of β-Lactam Antibiotics" (J. Elks, ed.), Spec. Publ. No. 28, p. 167. Chem. Soc., London.
Woodward, R. B. (1980). *Philos. Trans. R. Soc. London, Ser. B* **289,** 239.
Woodward, R. B., Heusler, K., Ernest, I., Burri, K., Friary, R. J., Haviv, F., Oppolzer, W., Paioni, R., Syhora, K., Wenger, R., and Whitesell, J. K. (1977). *Nouv. J. Chim.* **1,** 85.
Zimmermann, W. (1978). Res. Dep., Pharm. Div., CIBA-Geigy Ltd. Unpublished results.

6

Clavulanic Acid

PETER C. CHERRY AND CHRISTOPHER E. NEWALL

Chemistry and Biology of
β-Lactam Antibiotics, Vol. 2

I. Introduction

β-Lactamases are a major cause of bacterial resistance to penicillins and cephalosporins. They have been studied extensively and were classified by Richmond and Sykes (1973), who distinguished several classes according to their substrate and inhibition profiles. Subsequently, Sykes and Matthew (1976) classified gram-negative β-lactamases into two groups, chromosomally mediated β-lactamases and enzymes specified by R plasmids. The latter, notably class III β-lactamases such as the TEM-1 enzyme, are now of major clinical importance (Simpson *et al.,* 1980).

Bacterial resistance to antibiotics caused by these enzymes may be overcome in one of two ways—by the use of antibiotics that are stable to β-lactamases or by the coadministration of a β-lactamase inhibitor and a conventional β-lactam antibiotic such as ampicillin. The former strategy led to the development of cefamycins, such as cefoxitin, and alkoximino cephalosporins, such as cefuroxime. The second approach led to the use of β-lactamase-stable penicillins, e.g., methicillin and cloxacillin, as competitive enzyme inhibitors. Unfortunately, the protection afforded to sensitive substrates by these compounds was generally poor, and a search began for more effective agents.

A number of β-lactamases may be obtained in a relatively pure state, and thus it was possible to devise screening procedures for detecting and evaluating inhibitors. A recent example of such a screen uses the β-lactamase-sensitive chromogenic cephalosporin nitrocefin (Glaxo 87/312) (Uri *et al.,* 1978). During the early 1970s several β-lactamase inhibitors were reported; these were obtained from both synthetic and natural sources, and most were competitive inhibitors with little useful activity *in vivo*. However, in 1975 Beecham described a novel, potent inhibitor of β-lactamases that was effective synergistically with ampicillin or cephaloridine against β-lactamase-producing strains of gram-positive and gram-negative bacteria (Ger. Off. 2,517,316; Howarth *et al.,* 1976; Brown *et al.,* 1976a). This compound was clavulanic acid (**1**), the first example of a naturally occurring compound containing the clavam (1-oxadethia-penam) ring system (**2**, R = H).

II. Occurrence, Isolation, and Biological Activity of Clavulanic Acid

Clavulanic acid (MM 14151, BRL 14151) was isolated from *Streptomyces clavuligerus* NRRL 3585 (ATCC 27064) during a screening program which also afforded the olivanic acids MM 4550 and MM 13902 from *Streptomyces olivaceus* (Brown *et al., 1976a*). Another publication (Ger. Off. 2,604,697) has revealed that Glaxo independently isolated clavulanic acid from *S. clavuligerus*. The methyl ester of a compound isolated from *Streptomyces jumonjinensis* corresponds to methyl clavulanate (Neth. Pat. Appl. 76,03818), and *Streptomyces katsurahamanus* has also been reported to provide clavulanic acid (Jpn. Pat. Appl. 53,-104,796). The β-hydroxypropionyl derivative (3) of clavulanic acid has been isolated from *S. clavuligerus* fermentation (Ger. Off. 2,708,047).

Fermentation of *S. clavuligerus* may be conducted conventionally, as described by Nagarajan (1972), and clavulanic acid may be recovered from the broth in a number of ways. In one method the harvested culture liquor is clarified by centrifugation, chilled, and treated with *n*-butanol. The mixture is adjusted to pH 2 and stirred for several minutes; the organic phase is then stirred with Norit GSX carbon. After removal of the carbon the solution is diluted with deionized water and adjusted to pH 7 with sodium hydroxide. Concentration of the aqueous phase under vacuum and subsequent lyophilization afford crude sodium clavulanate. This may be partially purified by ion-exchange chromatography or converted directly to the benzyl ester by reaction with benzyl bromide in dimethylformamide (DMF). The benzyl clavulanate so formed may then be purified further by chromatography. An alternative isolation of benzyl clavulanate involves concentration and lyophilization of the culture filtrate; the residual solid, reported to contain ~1% w/w sodium clavulanate, is suspended in dry DMF and converted to benzyl clavulanate which is purified by chromatography as before (Ger. Off. 2,517,316).

An alternative procedure involves the isolation of lithium clavulanate (Ger. Off. 2,604,697). Thus the fermentation broth is adjusted to pH 5.45 with sulfuric acid, clarified by filtration, and applied to a column of Pittsburgh CAL charcoal. The column is eluted with aqueous acetone, and the eluate is concentrated under reduced pressure and loaded onto a column of IRA 68 ion-exchange resin (chloride form) which is eluted with 5% w/v aqueous lithium chloride. The eluate is concentrated under reduced pressure and stored at 4°C, whereupon crystals of lithium clavulanate are deposited.

Clavulanic acid is a progressive inhibitor of a wide range of β-lactamases including staphylococcal penicillinases and the enzymes identified by Richmond and Sykes (1973) as classes II, III, IV, and V. Many of these compounds are inhibited at very low concentrations, 50% inhibition (I_{50}) values often being less than 0.1 μg/ml (Reading and Cole, 1977; Hunter *et al.*, 1978). Clavulanic acid acts synergistically with β-lactamase-sensitive penicillins and cephalosporins, and in many instances clavulanic acid concentrations of 5 μg/ml or less decrease the minimum inhibitory concentrations (MICs) of these antibiotics against normally resistant bacteria to therapeutically useful levels. The synergy mainly results from the protection afforded to the sensitive antibiotic against inactivation by β-lactamases rather than by a contribution from the modest broad-spectrum antibacterial activity of clavulanic acid itself (MICs generally in the range 31–125 μg/ml). Good serum levels of clavulanic acid are observed in laboratory animals following subcutaneous or intramuscular administration. Oral absorption is good in several animal species, and in humans several pharmacokinetic parameters are reported to be similar to those of amoxicillin. Extensive clinical studies on a combination of clavulanic acid with amoxicillin have been made.

Three other bicyclic β-lactams structurally related to clavulanic acid have been isolated from *S. clavuligerus*. These are 2-hydroxymethylclavam (**2**, R = CH₂OH), 2-formyloxymethylclavam (**2**, R = CH₂OCHO), and clavam-2-carboxylic acid (**2**, R = CO₂H, isolated as its methyl ester); they possess antifungal activity against a variety of animal and plant pathogens (Belg. Pat. 855,467; Brown *et al.*, 1979).

III. Structure Determination and Chemical Degradation of Clavulanic Acid

The structure of clavulanic acid (**4**) was determined independently in at least two laboratories (Beecham and Glaxo) by a combination of spectroscopy and chemical transformations before being confirmed by X-ray analyses.

The mass spectrum of the methyl ester (**5**) derived from clavulanic acid shows a molecular ion corresponding to the empirical formula $C_9H_{11}NO_5$ with fragments attributable to the loss of hydroxyl from the allylic alcohol and of ketene from the β-lactam ring (Howarth *et al.*, 1976; Brown *et al.*, 1977a). Prominent absorptions at 1800, 1750, and 1695 cm^{-1} in the infrared (IR) spectrum of the ester are assigned to the highly strained β-lactam, the ester, and the enol ether, respectively. The ¹H nuclear magnetic resonance (NMR) spectrum of the methyl ester shows signals associated with the C-3 proton, the olefinic proton, the allylic methylene group, the methyl group, and the hydroxylic proton. However, the coupling constants of 2.8 Hz (cis) 0.8 Hz (trans) between the C-5 proton (δ 5.72 ppm) and the geminal protons ($J_{gem} = 17.5$ Hz) at C-6α (δ 3.54 ppm) and C-6β (δ 3.05 ppm) are unusually small when compared with those of 4 Hz (cis) and 2 Hz (trans) in the analogous sodium penicillanate (7). Similar small and near-zero coupling constants between the trans protons of β-lactam rings of fused β-lactam oxazolidines have been reported and ascribed to the greater electronegativity of oxygen compared with sulfur, or to distortion of the β-lactam ring (Stoodley and Watson, 1975). The point of attachment of the ethylidene group to the ring system was confirmed by the ^{1}H-NMR spectrum of the dihydro derivative (8) obtained by catalytic hydrogenation (Section IV) (Brown et al., 1977a).

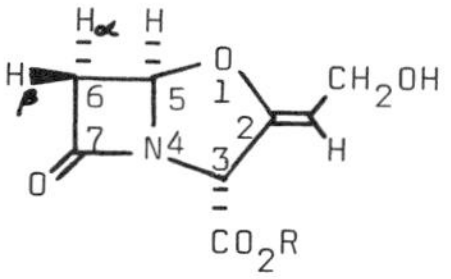

4: R = H
5: R = CH$_3$
6: R = Li

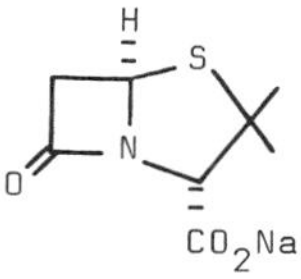

7

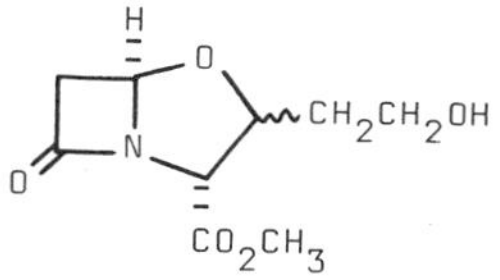

8

Methanolysis of lithium clavulanate resulted in a fundamental disruption of the molecule, the products of which assisted in confirming the β-lactam oxazolidine structure (6) (Glaxo, 1975). After standing in methanol for several hours or after refluxing for 2 min, lithium clavulanate was smoothly converted to the enamine (9), which on further heating cyclized to the pyrrole (10). The formation of the enamine is explained as shown below by methanolysis of the β-lactam ring (11) and concomitant (pathway a) or rapid subsequent fragmentation (pathway b + c or b + d) of the oxazolidine ring, followed by decarboxylation. The enamine had an ultraviolet (UV) maximum at 270 nm, which disappeared on acidification and reappeared at 264 nm on rebasification. These changes are accounted for by the acid hydrolysis of the enamine (9) to give the UV-inactive methyl formylacetate (12) and generation of the corresponding enolate salt (13) on basification.

The formation of the enamine on methanolysis of lithium clavulanate has an analogy in penicillin chemistry (Woodward et al., 1949). Thus on refluxing penicillin G sodium salt (14) in methanol, the initially formed penicilloate (15) is slowly converted to the penamaldic acid (16) (λ_{max} = 282 nm). Acidification of the penamaldate results in hydrolysis to the penaldate (17) with loss of UV activity, whereas rebasification generates the corresponding enolate salt (18) (λ_{max} = 270 nm). However, the rates of formation of the enamine (9) (<2 min) and the analogous penamaldic acid (**16**) (>6 days) are markedly different, reflecting the different stabilities of the putative oxazolidine intermediate (**19**) and the penicilloate (**15**).

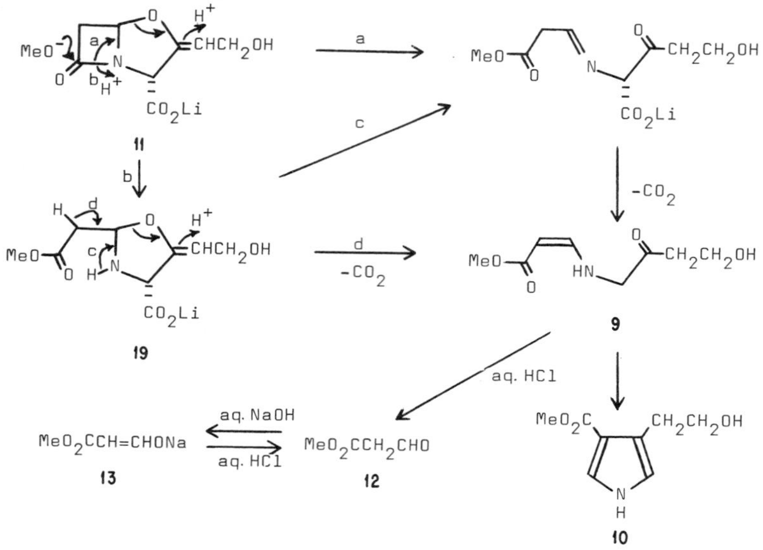

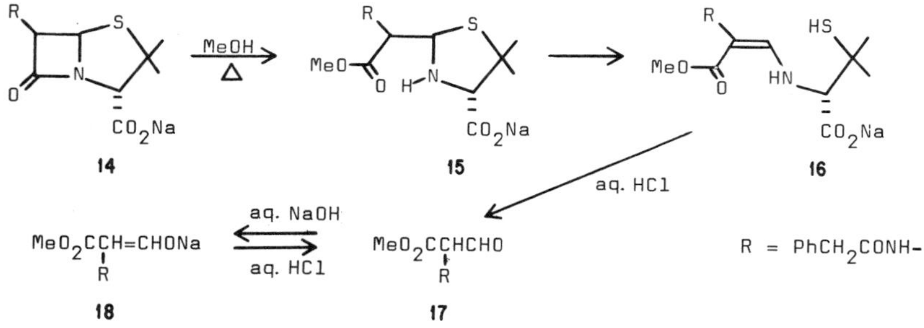

The instability of oxazolidine intermediates (e.g., **27**) resulting from nucleophilic attack at the β-lactam and their tendency to fragment further are general features of the chemistry of clavulanic acid and seem likely to be related to its unusual β-lactamase inhibitory properties (Section IX).

Similar breakdown pathways can be proposed for attack by other nucleophiles, but the products obtained may result from further reaction of enamines (**20**) analogous to those isolated from the methanolysis. Thus lithium clavulanate (**6**) has a half-life of less than 1 min in 0.1 *N* sodium hydroxide, as measured by the total loss of optical activity (Glaxo, 1975). Associated with the degradation is a UV maximum at 258 nm, the appearance of which over ~5 min corresponds to formation of the dianion of formylacetic acid (21). This reaction is of use in the quantitative estimation of clavulanic acid which contains no useful UV chromophore itself. Acidification of solutions of the dianion causes a disappearance of the maximum at 258 nm with the formation of formylacetic acid (22), whereas rebasification regenerates the dianion and the associated UV maximum. The formation of formylacetic acid was confirmed by trapping and isolating the corresponding 2,4-dinitrophenol (2,4-DNP) derivative. Neutralized aqueous solutions of the formylacetic acid give a purple coloration (λ_{max} = 550 nm) with ferric chloride, which can be used as the basis of an assay for clavulanic acid.

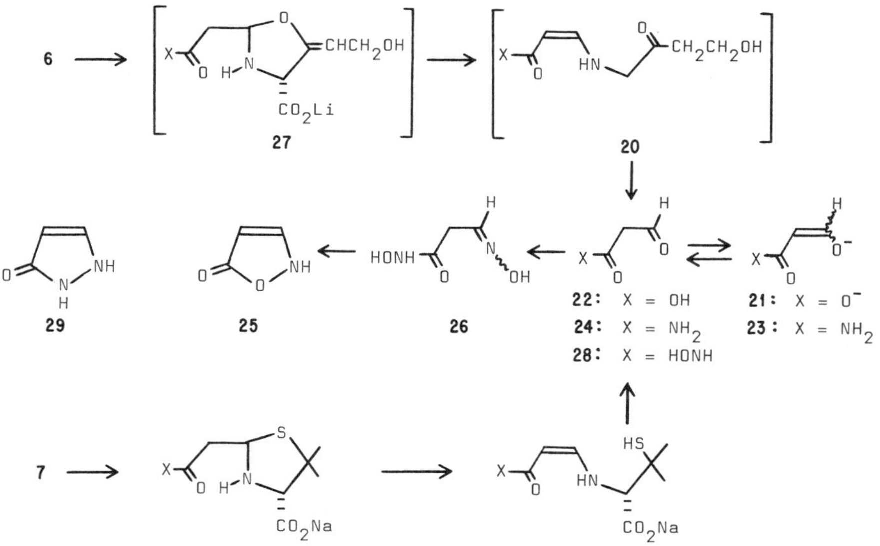

Reaction of clavulanic acid with ammonia and amines is analogous to the reaction with hydroxide ion. Thus, for example, the action of aqueous ammonia results in the somewhat slower appearance over ~20 min of a UV maximum at 268 nm corresponding to the anion of formylacetamide (23) (Glaxo, 1975). The peak disappears on acidification to give formylacetamide (24) and reappears on rebasification. The reaction with ammonia provides the basis of a convenient method of detecting the UV-inactive clavulanic acid on thin-layer chromatography (TLC) plates. A few-second exposure of a developed plate to ammonia vapor results in spots which can be immediately visualized by their strong quenching of UV fluorescence at 254 nm.

Reaction of clavulanic acid with the bidentate nucleophiles hydroxylamine and hydrazine affords five-membered heterocycles containing the three carbon atoms of the original β-lactam ring. On treatment with an excess of neutral aqueous hydroxylamine followed by ferric chloride, lithium clavulanate (6) fails to give the typical hydroxamic acid test for penicillins because of its rapid conversion to isoxazolin-5-one (25) (Glaxo, 1975). This product presumably results from cyclization of the aldoxime (26) following collapse of the oxazolidine (27, X = HONH) and unmasking of the aldehyde (28). The analogous pyrazolin-5-one (29) is rapidly formed by reaction of lithium clavulanate with hydrazine. Similar treatment of sodium penicillanate (7) with hydroxylamine and hydrazine also results in formation of the isoxazolinone (25) and the pyrazolinone (29), respectively, indicating a parallel reaction sequence. However, their rates of formation from the penicillanate are much slower because of the greater stability of the intermediate penicilloyl derivatives (30, X = HONH and X = H_2NNH) compared with the corresponding hypothetical oxazolidines (27, X = HONH and H_2NNH). In contrast to lithium clavulanate, sodium penicillanate gives a normal hydroxamic acid test with ferric chloride.

In addition to its instability to nucleophilic attack, clavulanic acid is very unstable under acidic conditions, with a half-life of ~5 min in 0.5 N hydrochloric acid as measured by the total loss of optical activity (Glaxo, 1975). The free acid (4) can be prepared in organic solution but on isolation has been obtained only as an oil which shows evidence of decomposition on standing. Acidification of aqueous solutions of lithium clavulanate (31) results in rapid and extensive hydrolysis with the evolution of carbon dioxide from decarboxylation of the α-amino-β-ketoacid (32) derived from the oxazolidine ring. Similar solutions of methyl clavulanate do not show the rapid loss of carbon dioxide, since an α-amino-β-ketoester is formed in this case. However, on standing, acidified solutions of both lithium clavulanate and the methyl ester evolve carbon dioxide from the rather slower decarboxylation of formylacetic acid (33) derived from the β-lactam ring. The resulting acetaldehyde has been trapped and identified as the 2,4-DNP derivative. Evidence from NMR studies suggests the presence of the expected 1-amino-4-hydroxybutan-2-one (34) in acidified solutions of clavulanic acid, and the corresponding 1-aminobutan-2-one (35) has been isolated as the hydrochloride salt from an analogous acidic hydrolysis of sodium deoxyclavulanate (36) (Section IV). Similar hydrolysis of sodium 2-ethylclavam-3-carboxylate (37) (Section IV) afforded 1-amino-2-hydroxypentanoic acid (38). This α-amino acid was shown to belong to the same "unnatural" D series as penicillamine (**39**), suggesting that clavulanic acid has the same absolute stereochemistry as penicillins (Glaxo, 1975).

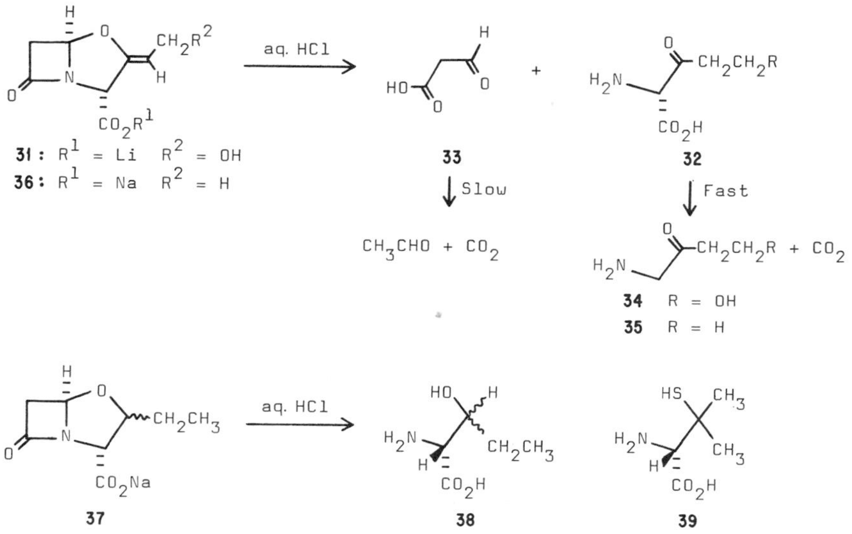

31: R^1 = Li R^2 = OH
36: R^1 = Na R^2 = H

33

32

CH$_3$CHO + CO$_2$

34   R = OH
35   R = H

37

38

39

The spectroscopic properties and degradation chemistry of clavulanic acid described above resulted in formulation of the correct gross structure (**1**) for the molecule, and this was confirmed by independent X-ray analyses of the *p*-nitrobenzyl ester (Howarth *et al.*, 1976) and of the lithium salt (Glaxo, 1975). In addition, the X-ray analyses showed the exocyclic double bond to have the Z configuration and the hydrogen atoms at the C-3 and C-5 positions to be on opposite faces of the molecule. The absolute configuration was confirmed to be 3*R*, 5*R* (i.e., the same as in naturally occurring penicillins) by X-ray analysis of the *p*-bromobenzyl ester (Howarth *et al.*, 1976).

IV. Derivatives of Clavulanic Acid Obtained by Hydrogenation and Hydrogenolysis

Depending on conditions, such as solvent, pH, catalyst ratio, and reaction time, hydrogenation of clavulanic acid and its derivatives over palladium on carbon (Pd–C) can result in isomerization about the double bond, hydrogenolysis of the allylic alcohol, or saturation of the double bond.

A.   Isomerization about the Double Bond

Initial investigations into the utility of the benzyl ester of clavulanic acid as a carboxyl-protected intermediate demonstrated that removal of the ester by hydrogenolysis in aqueous ethanolic sodium hydrogen carbonate over 10% Pd–C (substrate/catalyst ratio 3:1) resulted in sodium clavulanate (**40**, R = Na) which, prior to crystallization, contained ~10% by-product (Brown *et al.*, 1976b). Conversion of the mixture of sodium salts to *p*-bromobenzyl esters and chromatographic separation gave the minor ester which was identified spectroscopically and confirmed by X-ray analysis as the *E* isomer, *p*-bromobenzyl isoclavulanate (**41**, R = *p*-BrC$_6$H$_4$CH$_2$). On shaking with prehydrogenated 10% Pd–C under nitrogen (substrate/catalyst ratio 1:4) or with 10% Pd–C under hydrogen (substrate/catalyst ratio 2:1) for 20 min, sodium clavulanate in pH 7 buffer gave directly a mixture containing ~10% corresponding *E* isomer (**41**, R = Na) without detectable amounts of hydrogenolysis or hydrogenation products (Glaxo, 1975). Following selective precipitation of sodium clavulanate from ethyl acetate with sodium 2-ethylhexanoate, the resulting mixture (enriched in the *E* isomer) was converted to *p*-nitrobenzyl esters, and *p*-nitrobenzyl isoclavulanate (**41**, R = *p*-NO$_2$C$_6$H$_4$CH$_2$) was isolated by chromatography.

Photolytic irradiation of benzyl clavulanate in benzene provided an improved method for isomerizing the double bond, and benzyl isoclavulanate (**41**, R = PhCH$_2$) was isolated by chromatography in 40% yield together with 50% starting material. A similar attempt at photolytic isomerization of phenacyl clavulanate (**40**, R = PhCOCH$_2$) gave as a by-product the tetracyclic structure **42** which is reported to be a β-lactamase inhibitor (Brown *et al.*, 1977a; Ger. Off. 2,628,357).

Deprotection of benzyl isoclavulanate (**41**, R = PhCH$_2$) under the conditions used for benzyl clavulanate gave sodium isoclavulanate (**41**, R = Na) which was sometimes contaminated with the *Z* isomer (**40**, R = Na) as a result of reisomerization during the hydrogenolysis (Brown *et al.*, 1977a). Similarly, deprotection of the corresponding *p*-nitrobenzyl ester (**41**, R = *p*-NO$_2$C$_6$H$_4$CH$_2$) by catalytic hydrogenolysis or by reductive hydrolysis with iron powder and ammonium chloride in aqueous tetrahydrofuran resulted in sodium isoclavulanate containing 5–10% Z isomer (Glaxo, 1975). Spectroscopically, sodium isoclavulanate (**41**, R = Na) resembles the Z isomer (**40**, R = Na), the most characteristic differences being downfield shifts of δ ~0.3 ppm in the ^{1}H-NMR resonance of the olefinic and C-3 protons.

Sodium isoclavulanate has also been shown to be an antibacterial and an inhibitor of β-lactamases, but with only ~$\frac{1}{10}$ the activity shown by the natural isomer (Cole, 1980; Belg. Pat. 836,652).

B.   Hydrogenolysis of the Allylic Alcohol

During attempts to remove the benzyl protecting groups from benzyl clavulanate (**43**, R = H) and from the acetyl derivative (**43**, R = CH$_3$CO) in the presence of sodium hydrogen carbonate, hydrogenolysis of the hydroxyl and acetoxy groups was observed to give sodium deoxyclavulanate (**44**, R = Na) (Brown *et al.*, 1977a). The hydrogenolysis reaction was particularly favored if carried out under somewhat acidic conditions, for example, those occurring during deprotection of benzyl clavulanate in tetrahydrofuran in the absence of sodium hydrogen carbonate (Belg. Pat. 840,253). Similarly, hydrogenation of clavulanic acid itself in ethyl acetate solution over 10% Pd–C (substrate/catalyst ratio 2:3) resulted in complete conversion to the deoxy derivative (**44**, R = H) within 5–10 min and without significant reduction of the double bond (Glaxo, 1975). The product, which was isolated as the sodium salt, contained 10–15% corresponding E isomer (**45**, R = Na) resulting from isomerization about the double bond.

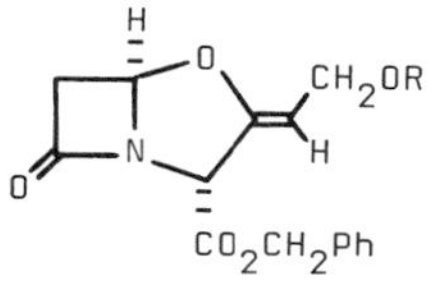

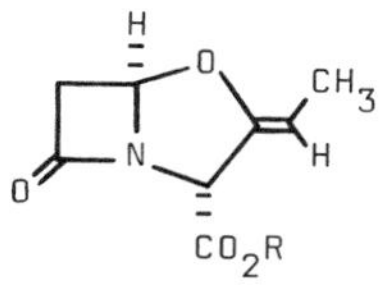

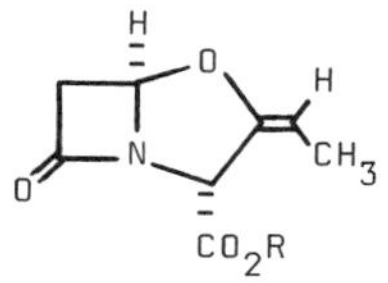

Sodium deoxyclavulanate (**44**, R = Na), which can be regarded as the unfunctionalized parent skeleton of clavulanic acid, shows biological properties very similar to those of clavulanic acid itself (Cole, 1979; Belg. Pat. 840,253).

C.   Saturation of the Double Bond

The resistance of the double bond of clavulanic acid to hydrogenation permitted the use of hydrogenolyzable esters such as benzyl and *p*-

nitrobenzyl as protecting groups for the carboxylic acid function (Brown *et al.*, 1976b, 1977a). However, saturation of the double bond could be achieved under appropriate conditions. Thus catalytic hydrogenation of methyl clavulanate (**40**, R = CH₃) in ethyl acetate over 10% Pd–C for 2 days afforded a mixture of epimeric dihydro derivatives **46a** and **47a** in the ratio 1:2 from which the major isomer was isolated by high-pressure liquid chromatography (HPLC) (Brown *et al.*, 1977a; Ger. Off. 2,547,698).

a:	R¹ = CH₃;	R² = OH
b:	R¹ = Na;	R² = OH
c:	R¹ = Na;	R² = H
d:	R¹ = CH₃;	R² = H

       46   **47**

    In contrast to the hydrogenation of clavulanic acid in ethyl acetate, hydrogenation of the lithium salt over 10% Pd–C (substrate/catalyst ratio 1:1) in pH 7 buffer for several hours resulted in saturation of the double bond without hydrogenolysis of the allylic alcohol. The product, isolated as a mixture of sodium salts **46b** and **47b**, gave on methylation a mixture of esters similar to that obtained directly from methyl clavulanate, but with the isomer ratio reversed (Glaxo, 1975). In the ¹H-NMR spectrum (CDCl₃) of the mixture of esters, the CH₂CH₂OH groups appeared as quartets (*J* = 6 Hz) at δ 1.73 and 2.02 ppm and were assigned to the 2*R* isomer (**46a**) and 2*S* isomer (**47a**), respectively, by analogy with the positions of the C-2 methyl groups in (2*R*)and (2*S*)-norpenicillin (Claes *et al.*, 1975). The signals for the C-5 protons were also characteristically different, appearing at δ 5.55 (dd, *J* = 3 and 1 Hz) in the 2*R* isomer (**46a**) and at δ 5.33 (dd, *J* = 3 and 0.5 Hz) in the 2*S* isomer (**47a**).

    The antibacterial activity of dihydroclavulanic acid (as mixture of the sodium salts **46b** and **47b**) is similar to that of clavulanic acid, but its β-lactamase inhibitory activity is considerably reduced.

    Acyl derivatives of dihydroclavulanic acid have been prepared as mixtures of epimers either by reduction of the appropriate acyl derivative of benzyl clavulanate or by acylation of methyl or benzyl dihydrocla-vulanate (Ger. Off. 2,547,698).

    Hydrogenation of the hydrogenolysis product, sodium deoxyclavulan-ate (**44**, R = Na), under the same neutral conditions used for lithium clavulanate gave the corresponding 2-ethylclavam as a 1:1 mixture of epimers (**46c** and **47c**) (Glaxo, 1975). A 1:2 mixture of the corresponding methyl esters (**46d** and **47d**) of the 2-ethylclavam has been derived from methyl clavulanate. The two epimers show ¹H-NMR signals for the

C-5 protons that are analogous to those of the above 2-hydroxyethyl-clavams (Kobayashi *et al.*, 1978).

V. Derivatives of Clavulanic Acid with a Modified CH$_2$OH Group

Comparison of the biological properties of the derivatives described above with those of clavulanic acid showed that geometrical changes in the skeleton, such as isomerization about the double bond and saturation of the double bond, resulted in a marked reduction in β-lactamase inhibitory activity. However, deoxyclavulanic acid (**44**, R = H) retained the activity of the natural product.

These observations focused attention on the allylic hydroxyl group as the best point for chemical modification, and derivative programs were started in both the Beecham and Glaxo laboratories. Most of the transformations described below were performed with esters of clavulanic acid in order to facilitate the modification, handling, or isolation of the compounds. The benzyl and *p*-nitrobenzyl esters were usually employed, the latter being particularly useful as it often conferred crystallinity and could easily be removed either by catalytic hydrogenation or chemical reduction. A number of other esters, such as the methyl esters, were found to be relatively amenable to controlled hydrolysis with lithium hydroxide. The methoxymethyl esters were particularly suitable in this respect, being cleaved in about 15 min at room temperature and pH 8.5 (Belg. Pat. 862,764). Other readily cleaved esters, such as the 2,2,2-trichloroethyl and tri-*n*-butylstannyl esters, have also been used.

Ester protecting groups are usually removed before biological testing, however, in some instances the final product is in the form of a metabolically labile ester. Metabolically labile ester groups may be used as protecting groups during a synthesis or be attached at the end of the reaction sequence. The biological activity of methyl clavulanate also may be due in part to slow conversion to the parent acid (Ger. Off. 2,517,316).

Most of the esters described above are readily prepared by conventional methods, e.g., by reaction of clavulanic acid with diazoalkanes or of salts of clavulanic acid with alkyl halides (Ger. Off. 2,517,316).

New derivatives are usually submitted for conventional antibacterial testing; in addition, β-lactamase inhibition and synergy with β-lactamase-sensitive antibiotics are studied. Enzyme inhibition is determined using cell-free partially purified β-lactamase preparations. The result of such a test is conveniently expressed as the I$_{50}$, the concentration of the test compound required to halve the rate of enzymic hydrolysis of a sensitive antibiotic such as penicillin G, ampicillin, or cephaloridine.

Synergy tests are intended to measure the extent to which an inhibitor improves the performance of sensitive antibiotics against β-lactamase-producing bacteria. The result of a synergy test is usually expressed as the MIC of the test antibiotic, e.g., ampicillin, in the presence of a specified concentration of the β-lactamase inhibitor.

A. O-Acyl and O-Alkyl Derivatives

Esters of clavulanic acid (**48a–d**) react with acyl halides or anhydrides (Belg. Pat. 834,645) and with isocyanates and isothiocyanates (Belg. Pat. 847,046) to give acyl (**49**), carbamoyl (**50**, X = O), and thiocarbamoyl (**50**, X = S) derivatives, respectively. The acyl derivatives may also be prepared by reacting an ester of clavulanic acid with a carboxylic acid in the presence of dicyclohexylcarbodiimide (DCC). These acylated derivatives are potent inhibitors of cell-free β-lactamases, having activity similar to that of clavulanic acid. However, their performance in synergy tests using gram-negative bacteria is generally poor; this may be due to their relative instability in aqueous media (Glaxo, 1975).

The esters **48a–d** react with diazomethane in the presence of Lewis acids, such as boron trifluoride etherate, to give the methyl ethers **51a–d**. The methyl ester **51c** may be prepared directly from clavulanic acid under these conditions. Other ether derivatives may be prepared by using higher or substituted diazoalkanes (Belg. Pat. 847,045; 849,475; Eur. Pat. Appl. 3,254). Alkylations of esters of clavulanic acid with trialkyloxonium fluoroborates (Belg. Pat. 861,716) or with alkyl halides in the presence of silver oxide (Belg. Pat. 864,607) have been described. Acetals may also be prepared; thus the reaction of p-nitrobenzyl clavulanate (**48b**) with dihydropyran and an acid catalyst gave the tetrahydropyranyl ether (**52b**) (Belg. Pat. 849,475). Substituted ethyl ethers have been prepared by reaction with N-acylaziridines (Belg. Pat. 870,405) or oxiranes (Eur. Pat. Appl. 2,370) in the presence of boron trifluoride etherate.

The ether derivatives are potent β-lactamase inhibitors; some of them perform well in synergy tests with intact bacteria and are also effective when coadministered with ampicillin to animals infected with ampicillin-resistant bacteria. A number of the ethers, including the methyl and ethyl ethers, are well absorbed in the rat or mouse following oral administration.

B. Halogen Derivatives

Replacement of the hydroxyl group of clavulanic acid by a halogen atom provides a very reactive allylic halide. This was accomplished by reacting p-nitrobenzyl clavulanate (**48b**) in ether–tetrahydrofuran with

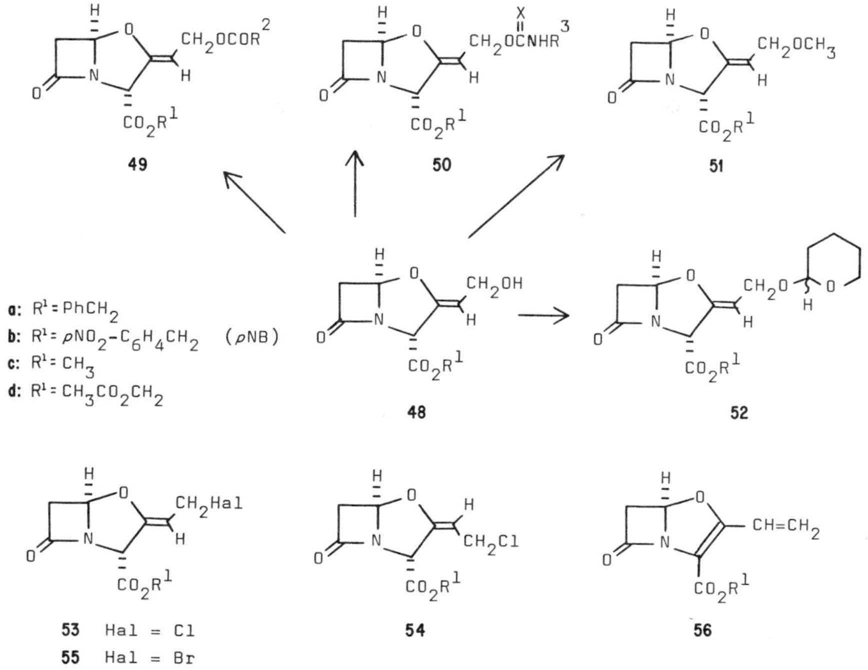

49

50

51

a: R^1 = PhCH$_2$
b: R^1 = pNO$_2$-C$_6$H$_4$CH$_2$ (pNB)
c: R^1 = CH$_3$
d: R^1 = CH$_3$CO$_2$CH$_2$

48

52

53 Hal = Cl
55 Hal = Br

54

56

thionyl chloride and pyridine at a reduced temperature; the crystalline Z isomer (53b) was obtained as the major product after dilution with ether (Cherry *et al.*, 1978a). A small amount of the E isomer (54b) was isolated from the mother liquor. The two isomers were readily distinguished by the characteristic positions of the vinylic and C-3 protons in their ^{1}H-NMR spectra. A similar reaction with thionyl bromide gave the allylic bromide (55b). Mesylation of p-nitrobenzyl clavulanate in the presence of a source of chloride ion provides an alternative method of preparing the chloride (53b) (Belg. Pat. 849,474).

The halides, especially the crystalline chloride (53b), are relatively stable in the solid state but in solution readily react with nucleophiles as described below. When treated with a nonnucleophilic base such as triethylamine (TEA), they rapidly eliminate hydrogen halide to give the diene (56), which is also a useful synthetic intermediate.

C. Nitrogen Derivatives

Reaction of the halide 53b or 55b with azide ion affords the azidoester (57b), catalytic hydrogenation of which gives the amino acid (58). Careful chemical reduction of **57b** with zinc and hydrochloric acid at pH 4.3 gives the azidoacid (**57c**), which can be isolated as its sodium salt. The benzyl ester of the azide (**57a**), prepared in an analogous manner from benzyl clavulanate (**48a**) via the chloride (**53a**), can be reduced to the amine benzyl ester (**59a**) with zinc and hydrochloric acid (Newall *et al.,* 1978; Belg. Pat. 855,375). The azides (**57**) can also be prepared directly from esters of clavulanic acid by reaction with hydrazoic acid in the presence of triphenylphosphine and an azodicarbonyl compound such as diethyl azodicarboxylate or azodibenzoyl (Ger. Off. 2,911,099).

The amines **58** and **59** may be acylated with acyl or thioacyl halides or with the anhydrides or active esters of carboxylic acids. Amino esters such as **59a** may be acylated by reaction with a carboxylic acid in the presence of DCC. Reactions with haloformates, isocyanates, isothio-cyanates, and sulfonyl halides give carbamates, ureas, thioureas, and sulfonamides, respectively. It was found that the reactions of the amines with reagents such as isocyanates and isothiocyanates were improved by the addition of tri-*n*-butyltin oxide to the reaction mixtures. Diacyl compounds, such as the phthalimido derivative (**60**), could also be pre-pared from the amino acid (**58**) (Newall *et al.,* 1978; Belg. Pat. 860,042).

Diacyl derivatives (**61**) may also be prepared by reacting esters of clavulanic acid with diacylamino compounds in the presence of triphen-ylphosphine and diethyl azodicarboxylate. Selective removal of one of the acyl groups affords the monoacyl derivative (e.g., **62**), and when both acyl substituents are benzyloxycarbonyl groups, they may be hy-drogenolyzed to give the parent amine (Belg. Pat. 866,496).

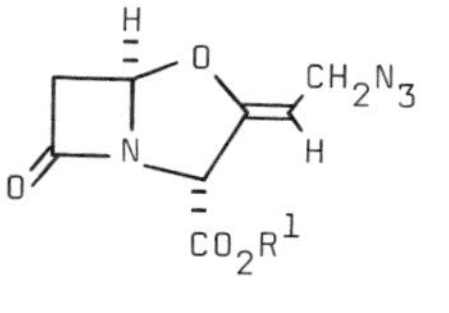

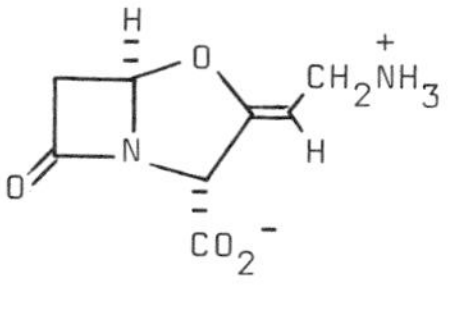

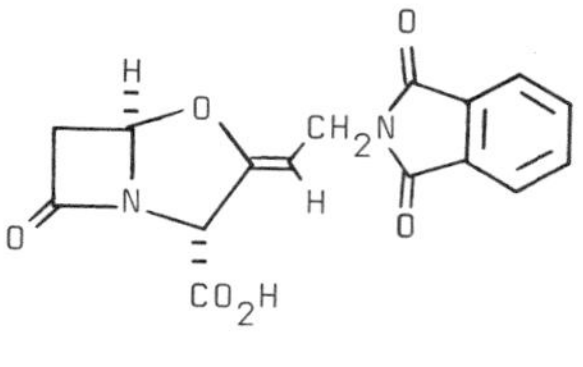

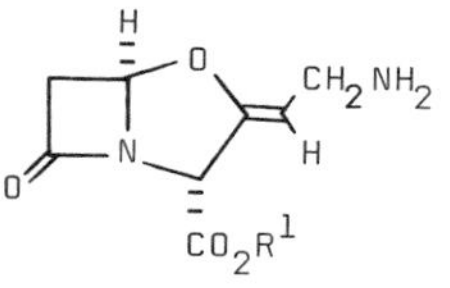

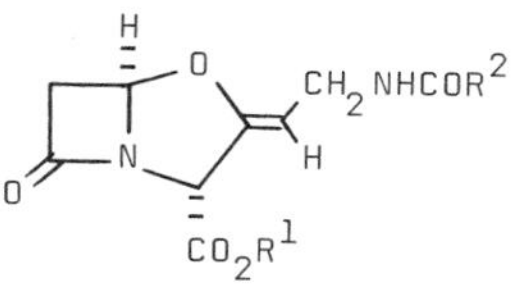

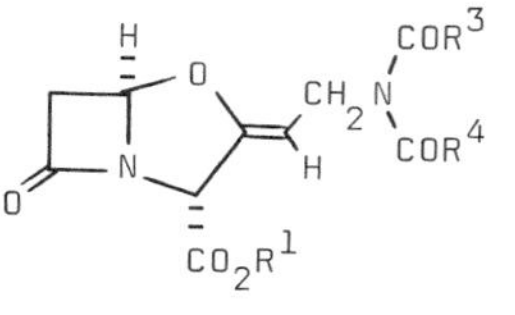

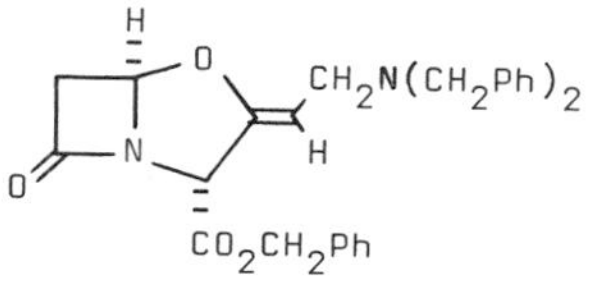

N-Alkylated compounds may be prepared in several ways. Thus the addition of dibenzylamine to the diene (56a) (prepared *in situ* from benzyl clavulanyl sulfate trimethylammonium salt) gave the tertiary amine (63) (Belg. Pat. 847,044). A similar reaction with diallylamine gave the *N,N*-diallyl derivative which was reduced to the *N,N*-dipropyl compound. *N*-Aryl derivatives (e.g., 64b, R^5 = Ph) may be prepared in low yield by the reaction of anilines with the bromide (55b) (Glaxo, 1977). Lower *N,N*-dialkyl compounds (e.g., 65) may also be prepared by hydrogenating the amino acid (58) in the presence of aldehydes such as formaldehyde and acetaldehyde (Glaxo, 1977). The tertiary amino derivatives may be further alkylated; thus 65 reacts with methyl iodide to give the betaine (66) (Glaxo, 1977). Reaction of the chloride (53b) with diallylamine provides another method of preparing the *N,N*-diallyl, hence the *N,N*-dipropyl compound (Br. Pat. Appl. 2,007,667).

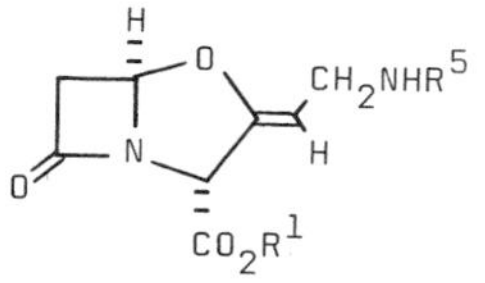

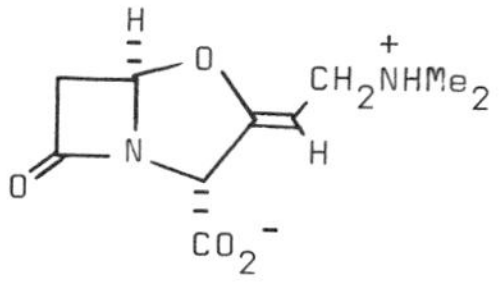

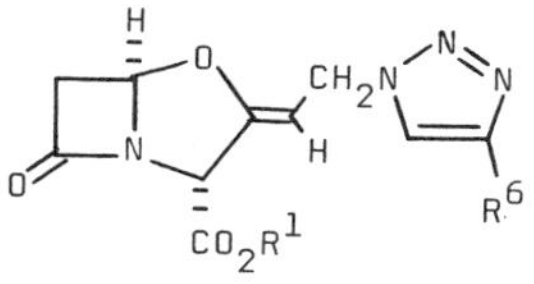

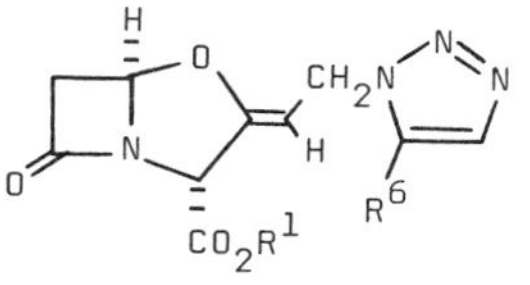

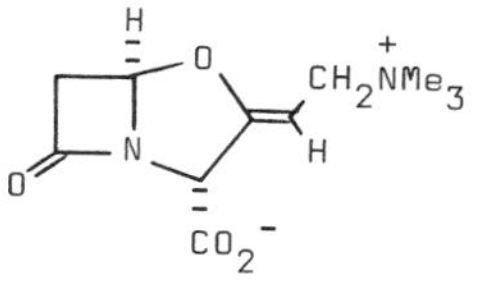

O-Acylated esters of clavulanic may also be used for the preparation of N-alkylated derivatives of the amine (59). Thus the reaction of the dichloroacetate of benzyl clavulanate with dibenzylamine in dry DMF at 0°C gave 63, selective debenzylation of which afforded the mono-*N*-benzyl compound (64c, R^5 = $PhCH_2$). Other secondary amino compounds have also been prepared, and some of these have subsequently been N-acylated (Belg. Pat. 866,276).

The azidoesters (57) react with acetylenes to give triazoles. With monosubstituted acetylenes the major product is the 4-substituted triazol-1-yl derivative (67), although small amounts of the 5-substituted derivative (68) may also be formed (Eur. Pat. Appl. 1,516). The triazoles are most readily formed with acetylenes carrying electron-withdrawing groups; however, acetylene itself reacts slowly to give the triazol-1-yl compound (67, R^6 = H).

The azido and amino acids (57c and 58) are powerful inhibitors of β-lactamases. This property is shared by most of their alkylated and acylated derivatives and by the triazolyl compounds. Antibacterial activity varies, with some of the compounds having modest activity against gram-negative organisms. However, a number of them, notably certain triazol-1-yl derivatives, are somewhat more active than clavulanic acid against many strains of bacteria. Several of the compounds are very effective as synergists with ampicillin, amoxicillin, or cephaloridine, and some of them are well absorbed following oral administration in animals.

D.   Sulfur Derivatives

Reaction of esters of clavulanic acid with thiols in the presence of a Lewis acid catalyst such as boron trifluoride etherate gives thioethers (69); these may be oxidized to the corresponding sulfoxides (70) and sulfones (71) (Belg. Pat. 850,779). The same compounds may also be prepared by reacting the halides (53 or 55) with thiolate or sulfinic acid salts (Cherry et al., 1978a; Belg. Pat. 851,821). This method can also be used to prepare acylthio, thioacylthio, carbamoylthio, and thiocarbamoylthio derivatives via displacement of halide ion with the appropriate sulfur nucleophile. These reactions proceed smoothly with the more acidic nucleophiles, but the presence of silver salts as reaction promoters is desirable with some of the less reactive alkyl thiolates. A number of arylthioethers were prepared by reacting clavulanic acid esters with sym-diaryl disulfides and tri-n-butylphosphine.

Reaction of the halide 53b with sodium trithiocarbonate followed by decomposition of the resulting hemitrithiocarbonate with dilute acid gave the thiol ester (72b). This compound was relatively stable to aerial oxidation but could be oxidized to the disulfide (73b) with iodine in pyridine. The thiol can also be prepared by reaction of the halide with hydrogen sulfide in methylene chloride in the presence of powdered potassium carbonate and 18-crown-6. Alkylation and acylation of the thiol (72) provide alternative methods of preparing the thioalkyl and thioacyl compounds described above.

Sulfur-substituted compounds may also be prepared by the addition of sulfur nucleophiles to the diene (56). The isolated products of these

reactions are identical with those of similar reactions using the halides
(**53** and **55**), the double bond having Z geometry and the C-3 carbon
atom having the R configuration. In some instances a careful examination
of the reaction mixtures reveals the presence of small amounts of the
thermodynamically less stable $3S$ isomers (Cherry *et al.*, 1980).

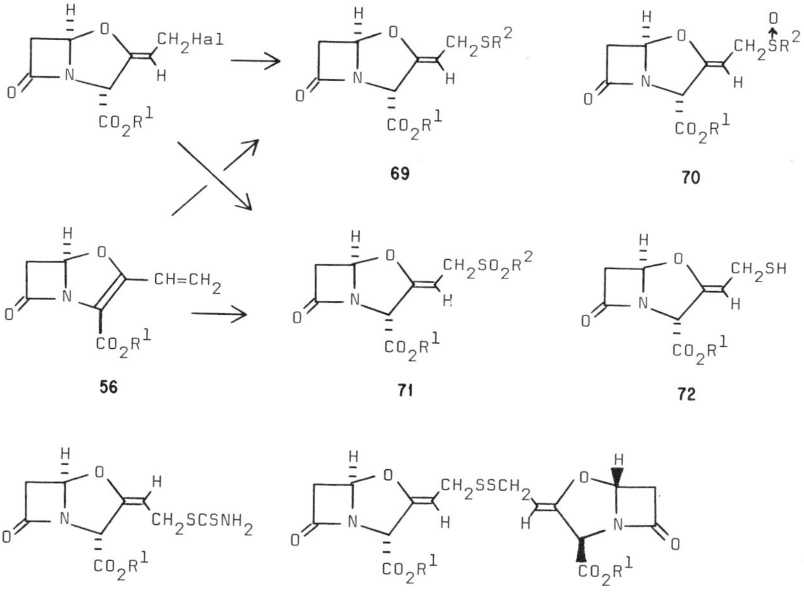

69   **70**   **56**   **71**   **72**   **74**   **73**

a: R^1 = $PhCH_2$
b: R^1 = pNB
c: R^1 = H

In many instances the conditions used for the 1,4-addition of a sulfur
nucleophile to the diene (**56b**) were very similar to those used for the
displacement of halide ion from **53b**. It was thus possible that reactions
starting with the latter could proceed via an elimination–addition mechanism with the diene as an intermediate. In order to distinguish between
these possibilities the chloroester (**53b**) and the diene (**56b**) were each
reacted with CH_3COSD and TEA in dry DMF, and the isolated products
were examined by ^1H-NMR spectroscopy and mass spectrometry (Cherry
et al., 1978a). The acetylthio compound (**69b**, R^2 = CH_3CO) obtained
from the haloester was only lightly deuterated at C-3 (<5% D), whereas
the material obtained from the diene was heavily deuterated (>60%).

Furthermore, reaction of the E isomer (**54b**) of the chloroester with ammonium dithiocarbamate gave only **74b**, no Z isomer (**69b**, $R^2 =$ H_2NCS) being detected. These observations indicate that the reactions of the haloesters with the soft sulfur nucleophiles proceed almost entirely by direct displacement rather than by a two-step mechanism with the diene as an intermediate.

A large number of compounds carrying a wide variety of acidic, basic, and neutral substituents have been prepared by the reaction sequences outlined above. They are potent inhibitors of β-lactamases, and many of them are much more active than clavulanic acid itself as inhibitors of staphylococcal penicillinase and the TEM-1 enzyme. A few of them, notably the isothiouronium, dithiobenzoyl, and methylsulfinyl derivatives, inhibit the chromosomally mediated cephalosporinase P99 of *Enterobacter cloacae,* which is resistant to clavulanic acid itself. Many of the compounds are active in synergy tests with ampicillin or amoxicillin, and selected compounds have been shown to be active when coadministered with these antibiotics to infected mice. The antibacterial activity of the sulfur derivatives is variable. Many possess the modest broad-spectrum activity shown by clavulanic acid itself, although some of them are much more active against gram-positive bacteria but have reduced activity against gram-negative organisms. A few of them, notably the dithiocarbamoyl (**69c**, $R^2 = H_2NCS$) and 1-methylpyridinium-4-thio derivatives, were significantly more active than clavulanic acid against most of the bacteria examined.

E. Carbon Derivatives

Reaction of the chloroester (**53b**) with carbanions derived from β-diketones, β-ketoesters, or similar compounds gives derivatives (**75**) with a carbon-linked substituent; the thallium salt of the β-dicarbonyl compound was a very effective reagent in these reactions. Alternatively the haloester may be reacted with the β-dicarbonyl compound in an aprotic solvent in the presence of potassium carbonate and 18-crown-6. The diene ester (**56**) can also be used to prepare **75** either by the latter method or under phase-transfer conditions with a β-dicarbonyl compound and tetra-*n*-butylammonium hydroxide (Ger. Off. 2,747,350).

Carbanions derived from nitroalkanes have been used in similar reactions. Thus addition of the diene (**56a**) to nitromethane and sodium hydride in DMF gave **76a** (Eur. Pat. Appl. 2,319). This compound, and others derived from α-nitroesters, may also be prepared under phase-transfer conditions or from the halo compounds (**53** or **55**) as described above (Glaxo, 1977). Reduction of the nitro group of **76b** and concomitant removal of the ester group gives **77**, the homolog of the amino acid (**58**).

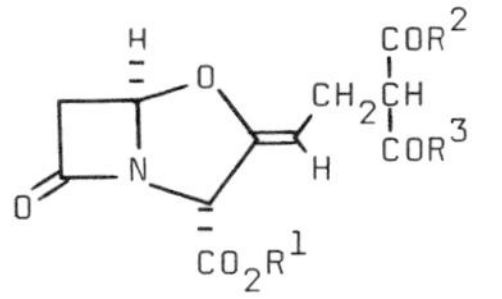

75

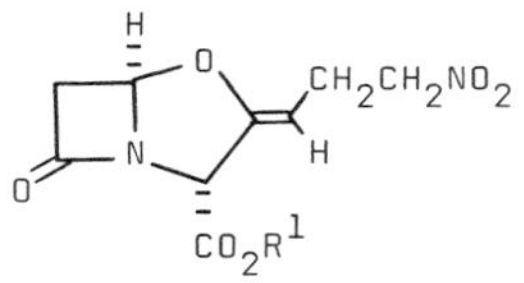

76

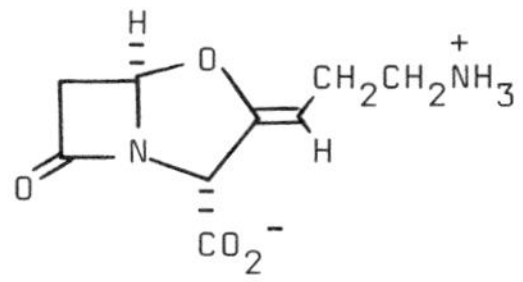

77

a: R^1 = $PhCH_2$

b: R^1 = pNB

F. Isoclavulanic Acid Derivatives

A number of derivatives of isoclavulanic acid have been described, thus O-acyl and O-alkyl derivatives can be prepared using the procedures described in Section V,A (Belg. Pat. 836,652; Ger. Off. 2,747,763). Other derivatives have been prepared from the E-isomeric chloroester (54b), and in general they are much less active than the corresponding Z isomers (Glaxo, 1976).

G. Biological Activity

Most of the data on the biological activity of these compounds remains unpublished and, although a certain amount of information is available from patents, it is often difficult to correlate. Quantitative structure–activity studies have been undertaken using the data obtained from a wide range of the analogs prepared in the Glaxo laboratories, and some generalizations can be made. Thus the antimicrobial activity against gram-negative bacteria and the ability to provide effective synergy with ampicillin or amoxicillin appear to be related to the hydrophilicity and size of the substituent replacing the hydroxyl group of clavulanic acid, the most active compounds being those with small hydrophilic substituents.

VI. Clav-2-ems (1-Oxadethiapen-2-ems) and Pen-2-ems

A. Clavudiene

Reaction of benzyl clavulanate with the Pfitzner–Moffat reagent (dimethyl sulfoxide–DCC–orthophosphoric acid in benzene) gave the diene (78), presumably by 1,4-elimination from the intermediate sulfonium salt, rather than the expected aldehyde (Section VII) (Corbett et al., 1977). Esters of the diene have also been formed from other compounds, notably by base-catalyzed 1,4-elimination from O-acyl derivatives of benzyl clavulanate (Belg. Pat. 849,308) or from the halogen derivatives described in Section V,B. In the latter case it was noted that, although treatment of the chloro compound (53b) with triethylamine at 0°C gave the crystalline diene (79) in an optically active form, similar reactions conducted at room temperature afforded racemic material (Cherry *et al.*, 1978a). The racemization of other clav-2-em compounds in the presence of base is discussed below. The preparation of derivatives of clavulanic acid by the 1,4-addition of carbon, nitrogen, and sulfur nucleophiles to the diene esters (e.g., 79) has been described in Section V,D.

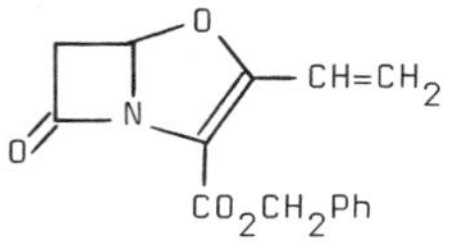

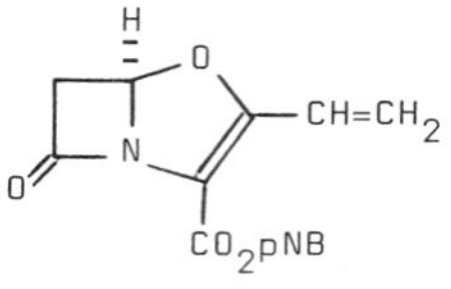

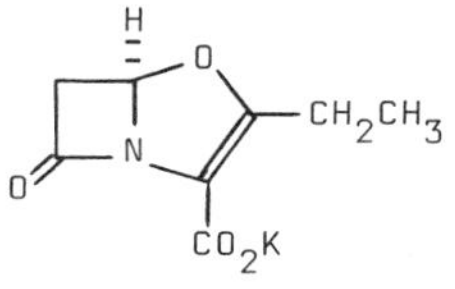

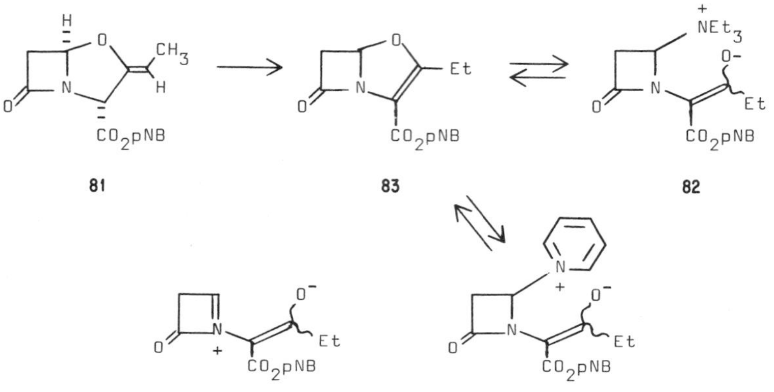

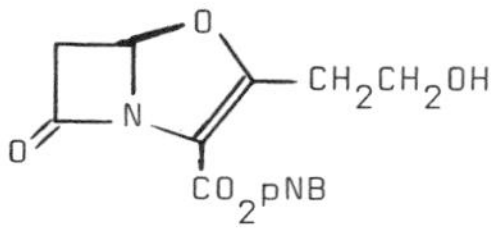

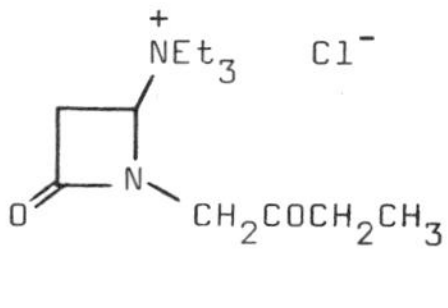

Deesterification of the diene (79) by catalytic hydrogenation in purified ethyl acetate gave the optically active 2-ethylclav-2-em acid, isolated as its potassium salt (80); failure to purify the solvent used for this reaction resulted in racemization. The salt (80) was a potent β-lactamase inhibitor in an *in vitro* test, being much more active than clavulanic acid against the staphylococcal penicillinase PC1 and the P99 cephalosporinase from *E. cloacae* (Cherry *et al.*, 1978a). It was, however, too unstable in aqueous solution to determine its antibacterial activity or its synergy with ampicillin against intact bacteria.

B. Preparation and Properties of Clav-2-ems Derived from Clavulanic Acid

The diene esters (**78** and **79**) described above represent a special case of the conversion of clavulanic acid derivatives to compounds with the clav-2-em ring system. Clav-2-ems (e.g., **80**), which are of particular interest because of their relationship with the pen-2-ems first reported by Woodward (1977a), would be expected to be readily available from clavulanic acid derivatives by base-catalyzed isomerization of the exocyclic double bond into the ring. An attempt to effect this isomerization by reacting *p*-nitrobenzyl deoxyclavulanate (**81**) with triethylamine in ethyl acetate at room temperature resulted in formation of the highly crystalline betaine (**82**) in good yield. When heated under reflux in ethyl acetate, **82** rapidly dissolved and within 2 min was converted to the desired 2-ethylclav-2-em (**83**) which was isolated as a crystalline solid in 78% yield (Cherry *et al.*, 1978b). It is believed that the betaine (**82**) is formed from the clavem (**83**) with which it is in equilibrium under the reaction conditions. However, because of its insolubility in ethyl acetate, the betaine crystallizes, displacing the equilibrium in its favor. In a solvent such as chloroform, from which **82** does not crystallize, an equilibrium mixture of **82** and **83** in a ratio of about 1:1 is established in the presence of triethylamine. This equilibrium may be approached from either side or from **81**.

The clavem (**83**) readily affords the betaine (**84**) when treated with pyridine. Under similar conditions the ethylideneclavam (**81**) fails to react, presumably because pyridine is too weak a base to isomerize **81** to **83**. However, the betaine (**84**) was formed when a catalytic amount of triethylamine was added to a solution of **81** in pyridine. This provides further evidence that formation of the betaines from *p*-nitrobenzyl deoxyclavulanate proceeds via the clavem (**83**).

Neither the clavem ester (**83**) nor the betaines (**82** or **84**) show any detectable rotation at the sodium D line, indicating that they are racemic. When the reaction of **81** with triethylamine in chloroform was followed polarimetrically, a rise in the rotation (~20%) was observed during the first hour; this was followed by racemization resulting in a gradual decrease in rotation to near zero after 24 hr. The initial rise in rotation indicates that chirality was retained by at least one of the initial products of the reaction, and it is suggested that the subsequent racemization may result from involvement of the achiral azetidinium salt (85) in the equilibrium between 82 and 83 (Cherry *et al.,* 1978b).

A number of 2-(2-substituted-ethyl) clavem esters and the corresponding betaines have been prepared from esters of clavulanic acid and various of its derivatives. The 2-hydroxyethylclav-2-em (86) has been converted to the racemic diene [(±)79] by mesylation and subsequent treatment with triethylamine (Belg. Pat. 858,516). The clavem esters (e.g., 83) may be deesterified by catalytic hydrogenolysis, however, deesterification of the betaine (82) was accompanied by decarboxylation, and the product isolated was the quaternary ammonium chloride (87) (Glaxo, 1976).

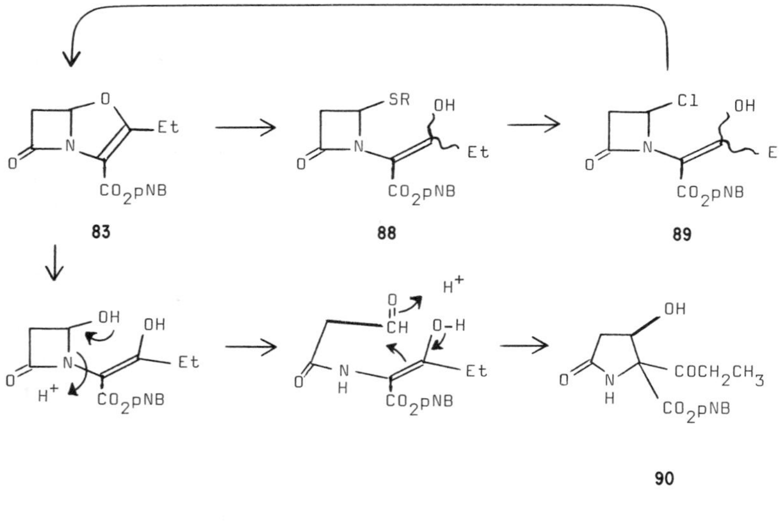

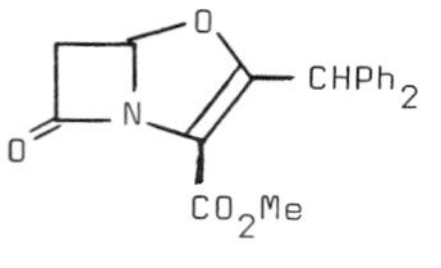

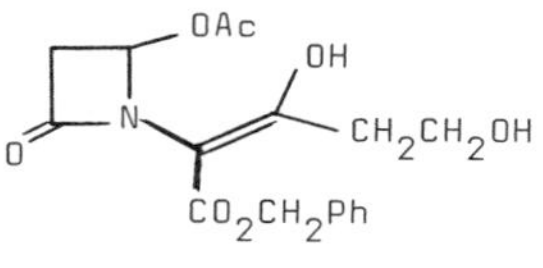

Reaction of the 2-ethylclav-2-em (83) with thiols afforded 88, the products of nucleophilic attack at C-5. Chlorinolysis of the thioethers (88) gave the chloro enol (89) which readily recyclized to the clavem (83) when treated with triethylamine. When 83 was heated in refluxing aqueous tetrahydrofuran, a more general rearrangement occurred, leading to formation of the hydroxypyrrolidone (90) (Glaxo, 1976). Analogous structures have been proposed for the products of the reactions of esters of the diene with aqueous DMF (Howarth, 1978) and of the totally synthetic clavem ester (91) with potassium carbonate, followed by an aqueous workup (Bentley *et al.*, 1977a). Howarth (1978) has described the reaction of benzyl 2-(2-hydroxyethyl)clav-2-em-3-carboxylate with acetic acid; the 4-acetoxyazetidinone (92) was among the products formed.

C. Synthesis of Pen-2-ems from Clavulanic Acid

The betaine (e.g., 82) and the chloro enols (e.g., 89) proved to be valuable as intermediates for the synthesis of 6,6-dihydropenems. Thus reaction of the 2-ethylclav-2-em (83) with *n*-butane thiol afforded 93, which was mesylated and then treated with chlorine to give 94. Reaction with hydrogen sulfide and triethylamine in tetrahydrofuran at 0°C resulted in ring closure, and *p*-nitrobenzyl 2-ethylpen-2-em-3-carboxylate (95) was isolated as a crystalline solid. Alternatively, mesylation of the betaine (82) gave the salt (96), which afforded the crystalline thiobetaine (97) when reacted with hydrogen sulfide and triethylamine in dichloroethane at 0°C. This compound smoothly cyclized to the pen-2-em (95) on brief heating in dichloroethane. The betaine (82) could conveniently be converted to the pen-2-em ester (95) in 60% yield without isolation of the intermediate mesylate or thiobetaine. Deprotection of 95 by catalytic hydrogenolysis gave the pen-2-em acid, isolated as its potassium salt (Cherry *et al.*, 1979). Analogous reaction sequences have been used to prepare a variety of 2-(2-substituted-ethyl)penems from clavulanic acid and its derivatives (Cherry *et al.*, 1979; Eur. Pat. Appl. 3,415; 10,358).

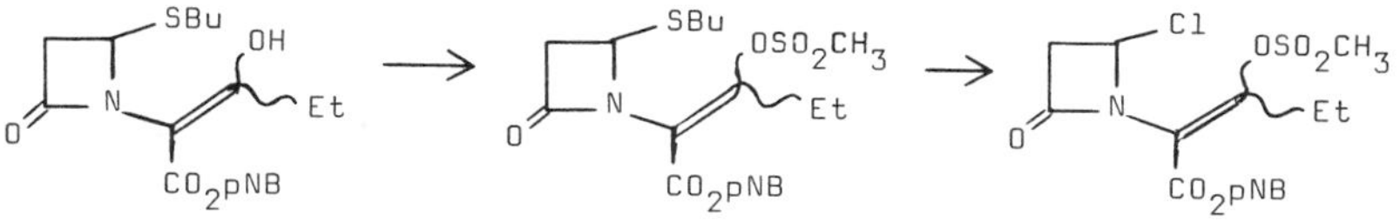

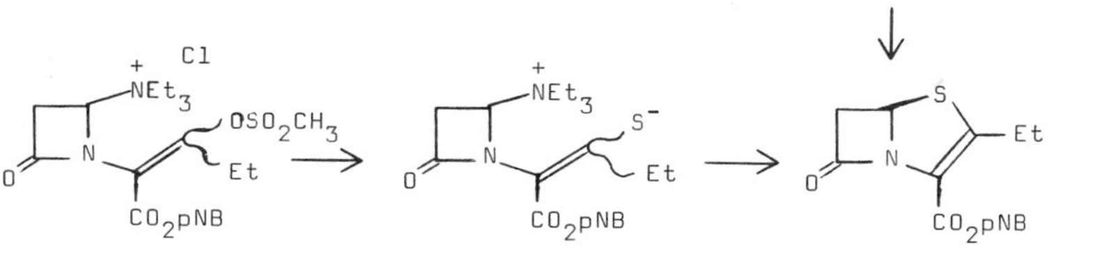

Mesylation of the 2-(2-hydroxyethyl)penem (**98**, R = HO) followed by treatment with triethylamine gave the 2-vinylpenem (**99**). Like racemic *p*-nitrobenzyl clavudiene, it readily underwent 1,4-additions with sulfur nucleophiles; thus reaction with thiophenol in the presence of potassium carbonate and 18-Crown-6 in dichloromethane at 20°C gave **100** (R = PhS), the structure and relative stereochemistry of which were confirmed by X-ray crystallography (Cherry *et al.*, 1980).

In a similar reaction with thioacetic acid conducted at 0°C two components were detected in the ratio 1:3. The major component was the expected 3*SR*, 5*RS*,*Z* isomer (**100**, R = CH$_3$COS) the minor component was assigned the structure of the thermodynamically less stable 3*RS*, 5*RS*,*Z* isomer (**101**, R = CH$_3$COS) on the basis of its ^{1}H-NMR spectrum. Treatment of the ethylidenepenam (**100**, R = CH$_3$COS) with triethylamine afforded the corresponding pen-2-em (**98**, R = CH$_3$COS).

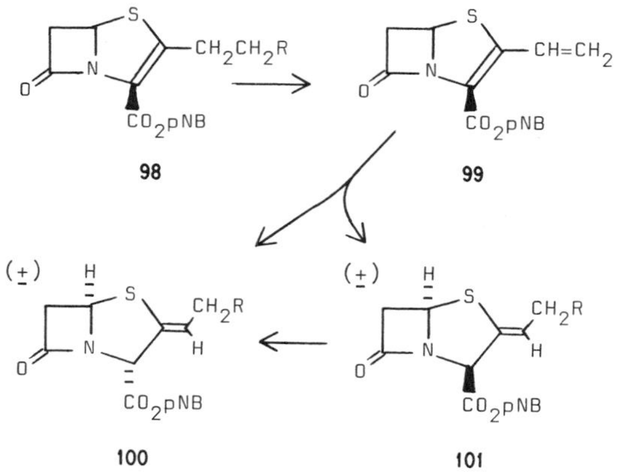

The penem acids and their salts exhibited good broad-spectrum antibacterial activity *in vitro,* as reported for other 6,6-dihydropenems by Woodward (1977b). However, their performance *in vivo* was disappointing, most of the compounds failing to protect mice against experimental infections. This lack of *in vivo* activity appeared not to be due to instability or poor pharmacokinetics but rather to a lack of bactericidal activity in the presence of serum proteins. They were poor inhibitors of most β-lactamases but showed some activity against the PC1 penicillinase and the P99 cephalosporinase. The potassium salt obtained by deprotection of the racemic acetylthioethylidenepenam (**100**, R = CH$_3$COS) exhibited little antibacterial activity and, in contrast to the corresponding derivative of clavulanic acid (**69**, R^2 = CH$_3$CO), was not a β-lactamase inhibitor.

VII.   Miscellaneous Derivatives of Clavulanic Acid

As indicated in Section VI, an attempt to oxidize benzyl clavulanate with the Pfitzner–Moffat reagent resulted in formation of the diene (78). However, oxidation with pyridinium chlorochromate gave the aldehyde (102), which was isolated as an inseparable mixture of E and Z isomers after chromatography (Corbett et al., 1977, Belg. Pat. 846,678). Oxidation of lithium clavulanate with Jones' reagent gave the aldehyde acid (103) which readily decarboxylated to form 104 (Glaxo, 1975). Ozonolysis of benzyl clavulanate provided the lactone (105) which inhibited β-lactamases (Belg. Pat. 849,109).

Dehydration of clavulanic acid with N,N-dimethylformamide dimethyl acetal in tetrahydrofuran was accompanied by decarboxylation, and 2-vinylclav-2-em (106) was isolated in good yield (Hunt, 1979). This formed Diels–Alder adducts (e.g., 107) with reactive dienophiles such as tetracyanoethylene. Hydrogenation of the diene (106) over Pd–C gave a mixture from which $(2S,5R)$-2-ethylclavam (108) and the E and Z isomers of $(5R)$-2-ethylideneclavam (109) were isolated following chromatography. The vinylclavem (106) and the ethylideneclavams (109) are reported to be β-lactamase inhibitors. The vinylclavem (106) undergoes 1,4-addition reactions with sulfur nucleophiles such as thiophenol to give products (e.g., 110) that are β-lactamase inhibitors and also exhibit antifungal activity (Br. Pat. Appl. 2,004,273).

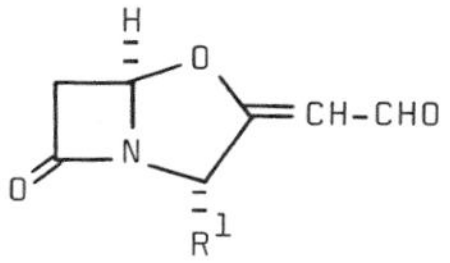

102 : R^1 = CO_2CH_2Ph
103 : R^1 = CO_2H
104 : R^1 =   H

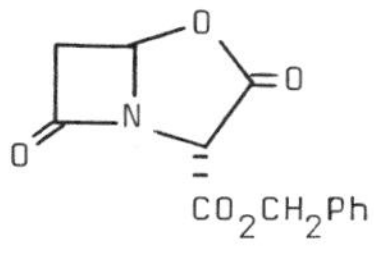

105

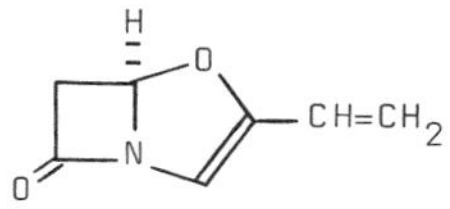

106

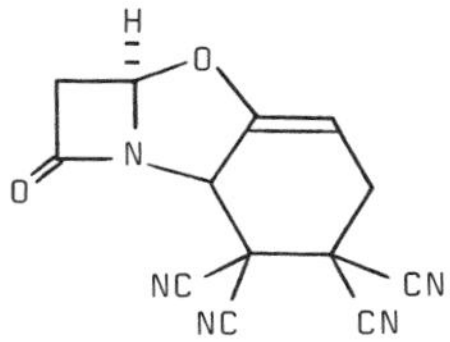

107

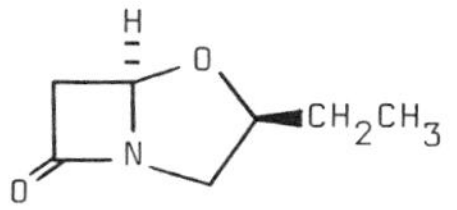

108

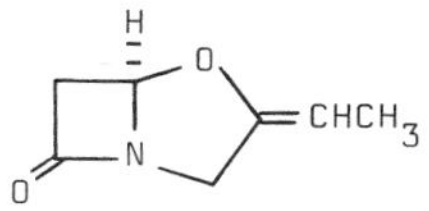

109

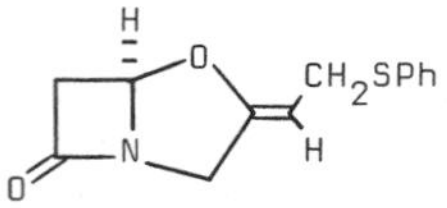

110 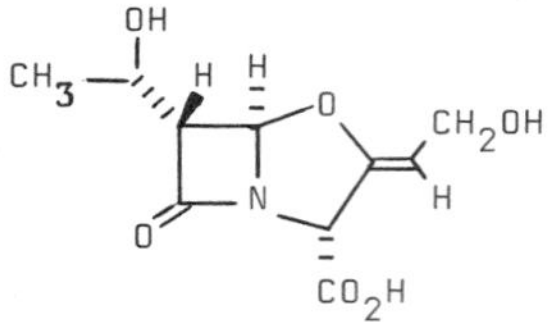   111 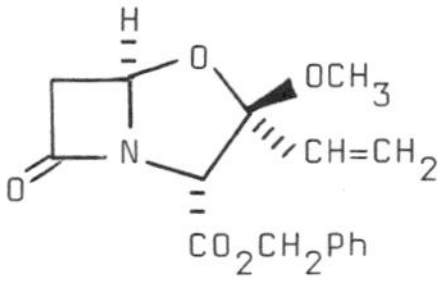   112

Functionalization of the 6-position has been achieved by the sequential reaction of esters of clavulanic acid with a strong nonnucleophilic base, such as lithium diisopropylamide, and an aldehyde or ketone. By this means salts of 6α-(1-hydroxyethyl)clavulanic acid (111) have been prepared (U.S. Pat. 4,076,826; Ger. Off. 2,822,001).

Reaction of O-acylated esters of clavulanic acid with alcohols proceeds with allylic rearrangement; thus with methanol the 2-methoxy-2-vinyl-clavam (112) was formed (Howarth, 1978). A similar rearrangement occurs during reaction of the haloester (53b) with methanol (Glaxo, 1975).

VIII.   Synthesis of Clavulanic Acid and Its Analogs

Prior to the isolation of clavulanic acid, there had already been interest in the preparation of oxygen analogs of penicillins. Treatment of the penicillin-derived β-lactam oxazoline (113) with the lithium salt of an alkane thiol had been reported to lead to oxapenicillin G (114) which showed antibacterial activity (Jpn. Pat. Appl. 49,007,263; Neth. Pat. Appl. 73,13896; Ger. Off. 2,356,862; U.S. Pat. 3,948,927). The Merck total synthesis of oxapenicillins had involved silver oxide–silver tetrafluoroborate-assisted cyclization of the chloroalcohol (115) (C-5–O closure) (Ger. Off. 2,411,856), but subsequent NMR correlations suggest that epimers with the unnatural configuration at C-3 may have been obtained (Alexander and Southgate, 1977). The oxapenam ring system (116) had also been obtained by photolytic cyclization of the diazoamide (117) (C-5–C-6 closure) (Golding and Hall, 1973, 1975).

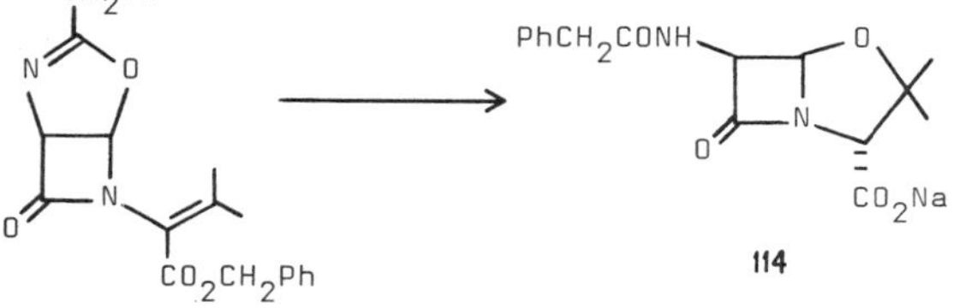

113   114

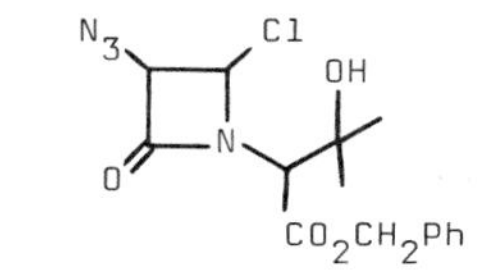

115 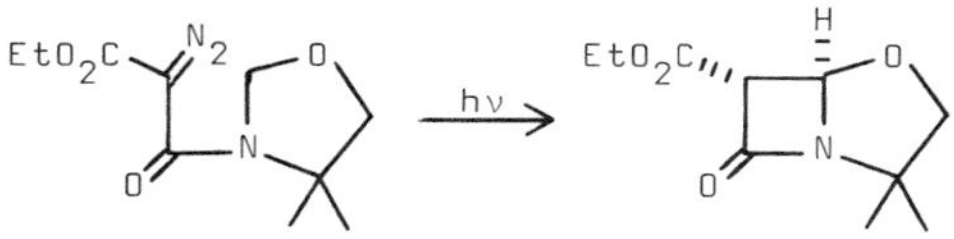   **117**   **116**

The isolation of clavulanic acid stimulated further interest in the ox-apenam (clavam) ring system, especially in the synthesis of 6-unsubsti-tuted derivatives. Photolytic cyclization of the *cis*(**118**) and *trans*- (**119**) diazoamides gave, respectively, the 2*R* isomer (**120**) and 2*S* isomer (**121**) of methyl 2-ethylclavam-3-carboxylate (Oida *et al.*, 1978). These products corresponded to the esters obtained by hydrogenation of methyl cla-vulanate (Section IV), confirming the more stable trans configuration of the hydrogen atoms at C-3 and C-5. The methyl ester (**122**), corresponding to the amino acid (**38**) derived by acidic hydrolysis of 2-ethylclavam-3-carboxylic acid (Section III), was synthesized and used to prepare the oxazolidines (**118** and **119**).

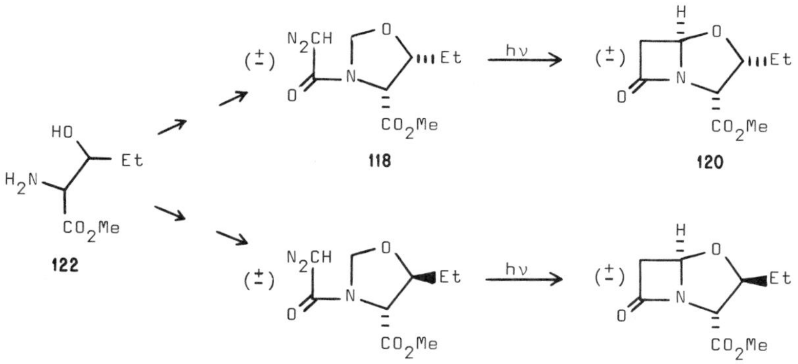

122   **118**   **120**

          119   **121**

The 2-ethylclavams (**123**) and their analogs (**124–126**) have been pre-pared by silver ion-assisted cyclizations of the chloroalcohols (**127**) de-rived from the readily available 4-acetoxyazetidin-2-one (**128**) (Kobayashi *et al.*, 1978; Jpn. Pat. Appl. 54,046,797). These products also had the more stable trans arrangement of hydrogen atoms at C-3 and C-5 but were usually mixtures of epimers at C-2. The esters (**123** and **124**) were less active than clavulanic acid as antibacterial agents and β-lactamase inhibitors. Analogous cyclization reactions have led to 6-substituted cla-vams (Ger. Off. 2,633,561).

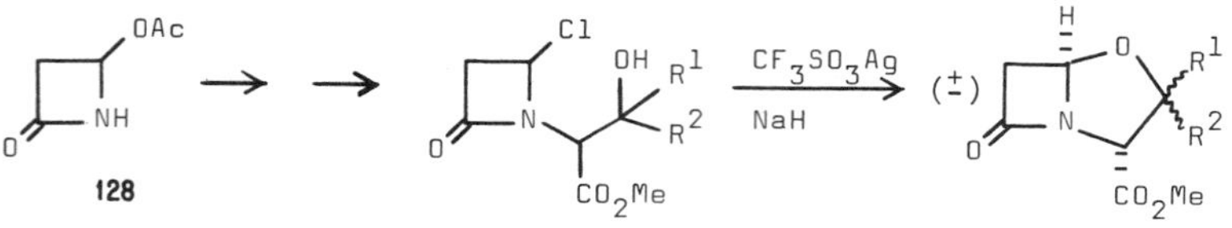

123: R^1 = Et R^2 = H
124: R^1 = Me R^2 = Me
125: R^1 = CH_2OCH_2Ph R^2 = H
126: R^1 = $CH_2CH_2OCH_2Ph$ R^2 = H

The clavam nucleus may also be made by closure of the C-3—N bond. Thus the α-bromoester (129) derived from 4-acetoxyazetidin-2-one (128) cyclized in the presence of benzyltrimethylammonium hydroxide to afford a separable mixture of the C-3 epimers (130 and 131, R = Me) which were distinguished by ^{1}H-NMR (Brown et al., 1977b; Ger. Off. 2,633,561). The natural C-3 epimers of penams and clavams (e.g., 130, R = Me) characteristically have the signal for the C-3 proton at δ~0.5 ppm downfield of the corresponding signal for the unnatural epimers (e.g., 131, R = Me). Base-catalyzed C-3 epimerization of the unnatural isomer (131, R = Me) showed the natural isomer (130, R = Me) to be thermodynamically more stable. The pair of 2-methylclavams (130 and 131, R = H) were obtained by a similar sequence, and 3-unsubstituted clavams have also been prepared (Belg. Pat. 850,593).

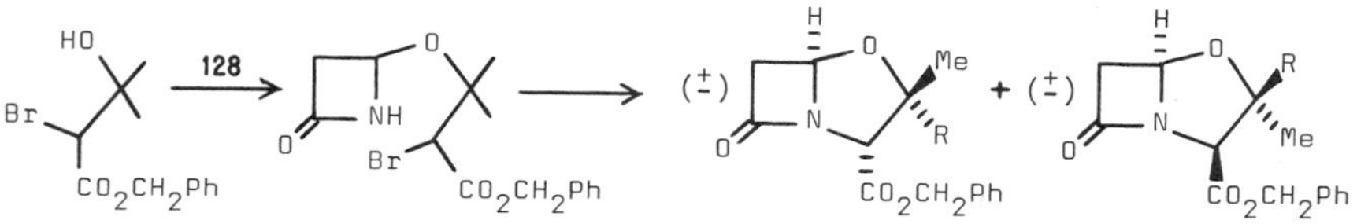

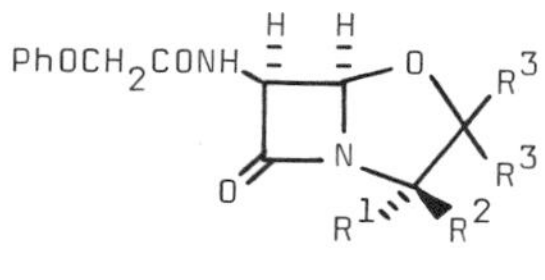

132: R^1 = CO_2CH_2Ph R^2 = H R^3 = Me
133: R^1 = H R^2 = CO_2CH_2Ph R^3 = Me
134: R^1 = CO_2CH_2Ph R^2 = H R^3 = H
135: R^1 = H R^2 = CO_2CH_2Ph R^3 = H

The above route has been applied to synthesis of the corresponding pairs of 6-substituted clavams (132 and 133) and (134 and 135) (Alexander and Southgate, 1977). The natural isomer (132) was separated and deprotected to afford the corresponding sodium salt which was considerably less active than penicillin V.

The analogous 6-phenylacetamido 2-unsubstituted clavams (136 and

137) have been prepared by total synthesis (Cama and Christensen, 1978). In this case, the C-3—N bond was formed by treatment of the diazoester (**138**) with rhodium acetate. Separation of the epimers and deprotection of the natural isomer (**136**) led to the corresponding racemic sodium salt which had limited aqueous stability and was much less active than penicillin G and bisnorpenicillin G as an antibacterial agent.

138

136: $R^1 = CO_2CH_2Ph$; $R^2 = H$
137: $R^1 = H$; $R^2 = CO_2CH_2Ph$

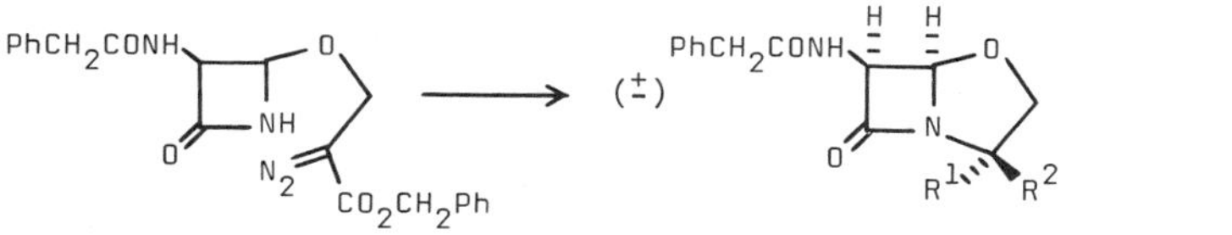

The enol (**89**) derived from clavulanic acid readily cyclizes to the clav-2-em (**83**) (Section IV,B). Similar clav-2-ems (**139** and **140**) have been synthesized via the corresponding chloroenols (**141**) prepared from 4-methylthioazetidin-2-one (**142**) (Bentley *et al.*, 1977a).

The unstable 6-substituted clav-2-em (**143**) has been prepared by an analogous route from the penicillin-derived azetidinone (**144**) and found to be only a weak inhibitor of β-lactamases (Eglington, 1977).

142

139: R = $CHMe_2$
140: R = Et

141

144

143

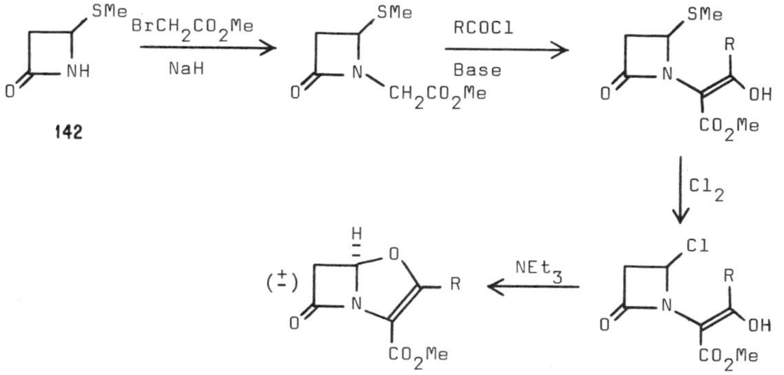

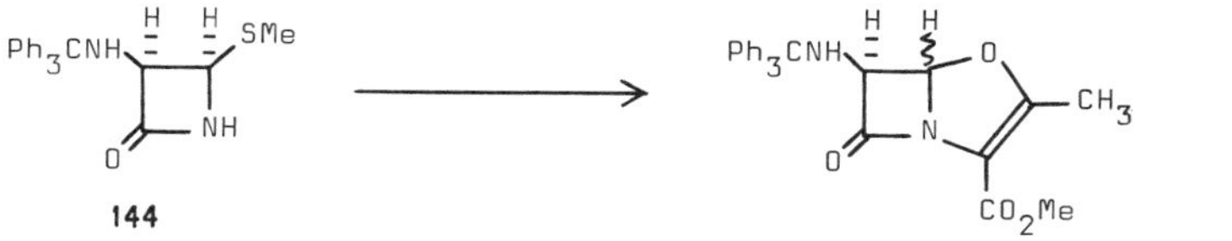

The ease with which clav-2-ems are formed by closure of chloroenols (e.g., **141**) makes them attractive intermediates for preparation of the isomeric 2-alkylideneclavams—more closely related structurally to clavulanic acid. However, as seen in Section VI, ethylideneclavams (e.g., **145**) are thermodynamically unstable with respect to the corresponding clav-2-ems (e.g., **146**) and are isomerized to these α,β-unsaturated esters in the presence of base. Thus attempts to isomerize the clav-2-ems **139** and **140** under basic conditions failed to provide the deconjugated esters (**147** and **148**) (Bentley *et al.*, 1977a).

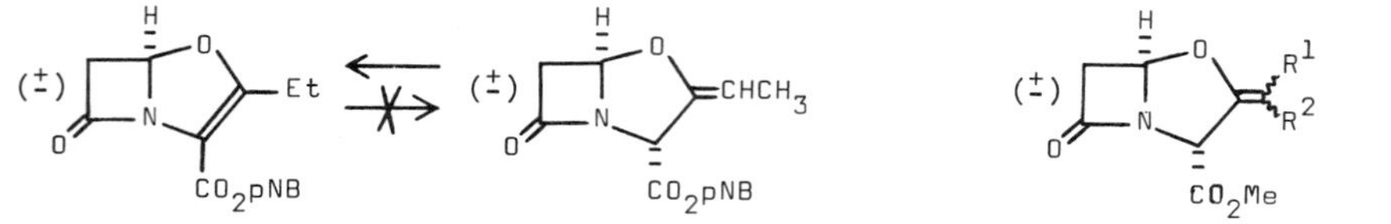

146   **145**   **147:** R^1 = Me; R^2 = Me
                                  148: R^1 = Me; R^2 = H

Exocyclic double-bond isomers have, however, been obtained by cyclization of suitable chloroenols containing a second group capable of conjugating with the enol. This additional group (X in **149–152**) may stabilize the enolate more effectively prior to cyclization and give directly the exocyclic double-bond isomer (**149 → 150 → 152**); alternatively isomerization of the double bond may occur after cyclization of the enolate (**149 → 151 → 152**).

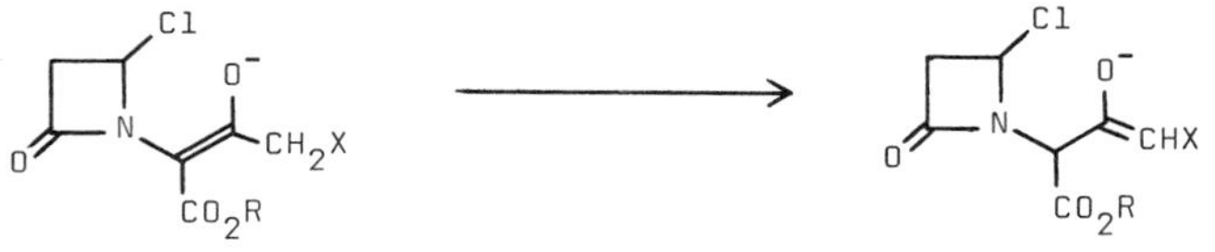

149   150

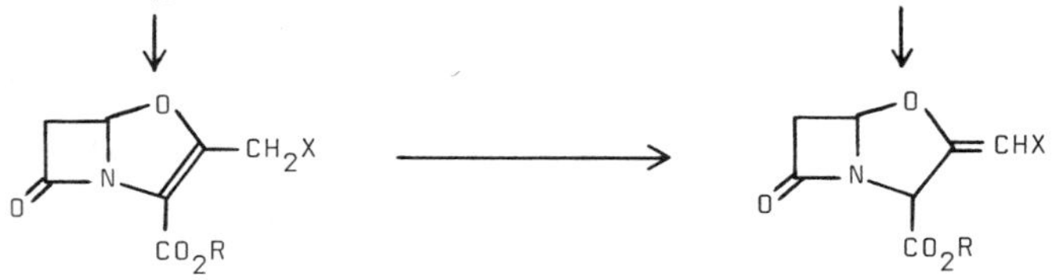

151   152

Using a second ester group as the alternative conjugating group, Bentley *et al.* (1977b) achieved the first total synthesis of (±)-methyl clavulanate. Thus alkylation of 4-methylthioazetidin-2-one (**142**) with dimethyl 2-bromo-3-oxoglutarate gave the enolized β-ketodiester (**153**).

Chlorinolysis followed by cyclization of the resulting chloroenol (154) with anhydrous potassium carbonate afforded the diester (155), the structure of which was confirmed by X-ray analysis. Cyclization of the chloroenol with triethylamine gave a mixture of the diester (155), the corresponding Z isomer (156), and the clavem (157). Reduction of the diester (155) with diisobutylaluminum hydride (DIBAL) gave a low yield of racemic methyl isoclavulanate (158), whereas photolytic isomerization gave a mixture of 155 and the corresponding Z isomer (156). The latter was too unstable to isolate, but reduction of the mixture of diesters with DIBAL gave a separable mixture of (±)-methyl isoclavulanate (158) and (±)-methyl clavulanate (159). (±)-Methyl clavulanate was also obtained by photolytic isomerization of the E isomer (158).

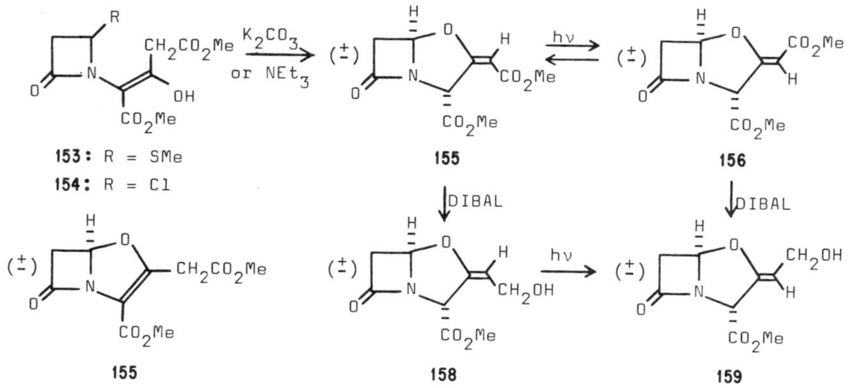

A number of 3-unsubstituted 2-ethylideneclavams (e.g., 160 and 161) have been prepared by analogous cyclization reactions on substrates containing ester (e.g., 162) or keto groups (e.g., 163) to ensure exocyclic double bonds in the products (Hunt et al., 1977; Bentley et al., 1979a; Belg. Pat. 850,942). Some of the 3-unsubstituted 2-ethylideneclavams (e.g., 160) are moderate inhibitors of β-lactamases.

In addition to the above use of ester and keto groups to stabilize the exocyclic double bond, aromatic and vinyl groups have also found application. Thus cyclization of the chloroenol (164) with triethylamine gave first the endocyclic isomer (165) but, on treatment with further triethylamine, this isomerized to the exo isomer (166) (Bentley et al., 1977a; Belg. Pat. 850,942). In the presence of potassium carbonate, the exo isomer was obtained directly from the chloroenol (164). The sodium salt corresponding to 166 is a potent inhibitor of several β-lactamases.

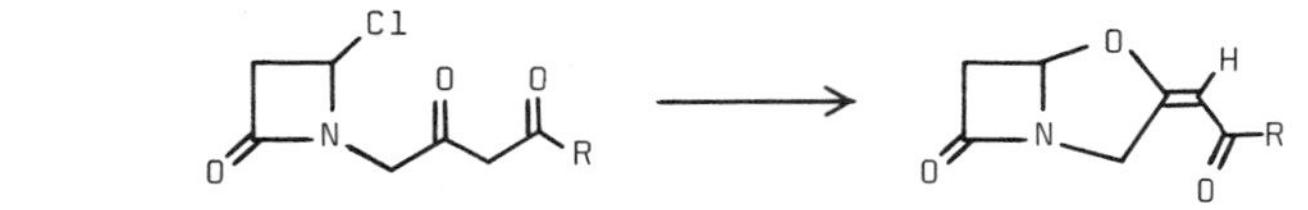

162: R = OMe   160: R = OMe
163: R = Me   161: R = Me

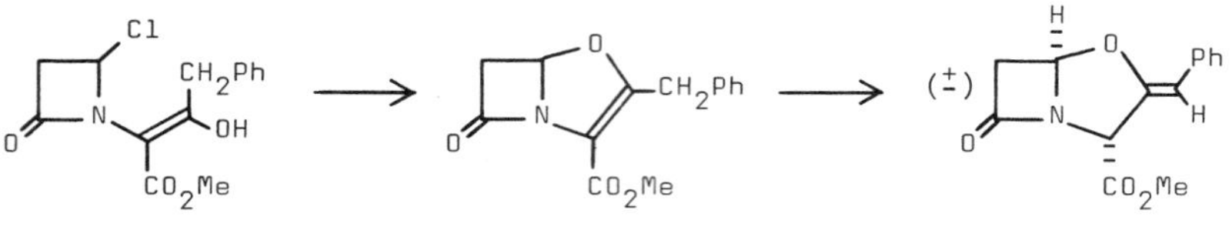

164   165   166

The second total synthesis of (±)-methyl clavulanate utilized a vinyl group to provide the exo isomer (Bentley *et al.*, 1979b). Thus cyclization of the chloroenol (167) gave the diene (168) which had the same stereochemistry about the double bond as clavulanic acid. Careful formation of the ozonide of the terminal double bond followed by catalytic hydrogenolysis afforded (±)-methyl clavulanate (159).

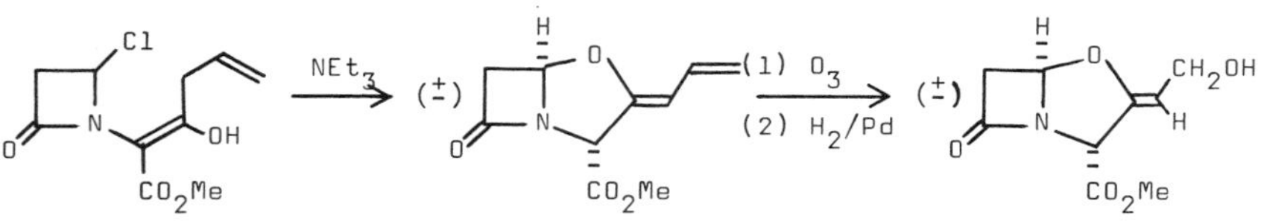

167   168   159

An alternative strategy for preparing 2-alkylideneclavams is to generate the unsaturation in the C-2 substituent after construction of the clavam ring system. The phenylseleno derivative (169) analogous to the oxazolidine (119) was prepared and cyclized photolytically to the clavam (170). Oxidative elimination of the phenylseleno group afforded the 2-methyleneclavam (171) (Oida *et al.*, 1978).

The same compound was obtained independently via the bromoesters (172 and 173) derived from a C-3—N ring-closure reaction (Bentley and Hunt, 1978a). The bromoester 172 failed to eliminate hydrogen bromide, but the mixture (172 and 173) was converted via the corresponding *o*-nitrophenylselenides and selenoxides into a mixture of the 2-methyleneclavam (171) and its C-3 epimer (174).

2-Alkylideneclavams have also been prepared by allylic rearrangement of 2-vinylclavams (Bentley and Hunt, 1978b). Silver ion-assisted cyclization of the chloroalcohol (175) provided the 2-vinylclavam (176) which on bromination afforded a mixture of the allylic bromides (177 and 178).

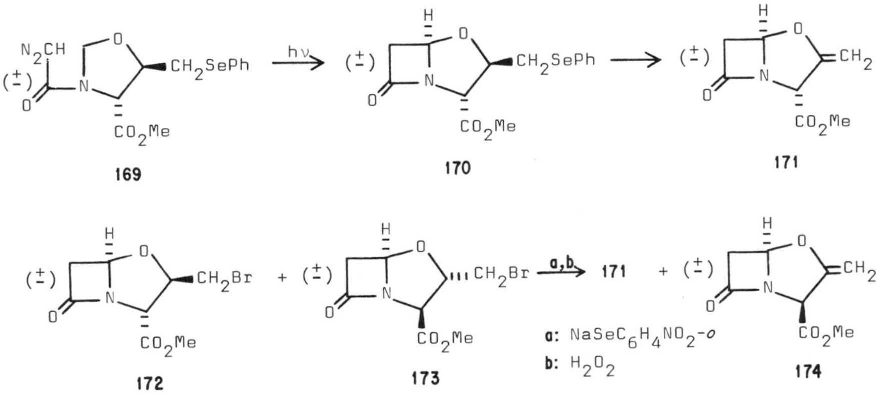

N_2CH ... CH_2SePh

$(\pm)$ ... CO_2Me

169

$\xrightarrow{h\nu}$

$(\pm)$ ... CH_2SePh

CO_2Me

170

$\longrightarrow$

$(\pm)$ ... CH_2

CO_2Me

171

$(\pm)$ ... CH_2Br

CO_2Me

172

$+$ $(\pm)$ ... CH_2Br $\xrightarrow{a,b}$ **171** $+$ $(\pm)$ ... CH_2

CO_2Me

173

a: $NaSeC_6H_4NO_2\text{-}o$
b: H_2O_2

CO_2Me

174

Treatment of this mixture with isopropanol and silver oxide gave the alkoxyethylideneclavam (**179**) as a mixture of *E* and *Z* isomers (1:5). Similar reactions with the 6-unsubstituted 2-vinylclavam (**180**) failed to give the corresponding alkoxyethylideneclavam.

$(\pm)$ Br, Br, Cl, OH ... CO_2Me

175

$\xrightarrow[AgBF_4]{Ag_2O}$

$(\pm)$ R, R, H ... CO_2Me

176: R = Br
180: R = H

$\downarrow$

$(\pm)$ Br, Br, H, R^1 ... CO_2Me

177 R^1 = Br

$+$

$(\pm)$ Br, Br, H ... $CHCH_2R^1$ ... CO_2Me

178: R^1 = Br
179: R^1 = O*i*-Pr

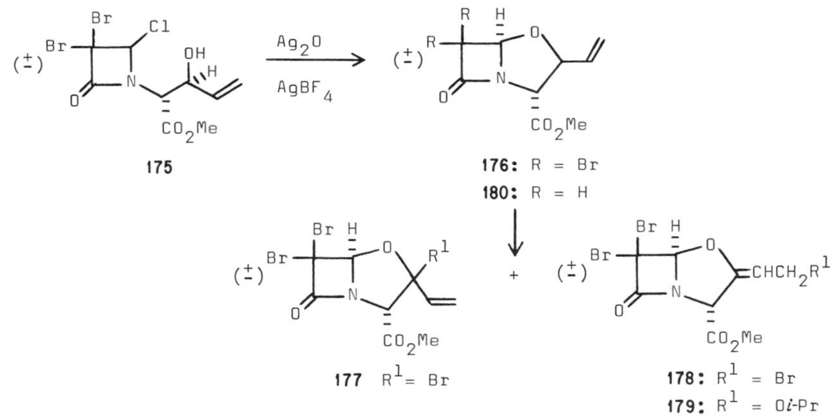

IX. Mechanism of Action of Clavulanic Acid and Related Inhibitors of β-Lactamases

Clavulanic acid acts as a progressive irreversible inhibitor of β-lactamases and thus differs fundamentally in its mode of action from previously reported competitive inhibitors such as methicillin, cloxacillin, and nafcillin. The detailed mechanism by which β-lactamases inactivate penicillins is unknown, but a favored possibility is cleavage of the β-lactam ring by a nucleophilic site to give an intermediate penicilloyl enzyme which is rapidly hydrolyzed to liberate a penicilloic acid and regenerate the β-lactamase. With 6β-bromopenicillanic acid as substrate, serine-44 of the lactamase I from *Bacillus cereus* has been implicated as the nucleophilic site (Knott-Hunziker *et al.*, 1979a; Orlek *et al.*, 1979), whereas a penicilloyl enzyme intermediate has been isolated from the hydrolysis of quinacillin by the β-lactamase from *Staphylococcus aureus* (Virden *et al.*, 1975). With clavulanic acid (**181**) as an analogous substrate for the β-lactamase, the expected acylenzyme intermediate would be the unstable oxazolidine (**182**). In contrast to formation of the corresponding penicilloyl enzyme, cleavage of clavulanic acid to the putative inter- mediate (**182**) would be accompanied by concurrent or rapid subsequent fragmentation to give a new acyl enzyme intermediate (e.g., **183**) resem- bling the product derived by methanolysis of clavulanic acid (Section III). Thus the cleavage of the β-lactam ring of clavulanic acid by a β- lactamase would trigger a secondary reaction which has no analogy in its hydrolysis of penicillins. It is thought that this secondary fragmen- tation and its consequences are responsible for the irreversible inhibition of the enzyme. Thus it has been suggested that the new acyl enzyme (e.g., **183**) may be more resistant to hydrolysis and release than a pen- icilloyl enzyme or that new reactive centers generated within the mol- ecule may interact with other nearby functional groups on the enzyme, disrupting the normal release of the substrate from the active site (Cart- wright and Coulson, 1979; Charnas *et al.*, 1978a; Durkin and Viswanatha, 1978; Labia and Peduzzi, 1978; Reading and Hepburn, 1979).

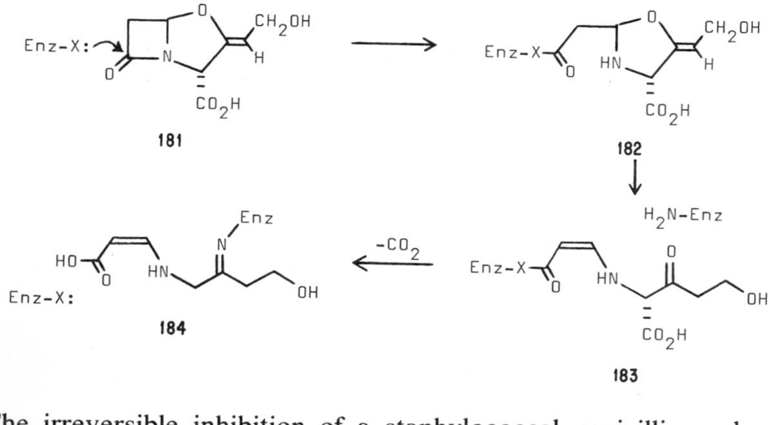

The irreversible inhibition of a staphylococcal penicillinase by cla- vulanic acid has been shown to have a stoichiometry of about 1:1 and to be associated with the appearance of a chromophore at 290 nm, which is more slowly converted to a maximum at 278 nm. The species corresponding to the chromophores are suggested to be cis and trans isomers of an enamine (e.g., **183**) and are analogs of the normal penicilloyl enzyme but are stabilized to hydrolysis by the α,β-unsaturation (Cartwright and Coulson, 1979). Independent studies on the inactivation of penicillinases have shown that the inhibition follows first-order kinetics and that the activity of the inhibited enzyme recovers slowly in the absence of clavulanic acid (Reading and Hepburn, 1979). These results were explained by formation of a relatively stable covalent intermediate (e-c) in the kinetic scheme

$$ e + c \leftrightarrows ec \rightarrow e\text{-}c \rightarrow e + p $$

where e is free enzyme, c is clavulanic acid, ec is the Michaelis complex, and p are products. The Schiff base (**184**), formed between the keto group of the acyl enzyme (**183**) and a neighboring amino group on the enzyme has been tentatively proposed as the covalent intermediate (e-c). The kinetics of inactivation of the β-lactamase from *Escherichia coli* R-TEM and β-lactamase I from *B. cereus* have been shown to be considerably more complex, involving at least two distinct steps in the inhibition (Durkin and Viswanatha, 1978; Labia and Peduzzi, 1978). Fisher *et al.* (1978) have represented the inhibition of the *E. coli* R-TEM β-lactamase by the minimal scheme:

$$
\begin{array}{c}
\text{e-i} \\
{\scriptstyle(3)}\uparrow \\
e + c \rightleftharpoons ec \xrightarrow{\;(2)\;} e\text{-}t \xrightarrow{\;H_2O\;} e + p^1 \\
{\scriptstyle(1)}\downarrow \; H_2O \\
e + p
\end{array}
$$

The Michaelis complex (ec) can react in three competing ways: (1) hydrolysis of the β-lactam with release of products (p) and regeneration of the enzyme, (2) formation of a transiently inhibited enzyme (e-t) which is then converted to products (p^1), liberating the enzyme to react with further clavulanic acid, or (3) somewhat slower conversion to irreversibly inactivated enzyme (e-i) at about one-third the rate of formation of the transient intermediate. The net result of these three concurrent processes is that, in the presence of an excess of clavulanic acid, all the enzyme eventually accumulates in the irreversibly inactivated state (e-i), though at the expense of the destruction of 115 molecules of clavulanic acid per molecule of enzyme.

The transiently inhibited enzyme (e-t) has been shown to be associated with a strong chromophore at 281 nm, which disappears if the catalytic activity is allowed to reappear (Charnas et al., 1978a). The irreversibly inhibited enzyme (e-i) was shown by isoelectric focusing to be an approximately equal mixture of three distinct components, one of which had a similar chromophore at 281 nm and on treatment with hydroxylamine regenerated the native enzyme with concomitant loss of its UV activity.

Although the exact nature of the transiently and irreversibly inactivated enzyme species is still unknown, the chromophores at 281 nm again suggest the possible involvement of enamine species (e.g., 183), and the covalent product (185) resulting from Michael addition of a neighboring nucleophilic center has been proposed inter alia as a possible inactivated enzyme species or intermediate (Charnas et al., 1978b). An analogous Michael addition to the α,β-unsaturated ketone (186) derived by dehydration of 183 is unlikely, since deoxyclavulanic acid (44, R = H), which cannot provide the same unsaturated intermediate, has inactivation kinetics very similar to those of clavulanic acid itself. Furthermore, radioactive labeling studies have shown that most, and perhaps all, of the inactivated enzyme species contain only the three carbon atoms originally constituting the β-lactam ring of clavulanic acid (i.e., C-5, C-6, and C-7). This observation also tends to rule out intermediates such as 187 but accords with the subsequent loss of 2-amino-3-keto-5-hydroxypentanoic acid from an intermediate such as 185.

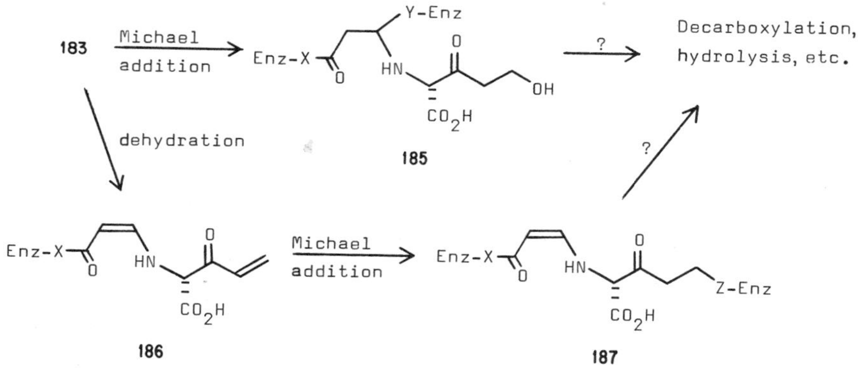

Despite the lack of detailed knowledge of the mechanism of action of clavulanic acid, the general requirements for an inhibitor based on the generation of an enamine species (e.g., 183) have been suggested to be (1) a β-lactam ring capable of acylating the enzyme, (2) a proton of sufficient acidity at the 6α position, (3) a good leaving group for an anti-β-elimination (e.g., at the C-5 position), and (4) an acyl enzyme intermediate sufficiently long-lived to allow inactivation before hydrolysis (Cartwright and Coulson, 1979; Knowles, 1980).

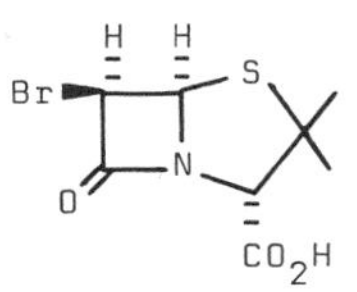

188 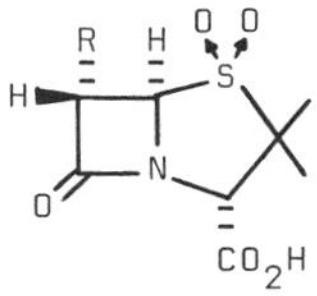   189: R = H   191
                       190: R = Cl

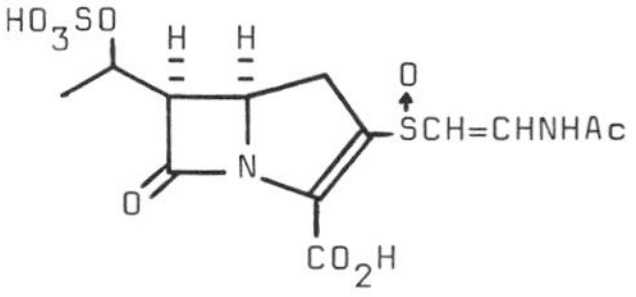

A number of derivatives of penicillanic acid have been prepared that appear to satisfy these requirements, causing similar irreversible inhibition of β-lactamases. They include 6β-bromopenicillanic acid (188), (Pratt and Loosemore, 1978; Knott-Hunziker et al., 1979b; Orlek et al., 1979), penicillanic acid sulfone (189) (English et al., 1978), 6α-chloropenicillanic acid sulfone (190) (probably reacting via the 6β isomer formed in solution) (Cartwright and Coulson, 1979), and the sulfones of methicillin and quinacillin (Knowles, 1980).

It has been suggested that the β-lactamase inhibitory properties of the naturally occurring olivanic acids (e.g., 191) might result from an analogous β-elimination of the side-chain sulfate group (Knowles, 1980). However, the olivanic acid MM 4550 (191) is reported to be principally a competitive inhibitor of β-lactamases (Cole, 1980), and so its main mode of action may be quite different from that of clavulanic acid.

In addition to being a potent β-lactamase inhibitor, clavulanic acid is also a modest antibacterial agent showing preferential binding to penicillin-binding proteins (PBP) 2 and 4 and least affinity for PBP 3 (Spratt et al., 1977; Horikawa and Ogawara, 1978). It remains to be seen whether the detailed mode of action is analogous to that for β-lactamase inhibition.

References

Alexander, R. G., and Southgate, R. (1977). *J.C.S. Chem. Commun.* 405–406.
Belgian Patent 834,645.
Belgian Patent 836,652.
Belgian Patent 840,253.
Belgian Patent 846,678.
Belgian Patent 847,044.

Belgian Patent 847,045.
Belgian Patent 847,046.
Belgian Patent 849,109.
Belgian Patent 849,308.
Belgian Patent 849,474.
Belgian Patent 849,475.
Belgian Patent 850,593.
Belgian Patent 850,779.
Belgian Patent 850,942.
Belgian Patent 851,821.
Belgian Patent 855,375.
Belgian Patent 855,467.
Belgian Patent 858,516.
Belgian Patent 860,042.
Belgian Patent 861,716.
Belgian Patent 862,764.
Belgian Patent 864,607.
Belgian Patent 866,276.
Belgian Patent 866,496.
Belgian Patent 870,405.
Bentley, P. H., and Hunt, E. (1978a). *J.C.S. Chem. Commun.* 518–519.
Bentley, P. H., and Hunt, E. (1978b). *J.C.S. Chem. Commun.* 439–441.
Bentley, P. H., Brooks, G., Gilpin, M. L., and Hunt, E. (1977a). *J.C.S. Chem. Commun.* 905–906.
Bentley, P. H., Berry, P. D., Brooks, G., Gilpin, M. L., Hunt, E., and Zomaya, I. I. (1977b). *J.C.S. Chem. Commun.* 748–749.
Bentley, P. H., Brooks, G., Gilpin, M. L., Hunt, E., and Zomaya, I. I. (1979a). *Tetrahedron Lett.* 391–392.
Bentley, P. H., Brooks, G., Gilpin, M. L., and Hunt, E. (1979b). *Tetrahedron Lett.* 1889–1890.
British Patent Application 2,004,273.
British Patent Application 2,007,667.
Brown, A. G., Butterworth, D., Cole, M., Hanscomb, G., Hood, J. D., Reading, C., and Rolinson, G. N. (1976a). *J. Antibiot.* 29, 668.
Brown, A. G., Howarth, T. T., Stirling, I., and King, T. J. (1976b). *Tetrahedron Lett.* 4203–4204.
Brown, A. G., Goodacre, J., Harbridge, J. B., Howarth, T. T., Ponsford, R. J., Stirling, I., and King, T. J. (1977a). *In* "Recent Advances in the Chemistry of β-Lactam Antibiotics" (J. Elks, ed.), Spec. Publ. No. 28, pp. 295–298. Chem. Soc., London.
Brown, A. G., Corbett, D. F., and Howarth, T. T. (1977b). *J.C.S. Chem. Commun.* 359–360.
Brown, D., Evans, J. R., and Fletton, R. A. (1979). *J.C.S. Chem. Commun.* 282–283.
Cama, L. D., and Christensen, B. G. (1978). *Tetrahedron Lett.* 4233–4236.
Cartwright, S. J., and Coulson, A. F. W. (1979). *Nature (London)* 278, 360–361.
Charnas, R. L., Fisher, J., and Knowles, J. R. (1978a). *Biochemistry* 17, 2185–2189.
Charnas, R. L., Fisher, J., and Knowles, J. R. (1978b). *In* "Enzyme-Activated Irreversible Inhibitors" (N. Seiler, M. J. Jung, and J. Koch-Weser, eds.), pp. 315–322. Elsevier/North-Holland, Amsterdam.
Cherry, P. C., Gregory, G. I., Newall, C. E., Ward, P., and Watson, N. S. (1978a). *J.C.S. Chem. Commun.* 467–468.

Cherry, P. C., Newall, C. E., and Watson, N. S. (1978b). *J.C.S. Chem. Commun.* 469–470.
Cherry, P. C., Newall, C. E., and Watson, N. S. (1979). *J.C.S. Chem. Commun.* 663–664.
Cherry, P. C., Evans, D. N., Newall, C. E., Watson, N. S., and Murray-Rust, P. (19(?)). *Tetrahedron Lett.* **21**, 561–564.
Claes, P. J., Hoogmartens, J., Janssen, G., and Vanderhaeghe, H. (1975). *Eur. J. Med. Chem.—Chim. Ther.* **10**, 573–577.
Cole, M. (1980). *Phil. Trans. R. Soc. Lond.* **B289**, 207–223.
Corbett, D. F., Howarth, T. T., and Stirling, I. (1977). *J.C.S. Chem. Commun.* 808.
Durkin, J. P., and Viswanatha, T. (1978). *J. Antibiot.* **31**, 1162–1169.
Eglington, A. J. (1977). *J.C.S. Chem. Commun.* 720.
English, A. R., Retsema, J. A., Girard, A. E., Lynch, J. E., and Barth, W. E. (1978). *Antimicrob. Agents Chemother.* **14**, 414–419.
European Patent Application 1,516.
European Patent Application 2,319.
European Patent Application 2,370.
European Patent Application 3,254.
European Patent Application 3,415.
European Patent Application 10,358.
Fisher, J., Charnas, R. L., and Knowles, J. R. (1978). *Biochemistry* **17**, 2180–2184.
German Offenlegungsschrift 2,356,862.
German Offenlegungsschrift 2,411,856.
German Offenlegungsschrift 2,517,316.
German Offenlegungsschrift 2,547,698.
German Offenlegungsschrift 2,604,697.
German Offenlegungsschrift 2,628,357.
German Offenlegungsschrift 2,633,561.
German Offenlegungsschrift 2,708,047.
German Offenlegungsschrift 2,747,350.
German Offenlegungsschrift 2,747,763.
German Offenlegungsschrift 2,822,001.
German Offenlegungsschrift 2,911,099.
Glaxo Group Research Ltd. (1974–1979). Unpublished results.
Golding, B. T., and Hall, D. R. (1973). *J.C.S. Chem. Commun.* 293–294.
Golding, B. T., and Hall, D. R. (1975). *J.C.S. Perkin I* 1517–1521.
Horikawa, S., and Ogawara, H. (1978). *J. Antibiot.* **31**, 1283–1291.
Howarth, T. T. (1978). *Am. Chem. Soc. Natl. Meet., 176th, Miami Beach, Fla.* Pap. No. MEDI 9 (Abstr.).
Howarth, T. T., Brown, A. G., and King, T. J. (1976). *J.C.S. Chem. Commun.* 266–267.
Hunt, E. (1979). *J.C.S. Chem. Commun.* 686–687.
Hunt, E., Bentley, P. H., Brooks, G., and Gilpin, M. L. (1977). *J.C.S. Chem. Commun.* 906–907.
Hunter, P. A., Reading, C., and Witting, D. A. (1978). *Curr. Chemother., Proc. Int. Congr. Chemother., 10th, Zurich, 1977* pp. 478–480.
Japanese Patent Application 49,007,263.
Japanese Patent Application 53,104,796.
Japanese Patent Application 54,046,797.
Knott-Hunziker, V., Waley, S. G., Orlek, B. S., and Sammes, P. G. (1979a). *FEBS Lett.* **99**, 59–61.
Knott-Hunziker, V., Orlek, B. S., Sammes, P. G., and Waley, S. G. (1979b). *Biochem. J.* **177**, 365–367.

Knowles, J. R. (1980). *Phil. Trans. R. Soc. Lond.* **B289**, 309–319.

Kobayashi, T., Iwano, Y., and Hirai, K. (1978). *Chem. Pharm. Bull.* **26**, 1761–1767.

Labia, R., and Peduzzi, J. (1978). *Biochim. Biophys. Acta* **526**, 572–579.

Nagarajan, R. (1972). *In* "Cephalosporins and Penicillins: Chemistry and Biology" (E. H. Flynn, ed.), pp. 640–642. Academic Press, New York.

Netherlands Patent Application 73,13896.

Netherlands Patent Application 76,03818.

Newall, C. E., Cherry, P. C., Gregory, G. I., Tonge, A. P., Ward, P., and Watson, N. S. (1978). *Am. Chem. Soc. Natl. Meet., 176th, Miami Beach, Fla.* Pap. No. MEDI 15 (Abstr.)

Oida, S., Yoshida, A., and Ohki, E. (1978). *Chem. Pharm. Bull.* **26**, 448–455.

Orlek, B. S., Sammes, P. G., Knott-Hunziker, V., and Waley, S. G. (1979). *J.C.S. Chem. Commun.* 962–963.

Pratt, R. F., and Loosemore, M. J. (1978). *Proc. Natl. Acad. Sci. U.S.A.* **75**, 4145–4149.

Reading, C., and Cole, M. (1977). *Antimicrob. Agents Chemother.* **11**, 852–857.

Reading, C., and Hepburn, P. (1979). *Biochem. J.* **179**, 67–76.

Richmond, M. H., and Sykes, R. B. (1973). *Adv. Microb. Physiol.* **9**, 31–88.

Simpson, I. N., Harper, P. B., and O'Callaghan, C. H. (1980). *Antimicrob. Agents Chemother.* **17**, 929–936.

Spratt, B. G., Jobanputra, V., and Zimmermann, W. (1977). *Antimicrob. Agents Chemother.* **12**, 406–409.

Stoodley, R. J., and Watson, N. S. (1975). *J.C.S. Perkin I* 883–888.

Sykes, R. B., and Matthew, M. (1976). *J. Antimicrob. Chemother.* **2**, 115–157.

United States Patent 3,948,927.

United States Patent 4,076,826.

Uri, J. V., Actor, P., and Weisbach, J. A. (1978). *J. Antibiot.* **31**, 789–791.

Virden, R., Bristow, A. F., and Pain, R. H. (1975). *Biochem. J.* **149**, 397–401.

Woodward, R. B. (1977a). *In* "Recent Advances in the Chemistry of β-Lactam Antibiotics" (J. Elks, ed.), Special Publication No. 28, pp. 167–180. Chem. Soc., London.

Woodward, R. B. (1977b). *Acta Pharm. Suec.* **14**, Suppl., 23–25.

Woodward, R. B., Neuberger, A., and Trenner, N. R. (1949). *In* "The Chemistry of Penicillin" (H. T. Clarke, J. R. Johnson, and R. Robinson, eds.), pp. 415–439. Princeton Univ. Press, Princeton, New Jersey.

Index